Mike Mackenzie.
01706 341100.
07810 892 667.

MUSCULOSKELETAL IMAGING

Each volume of **The Core Curriculum Series** examines one key area in radiology and focuses on the essential information readers need for rotations and later, their written board exams. Readers will appreciate the easy-to-follow format, the abundant high-quality illustrations, and the full complement of learning tools—including chapter outlines, bulleted lists, tables, summary boxes, margin notes, and points for review. Please contact the publisher for additional information on existing and upcoming titles.

Other titles in **The Core Curriculum Series**...

Brant: *Ultrasound*
Cardenosa: *Breast Imaging*
Castillo: *Neuroradiology*
Kazerooni and Gross: *Cardiopulmonary Imaging*

The Core Curriculum

MUSCULOSKELETAL IMAGING

FELIX S. CHEW, M.D.

Professor of Radiologic Sciences–Radiology
Section Head of Musculoskeletal Radiology
Vice Chairman for Education
Department of Radiology
Wake Forest University School of Medicine
Winston-Salem, North Carolina

With contributions by

LIEM T. BUI-MANSFIELD, M.D.

Lieutenant Colonel, U.S. Army Medical Corps
Section Head of Musculoskeletal Radiology
Brooke Army Medical Center
San Antonio, Texas
Clinical Adjunct in Radiology
Wake Forest University School of Medicine
Winston-Salem, North Carolina

MITCHELL J. KLINE, M.D.

Clinical Adjunct in Radiology
Department of Radiology
University of Louisville School of Medicine
Louisville, Kentucky

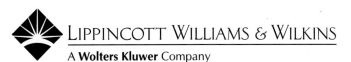

LIPPINCOTT WILLIAMS & WILKINS
A **Wolters Kluwer** Company
Philadelphia • Baltimore • New York • London
Buenos Aires • Hong Kong • Sydney • Tokyo

Acquisitions Editor: Beth Barry
Developmental Editor: Lisa Consoli
Supervising Editor: Steven P. Martin
Production Editor: Amanda Waltman Yanovitch, Silverchair Science + Communications
Manufacturing Manager: Colin Warnock
Cover Designer: Karen Quigley
Compositor: Silverchair Science + Communications
Printer: Maple Press

Library of Congress Cataloging-in-Publication Data

Chew, Felix S.
    Musculoskeletal imaging / Felix S. Chew, Liem T. Bui-Mansfield, Mitchell J. Kline.
        p. ; cm. -- (The core curriculum)
    Includes bibliographical references and index.
    ISBN 0-7817-3797-4
        1. Musculoskeletal system--Imaging. I. Bui-Mansfield, Liem T. II. Kline, Mitchell J. III.
Title. IV. Series.
    [DNLM: 1. Musculoskeletal Diseases--radiography. 2. Diagnostic Imaging--methods.
WE 141 C5289m 2003]
    RC925.7.C45 2003
    616.7'0754--dc21

                                                                    2002043366

Care has been taken to confirm the accuracy of the information presented and to
describe generally accepted practices. However, the authors, editors, and publisher are
not responsible for errors or omissions or for any consequences from application of the
information in this book and make no warranty, expressed or implied, with respect to
the currency, completeness, or accuracy of the contents of the publication. Application
of this information in a particular situation remains the professional responsibility of the
practitioner.

    The authors, editors, and publisher have exerted every effort to ensure that drug
selection and dosage set forth in this text are in accordance with current recommenda-
tions and practice at the time of publication. However, in view of ongoing research,
changes in government regulations, and the constant flow of information relating to
drug therapy and drug reactions, the reader is urged to check the package insert for each
drug for any change in indications and dosage and for added warnings and precautions.
This is particularly important when the recommended agent is a new or infrequently
employed drug.

    Some drugs and medical devices presented in this publication have Food and Drug
Administration (FDA) clearance for limited use in restricted research settings. It is the
responsibility of health care providers to ascertain the FDA status of each drug or device
planned for use in their clinical practice.

                                            10 9 8 7 6 5 4 3 2 1

*To our families, without whom nothing
would be possible, worthwhile, or meaningful*

Contents

Joint Disease

Miscellaneous Topics

FOREWORD

The initial publication in 1989 of Felix S. Chew's *Skeletal Radiology: The Bare Bones* filled a long-standing need for a concise, introductory primer to the imaging of musculoskeletal diseases. In *The Core Curriculum: Musculoskeletal Imaging*, Dr. Chew is joined in authorship by Drs. Liem Bui-Mansfield and Mitch Kline, two outstanding young musculoskeletal radiologists trained by Dr. Chew and his associates at the Wake Forest University School of Medicine. Together, they have thoroughly updated the information available in *The Bare Bones*; their new work includes considerably more magnetic resonance imaging as well as an entire chapter devoted to diagnostic and interventional procedures, a subject of growing importance in the diagnosis and treatment of musculoskeletal disease.

Medical school curricula do not often include a serious study of afflictions of the bones and joints. Even the most common conditions—trauma, osteoporosis, bone metastases, and degenerative joint disease—receive scant attention. Therefore, most residents first encounter radiology with a limited knowledge of the musculoskeletal system. With this background, they are suddenly thrust into a clinical setting where an entirely new vocabulary is used to describe a vast array of unfamiliar disease processes, a perplexing variety of normal variants, and the detailed radiologic and surgical anatomy of several different body regions. The prospect is daunting.

Where can a resident or medical student turn to acquire a firm foundation for musculoskeletal imaging? One should turn to *The Core Curriculum: Musculoskeletal Imaging*. Dr. Chew's initial goal, admirably achieved, was to provide the uninitiated with a working knowledge of skeletal disease and an awareness of the role and value of imaging in its discovery, analysis, and confirmation. He has done so. In stripping skeletal radiology to its essentials, Dr. Chew and his new coauthors have actually left considerable flesh on the bones. They describe and illustrate all of the essential aspects of the most common skeletal diseases. They do so by synthesizing the current knowledge regarding the clinical, pathologic, and physiologic features of each disease, and then outlining the proper approach to the interpretation of radiographs, computed tomographic scans, magnetic resonance imaging scans, and skeletal scintigrams. The essential features of each disorder are demonstrated with exceptional illustrations, augmented as necessary by excellent diagrams, and frequently summarized in tables. The book then concludes with a highly informative chapter on diagnostic interventional procedures. It is a masterful approach that is consistently applied with excellent results.

The book is divided into four parts. The six chapters of Part I are devoted to trauma, properly reflecting the frequency with which skeletal injuries are encountered and the overriding importance of imaging in the diagnosis and management of fractures and dislocations. The first chapter gives an excellent background to the clinical and biomechanical considerations. The next three chapters address injuries of the upper extremity; spine, thoracic cage, and pelvis; and lower extremity, respectively. Chapter 5 describes the distinctive nature of skeletal trauma in children, and Chapter 6 describes imaging of fracture treatment and healing. Part II begins with a discussion of the clinical features and imaging approach to lesions of bone. These lesions are then enumerated individually and described in separate chapters on malignant and benign lesions. The final chapter is justifiably devoted to the frequently encountered clinical problem of metastatic disease to the skeleton, and it emphasizes the primary role of imaging techniques in detection and management. Part III covers joint disease, beginning with a description of basic clinical and pathologic features. An overall approach to the radiology of arthritis is presented, followed by chapters on inflammatory arthritis and noninflammatory joint disease. In separate chapters, Part IV describes developmental and congenital conditions; metabolic, endocrine, and nutritional conditions; and infections of the bones, joints, and soft tissues. There follows a chapter on postsurgical imaging that includes a thorough discussion of the use of imaging in joint replacement, a topic of particular interest to Dr. Chew, with a concluding chapter on diagnostic and interventional procedures.

It is all here. I commend this book to all residents in diagnostic radiology, indeed to all students of skeletal disease. Medical students with an interest in diagnostic radiology, orthopedic surgery, or rheumatology would certainly benefit from its contents. Experienced radiologists will find it a great refresher and undoubtedly gain new insights into musculoskeletal diseases and pick up several useful pointers on musculoskeletal imaging along the way. Teachers of skeletal radiology will discover that the approaches developed and the excellent tables and figures can be of considerable value in preparing their own presentations.

Dr. Chew's first edition of *The Bare Bones* was outstanding. The second edition was better, and *The Core Curriculum: Musculoskeletal Imaging* is even better. I congratulate Drs. Chew, Bui-Mansfield, and Kline. You, the reader, have in your hands a superb contribution to musculoskeletal radiology.

—Lee F. Rogers, M.D.
Editor-in-Chief, *American Journal of Roentgenology*
Isadore Meschan Distinguished Professor of Radiologic Sciences–Radiology
Department of Radiology
Wake Forest University School of Medicine
Winston-Salem, North Carolina

PREFACE

The ranges of pathology and individual variation in the skeleton are too vast for sheer memorization and pattern recognition. One is better able to appreciate abnormalities on images when one understands how the radiologic findings mirror the underlying conditions. For trauma, this requires some familiarity with biomechanics; for oncology, an appreciation of radiologic–pathologic correlation; and for developmental conditions, an understanding of skeletal growth, maturation, and functional adaptation. In the 14 years since the publication of my first textbook of skeletal radiology, the wider application and further refinement of MRI and CT have continued to reduce the role of radiography in musculoskeletal imaging. Inferential diagnosis on the basis of radiologic signs has lost ground to the deliberate demonstration of specific anatomic and pathophysiologic features of disease. The choice and specific performance of examinations has become particularly dependent on clinical context. It is no longer sufficient to react to an image with a list of differential diagnoses; rather, one must consider the clinically relevant possibilities and devise strategies for distinguishing among them with certainty.

The Core Curriculum: Musculoskeletal Imaging is a single unified textbook that teaches general principles of skeletal radiology that are applicable regardless of imaging modality. Organized into four parts, this book presents the core knowledge base in musculoskeletal imaging necessary for a radiology resident. Part I covers musculoskeletal trauma, beginning with an approach to trauma and concluding with separate chapters describing trauma to the upper and lower extremities in adults, trauma to the adult spine, trauma in children, and fracture healing and treatment. Part II covers tumors and tumor-like lesions, beginning with an approach to bone lesions and concluding with separate chapters on malignant and aggressive tumors, benign lesions, and metastatic tumors. Part III covers joint disease, beginning with an approach to joint disease and concluding with separate chapters on inflammatory arthritis and noninflammatory joint disease. Part IV covers miscellaneous topics, including chapters on developmental and congenital conditions; metabolic, endocrine, and nutritional conditions; infection and marrow disease; and postsurgical musculoskeletal imaging. The final chapter covers interventional procedures in musculoskeletal radiology. Although this book is intended specifically for radiologists and radiologists in training, it is also suitable for practitioners and trainees in all fields who deal with the diagnosis and management of musculoskeletal disease.

The images in this textbook were selected from the teaching files and clinical case material at Upstate Medical Center in Syracuse, New York; the Massachusetts General Hospital in Boston, Massachusetts; Wake Forest University Baptist Medical Center in Winston-Salem, North Carolina; Keller Army Community Hospital in West Point, New York; and The Cleveland Clinic Foundation in Cleveland. Friends and colleagues who have graciously provided additional case material include Drs. Carol Boles, William Enneking, Heather Hardie, Terry Hudson, Linda Hughes, Wendy Jones, Susan Kattapuram, Michelle Kraut, Susan Leffler, Leon Lenchik, Mark Levinsohn, Gwilym Lodwick, Catherine Maldjian, Henry Mankin, Kevin McEnery, Michael Mulligan, Robert Novelline, William Palmer, Catherine Roberts, Lee Rogers, Daniel Rosenthal, Dempsey Springfield, and others whom I may have unintentionally overlooked at the moment of this writing. Dr. Catherine Roberts reviewed the entire manuscript and made invaluable suggestions. The line illustrations were drawn by Crisianee Berry. Additional assistance with the preparation of the manuscript was provided by Jamie Cheung, Kim McKenzie, and Sharon Meister.

—Felix S. Chew, M.D.

FIGURE CREDITS

Figures 8.10A, 8.10B, and 8.10C from Chew FS, Disler DG. Chondrosarcoma. *AJR Am J Roentgenol* 1991;156:1016.

Figures 8.24A and 8.24B from Chew FS, Schellingerhout D, Keel SB. Primary lymphoma of skeletal muscle. *AJR Am J Roentgenol* 1999;172:1370.

Figures 8.35A, 8.35B, and 8.35C from Ramsdell MG, Chew FS, Keel SB. Myxoid liposarcoma of the thigh. *AJR Am J Roentgenol* 1998;170:1242.

Figures 16.2A and 16.2B from Chew FS, Schulze ES, Mattia AR. Osteomyelitis. *AJR Am J Roentgenol* 1994;162:942.

Figures 17.26A and 17.26B from Chew FS, Ramsdell MG, Keel SB. Metallosis after total knee replacement. *AJR Am J Roentgenol* 1998;170:1556.

Figures 1.1 through 8.9, 8.11 through 8.23, 8.25 through 8..34, 8.36 through 16.1, 16.3 through 17.25, and 17.27 through 18.35 have been used with permission from the following sources: Chew FS. *Skeletal radiology: the bare bones*. Rockville, MD: Aspen Publishers, 1989; Chew FS. *Skeletal radiology: the bare bones teaching collection*. St. Paul, MN: Image PSL, 1991; Chew FS. *Skeletal radiology: the bare bones*, 2nd ed. Baltimore, MD: Williams & Wilkins, 1997; Chew FS. *Skeletal radiology interactive*. Baltimore, MD: Williams & Wilkins, 1998; Chew FS, Maldjian C, Leffler SG. *Musculoskeletal imaging: a teaching file*. Philadelphia, PA: Lippincott Williams & Wilkins, 1999; Chew FS, Kline MJ, Whitman GJ (eds). *iRAD: Interactive radiology review and assessment*. Philadelphia, PA: Lippincott Williams & Wilkins, 2000; Chew FS. *Skeletal radiology interactive*, 2nd ed. Winston-Salem, NC: Bubbasoft of North Carolina, 2002.

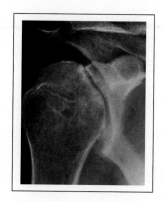

TRAUMA

APPROACH TO TRAUMA

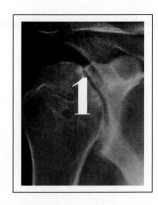

Trauma to the human frame may cause deformation and breakage. The radiology of musculoskeletal trauma is more than a search for broken bones; it is an analysis of the effect of traumatic forces on a particular patient. It requires an understanding of the ways in which various forces affect the body: how they are applied, where they concentrate, and how they cause the body to lose its structural integrity. One must always remember that fractures are but one manifestation of trauma and that injuries to other organ systems may be present.

EPIDEMIOLOGY

Fractures are not isolated phenomena; rather, they occur in the context of individual patients. Characteristics that affect the frequency, severity, location, and type of fracture include age, gender, activity, and health of the musculoskeletal system. The incidence of fractures of the extremities has a bimodal distribution with respect to age. In men, there is a first peak, between 10 and 20 years of age, that is related to immaturity of the skeleton and a second peak, beginning at approximately 70 years of age, that is related to involutional osteoporosis. In women, there is a first peak at 10 years of age, again related to immaturity of the skeleton, and a second peak, beginning at approximately 50 years of age, that is related to postmenopausal osteoporosis. The skeleton is weak when it is growing, gains strength as it matures, and weakens again as it ages. In patients younger than 50 years of age, the incidence of fractures in men is nearly twice that of females, but in patients older than 50 years of age, the incidence in women becomes much greater. Some of these differences may be accounted for by gender differences in recreational and occupational activities and differences in accident rates.

> Under the age of 50 years, fractures are more common in men, but over the age of 50 years, fractures are more common in women.

In adolescents and young adults, the most common sites of fractures in the extremities are the phalanges and metacarpals of the hand, the distal humerus, the shaft of the tibia, the clavicle, the distal radius, and the phalanges of the foot (Table 1.1). In adults older than 50 years of age, the most common sites of fractures in the extremities are the proximal femur, the proximal humerus, the distal radius, and the pelvis (Table 1.2).

BONE BIOMECHANICS

Bone responds to trauma in predictable ways. From knowledge of the anatomic site involved and the forces applied, one can often predict the fractures that result. Conversely, knowing

Table 1.1: Most Common Sites of Fractures in Young Adults

Phalanges of the hand and foot
Metacarpals
Distal humerus
Tibia
Clavicle
Distal radius

Table 1.2: Most Common Sites of Fractures in Adults Older Than 50 Years

Proximal femur
Proximal humerus
Distal radius
Pelvis

the site and morphology of a particular fracture frequently allows one to infer the forces that caused it. Such knowledge has practical applications to diagnosis and management.

FORCE AND DEFORMATION

Application of external force to bone is called *loading*. Bone is physically deformed (i.e., undergoes strain) when it is placed under a load (Fig. 1.1). At physiologic levels of loading, bone undergoes elastic deformation as it absorbs and stores the energy imparted by the loading. When the load is removed, the stored energy is dissipated by elastic recoil, the bone recovers its preloaded shape, and no damage is sustained. Loading has a linear relationship to elastic deformation called *stiffness*. The stiffer the material, the less it deforms under a given load. When the severity of loading exceeds the level at which elastic recoil is possible, the bone sustains plastic (also called *ductile*) deformation. The absorbed energy from loading is expended in the work of

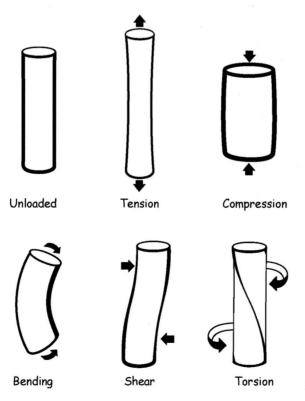

Figure 1.1 Various modes of loading.

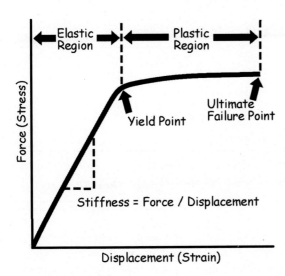

Figure 1.2 The relationship between stress and strain. Strain increases linearly with stress until the yield point is reached. Beyond this point, permanent deformation takes place with only small increments of additional stress.

permanently deforming the bone. The *ductility* of a material describes the degree to which it can sustain plastic deformation without breaking. At even greater levels of loading, the bone fails completely, and the imparted energy is expended in fracturing the bone and displacing the fragments. If loading continues, other body parts may sustain injury. Excessive loading results in injury; in general, the greater the amount of loading and the more rapidly it is applied, the more severe the injury. The relationship between force and deformation can be represented graphically (Fig. 1.2).

The external force of loading involves three fundamental components: compressive, tensile, and shear. The compressive component acts inwardly and squashes the bone together, the tensile component acts outwardly and pulls the bone apart, and the shear component acts parallel to the direction of force and sends different points in the bone past each other (Fig. 1.3). Bone subjected to tensile loading tends to elongate; mechanical failure occurs when cement lines debond and the osteons are pulled apart. Bone subjected to compressive loading tends to shorten; mechanical failure occurs when individual osteons sustain oblique cracking. Bone subjected to shear loading undergoes angular deformity. Both tensile and compressive loading have shear as a component because angular deformity occurs as bone elongates or shortens.

Bone is a diphasic material comprised of a rigid calcium hydroxyapatite crystalline structure that is resistant to compressive forces and a collagenous matrix of flexible fibrils and ground substance that is resistant to tensile forces. In compact bone (also referred to as *lamellar bone* or *cortical bone*), the material of bone is organized into concentric layers around the neurovascular supply to form osteons (haversian systems). Osteons are the basic functional and structural unit of compact bone. In cancellous bone (trabecular bone), the material of bone is organized into a

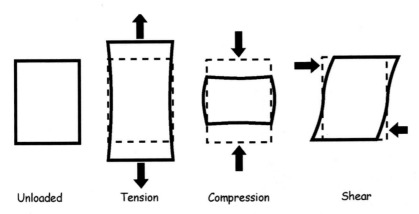

Figure 1.3 Diagrammatic representation of stress and strain.

Table 1.3: Types of Loading

Direct loading
   Crush
   Penetrating
   Tapping
Indirect loading
   Tension
   Compression
   Shear
   Torsion
   Angulation

three-dimensional lattice-like system of plates and columns (trabeculae), with the neurovascular supply passing between trabeculae. Compact bone is stiffer than cancellous bone, but cancellous bone is more ductile. The functional architecture of mature bone reflects a continuing process of remodeling to accommodate the type, magnitude, and direction of physiologic loading. In general, bone resists compression better than tension, and tension better than shear.

LOADING AND FRACTURES

Direct loading causes injuries at the site of loading. The morphology of fractures caused by direct loading tends to be unpredictable and irregular.

Loading can be direct or indirect (Table 1.3). Direct loading causes injuries at the site of loading. The morphology of fractures caused by direct loading—although related to the site, direction, and amount of force applied—tends to be unpredictable and bizarre. Such injuries may be classified as crushing, penetrating, or tapping. A crushing injury results from the application of a large force over a large area, for example, a building collapsing on an individual. Crushing force results in comminuted or transverse fractures and extensive soft tissue damage. A penetrating injury results from a large force being applied to a small area, for example, a gunshot wound. Penetrating force usually results in comminuted fractures; the degree of comminution depends on the energy of the penetrating projectile (Fig. 1.4). A tapping injury results from a small force

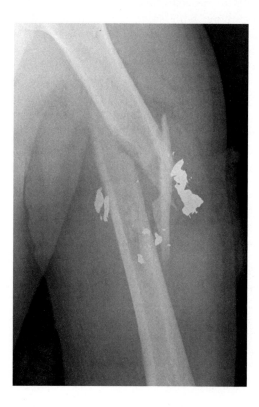

Figure 1.4 Low-velocity gunshot wound causing comminuted fractures of the humeral shaft. The bullet fragmented on impact.

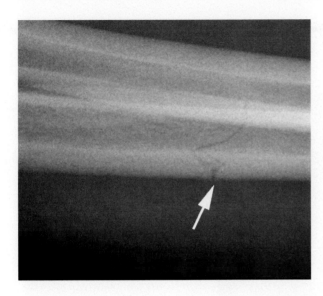

Figure 1.5 Tapping fracture (*arrow*) of the ulnar shaft (nightstick fracture).

being applied to a small area, for example, a blow to the forearm from a nightstick. Tapping force results in a transverse or stellate fracture at the site of impact (Fig. 1.5). Bones without much soft tissue coverage, such as the ulna or tibia, are more vulnerable to direct trauma than bones such as the humerus or femur.

Indirect loading causes injuries at a distance from the site of loading. The morphology of fractures caused by indirect loading tends to be predictable and regular, although it is also related to the site, direction, and amount of force applied. Loading under tension (pulling apart), compression (squashing together), shearing (pulling across the grain), torsion (twisting), angulation (bending), and certain combinations of these produce fractures with predictable shapes that often occur at specific sites (Fig. 1.6). The soft tissues may modify indirect loading—for example, muscles can reduce tensile loads on bones by contracting and supplying an opposing compressive force.

Traction or tension fractures occur as a result of traction on a bone by a tendon or ligament. The bone is pulled apart, or avulsed, and the fracture line is transverse to the direction of force as the bone fibers fail under tension. The patella, for example, may be pulled apart if the knee is forcibly flexed while the extensor muscles are contracting (Fig. 1.7). The size of the avulsed fragment may range from large to tiny. A large fragment may comprise a full-thickness piece of the bone; a small fragment may represent a mere fraction of the cortex. Tension fractures are most common in cancellous bone.

Indirect loading causes injuries at a distance from the site of loading. The morphology of fractures caused by indirect loading tends to be predictable and regular.

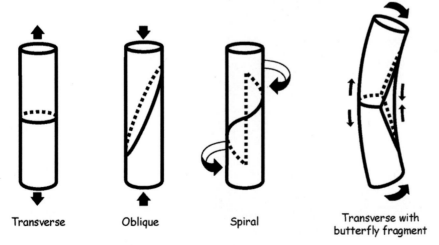

Transverse   Oblique   Spiral   Transverse with butterfly fragment

Figure 1.6 Types of loading correlated with direction of fracture lines.

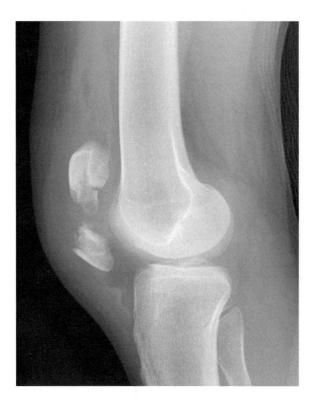

Figure 1.7 Tension fracture of the patella.

When a long bone is angulated, the convex side is placed under tension, and the concave side is placed under compression. Because bone fails first under tension, a transverse fracture propagates across the bone from the convex side. On the concave side, the bone may fail under compressive and shearing forces and splinter. Alternatively, a triangular fragment may shear off at an angle to the main fracture line. This results in comminution with a butterfly fragment on the concave side of the bend (Fig. 1.8).

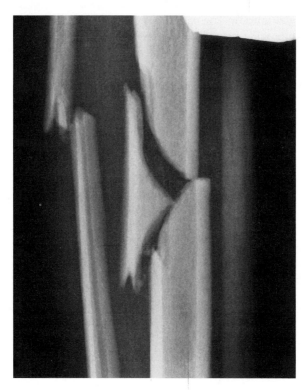

Figure 1.8 Transverse fracture of the tibia with butterfly fragment.

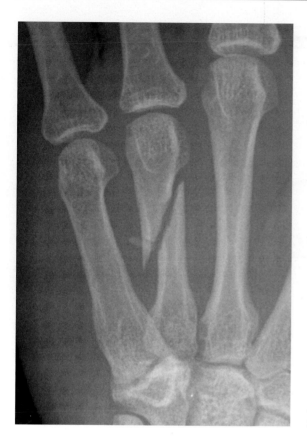

Figure 1.9 Oblique fracture of the fourth metacarpal shaft of the hand.

Longitudinal compressive loading of the shaft of a long bone results in an oblique fracture caused by osteons being forced past each other and shearing off (Fig. 1.9). Compressive loading of a whole bone often results in T- or Y-shaped fractures as the hard cortical bone of the shaft is driven into the softer cancellous metaphysis. Such fractures are common at the ends of the humerus or femur and in the hands and toes.

Rotational loading (torsion or twisting) causes horizontal shearing with compressive and tensile components at an angle to the long axis of the shaft (Fig. 1.10). These stresses lead to a spiral fracture that curves around the circumference of the bone, representing a failure in tension, as the bone is pulled apart. The fracture line makes one complete rotation around the circumference of the bone and has sharp pointed ends joined by a vertical component (Fig. 1.11). The vertical fracture acts as a hinge, with the fracture fragments separating on the opposite side along the curved component.

Many fractures are produced by a combination of forces. Angulation with axial compression results in a curved fracture line with oblique and transverse components and sometimes a butterfly fragment. Angulation with rotation results in an oblique fracture with short, blunted ends.

BONE BRUISES

Bone bruises are traumatic injuries to cancellous bone in which hemorrhage and edema displace the normal marrow. These injuries, which involve microfractures of individual trabeculae and disruption of small vessels, are evident only on MRI. The mechanism of injury is typically compression, either from direct impact or indirect loading, with the impact transmitted through an adjacent bone. When the mechanism is direct impact, the bone bruise is usually isolated. When the mechanism is through indirect, transmitted impact, additional significant injuries may be present elsewhere in the anatomic region (Fig. 1.12). The pattern of bone bruises may help to identify associated injuries and suggest the mechanism of injury. Bone bruises typically revert to nor-

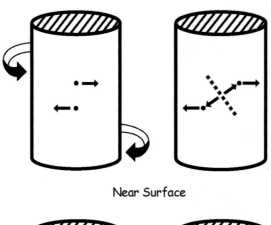

Near Surface

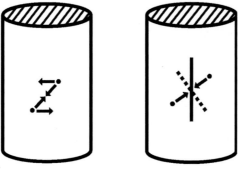

Far Surface

Figure 1.10 Diagrammatic representation of spiral fracture. On the near cortex of the bone, under torsion, horizontal shear stress forces points in the bone past each other. Tensile stress is present because these points are at the same time pulled apart, leading to an obliquely oriented tension fracture around the circumference of the bone. On the far cortex of the bone, compressive forces are present, leading to a vertical fracture that joins the spiral fracture lines.

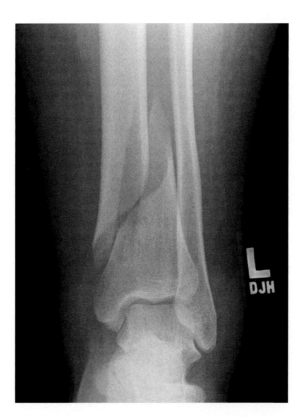

Figure 1.11 Spiral fracture of the tibial shaft.

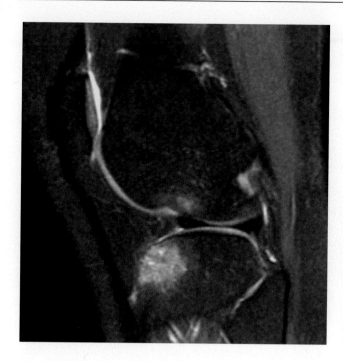

Figure 1.12 Bone bruises caused by indirect impact during hyperextension injury of the knee. Sagittal T2-weighted MR image shows a bone bruise in the anterior aspect of the lateral tibial plateau and a matching impaction fracture of the lateral femoral condyle.

mal on follow-up MRI within several months; typically, the radiograph remains normal throughout the episode.

IMAGING FRACTURES

Although some fractures can be identified on virtually any imaging modality, radiography dominates the imaging evaluation for acute fractures. CT has a supporting role in characterizing complex fractures in preparation for possible surgery and occasionally in identifying fractures when radiographs are equivocal. In the spine, CT is sometimes used to screen for fractures in the setting of blunt trauma. MRI is used more commonly for soft tissue and joint injuries rather than for fractures, but unsuspected fractures are often present. MRI is also used for identifying fractures when radiographs are negative or equivocal and for identifying stress fractures. The radionuclide bone scan may be used for identifying stress fractures.

Most radiographs of the skeleton are made to search for fractures in traumatized limbs. Radiographs are a diagnostic supplement to the history and physical examination; care of the patient should not be secondary to performing the radiographic examination. Splinting an injured limb, for example, can alleviate pain without interfering with subsequent radiologic examinations.

On radiographs, fractures of cortical bone are definitively recognized as focal discontinuities in the structure of bone, particularly when displacement is present. Impacted fractures of cortical bone may be recognized as focal alterations in the contour of the bone, typically an abrupt change in what should otherwise be a smooth contour. Compression fractures in cancellous bone may have a discontinuity in cortex, a change in shape, a linear region of sclerosis, or any combination of these features. Avulsion fractures occur when tension on the attachment of a tendon, ligament, or capsule pulls off a fragment of bone. These fractures may be recognized as a displaced fragment that may range in size from less than 1 mm in thickness to several centimeters.

On CT scans, the features of fractures are similar to those seen on radiography, but the ability to display the features is greatly enhanced by axial cross sections and multiplanar reconstructions (Fig. 1.13).

On MRI, fracture lines are dark on T1-weighted images, with surrounding intermediate signal that may involve the adjacent marrow and soft tissues, corresponding

Radiography dominates the imaging evaluation for acute fractures.

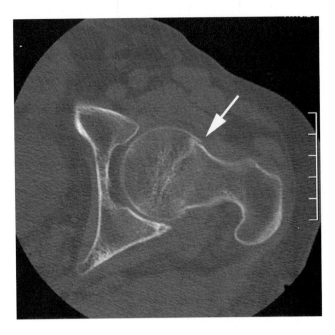

Figure 1.13 Subtle fracture on CT. Axial CT scan shows subtle discontinuity in the anterior femoral cortex with slight impaction (*arrow*), corresponding to a minimally impacted subcapital fracture of the femoral neck.

to hemorrhage and edema (Fig. 1.14). On T2-weighted images, the surrounding edema and hemorrhage generally have high signal, while the fracture line remains dark. In compression fractures of cancellous bone, the fracture line may be absent, but the change in signal will be present if the fracture is acute. Avulsion fracture fragments may be difficult to identify on MRI, as the fragment itself may have the same dark signal on T1- and T2-weighted images as the soft tissue structure that pulled it off. Surrounding edema and hemorrhage should be present. Fractures caused by compressive loading tend to have greater amounts of adjacent marrow edema than fractures caused by tensile loading.

On MRI, fracture lines are dark and often surrounded by edema and hemorrhage.

On radionuclide bone scans, fractures are evident as regions of focal accumulation of radioactivity. However, because the accumulation of the radioactive tracer depends on increased bone metabolism, radionuclide bone scans are useful only after the healing process has begun and are not used in imaging acute trauma.

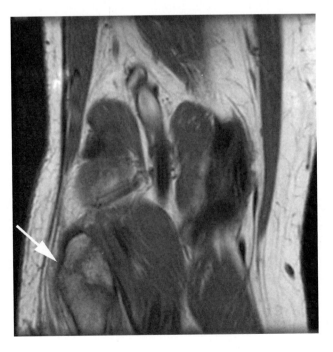

Figure 1.14 Nondisplaced fracture on MRI that was unapparent on radiographs. T1-weighted coronal MR image shows dark fracture lines (*arrow*) in the fibular head.

Table 1.4: Grading of Sprains and Strains

		Clinical Signs	
Grade	Injury	Ligament	Muscle-Tendon
1	Failure of a few fibers	No laxity	No weakness
2	Partial failure	Laxity	Weakness
3	Complete rupture	Frank instability	No muscle action

SOFT TISSUE BIOMECHANICS

Similar to bone, the soft tissue structures of the musculoskeletal system deform when loaded, but they do so in different ways. In addition to recoverable or elastic deformation, the soft tissues may also sustain nonrecoverable or nonelastic deformation. *Creep* is continuous deformation under an applied load, and *stress relaxation* is the decrease in internal load over time at a constant deformation. These *viscous effects* vary with time and the rate of loading, and the structure does not instantaneously recover its original size and shape when the load is removed. When a soft tissue structure is loaded rapidly, it deforms elastically and perhaps fails if the load is great enough; if the same load is applied more slowly, creep and stress relaxation allow the structure to deform to a greater extent, permitting it to absorb more energy without failing. For these reasons, ligaments and tendons are stronger under tensile loading when the load is applied slowly rather than rapidly. Where they attach to bone, it is generally the rate of loading and the strength of the soft tissues relative to the bone that determine whether a soft tissue or a bony injury is sustained. In general, rapid rates of loading cause the soft tissues to fail, whereas slower rates of loading avulse the bone. Injuries of tendons or muscle-tendon units are called *strains*; injuries of ligaments are called *sprains*. Injuries of either may also be called *tears*. Strains and sprains are classified by severity, with grade 1 being a mild injury and grade 3 being a severe, complete discontinuity (Table 1.4). Injuries to soft tissue alone without associated fractures are common and may be difficult to detect on radiographs. Because MRI and sonography can directly image soft tissue injuries, diagnostic imaging has been gaining importance in this clinical area.

Collateral soft tissue injury always accompanies bony injury. Damage may range from superficial abrasions and minimal contusions at the site of injury to massive devitalization involving major segments of the limbs. Direct trauma may cause abrasion, contusion, or crushing of soft tissues (Fig. 1.15). Subcutaneous avulsion of the cutis,

Injuries of tendons or muscle-tendon units are called *strains*. Injuries of ligaments or joint capsules are called *sprains*.

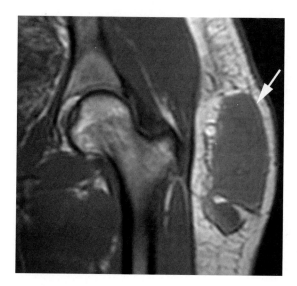

Figure 1.15 Soft tissue contusion from a mountain-biking accident. Coronal T1-weighted MRI shows a hematoma (*arrow*) in the subcutaneous tissues of the hip. (Courtesy of Catherine C. Roberts, MD.)

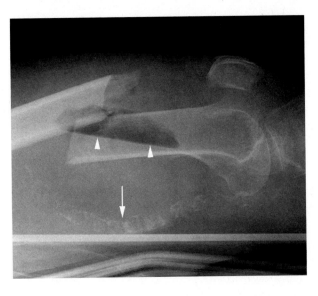

Figure 1.16 Hematoma and sterile collection of bone marrow spilling into the soft tissues adjacent to a displaced femoral shaft fracture. Note the fat-fluid level (*arrowheads*) on this horizontal beam radiograph and the posterior displacement of the calcified popliteal artery (*arrow*) by the collection.

compartment syndrome, and major vascular injury may be caused by indirect mechanisms. For example, displacing fragments from a fracture caused by high-energy indirect loading may slice through the adjacent neurovascular structures and surrounding soft tissues like a meat grinder. In the forearm and lower leg, hemorrhage and acute inflammation from soft tissue injuries may lead to a compartment syndrome in which increased hydrostatic pressure within a fascial compartment may compromise the circulation and cause ischemic necrosis. Strains of adjacent musculature are common accompaniments to fractures, and sharp bony fragments may lacerate adjacent muscles. Complete fractures of long bones may result in hematomas and sterile collections when the bone marrow spills into the adjacent soft tissues (Fig. 1.16).

The articular cartilage that covers the ends of bones in joints is usually loaded in compression because the coefficient of friction at the surface is too low to generate significant shearing forces. With compressive loading, usually indirect blunt impact transferred through the bone, the structure of the extracellular matrix may sustain damage. With more severe loading, the chondrocytes may die, and the cartilage may crack apart and become fissured. Fibrocartilage articular structures such as articular discs, menisci, and labra may be injured by a variety of mechanisms.

IMAGING SOFT TISSUE INJURIES

Although radiography is typically the first imaging study used for evaluation of soft tissue injuries, it is performed principally to look for associated fractures. CT is sometimes used in the same way, particularly in the spine. MRI is the best imaging modality for identifying and characterizing soft tissue and joint injuries. The radionuclide bone scan is not useful in recognizing sprains and strains. Ultrasound is gaining more of a foothold in musculoskeletal soft tissue imaging in the United States.

On radiographs, injuries of ligaments and joint capsules (sprains) and of muscle-tendon units (strains) may be recognized indirectly, evident as soft tissue swelling or the loss of anatomic positioning of bony structures. Stress views or kinematic observation under fluoroscopy may be helpful (Fig. 1.17). For example, when bony structures stabilized by a ligament are displaced from their usual positions, injury to the ligament may be inferred. Soft tissue swelling, particularly when focal, may also indicate a sprain or a strain.

On CT, the ability to identify soft tissue structures is improved compared with radiographs, but soft tissue injuries remain difficult to identify directly. As with radiography, indirect signs such as displacement of bony structures or soft tissue swelling may allow one to infer the presence of a sprain or strain.

Sprains and strains may be directly imaged by MRI.

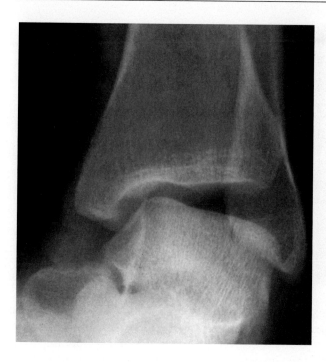

Figure 1.17 Chronic lateral ankle sprain with subluxation on AP stress radiograph.

On MRI, sprains and strains may be directly imaged. Complete tears (grade 3 sprains) of ligaments may be evident as absence of the structure, displacement of the structure, discontinuity of the structure, or abnormal signal intensity. When tears are acute, displacement and discontinuity with surrounding hemorrhage and edema allow a definitive diagnosis. Partial tears (grade 1 or 2 sprains) may be evident as focally increased signal on T2-weighted images with surrounding hemorrhage and edema; at least some portions of the ligament remain in continuity. Complete tendon tears (grade 3 strains) are usually evident as discontinuity of the tendon with retraction in the direction of the muscle belly. Hemorrhage and edema are typically present in the acute phase but may be absent if the injury is chronic. When tears are partial (grade 1 or 2 strains), focally increased signal on T2-weighted images is present, sometimes with surrounding edema and hemorrhage. Abnormal intrasubstance signal and swelling are generally present in all tendon tears. Fluid within the tendon sheath is also a typical finding in both complete and partial tendon tears. Muscle tears are evident as high signal on T2-weighted images, corresponding to edema and hemorrhage (Fig. 1.18). The abnormal signal is distributed along fascial planes and may be interdigitated within muscle fascicles.

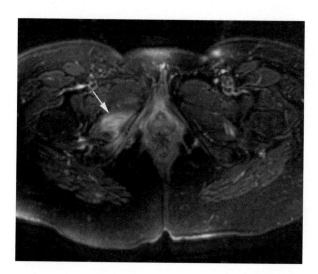

Figure 1.18 Muscle strain accompanying fracture. Axial T2-weighted MRI of the pelvis at the level of the inferior pubic rami shows high signal (*arrow*) in the right obturator internus and obturator externus muscles, along with high signal in the right inferior pubic ramus.

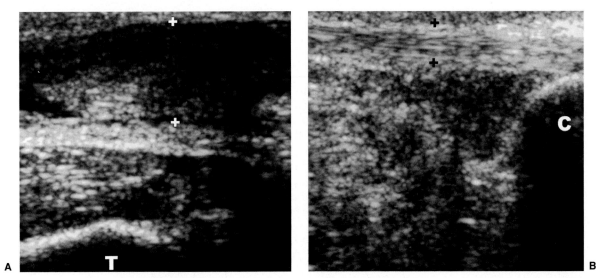

Figure 1.19 Ultrasound of Achilles tendon partial tear. *A.* Longitudinal scan shows markedly thick-ened tendon (marked by cursors) with heterogeneous echogenicity. T, posterior tibia. *B.* Longitudinal scan on normal contralateral side shows tendon of normal thickness (marked by cursors) with well-ordered echogenicity. C, calcaneus.

On ultrasound, complete tendon tears may be recognized by discontinuity of the ten-don with the two ends separated by hypoechoic blood, fluid, or granulation tissue. Some-times, the structure is simply absent from its expected location. Partial tears may be recognized as focal hypoechoic defects within the substance of the tendon or focal thinning (Fig. 1.19). If a tendon sheath is present, fluid within the tendon sheath will be interposed between the torn fragments of either complete or partial tears.

OPEN FRACTURES

Open fractures involve a break in the skin. These are also called *compound fractures* and are distinguished from closed fractures, in which the skin remains intact. The presence of a skin wound is often an indication of extensive soft tissue injury. Traumatized, devitalized soft tissues pose a grave threat of infection; exposed bone will not heal. Radiographic signs indicative of an open fracture include a soft tissue defect, a bone fragment protruding beyond the soft tissues, gas in the soft tissues or within an adjacent joint, the presence of a foreign body, and missing bone fragments.

Gas within a joint that is adjacent to a fracture is an indication of an open fracture.

Open fractures can be classified on the basis of the energy of the injury and consequent extent of soft tissue devitalization (Tables 1.5 and 1.6). Type I open fractures are low-

Table 1.5: Causes of Open Fractures		
Motor vehicle accidents		64%
Motorcycle	28%	
Automobile	24%	
Pedestrian	12%	
Falls		13%
Crush injuries of various causes		8%
Firearms		2%
Miscellaneous		13%
Adapted from Dellinger EP, Miller SD, Wertz MJ, et al. Risk of infection after open fracture of the arm or leg. *Arch Surg* 1987;123.		

Table 1.6: Classification of Open Fractures

Type	Energy of Injury	Skin Wound (cm)	Contamination	Soft Tissue Injury	Fracture
I	Low	<1	Clean	Minimal	Simple, minimal comminution, if any
II	Medium	>1	Moderate 2% infection rate	Moderate, some muscle damage	Moderate comminution
III-A	High	Usually >10	High 18% infection rate	Severe with crushing	Widely displaced, comminuted, and/or segmental
III-B	High	Usually >10	High >50% infection rate	Severe with crushing, extensive soft tissue loss	Widely displaced, comminuted, and/or segmental
III-C	High	Usually >10	High >50% infection rate	Severe with crushing, major vascular disruption	Widely displaced, comminuted, and/or segmental

Adapted from Chapman MW. Open fractures. In: Rockwood CA Jr, Green DP, Bucholz RW, eds. *Rockwood and Green's fractures in adults*, 3rd ed. Philadelphia: Lippincott, 1991.

energy wounds with a skin wound that is typically 1 cm or less in length. A sharp bone fragment piercing the skin from the inside out usually causes the skin wound, which is generally clean. Muscle and soft tissue damage is minimal or absent. These injuries are usually débrided and closed. The risk of infection under ideal management is low. Type II open fractures are usually penetrating wounds with fractures (Fig. 1.20). The extent of soft tissue injury is relatively localized, but the skin wound is greater than 1 cm in length. These

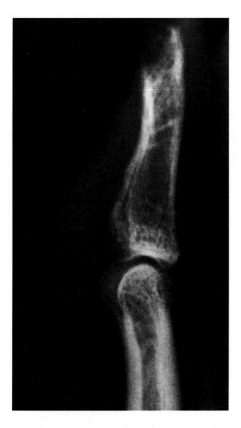

Figure 1.20 Partial amputation of a fingertip (type II open fracture).

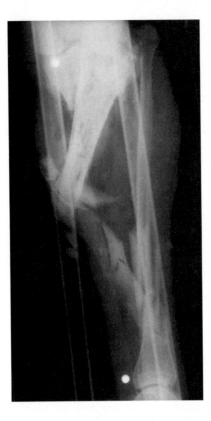

Figure 1.21 Comminuted open fracture of the tibia from crush injury (type III-C).

injuries may be débrided and closed or left open, depending on circumstance. The infection rate is approximately 2%. Type III open fractures are severe high-energy wounds with gross disruption of skin, soft tissues, and bone. Extensive muscle devitalization and soft tissue disruption or gross contamination are present, and the skin wound is generally 10 cm

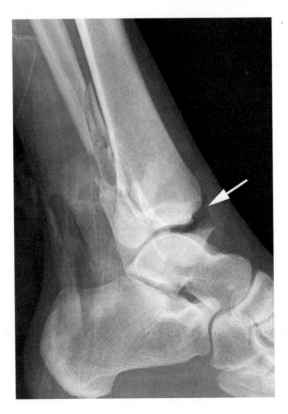

Figure 1.22 Open, comminuted fracture-dislocation of the ankle. Lateral radiograph shows fractures with air within the ankle joint (*arrow*). The joint had been reduced at the scene of the injury before transport.

or more in length. The associated fractures are widely displaced, segmental, or badly comminuted, as one would expect with a high-energy injury (Fig. 1.21). Type III open fractures can be further classified into type III-A, in which there is only limited stripping of the periosteum and soft tissues from the bone; type III-B, in which there is extensive soft tissue loss and gross exposure of bone; and type III-C, in which there is a major vascular disruption. The infection rate is approximately 18% for type III-A open fractures but is more than 50% for types III-B and III-C open fractures. Paradoxically, as techniques of surgical management have improved, the infection rate of open fractures has increased. The explanation lies in the attempted salvage of more severely traumatized limbs that previously would have simply been amputated. The spectrum of infecting organisms has also been changing.

Open fractures that involve a joint often require special care. Gas within a joint that is adjacent to a fracture is an indication that the joint may be contaminated and requires débridement and repair (Fig. 1.22). If the joint was dislocated as well as opened to the environment, contamination may be gross.

Gunshot Wounds

Gunshot wounds pose a public health problem of considerable magnitude, particularly among young adult men. The proliferation of handguns in the civilian population contributes to the increasing rate of injuries, and gun control has been advocated as a method for reducing it. The cost of the medical care of gunshot patients is borne almost completely by society at large, either through governmental funds and subsidies or as bad debts ultimately shared by the public.

The overall mortality rate of civilian gunshot wounds is approximately 10%. Mortality is related to the site of injury, the type and number of projectiles (whether low-velocity or high-velocity), and the delay between the time of injury and definitive medical care. Bullets produce open wounds; contaminated material such as clothing and skin is carried deep into the wound. Because insufficient heat is generated during firing and flight, bullets are not bacteriologically sterile. A bullet with a full metal jacket does not fragment in tissue, but partially jacketed or unjacketed bullets tend to expand, deform, and fragment, increasing the volume of the injury. As established by convention, military small arms use fully jacketed ammunition, but civilian small arms may use partially jacketed or unjacketed ammunition. Many police departments use unjacketed, hollow-point bullets in their weapons to reduce the likelihood of a bullet passing through an intended target and striking a bystander.

Firearms may cause contaminated, open fractures.

Low-velocity gunshot wounds are caused by pistols and many small-bore civilian rifles (muzzle velocities of less than 1,000 ft per second or 305 m per second). Tissues are lacerated and crushed as the bullet strikes and passes into the body. The entire energy of the projectile often is absorbed at the site of impact, and the bullet itself frequently comes to rest in the body, its energy spent (Fig. 1.4). Low-velocity gunshot wounds that involve bone are generally type II open fractures. The extent of soft tissue injury is restricted to the immediate path of the projectile (Fig. 1.23). The path of the bullet in the body may be erratic, following anatomic tissue planes and other paths of low resistance. A trail of small metallic fragments is usually deposited along its trajectory within the body. A bullet that comes to rest in a body cavity or lumen may migrate or embolize. The size of a bullet on radiographs depends on its actual size, the radiographic projection, and the degree of magnification. CT may be helpful in localizing the bullet.

Military weapons such as assault rifles and some civilian hunting rifles cause high-velocity wounds (muzzle velocities of greater than 2,000 ft per second or 610 m per second). Because kinetic energy increases with the square of the velocity of a projectile, projectiles from high-velocity weapons generally cause severe type III open wounds. On impact, kinetic energy is rapidly transferred from the missile to the tissue. In addition to crushing and lacerating the tissues, shock waves and cavitation from high-velocity projectiles result in additional and possibly more significant damage. As a high-velocity projectile passes through the body, it compresses the tissues along its path, creating a transient shock wave. Shock waves can cause gas-filled organs to rupture but cause little if any damage to muscle or bone. A temporary vacuum cavity forms behind a high-velocity projectile, similar to the turbulence that forms

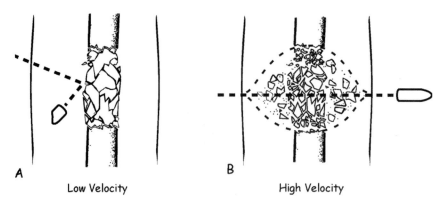

Low Velocity   High Velocity

Figure 1.23 Gunshot wounds. *A.* Low-velocity projectile causes direct damage along its trajectory. *B.* High-velocity projectile is associated with a temporary vacuum cavity (*dashed lines*) and extensive damage. The projectile often has enough energy to pass completely through the body.

behind a hand as it is moved rapidly through water. The pressure within the temporary cavity is subatmospheric, causing debris to be sucked into the wound. The cavity oscillates violently and rapidly as it collapses, damaging an extensive volume of tissue. If the bullet strikes bone, the bone shatters and comminutes widely. Vascular and neural structures may be extensively damaged, and a broad area of tissue and muscle may be devitalized. Even if not hit directly, soft tissue may be pulped, small blood vessels disrupted, and bone shattered. Large vessels may be pushed aside, but intimal damage may lead to thrombosis. The projectile often has so much energy that it passes completely through the body, creating both entrance and exit wounds of highly variable size in the skin (Fig. 1.24). The area of tissue devitalization may extend around the path of the missile for several centimeters in all directions.

Although shotguns have low muzzle velocity, the aggregate mass of the projectiles may be ten times greater than a single bullet, resulting in proportionally greater wounding power, especially at close range (Fig. 1.25). Multiple projectiles spread over a contiguous area can devitalize a large volume of tissue. Shotgun wounds are considered type III open fractures.

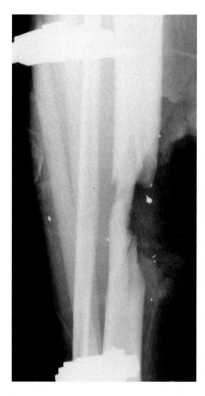

Figure 1.24 High-velocity gunshot wound to the lower leg. AP radiograph shows extensive medial bone and soft tissue loss. The bullet passed completely through.

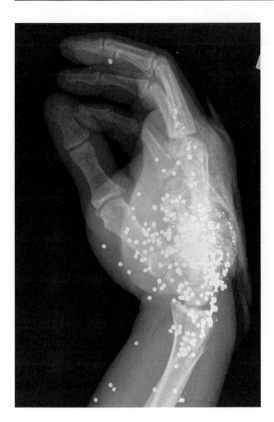

Figure 1.25 Shotgun wound to the hand.

Plastic and rubber bullets from firearms and BBs or small pellets from air guns are inaccurate low-velocity missiles that still have the potential to maim or kill. Blank rounds of ammunition are cartridges with gunpowder but no projectile; however, the explosive force of blank ammunition may kill or injure at close range.

STRESS INJURIES

Stress fractures may be divided into *fatigue fractures*, in which normal bone fractures in response to abnormal loads, and *insufficiency fractures*, in which abnormal bone fractures in response to normal loads. Fractures through focal lesions such as tumors are called *pathologic fractures* and are discussed in Chapter 10.

Fatigue fractures or stress fractures in normal bone are the result of repetitive physical activity, usually occupational or recreational. The individual loads themselves are insufficient to cause fracture, but frequent cyclic loading may initiate a process that leads to fracture. An increase or change in physical activity stimulates changes in the musculoskeletal system. Bone responds to repetitive loading by remodeling, with the quality and location of the remodeling depending on the magnitude and direction of the loading (Wolff's law). The result is bony hypertrophy. Because cortical bone remodels by a process of resorption first and then replacement, there is a vulnerable period during increases in physical activity when the bone has been weakened by resorption but not yet strengthened by replacement. The level and frequency of activity determine the duration of vulnerability. Muscular fatigue is also thought to have a role in the generation of stress fractures. With repetitive exercise to near exhaustion of muscles, decreased stress shielding by muscle action may increase the loads placed on the bones. The site of a stress fracture depends on the type of activity (Table 1.7). In runners, for example, common sites include the metatarsal shafts, the tibial shaft, the sesamoids of the foot, the medial femoral cortex, and the inferior pubic ramus. Students with heavy book bags and other occupational or recreational backpackers may sustain stress fractures involving the clavicle or upper ribs. Stress

Table 1.7: Stress Fractures by Sporting Activity

Sport/Athletic Activity	Bone Commonly Involved
Running	Femoral neck, sacral ala, metatarsal, pubic ramus, tarsal navicular, fibula
Hiking	Metatarsal, pelvis
Backpacking	Upper ribs, clavicle
Jumping	Pelvis, femur
Tennis	Ulna, metacarpal
Baseball	
Pitching	Humerus, scapula, first rib, ulna
Batting	Rib
Catching	Patella
Basketball	Patella, tibia, os calcis, sacrum, tarsal navicular
Javelin	Ulna
Soccer	Tibia, pubis
Swimming	Tibia, metatarsal
Skating	Fibula, metatarsal, tibia
Curling	Ulna
Aerobics	Fibula, tibia
Ballet dancing	Metatarsal, tibia, spine
Cricket	Humerus, spine
Golf	Lower ribs, ulna, sternum, tibia, hook of the hamate
Fencing	Pubis
Handball	Metacarpal
Water skiing	Pars interarticularis
Rowing	Lower ribs
Trap shooting	Coracoid process
Volleyball	Pisiform

Adapted from Knapp TP, Garrett WE Jr. Stress fractures: general concepts. *Clin Sports Med* 1997;16:339–356.

fractures are typically identified while they are still incomplete; therefore, the prognosis for healing is excellent.

A similar process of cyclic loading may cause insufficiency fractures, in which abnormally weak bone fractures in response to normal loads. Such fractures may occur, for example, in older, osteoporotic patients who suddenly become more mobile after joint replacement surgery or podiatric surgery or in patients with metabolic bone disease and decreasing bone strength.

On radiographs and CT, stress fractures of long bones are typically evident as thin, transverse, radiolucent lines that involve only a portion of the cortex. By the time most cortical stress fractures are visible on radiographs, healing fracture callus is usually present (Fig. 1.26). Sometimes the callus is visible, but the fracture line itself cannot be seen. A lucent line that is completely surrounded by sclerotic bone represents a stress fracture with failure to heal or nonunion (Fig. 1.27). Stress fractures may also be oriented longitudinally, along the long axis of the bone. In such cases, radiographs are often negative, but CT or MRI may demonstrate the fracture (Fig. 1.28). Stress fractures through cancellous bone are apparent as fuzzy linear densities oriented perpendicular to the direction of compressive stress (Fig. 1.29). As these injuries heal, increasing sclerosis with subsequent remodeling is seen. Depending on the orientation of the fracture line and the presence or absence of fracture callus, stress fractures may be unapparent on CT.

On radionuclide bone scan, stress fractures are focal "hot spots" (Fig. 1.30). Periosteal new bone formation and endosteal thickening in the absence of a demonstrable fracture line usually represent stress reaction, a healing process that occurs in the presence of stress microfractures. The condition is also called *traumatic periostitis*. In traumatic periostitis,

Fracture callus may be the only indication of a stress fracture on radiographs.

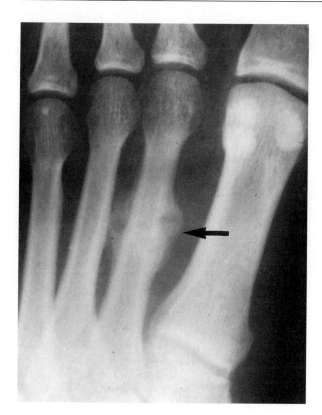

Figure 1.26 Healing stress fracture of the second metatarsal (*arrow*) in a runner.

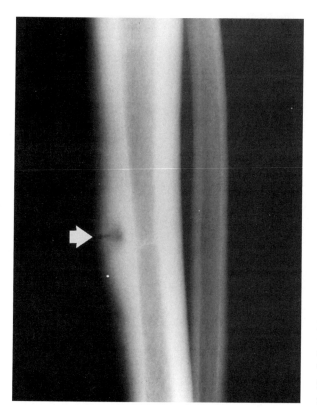

Figure 1.27 Tibial stress fracture (*arrow*) extending incompletely through a thickened anterior cortex. The sclerotic bone that surrounds the fracture and the lack of callus indicate nonunion.

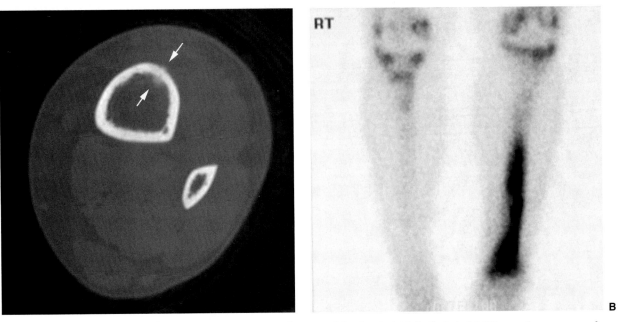

Figure 1.28 Longitudinal stress fracture of the distal tibial shaft. *A.* Axial CT scan shows a vague fracture line in the sagittal plane through the anterior cortex of the distal tibia, with a small amount of periosteal and endosteal fracture callus (*arrows*). *B.* Radionuclide bone scan shows the longitudinal stress fracture in the distal tibia. Radiographs were normal. RT, right.

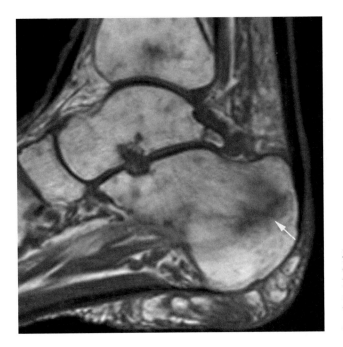

Figure 1.29 Stress fracture of the calcaneus. Sagittal T1-weighted MRI shows the fracture line (*arrow*) through the cancellous bone, without involvement of the cortex.

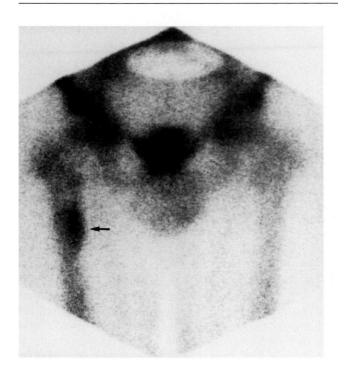

Figure 1.30 Femoral stress fracture. Radionuclide bone scan shows tracer accumulation at medial proximal femoral cortex (*arrow*). Radiographs were normal at the time of scanning.

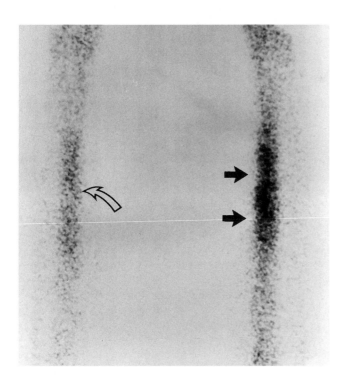

Figure 1.31 Bone scan shows traumatic periostitis, greater on the right (*solid arrows*) than the left (*open arrow*). Radiographs were normal.

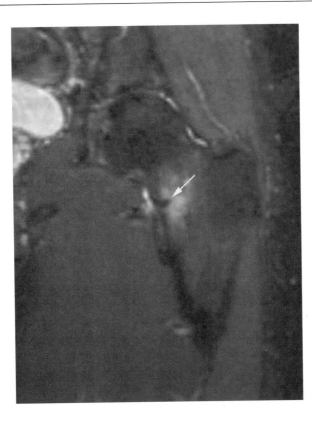

Figure 1.32 Femoral neck stress fracture. Coronal T2-weighted MRI with fat suppression shows a focus of marrow edema adjacent to the medial cortex of the femoral neck, traversed by a dark fracture line (*arrow*). A small amount of periosteal edema is also present.

the region of abnormal activity on radionuclide bone scan is typically larger and less intense than that of stress fractures (Fig. 1.31).

On MRI, stress fractures may show extensive endosteal and periosteal edema and evidence of bone healing. The fracture line will be dark on all pulse sequences and surrounded by edema (Fig. 1.32). In many cases, the edema will be present, but an actual fracture line will not be seen (Fig 1.33). The bone scan and MRI are far more sensitive than radiographs for detecting stress reaction and stress fractures.

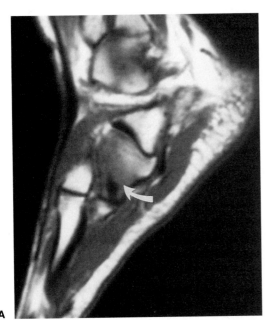

A

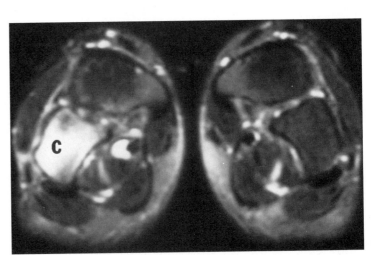

B

Figure 1.33 Cuboid stress fracture. *A.* Sagittal T1-weighted MRI shows low signal in the marrow of the cuboid (*arrow*). *B.* Coronal T2-weighted MRI shows extensive edema in and around the cuboid (C).

Correlation of the diagnostic images with the history and physical examination of the patient is often necessary for accurate diagnosis of stress fractures. With stress fractures, point tenderness is present at the site of injury, and the symptoms worsen with activity but improve with rest.

Stress fractures typically present with point tenderness and worsening symptoms during activity.

THERMAL TRAUMA

BURNS

Burns cause coagulative tissue necrosis. The depth of the injury is related to the severity and duration of the applied heat. Initially, one can see soft tissue loss and soft tissue edema (Fig. 1.34). Osteoporosis and periostitis may occur in the weeks that follow. Periarticular osseous excrescences are common after extensive burns and may be seen 2 to 3 months after injury (Fig. 1.35). The range of motion of involved joints will be limited mechanically. The exact pathogenesis of these ossifications is unknown and seems not to correlate with the severity of the burn.

Heterotopic bone formation commonly follows burn injuries.

COLD INJURY

Cold injuries are essentially vascular injuries. In chilblains or immersion foot, prolonged exposure to low but nonfreezing temperatures causes vasoconstriction and hypoxic damage. Leakage of physiologic fluids from damaged small vessels leads to pain and edema. An intense hyperemic and inflammatory response develops; this is usually painful and often lasts for days to weeks. Ultimate recovery is common, but the affected part typically remains more sensitive to cold than before the exposure. Damp cold has a greater effect than cold at low humidity. In freezing injuries or frostbite—to which the digits, nose, and ears are most vulnerable—the formation of ice crystals within the tissues may cause permanent damage. Autoamputation of soft tissue and bone may be the ultimate result. On radiographs, one may see soft tissue edema, osteoporosis, and periostitis. Soft tissue and even bone loss from tuftal resorption may occur in the fingers and toes (Fig. 1.36). Cartilage damage may result in secondary degenerative joint disease. Acute evaluation of cold injuries may include arteriography or radionuclide perfusion studies. In children, frostbite may damage the growth plates of fingers or toes, with subsequent growth deformity.

Cold injuries may damage articular cartilage and lead to degenerative joint disease.

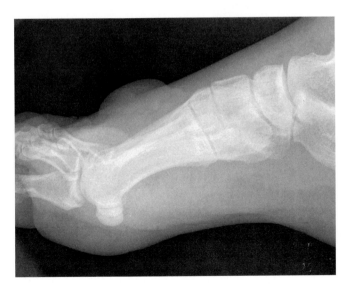

Figure 1.34 Acute scalding injury to the dorsum of the foot, resulting in a bleb.

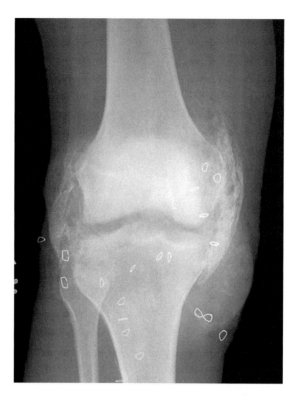

Figure 1.35 Soft tissue ossification at the knee after severe burns. Skin grafting has also been performed.

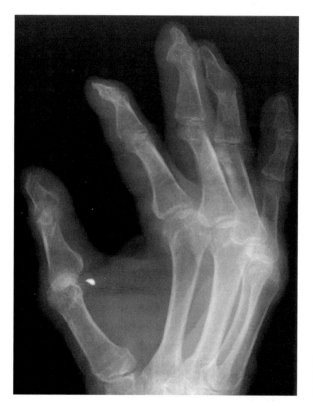

Figure 1.36 Acro-osteolysis caused by frostbite in a homeless man. (Courtesy of Catherine C. Roberts, MD.)

DESCRIBING FRACTURES AND DISLOCATIONS

Precise use of language in describing fractures and dislocations is imperative for patient care. The most important fact about a fracture is its site within the skeleton. The location within the involved bone should be precisely noted. In the long bones, it is conventional to divide the shaft into thirds and to indicate which third is involved (proximal, middle, or distal). A fracture site can also be located at the junction of the proximal and middle thirds or the junction of the middle and distal thirds. If anatomic landmarks are present, they may be used for reference; some anatomic regions have specific terminology.

> The most important fact about a fracture is its site within the skeleton.

Fractures may be closed or open and complete or incomplete. The morphology of the fracture should be described in terms of the principal fracture line: transverse, spiral, or oblique, and so forth. Simple fractures have one fracture plane and two major fragments. Comminuted fractures have two or more fracture planes and three or more major fragments. Examples of comminuted fractures include transverse fractures with butterfly fragments and segmental fractures (transverse fractures at different levels of a shaft that isolate a segment of bone) (Fig. 1.37).

Alignment refers to the long axis of the fragments; *angulation* is a change from the normal alignment and refers specifically to the angle between the long axes of the major fragments. The direction of angulation of a fracture reflects the direction of loading. By convention, varus or medial angulation of the distal fragment is deviation of the distal part toward the midline of the body; valgus or lateral angulation of the distal fragment is deviation of the distal part away from the midline of the body (Fig. 1.38). Angulation can also be anterior or posterior. An alternative method of reporting fracture angulation is to describe the direction of the apex of the angle formed by the major fragments. A fracture with valgus (lateral) angulation of the distal fragment would be described as apex medial.

Position refers to the relationship of the fracture fragments to their normal anatomic location. Loss of position is called *displacement*. Fragments that are completely separated from each other are completely displaced. Fragments that maintain partial contact with their anatomic location are partially displaced; partial displacement of cortical fractures is usually described in terms of a proportion of the shaft width. In nondisplaced fractures, the fragments remain in

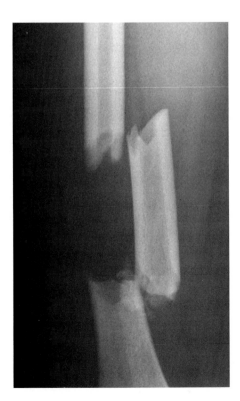

Figure 1.37 Segmental fracture of the femoral shaft with complete displacement.

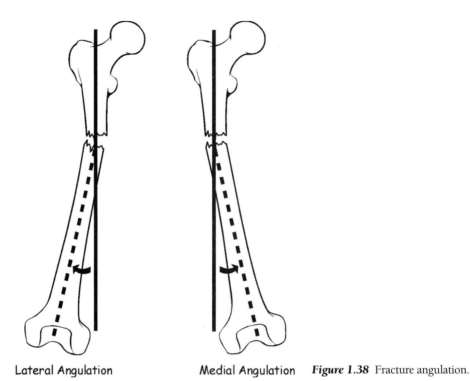

Lateral Angulation   Medial Angulation   *Figure 1.38* Fracture angulation.

their normal anatomic location. In rotary displacement, the fragments turn away from each other; documentation of rotary displacement requires a single film that includes both ends of the fractured bone. *Shortening* is the overlap of fragments along the axis of the limb, and *distraction* is separation of fragments along the axis of the limb. Loss of position by articulating bones is called *dislocation* or *luxation* if there is no remaining contact between the articulating bones and *subluxation* if partial contact has been maintained (Fig. 1.39).

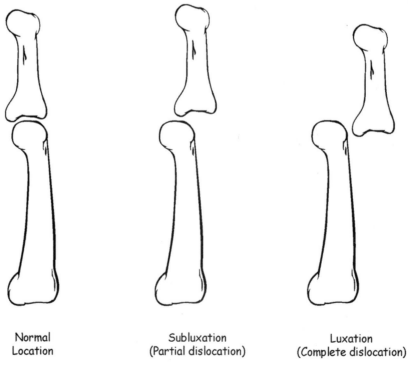

Normal   Subluxation   Luxation
Location   (Partial dislocation)   (Complete dislocation)

Figure 1.39 Normal and abnormal joint location.

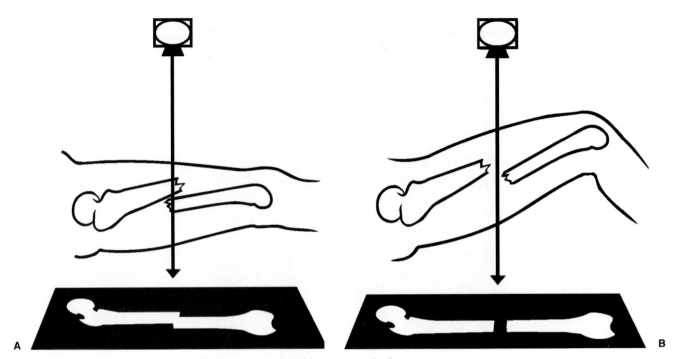

Figure 1.40 Radiographic projection affecting appearance of fracture. *A.* The fragments appear overlapped. *B.* The fragments appear distracted.

The apparent position and alignment of bones and fragments on radiographs can vary with positioning of the part relative to the x-ray apparatus (Fig. 1.40). In general, two views obtained 90 degrees to each other is the minimum necessary to determine the relative position and alignment of fracture fragments in three dimensions. Sequential measurements of fracture position and angulation on films are often not possible unless great care is taken to obtain films in the same projection.

Intra-articular fractures are those at the end of a bone in which the fracture line extends into the articulating portion of the bone, although not necessarily into the articular surface itself. Osteochondral fractures are intra-articular fractures that extend through both bone and articular cartilage. On radiographs, the presence of the cartilage fragment may be inferred from the donor site of the bony fragment (Fig. 1.41). Cartilage injuries may be imaged directly by MRI (Fig. 1.42).

Avulsion fractures are traction fractures from tensile loading of tendons or ligaments and range from large transverse fractures to tiny flecks of cortex at the insertion or origin of the involved muscle or tendon. These fractures indicate disruption of the bone-tendon

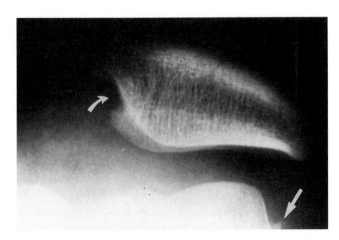

Figure 1.41 Osteochondral fracture of the patella leaving a defect in the medial facet (*curved arrow*). The fracture fragment (*arrow*) consists of articular cartilage with an attached segment of subchondral bone.

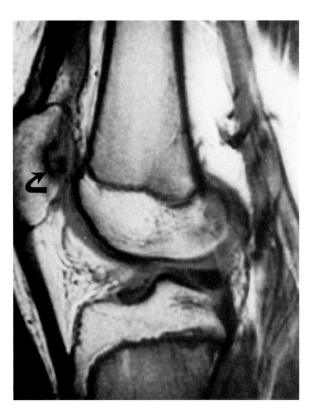

Figure 1.42 Sagittal PD MRI shows an osteochondral fracture of the patella (*arrow*).

or bone-ligament complex and have great clinical significance. They also imply that the soft tissue structure—the tendon or ligament that has pulled off the bone fragment—is itself still intact.

Dislocations and subluxations should be described by the location of the distal part relative to the proximal part. For example, in an anterior glenohumeral dislocation, the humerus has dislocated to a position that is anterior to the glenoid; conversely, in a posterior glenohumeral dislocation, the humerus has dislocated to a position that is posterior to the glenoid.

RADIOLOGIC REPORTING

The ultimate work product of diagnostic radiology is information for clinical decision making. The work is not complete until that information is transferred to those who are attending the patient. The information that the radiologist obtains from the images is documented in the radiologic report and should be sufficient to satisfy the clinical imperative for the radiologic examination. The radiologist's report becomes part of the patient's medical record. It should be composed with care and diligence and rendered in a timely fashion. Direct communication between radiologist and attending physician by telephone or in person is often appropriate.

The radiologist's report becomes part of the patient's medical record.

A radiologic report of a fracture should begin with the date (time) of the examination, the type of examination (portable or not), the date of the report, the body part examined, the projections obtained, and the appliances present (e.g., casts or splints). A description of the fracture is the body of the report and should include as a minimum the location, direction, position, and alignment. Additional descriptive and diagnostic observations are included as appropriate. In radiologic reports, unless otherwise specified, fractures can be assumed to be acute, complete, not comminuted, not displaced, not angulated, extra-articular, nonpathologic, and closed.

There are many different systems of classification for fractures in most regions of the body, often devised for different purposes by practitioners with different interests. The best classifications are those that provide a conceptual basis for understanding patterns of injuries, facilitate clinical management decisions, or correlate with prognosis. Descriptive and anatomic classifications are useful in radiology, but classification of a fracture based on prognosis and management is best left to the patient's attending physician. For complex systems of fracture classification, observer variability may be quite high. Rather than guess the classification scheme that the referring clinician may be using, the radiologist should strive to describe the injuries (present and absent) in sufficient detail for any classification system to be applied on the basis of the radiologic report.

SOURCES AND READINGS

Arendt EA, Griffiths HJ. The use of MR imaging in the assessment and clinical management of stress reactions of bone in high-performance athletes. *Clin Sports Med* 1997;16:291–306.

Bartlett CS, Helfet DL, Hausman MR, et al. Ballistics and gunshot wounds: effects on musculoskeletal tissues. *J Am Acad Orthop Surg* 2000;8:21–36.

Barton KL, Kaminsky CK, Green DW, et al. Reliability of a modified Gartland classification of supracondylar humerus fractures. *J Pediatr Orthop* 2001;21:27–30.

Bartonicek J. Pauwels' classification of femoral neck fractures: correct interpretation of the original. *J Orthop Trauma* 2001;15:358–360.

Bennell K, Matheson G, Meeuwisse W, et al. Risk factors for stress fractures. *Sports Med* 1999;28:91–122.

Bergman AG, Fredericson M. MR imaging of stress reactions, muscle injuries, and other overuse injuries in runners. *Magn Reson Imaging Clin N Am* 1999;7:151–174.

Brooks AA. Stress fractures of the upper extremity. *Clin Sports Med* 2001;20:613–620.

Browner BD, Levine AM, Jupiter JB, et al., eds. *Skeletal trauma: fractures, dislocations, ligamentous injuries*, 2nd ed. Philadelphia: Saunders, 1998.

Bucholz RW, Heckman JD, eds. *Rockwood and Green's fractures in adults*, 5th ed. Philadelphia: Lippincott Williams & Wilkins, 2001.

Buckwalter JA, Einhorn TA, Simon SR. *Orthopaedic bioscience: biology and biomechanics of the musculoskeletal system*, 2nd ed. American Academy of Orthopaedic Surgeons, 2000.

Dellinger EP, Miller SD, Wertz MJ, et al. Risk of infection after open fracture of the arm or leg. *Arch Surg* 1987;123:1320–1327.

DeLong WG Jr, Born CT, Wei SY, et al. Aggressive treatment of 119 open fracture wounds. *J Trauma* 1999;46:1049–1054.

Deutsch AL, Coel MN, Mink JH. Imaging of stress injuries to bone: radiography, scintigraphy, and MR imaging. *Clin Sports Med* 1997;16:275–306.

Folk JW, Starr AJ, Early JS. Early wound complications of operative treatment of calcaneus fractures: analysis of 190 fractures. *J Orthop Trauma* 1999;13:369–372.

Frandsen PA, Andersen PE, Madsen F, et al. Garden's classification of femoral neck fractures. *J Bone Joint Surg Br* 1988;70B:588–590.

Gibbon WM, Long G. Imaging of athletic injuries. *Curr Orthopaed* 2000;14:424–434.

Grieco A, Molteni G, De Vito G, et al. Epidemiology of musculoskeletal disorders due to biomechanical overload. *Ergonomics* 1998;41:1253–1260.

Howard M, Court-Brown CM. Epidemiology and management of open fractures of the lower limb. *Br J Hosp Med* 1997;57:582–587.

Ishibashi Y, Okamura Y, Otsuka H, et al. Comparison of scintigraphy and magnetic resonance imaging for stress injuries of bone. *Clin J Sport Med* 2002;12:79–84.

Kellermann A, Heron S. Firearms and family violence. *Emerg Med Clin North Am* 1999;17:699.

Knapp TP, Garrett WE Jr. Stress fractures: general concepts. *Clin Sports Med* 1997;16:339–356.

Kumar S. Theories of musculoskeletal injury causation. *Ergonomics* 2001;44:17–47.

Lanoix R, Gupta R, Leak L, et al. C-spine injury associated with gunshot wounds to the head: retrospective study and literature review. *J Trauma* 2000;49:860–863.

Ludwig J, Cook PJ. Homicide and suicide rates associated with implementation of the Brady Handgun Violence Prevention Act. *JAMA* 2000;284:585–591.

Miller M, Azrael D, Hemenway D. Community firearms, community fear. *Epidemiology* 2000;11:709–714.

Nordin M, Frankel VH. *Basic biomechanics of the musculoskeletal system*, 3rd ed. Philadelphia: Lippincott Williams & Wilkins, 2001.

Ordog G, ed. *Management of gunshot wounds*. New York: Elsevier, 1988.

Pope MH, DeVocht JW. The clinical relevance of biomechanics. *Neurol Clin* 1999;17:17–41.

Roebuck JD, Finger DR, Irvin TL. Evaluation of suspected stress fractures. *Orthopedics* 2001;24:771–773.

Rogers LF. *Radiology of skeletal trauma*, 3rd ed. Philadelphia: WB Saunders, 2002.

Rosenfeld JV. Gunshot injury to the head and spine. *J Clin Neurosci* 2002;9:9–16.

Sanders TG, Medynski MA, Feller JF, et al. Bone contusion patterns of the knee at MR imaging: footprint of mechanism of injury. *Radiographics* 2000;20:S135–S151.

Schultz RJ. *The language of fractures*, 2nd ed. Baltimore: Williams & Wilkins, 1990.

Siebenrock KA, Gerber C. The reproducibility of classification of fractures of the proximal end of the humerus. *J Bone Joint Surg Am* 1993:75A:1751–1755.

Skaggs DL, Kautz SM, Kay RM, et al. Effect of delay of surgical treatment on rate of infection in open fractures in children. *J Pediatr Orthop* 2000;20:19–22.

Sloan JH, Kellermann AL, Reay DT, et al. Handgun regulations, crime, assaults, and homicide: a tale of two cities. *N Engl J Med* 1988;319:1256–1262.

Tejan J, Lindsey RW. Management of civilian gunshot injuries of the femur. A review of the literature. *Injury* 1998;29:SA13–SA22.

Templeman DC, Gulli B, Tsukayama DT, et al. Update on the management of open fractures of the tibial shaft. *Clin Orthop* 1998;350:18–25.

Tencer AF, Johnson KD. *Biomechanics in orthopedic trauma: bone fracture and fixation*. Philadelphia: JB Lippincott Co, 1994.

Thomsen NO, Jensen CM, Skovgaard N, et al. Observer variation in the radiographic classification of fractures of the neck of the femur using Garden's system. *Int Orthop* 1996;20:326–329.

Wainwright AM, Williams JR, Carr AJ. Interobserver and intraobserver variation in classification systems for fractures of the distal humerus. *J Bone Joint Surg Br* 2000;82:636–642.

Wiss DA, Gellman H. Gunshot wounds to the musculoskeletal system. In: Browner BD, Jupiter JB, Levine AM, et al., eds. *Skeletal trauma*. Philadelphia: WB Saunders, 1992:367–400.

Yao L, Johnson C, Gentili A, et al. Stress injuries of bone: analysis of MR imaging staging criteria. *Acad Radiol* 1998;5:34–40.

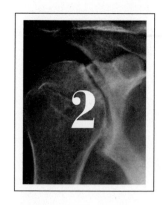

Trauma in Adults: Upper Extremity

This chapter describes the radiology of many common injuries to the upper extremities in adults.

HAND

Fractures of the metacarpals and phalanges of the hand are approximately three times more common in men than in women. These injuries have a peak incidence in young men and decrease in incidence with increasing age.

FINGERS

Avulsion injuries of the phalanges involve tensile failure of ligamentous or musculotendinous units. These injuries result when excessive loading occurs while the tendon or ligament is already under tension. The substance of a tendon or ligament may tear, or there may be avulsion of its bony insertion. For example, sudden, forcible flexion of the distal interphalangeal (DIP) joint of an extended finger, as occurs when an outstretched finger is struck by a baseball, may result in tensile failure of the extensor mechanism of the distal phalanx. The injury is called a *baseball finger*, and the resulting clinical deformity is called a *mallet finger*, in which the DIP joint is maintained in flexion and cannot be extended. An avulsion fracture of the dorsal proximal corner of the distal phalanx is present in 25% of cases of baseball finger (Fig. 2.1); thus, most of these injuries are tendinous. An avulsed bone fragment can be retracted by muscle pull. The converse injury occurs with forcible extension of the DIP joint of a flexed finger or with forcible hyperextension at the DIP joint. In this case, the volar plate of the distal phalanx at the flexor digitorum profundus tendon insertion may be avulsed; alternatively, the tendon may tear. Similar injuries may occur at the proximal interphalangeal (PIP) joint.

Purely ligamentous and tendinous injuries are more common than bony avulsions in the fingers, so radiographs may show only soft tissue swelling or deformities of alignment. Avulsion fractures at the base of a phalanx from the volar edge indicate disruption of the

Avulsion injuries in the hand are caused by tensile loading.

Ligamentous and tendinous injuries are more common than avulsion fractures.

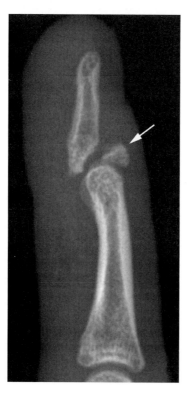

Figure 2.1 Avulsion fracture at the extensor insertion of the distal phalanx (*arrow*).

attachment of the volar plate. Avulsions from the lateral edge indicate disruption of the attachments of collateral ligaments (Fig. 2.2). Avulsions from the dorsal edge indicate disruption of the extensor tendon. The avulsed fragments always contain the tendinous or ligamentous insertion (enthesis) and may range in size from a tiny sliver of cortical bone to a large intra-articular fragment. If the intra-articular fragment involves one-third or more of the articular surface, the joint may subluxate and require operative fixation. A bony defect should be present where the fragment originated, and although one margin of the fragment

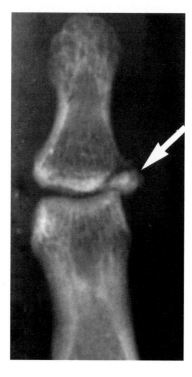

Figure 2.2 Avulsion fracture at the collateral ligament insertion of the distal phalanx (*arrow*).

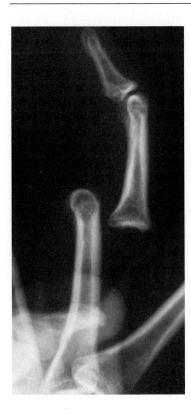

Figure 2.3 Dorsal proximal interphalangeal joint dislocation.

has cortex, one portion does not. In contrast to the situation with fracture fragments, accessory ossicles and sesamoid bones invariably are completely corticated, and no donor site should be present. Deformities of alignment reflect the function of the injured unit. In some cases, stress views may be necessary to demonstrate the loss of function.

The most common dislocation occurs at the PIP joint and is often associated with injury to the collateral ligaments (Fig. 2.3). Nonmedical personnel often reduce PIP joint dislocations, and many fracture-subluxations are actually reduced fracture-dislocations. After reduction, if there are no fractures, one may see only soft tissue swelling. Dorsal dislocations are common, lateral dislocations are less common, and volar dislocations are rare.

Fractures involving the phalangeal tufts are the result of direct sharp or blunt trauma. Phalangeal tuft injuries are commonly the result of occupational accidents.

The most common metacarpal fracture is an impacted fracture of the fifth metacarpal neck with volar angulation (boxer's fracture). It is sustained by bending and axial loading when the closed fist strikes an object (e.g., a wall or chin). In severe cases, the fourth metacarpal neck may also be fractured.

THUMB

Ligamentous disruption of the ulnar collateral ligament of the thumb's metacarpophalangeal joint, or gamekeeper's thumb, is sustained during downhill skiing when an improperly planted pole places sudden valgus stress on the thumb. Similar mechanisms of injury may also occur in sports such as football, hockey, wrestling, and basketball. Unless there is avulsion of a fragment of bone, stress views are necessary to show this injury on radiographs (Figs. 2.4 and 2.5). On MRI, the torn ulnar collateral ligament may be imaged directly. The adductor pollicis aponeurosis is normally superficial to the ulnar collateral ligament. Interposition of the adductor pollicis aponeurosis between the ruptured ulnar collateral ligament and its distal attachment is called a *Stener lesion* (Fig. 2.6). A Stener lesion will prevent healing of the ligament and result in chronic instability.

The exceptional mobility of the thumb in opposing the other digits is possible in part because of a shallow saddle-shaped articulation between the first metacarpal and the trape-

Gamekeeper's thumb is a common injury in downhill skiers.

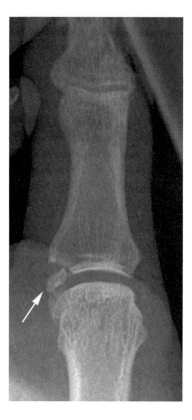

Figure 2.4 Avulsion fracture (*arrow*) at the proximal phalanx of the thumb by the ulnar collateral ligament (gamekeeper's thumb).

zium. Axial loading of a partially flexed first metacarpal can produce a simple intra-articular fracture. The adductor pollicis and abductor pollicis longus muscles pull the metacarpal base and shaft proximally, but the anterior lip remains attached to the trapezium by its ligaments (Bennett fracture) (Fig. 2.7). These intra-articular fractures usually require opera-

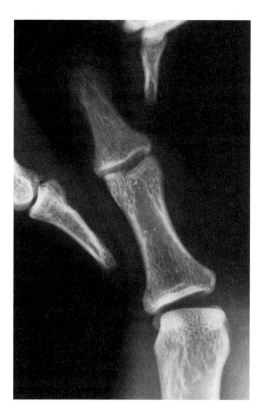

Figure 2.5 Ligamentous disruption of the ulnar collateral ligament, allowing the ulnar aspect of the thumb's metacarpophalangeal joint to widen with stress (gamekeeper's thumb).

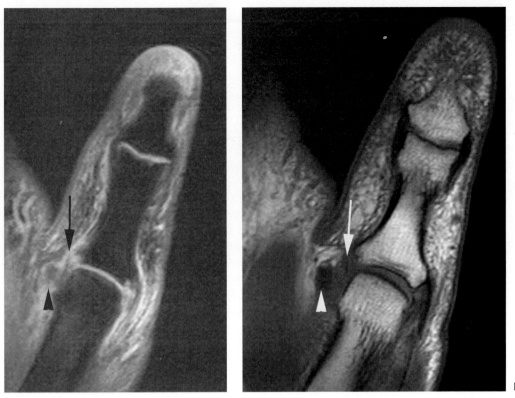

Figure 2.6 Stener lesion. *A.* Coronal STIR and (*B*) coronal T1-weighted MRI show a torn ulnar collateral ligament with proximal retraction (*arrowhead*). The adductor pollicis aponeurosis (*arrow*) is interposed between the torn ligament and its distal site of attachment.

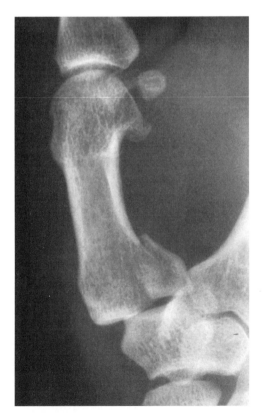

Figure. 2.7 Intra-articular fracture of the base of the first metacarpal with subluxation (Bennett fracture).

tive reduction and fixation. If a T- or Y-shaped comminuted fracture (Rolando fracture) rather than a simple fracture is sustained, anatomic reduction and fixation may become problematic. Posttraumatic degenerative arthritis may follow. In contrast to these injuries, extra-articular fractures of the first metacarpal shaft present few problems in management because muscle origins along the length of the shaft prevent displacement.

WRIST

BIOMECHANICS

The wrist positions the hand in space, transmits power to the hand from muscles in the forearm, and transmits mechanical force between the hand and the forearm. Its range of motion is magnified in flexion and extension and in radial and ulnar deviation by a dual articulation: one between the radius and lunate and one between the lunate and capitate. With ulnar and radial deviation of the hand, the distal carpal row rotates as well as turns. The carpus can be envisioned as having a central column that consists of the lunate and the capitate. Flexion and extension and the transmission of mechanical force occur through the central column. The capitate, distal carpal row, and hand compose a single functional unit. The lunate is an intercalated segment between the capitate and the radius that has no direct muscular control (no muscles insert on the lunate). The scaphoid flanks the lunate on one side and functions as a connecting rod alongside the capitate and lunate, providing stability during motion. The triquetrum acts as a pivot for intercarpal rotation through a sloping, helicoid articulation with the hamate.

> The lunate and capitate form the central column of the carpus.

Ligaments of the wrist limit motion when they become taut at their maximum excursion. The volar carpal ligaments are strong and form a sling that suspends the carpus from the radius and triangular fibrocartilage complex (TFCC) (Fig. 2.8). The dorsal ligaments are weaker. Interosseous ligaments bind adjacent carpal bones to each other; those of clinical importance are the scapholunate and lunotriquetral ligaments. The scaphoid and triquetrum flank the lunate on either side and have strong ligamentous attachments to the distal carpal row as well

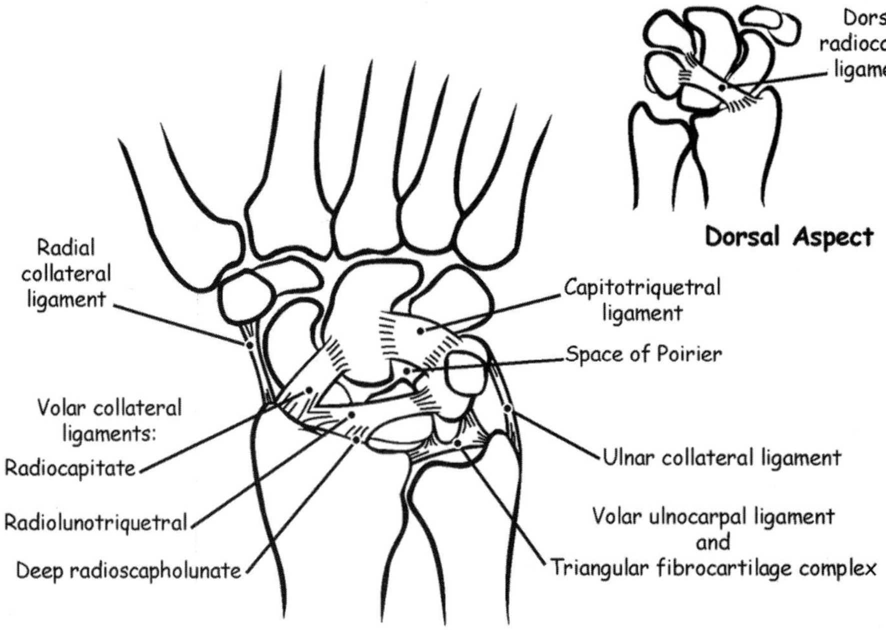

> The volar carpal ligaments are stronger than the dorsal ligaments.

Figure 2.8 Ligaments of the wrist. The strong ligaments are on the volar aspect of the wrist and form a sling that suspends the carpus from the distal forearm. The space of Poirier exists because there is no strong ligamentous attachment of capitate to lunate. Many indirect injuries of the carpus involve a carpal sling disruption that extends into the space of Poirier.

as attachments to the lunate and to the distal forearm. Because no strong ligaments connect the capitate and lunate to each other, the stability of that articulation depends on the integrity of the adjacent scaphoid and triquetrum and their ligamentous attachments. The gap in the volar ligamentous sling at the lunate-capitate articulation is called the *space of Poirier*.

Radiographic evaluation of the wrist is based primarily on the appearance of each bone and its relationship with the other bones. The arcs made by the proximal articular surfaces of the proximal carpal row, the distal articular surfaces of the proximal carpal row, and the proximal articular surfaces of the distal carpal row are helpful anatomic landmarks. The positions of the scaphoid fat stripe and the pronator quadratus fat pad are occasionally helpful indirect signs of wrist fracture.

SCAPHOID FRACTURES

Scaphoid fractures account for approximately 85% of all isolated carpal bone fractures. The scaphoid bridges the lunate-capitate articulation. With extreme, forceful dorsiflexion between the lunate and capitate and perhaps impingement of the scaphoid on the dorsal radial rim, the scaphoid starts to bend, and the fracture line begins on its volar aspect under tensile loading, propagating transversely through the narrowest region (the scaphoid waist). Most scaphoid fractures have no comminution (70% of cases). Less common are fractures through the proximal (10%) or distal (20%) poles. The scaphoid may also fracture during perilunate injuries (discussed later in this chapter). Many scaphoid fractures are nondisplaced and difficult to recognize without special scaphoid views (Fig. 2.9). Indirect signs of scaphoid fracture are obscuration or lateral displacement of the scaphoid fat stripe and soft tissue swelling over the dorsum of the wrist. Sometimes it is worthwhile for the radiologist to examine the patient directly. Early examination with either MRI or scintigraphy has been advocated for evaluation of suspected occult fracture of the scaphoid and may be cost-effective. Because the blood supply to the proximal pole of the scaphoid enters the distal pole and courses proximally across the waist, posttraumatic osteonecrosis of the proximal pole with nonunion is a common complication seen in up to 30% of cases. Osteonecrosis of the scaphoid may be directly imaged with MRI. The ultimate prognosis of complicated scaphoid fractures after surgical intervention is favorable. Wrist instability is a common sequela of scaphoid nonunion.

The scaphoid is the most commonly fractured carpal bone.

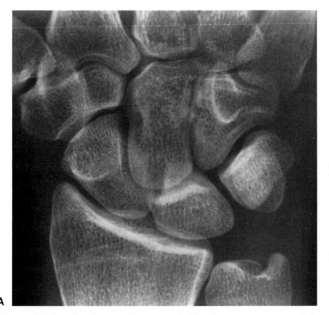 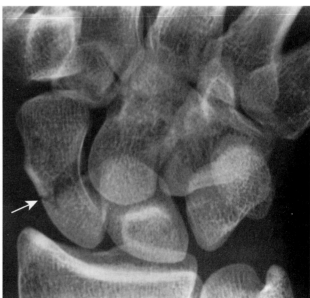

Figure 2.9 Scaphoid wrist fracture. *A.* The fracture is not visible on the standard PA radiograph. *B.* Special scaphoid radiograph shows the fracture (*arrow*).

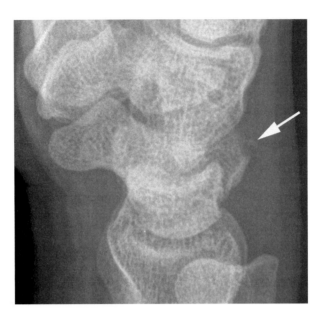

Figure 2.10 Triquetral fracture. Slightly oblique lateral radiograph shows displaced avulsion fragment (*arrow*) with overlying soft tissue swelling.

OTHER ISOLATED CARPAL FRACTURES

CT is often helpful in demonstrating carpal bone fractures.

Isolated fractures of carpal bones other than the scaphoid are relatively uncommon. Isolated triquetral fractures usually involve the dorsal surface and are seen best on lateral or slightly oblique radiographs (Fig. 2.10). Isolated lunate fractures usually involve the dorsal or volar surface and are ligamentous avulsions. Pisiform fractures may occur with direct trauma and are best seen on oblique radiographs. Hamate fractures may involve any part, but fractures of the hook of the hamate become displaced by the insertion of the transverse carpal ligament. These may follow falls or direct trauma from the handle of a racquet, golf club, or baseball bat. Complications include nonunion, osteonecrosis, and ulnar or median nerve injury, and most are treated surgically. Dorsal fracture-dislocations may also occur at the articulation of the hamate with the bases of the fourth and fifth metacarpals (Fig. 2.11). CT is often helpful in demonstrating carpal bone fractures.

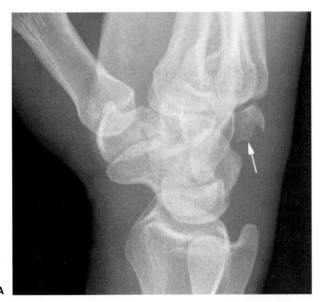

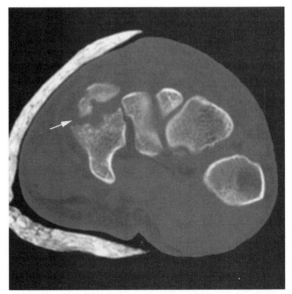

A

B

Figure 2.11 Fracture-dislocation of the hamate. A. Radiograph shows dorsal fracture-dislocation (*arrow*) involving the articulations of the fourth and fifth metacarpals with the hamate. B. Axial CT scan shows the displaced, comminuted hamate fracture (*arrow*).

Table 2.1: Perilunate Injuries of the Wrist

Stage	Injury
1	Rotary subluxation of the scaphoid (scapholunate dissociation)
2	Perilunate dislocation
3	Midcarpal dissociation (triquetral dislocation)
4	Lunate dislocation

PERILUNATE INJURIES

A consistent pattern of injuries is sustained around the lunate when the hand is extended to break a backward fall. On impact, the hand and wrist undergo hyperextension, ulnar deviation, and intercarpal supination (rotary motion between the proximal and distal carpal rows). The ligamentous sling of the carpus is loaded in tension from the radial side, and a sequence of injuries may ensue (Table 2.1). In stage 1, scapholunate dissociation or rotary subluxation, there is rupture of the proximal ligamentous attachments of the scaphoid, opening the space of Poirier on the radial side. The separation of the scaphoid from the middle column leaves scapholunate dissociation. Disruption of the ligaments of the scaphoid allows it to rotate about its short axis in a volar direction (Fig. 2.12). This mechanism of loading may also fracture the scaphoid. In stage 2, perilunate dislocation, the capitate dislocates from the lunate dorsally, taking with it the hand and the scaphoid (Fig. 2.13). The space of Poirier opens on the radial side, but the triquetral ligaments remain intact. In stage 3, midcarpal dissociation or triquetral dislocation, under continued loading the triquetral ligaments fail by tear or avulsion of insertions, separating the triquetrum from the lunate. Although the lunate remains in place, the rest of the carpus is dislocated dorsally, coming to rest on the dorsal surface of the lunate. The lunate is subluxated and tilted volarly but is not completely dislocated (Fig. 2.14). Lunate dislocation (stage 4) occurs if there is sufficient force to tear the dorsal radiocarpal ligament, allowing the dorsally dislocated carpus to eject the lunate from the radius volarly. The capitate comes to rest in the radial articular surface. The dislocated lunate is also rotated 90 degrees volarly, still held to the radius by its volar ligaments (Fig. 2.15). Avulsion fractures instead of ligamentous ruptures may occur, including avulsion and tension fractures of the carpal bones (especially the scaphoid) and of the distal radius and ulna. The radiographic signs of reduced perilunate injuries may be subtle, particularly in the absence of bony involvement.

TRIANGULAR FIBROCARTILAGE COMPLEX AND ULNAR-SIDED INJURIES

The TFCC is a biconcave fibrocartilage disc interposed between the proximal carpal row and the ulna and suspended by dorsal and volar radioulnar ligaments that extend from the medial aspect of the distal radius to the ulnar styloid process. The TFCC extends the articular surface of the distal radius across the distal ulna, separating the radiocarpal compartment of the wrist from the distal radioulnar joint. Tears of the TFCC may be traumatic or degenerative. Most tears occur through the central portion of the disc where it is thinnest, leading to ulnar-sided wrist pain (Fig. 2.16). Tears that involve the radioulnar ligaments may result in instability of the distal radioulnar joint. Disruption of other carpal ligaments on the ulnar side of the wrist may occur with or without injury to the TFCC. The mechanism and classification of these injuries are not well established.

Tears of the triangular fibrocartilage complex may be traumatic or degenerative.

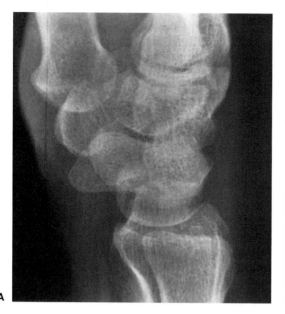

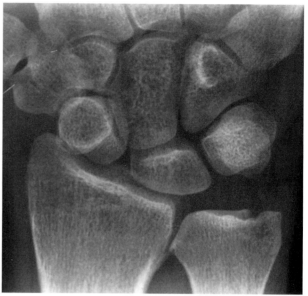

A

B

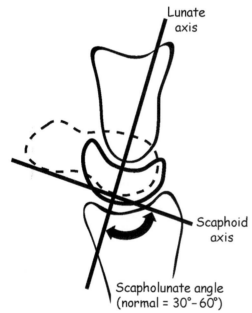

C   Lateral Projection

Figure 2.12 Rotary subluxation of scaphoid. *A.* Lateral radiograph shows volar rotary subluxation of the scaphoid. The scapholunate angle is nearly 90 degrees. *B.* PA radiograph shows foreshortening of the scaphoid with a cortical ring sign over its distal pole. *C.* Scapholunate (SL) angle measurement. Normal SL angle is 30 to 60 degrees.

CARPAL INSTABILITY

Ligamentous injuries of the wrist are often overlooked if fractures are present.

The seriousness of ligamentous injuries of the wrist is often overlooked during the acute clinical presentation, particularly if fractures are absent and dislocations have been reduced. When untreated, patients with "wrist sprains" often return with chronic, disabling wrist symptoms, including instability, pain, decreased grip strength, post-traumatic arthritis, and painful "clicks." Fractures of the distal radius may be associated with more serious carpal ligament injuries that are ignored once the radial fractures have healed. There are six recognized types of carpal instability. When the normal wrist is held in neutral position, the axes of the radius, lunate, and capitate are collinear on lateral radiographs. With flexion or extension, approximately half the

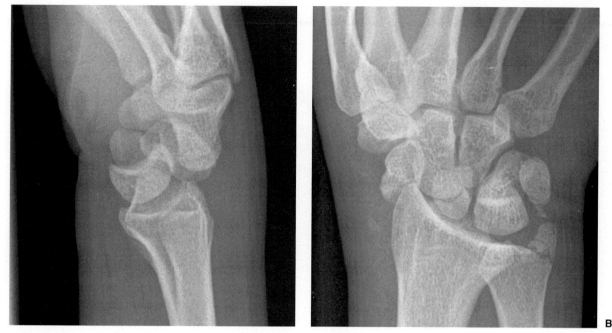

A   B

Figure 2.13 Transscaphoid perilunate dislocation. *A.* Lateral radiograph shows complete dorsal dislocation of the capitate with normal location of the lunate. *B.* PA radiograph shows the overlap of the
scaphoid and capitate but not the triquetrum. The scaphoid is fractured.

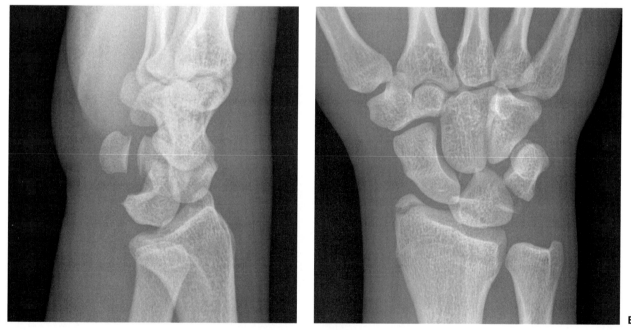

A   B

Figure 2.14 Midcarpal dislocation. *A.* Lateral radiograph shows complete dorsal dislocation of the capitate and volar subluxation of the lunate. *B.* PA radiograph shows separation of the scaphoid, capitate,
and triquetrum from the lunate. Avulsion fractures of the triquetrum and radial styloid are present.

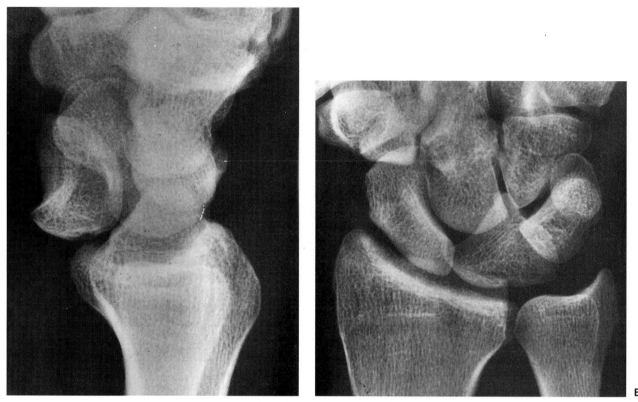

Figure 2.15 Lunate dislocation. *A.* Lateral radiograph shows volar dislocation of the lunate with 90 degrees rotary displacement. The capitate occupies the normal position of the lunate. *B.* PA radiograph shows the lunate as an overlapping triangular structure.

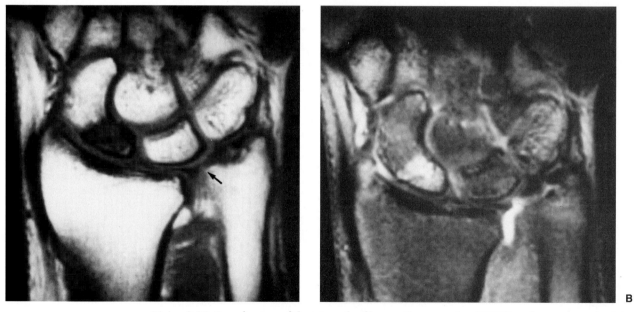

Figure 2.16 Complex tear of the triangular fibrocartilage complex (TFCC) and osteonecrosis of the proximal pole of the scaphoid. *A.* Coronal T1-weighted MR image shows the TFCC tear (*arrow*) and low signal in proximal pole. *B.* Coronal T2-weighted MR image shows fluid in the distal radioulnar joint outlining the tear and high signal in the proximal pole.

Table 2.2: Patterns of Carpal Instability

Type	Scapholunate Angle (degrees)	Capitolunate Angle (degrees)
Normal	30–60	≤20
Dorsal intercalated segment instability	>60	>20
Volar intercalated segment instability	<30	>20
Rotary subluxation of the scaphoid	>60	<20

motion occurs between the lunate and radius, and half between the capitate and lunate. The scapholunate angle and the capitolunate angle may be helpful in identifying patterns of carpal instability (Table 2.2). In dorsiflexion instability (also called *dorsal intercalated segment instability*, or DISI), the axes of the radius, lunate, and capitate assume a zigzag configuration with dorsal angulation of the lunate (relative to the radius) and volar angulation of the capitate (relative to the lunate). Dorsiflexion instability may be associated with rotary subluxation of the scaphoid. In volar flexion instability (also called *volar intercalated segment instability*, or VISI), the zigzag is the reverse, with volar angulation of the lunate (relative to the radius) and dorsal angulation of the capitate (relative to the lunate). Volar flexion instability may be associated with dorsally angulated distal radius fractures. Ulnar translocation is subluxation of the entire carpus on the radius in the ulnar direction, seen best on the PA view. Dorsal and volar carpal subluxations may involve the radiocarpal or the lunatocapitate joints. These are usually not evident on static radiographs and often require stress lateral views under fluoroscopy for demonstration. The final type of carpal instability, rotary subluxation of the scaphoid, has been described earlier. MRI, wrist arthrography, and dynamic motion studies under fluoroscopy may be required to document carpal instability or the underlying ligamentous injuries (Fig. 2.17). The treatment of carpal instability is usually intercarpal arthrodesis.

The six types of carpal instability are DISI, VISI, ulnar translocation, dorsal carpal sublaxation, volar carpal sublaxation, and rotary sublaxation of the scaphoid.

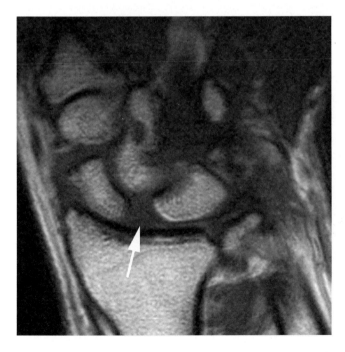

Figure 2.17 Scapholunate ligament tear. Coronal T1-weighted MR image shows absence (*arrow*) of the normal ligament between the scaphoid and lunate.

DISTAL RADIUS AND FOREARM

Fractures of the distal radius usually occur from falls on the outstretched hand. A Colles fracture is a nonarticular transverse fracture of the distal radial metaphysis with dorsal displacement, dorsal angulation, and dorsal impaction (Fig. 2.18). This injury—common in older persons with osteoporosis, particularly women—is sustained during a fall forward onto an outstretched, dorsiflexed hand with the impact force aligned to the long axis of the radius. The fracture results from tensile failure of cancellous metaphyseal bone on the volar side and compressive failure on the dorsal side. The distal radial articular surface and the carpus are spared. In 60% of cases, the ulnar styloid is avulsed by the TFCC. Alternatively, the TFCC may tear, the distal radioulnar joint may dislocate, or the distal ulnar shaft may fracture. Because the radial fracture traverses the spongy bone of the metaphysis, healing is generally prompt with closed treatment, but associated ulnar styloid fractures frequently do not unite. Residual, posttraumatic dorsal tilt of the distal radial articular surface may result in instability of the wrist. A transverse radial metaphyseal fracture that displaces and angulates volarly is called a *reverse Colles fracture* or a *Smith fracture*.

> Fractures of the distal radius are common in osteoporotic women.

Simple intra-articular fractures of the distal radius that involve either its dorsal or volar margin are called *Barton fractures*.

Complex intra-articular fractures of the distal radius may be caused by high-energy axial compression forces transmitted through the lunate to the medial half of the radial articular surface. The articular surface usually splits into three major fragments: the radial styloid and two medial fragments, one dorsal and one volar. The medial fragments may be angulated dorsally or volarly, depending on the degree of flexion or extension of the wrist at the time of injury (Fig. 2.19). Additional impaction and comminution may be present depending on the magnitude of the loading. Most patients with these fractures also have intracarpal soft tissue injuries, including ligament tears and TFCC injuries. The distal radi-

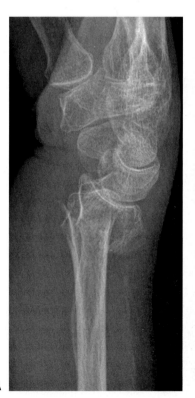
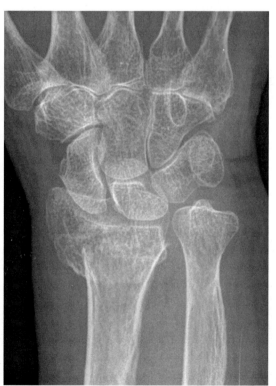

A   B

Figure 2.18 Transverse fracture of the distal radial metaphysis with dorsal displacement and angulation in an elderly woman (Colles fracture). *A.* Lateral radiograph. *B.* PA radiograph.

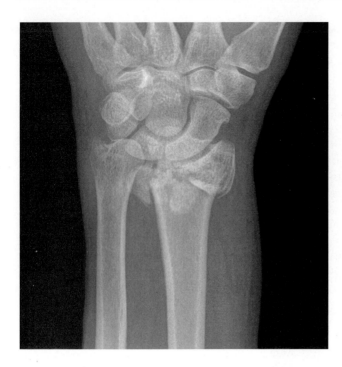

Figure 2.19 Intra-articular fracture of the distal radius with volar angulation and displacement.

oulnar joint is disrupted, and the ulnar styloid may be fractured. These injuries are typically treated surgically.

Isolated avulsion fractures of the radial styloid may follow avulsions of the radial collateral ligament. Compressive forces transmitted through the scaphoid may cause isolated shear fractures of the radial styloid; these may be associated with avulsion fractures of the ulnar styloid. Simple intra-articular fractures of the distal radius that involve the radial styloid process are sometimes called *Hutchinson* or *chauffer's fractures*.

Dislocation or subluxation of the distal radioulnar joint may occur in association with other fractures of the radius or in isolation. Because this injury is often overlooked and difficult to document on radiographs, CT may be required for the definitive diagnosis (Fig. 2.20). Often, an unstable distal radioulnar joint reduces in neutral or supination and subluxates in pronation. Therefore, the CT examination should be performed in pronation, if not both pronation and supination. Chronic dislocation or instability of the distal radioulnar joint may result in posttraumatic wrist disability.

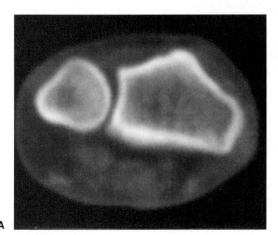
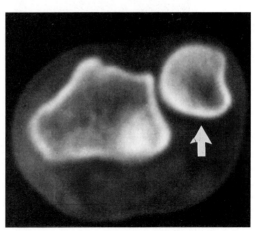

A   B

Figure 2.20 Subluxation of the left distal radioulnar joint demonstrated by CT. *A.* The right distal radioulnar joint is normal. *B.* In pronation, the left distal radioulnar joint is subluxated dorsally (*arrow*).

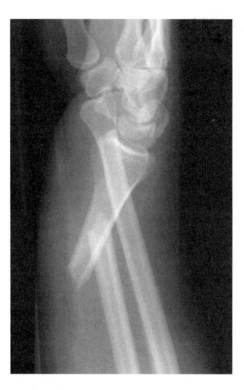

Figure 2.21 Angulated, displaced fracture of the distal radial shaft at the junction of the middle and distal thirds with dislocation of the distal radioulnar joint (Galeazzi fracture).

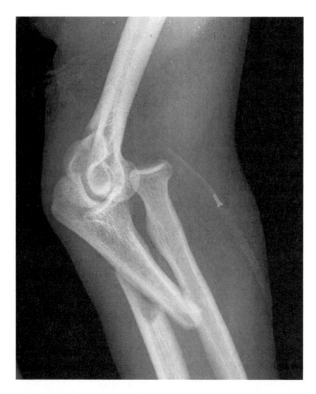

Figure 2.22 Apex anterior fracture of the ulnar shaft with anterior dislocation of the radial capitellar joint (Monteggia fracture, Bado type I).

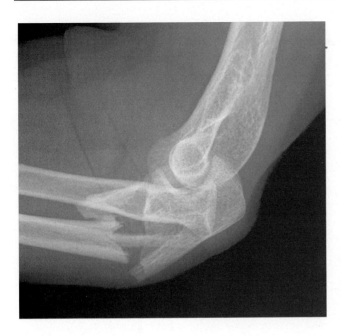

Figure 2.23 Apex posterior fracture of the ulnar shaft with posterior dislocation of the radial-capitellar joint (Monteggia fracture, Bado type II).

Most fractures of the forearm (60%) involve both radius and ulna. Less common are isolated fractures of the ulna with or without radial dislocation (25%), and the least common are isolated fractures of the radius with or without ulnar dislocation (15%). The greater the loading, the more likely it is that both bones are fractured. Raising the forearm to ward off a blow by a blunt instrument such as a nightstick may result in a nondisplaced tapping fracture from direct loading of the ulnar shaft (see Fig. 1.5).

A fracture of the radial shaft with dislocation of the distal radioulnar joint is called a *Galeazzi fracture* or a *Piedmont fracture* (Fig. 2.21). An impacted or comminuted fracture of the radial head with dislocation of the distal radioulnar joint is called an *Essex-Lopresti fracture*. A fracture of the ulnar shaft with dislocation of the radial head is called a *Monteggia fracture* (Fig. 2.22). Monteggia fractures are described using the Bado classification. The common type of Monteggia fracture is an angulated fracture of the proximal ulnar shaft with apex anterior along with anterior dislocation of the radial-capitellar joint (Bado type I). Less common types may also occur, including apex posterior angulation of the ulnar shaft fracture with posterior dislocation of the radial-capitellar joint (Bado type II) (Fig. 2.23), apex lateral angulation of the ulnar shaft fracture with lateral dislocation of the radial-capitellar joint (Bado type III), and fractures of both the proximal ulnar and radial shafts with radial-capitellar dislocation (Bado type IV). To detect these fracture-dislocations, both elbow and wrist should be included in examinations of the forearm.

> To detect fracture-dislocations, both elbow and wrist should be included in examinations of the forearm.

ELBOW

The most common elbow fractures in adults involve the radial head or neck. Radial head and neck fractures are sustained during falls onto an outstretched hand, impacting the radial head against the capitellum. One of two types of fractures is typically sustained: a linear shear fracture through the radial head (Fig. 2.24) or an impaction fracture of the radial neck (proximal radial metaphysis) (Fig. 2.25). Because they are intra-articular, a fat pad sign is often present. Approximately half of these fractures are nondisplaced and may require oblique views for demonstration. More severe fractures have displacement and comminution and may even involve the capitellum.

An intra-articular olecranon process fracture may be caused by a fall onto an outstretched hand with the elbow in flexion. The combination of axial compression with tension from contraction of the triceps produces oblique or transverse fractures through the

> A fat pad sign is often present in adults with elbow fractures.

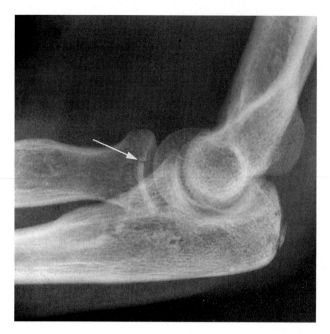

Figure 2.24 Nondisplaced radial head fracture (*arrow*).

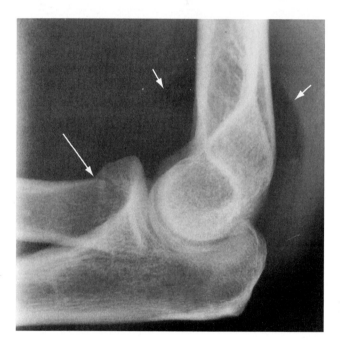

Figure 2.25 Impacted radial neck fracture (*long arrow*) with fat pad sign (*short arrows*).

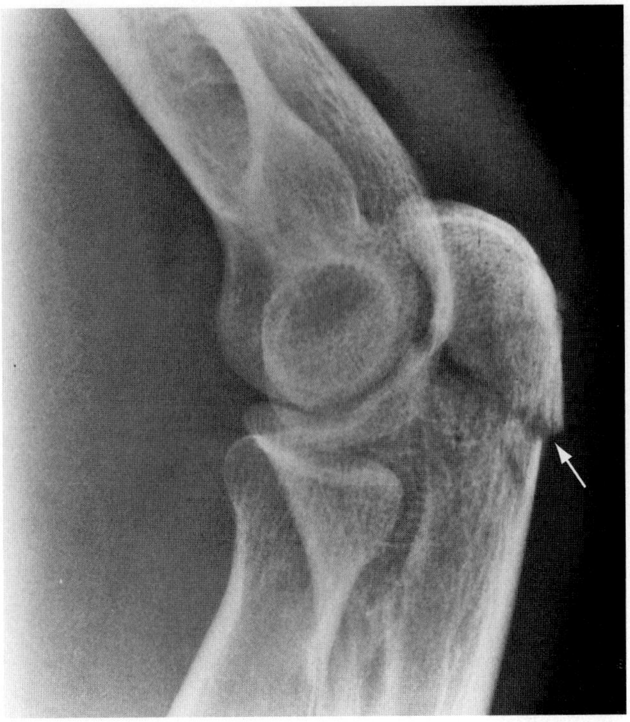

***Figure* 2.26** Fracture of the olecranon process (*arrow*).

semilunar notch (Fig. 2.26). Fractures may also be caused by direct falls onto the flexed elbow. In the elderly, triceps contraction may avulse a fragment of the olecranon.

Most acute dislocations of the elbow result from falls or sports-related mishaps. Typically, the ulna dislocates posteriorly relative to the humerus, taking the radius with it. In many cases, there are no associated fractures. When there are fractures associated with elbow dislocations, the fragments are most commonly avulsions from the coronoid process of the ulna (Fig. 2.27). Although posterior elbow dislocations are the most common, dislocation in other directions may occur. Elbow dislocations are more common in children than adults (see Chapter 5).

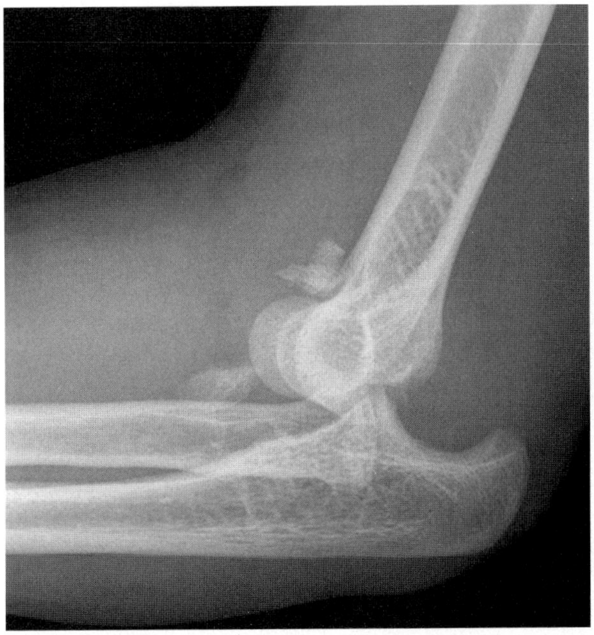

***Figure* 2.27** Posterior elbow fracture-dislocation.

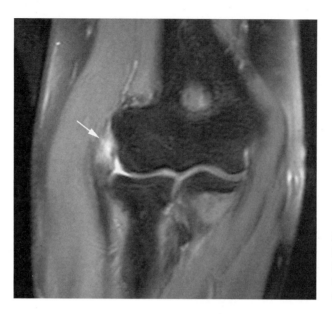

Figure 2.28 Lateral epicondylitis. Coronal STIR MRI shows thickening and high signal at the extensor musculature origin at the lateral epicondyle (*arrow*).

Intercondylar fractures of the distal humerus involve impaction of the ulna into the trochlear groove, where it splits the distal humerus like a wedge, often separating the medial and lateral fragments with a T- or Y-shaped fracture line. Comminution and displacement are common. These fractures are treated with open reduction and internal fixation.

Soft tissue injuries of the elbow in adults may occur on the lateral (radial), medial (ulnar), anterior, or posterior aspects. Lateral epicondylitis is a stress injury of the origin of the common extensor tendon at the lateral epicondyle that can be caused by a discrete injury or by repetitive stress. Also called *tennis elbow* because of its association with the backhand stroke in tennis, the condition may be demonstrated on MRI as high signal on T2-weighted images and thickening of the extensor carpi radialis brevis muscle origin (Fig. 2.28). The lateral ligamentous complex may be injured acutely or chronically and consists of tears of the radial collateral ligament and the extensor-pronator muscle group origin (Fig. 2.29). On the medial aspect of the elbow, tears of the ulnar collateral ligament may accompany activities such as baseball pitching. These injuries are best dem-

Lateral epicondylitis may be demonstrated on MRI.

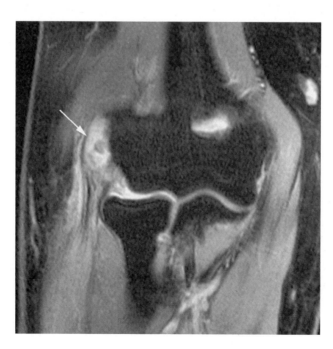

Figure 2.29 Lateral complex elbow injury. Coronal STIR MRI shows tears of the radial collateral ligament and the extensor muscle group origin (*arrow*).

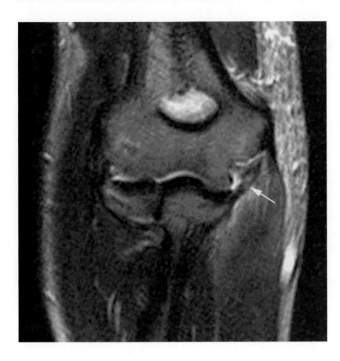

Figure 2.30 Ulnar collateral ligament tear. Coronal T2-weighted MRI shows high signal and disruption of the ulnar collateral ligament (*arrow*). Note that the flexor muscle origin is intact.

onstrated on MRI (Fig. 2.30); MR arthrography often increases the conspicuity of the abnormality. At the anterior aspect of the elbow, tears of the biceps tendon from its insertion at the bicipital tuberosity of the radius may occur. On radiographs, a complete tear is manifested by proximal retraction of the muscle belly, giving a "Popeye-the-sailor-man" (cartoon character from the 1950s) appearance (Fig. 2.31). On clinical examina-

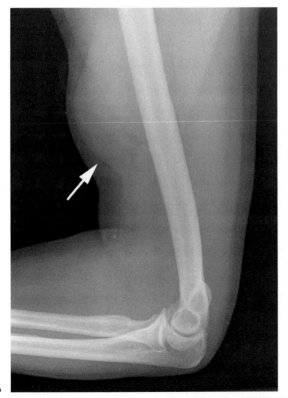

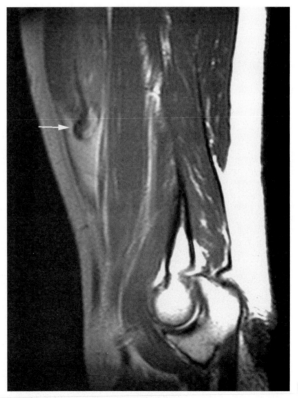

A

B

Figure 2.31 Biceps tendon tear. *A.* Lateral radiograph of the arm shows a focal bulge of the biceps muscle (*arrow*). *B.* Sagittal T1-weighted MRI shows the retracted biceps tendon (*arrow*).

tion, weakness in elbow flexion when the hand is supinated is present, along with the bulging biceps muscle belly. MRI demonstrates complete as well as partial tears of the distal biceps tendon. At the posterior aspect of the elbow, tears of the triceps tendon may occur but are relatively rare compared with the soft tissue injuries on the other aspects of the elbow.

SHOULDER AND ARM

HUMERUS

Fractures of the proximal humerus usually occur through the shaft at the surgical neck (Fig. 2.32). The rotator cuff abducts and rotates the proximal fragment. The greater or lesser tuberosities may also be fractured, and in very severe injuries, the anatomic head may be dislocated. Anatomic neck fractures are rare and have a poor prognosis because the blood supply to the humeral head is disrupted. Fractures of the humeral shaft are laterally and posteriorly angulated when the fracture separates the insertions of the pectoralis major and the deltoid, allowing the pectoralis major to adduct the proximal fragment. A fracture below the deltoid insertion allows it to abduct the proximal fragment, resulting in medial angulation. Most simple humeral shaft fractures are treated by closed means; occasionally, screws, plates, or rods are used.

Isolated fractures of the greater tuberosity may occur in falls or other trauma. Because the supraspinatus and infraspinatus tendons of the rotator cuff have their insertion on the greater tuberosity, patients may present with signs and symptoms of rotator cuff tears. MRI is the preferred method for identifying radiographically occult greater tuberosity fractures (Fig. 2.33) as well as identifying rotator cuff tears and other causes of shoulder pain.

GLENOHUMERAL JOINT ANATOMY

The glenohumeral joint is highly mobile and is the most common site of subluxation or dislocation. The glenoid fossa is the shallow depression in the articular surface of the glenoid process, made deeper and larger by a circular rim of fibrocartilage, the glenoid labrum.

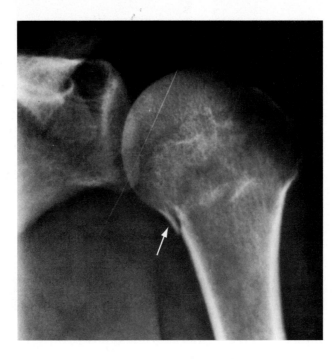

Figure 2.32 Surgical neck fracture of the humerus (*arrow*).

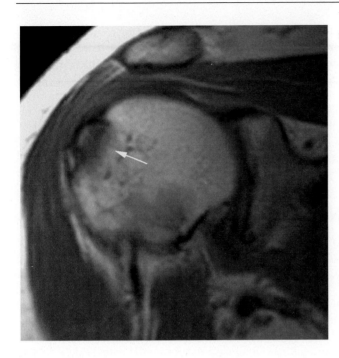

Figure 2.33 Greater tuberosity fracture. Oblique coronal T1-weighted MRI shows low signal in the greater tuberosity (*arrow*) with a nondisplaced fracture line. The rotator cuff is intact.

A distinct circular area of thinning is often seen in the center of the glenoid cavity. This bare area is related to the region's greater contact with the humeral head and is also related to age (Fig. 2.34). This normal variant may be mistaken for a glenolabral articular disruption (GLAD) or an osteochondral defect of the glenoid (see below). The rotator cuff tendons surround the glenohumeral joint and represent the major dynamic stabilizers of the joint. The supraspinatus and infraspinatus tendons cover the superior aspect of the joint and insert along the greater tuberosity of the humerus. The subscapularis tendon covers the anterior aspect of the joint and inserts on the lesser tuberosity of the humerus. The teres minor tendon covers the posterior aspect. The rotator cuff interval is a gap between the supraspinatus and subscapularis tendons, through which the long head of the biceps tendon passes to insert along the superior aspect of the glenoid labrum. The superior glenohumeral and the middle glenohumeral ligaments extend from the humerus to the superior

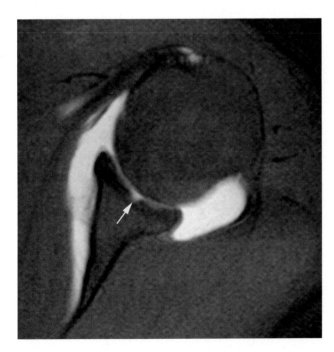

Figure 2.34 Bare area of the glenoid fossa. Axial T1-weighted MR arthrographic image with fat suppression shows a shallow central depression filled with contrast medium (*arrow*).

and anterior aspects of the glenoid labrum, respectively. The inferior glenohumeral ligament, a primary static stabilizer of the shoulder joint, passes from the medial aspect of the proximal humeral shaft in anterior and posterior cords to attach to the inferior glenoid labrum anteriorly and posteriorly. The presence, size, and attachments of the glenohumeral ligaments are variable from patient to patient. The shoulder has a strong joint capsule. In the acute setting, radiographs and CT are the primary means of imaging the shoulder; in the subacute and chronic setting, MRI is the primary means. Because the articular surface of the glenoid is oriented obliquely, the radiographic examination should always include a lateral view (axillary, transscapular, or transthoracic) when shoulder dislocation is suspected.

In the acute setting, radiographs and CT are the primary means of imaging the shoulder; in the subacute and chronic setting, MRI is the primary means.

GLENOHUMERAL JOINT DISLOCATIONS

Shoulder dislocations are anterior in 95% of cases.

In approximately 95% of cases of glenohumeral dislocation, the humeral head dislocates anteriorly and ends up anterior, inferior, and medial to the glenoid process in a subcoracoid location (Figs. 2.35 and 2.36). Abduction and external rotation of the arm cause the acromion to come in contact with the surgical neck of the humerus, and the humeral head can be levered out of the glenoid fossa. A direct blow to the back of the shoulder can eject the humeral head, and traction on the limb can pull it out. Impaction of the anterior-inferior surface of the glenoid labrum on the posterolateral aspect of the humeral head after it dislocates may cause a depressed humeral head fracture called the *Hill-Sachs lesion* (Fig. 2.37). Less dramatic but perhaps more important than the dislocation itself is the concomitant detachment of the labrum and capsule from the anterior glenoid process (Bankart lesion) sometimes associated with an avulsion fracture (Fig. 2.38). These injuries often result in posttraumatic anterior shoulder instability or recurrent dislocations. In approximately 5% of shoulder dislocations, the humeral head comes to rest posterior to the glenoid process, and the dislocation may be difficult to recognize on standard AP views (Fig. 2.39). After relocation of a posterior dislocation, an impaction fracture of the anterior aspect of the humeral head may be present (Fig. 2.40). Posterior shoulder dislocations may occur in the setting of tonic-clonic seizures. Other types of shoulder dislocations are rare. Acute dislocations are treated with closed reduction; associated soft tissue or glenoid rim injuries may require surgical repair.

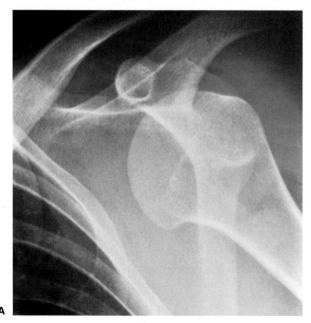 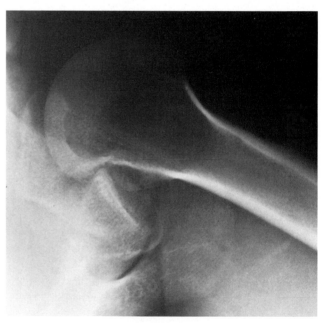

A   B

Figure 2.35 Anterior shoulder dislocation. *A.* AP radiograph shows the humeral head dislocated medially and inferiorly. *B.* Axillary radiograph shows the humeral head dislocated anteriorly.

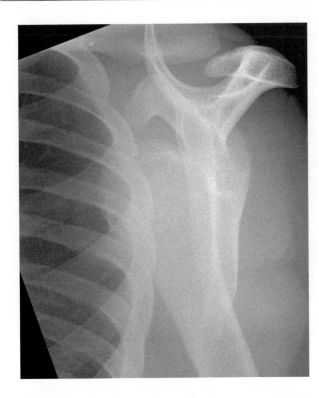

Figure 2.36 Anterior shoulder dislocation demonstrated on transscapular radiograph (Y-view).

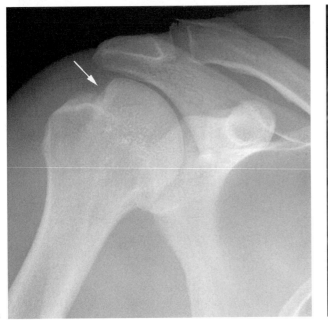

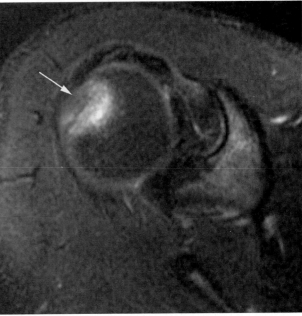

A

B

Figure 2.37 Hill-Sachs lesion. *A.* Internally rotated AP radiograph of the shoulder shows that an impaction fracture (*arrow*) of the humeral head was sustained during previous anterior dislocation. *B.* Axial T2-weighted fat-suppressed MRI shows high signal (*arrow*) at the site of impaction.

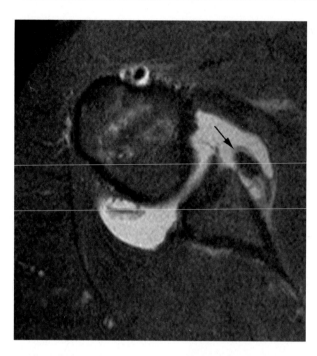

Figure 2.38 Avulsion fracture of the glenoid rim (osseous Bankart injury) after anterior shoulder dislocation. Axial T2-weighted fat-suppressed MRI shows a displaced fragment of bone (*arrow*) from the anterior glenoid process with attached labrum and capsule.

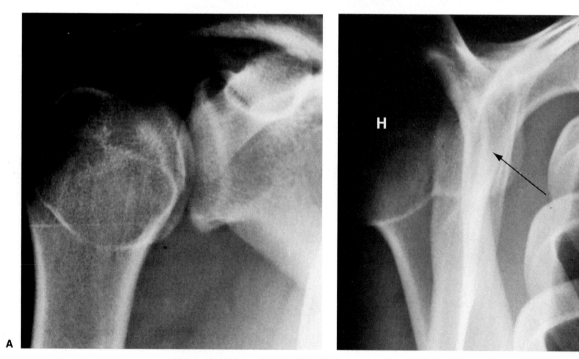

Figure 2.39 Posterior shoulder dislocation. *A.* AP radiograph shows internal rotation of the humeral head. *B.* Transscapular radiograph (Y-view) shows posterior location of humeral head (H) relative to center of glenoid fossa (*arrow*).

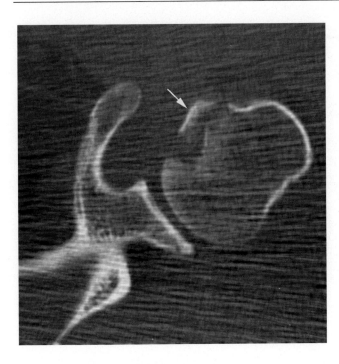

Figure 2.40 Reduced posterior shoulder dislocation with impaction fracture of humeral head and avulsion fracture of the lesser tuberosity (*arrow*).

ROTATOR CUFF INJURIES

The tendons of the rotator cuff may tear as a result of acute or repetitive trauma, mechanical impingement, degeneration, focal ischemia, or some combination of these. Rotator cuff tears may also be associated with rheumatoid arthritis. More than 90% of rotator cuff tears present with chronic weakness and pain. A minority of rotator cuff tears presents after a discrete episode of trauma; however, many patients with chronic presentations have a history of glenohumeral dislocation or other shoulder trauma. Full-thickness rotator cuff tears result in a discontinuity that may fill with fluid or granulation tissue; the involved muscle belly may retract. Partial-thickness tears may involve either the inferior or superior surfaces of the cuff or may be entirely within the substance of the tendons. The most common rotator cuff tear is an isolated tear of the supraspinatus tendon at its insertion at the greater tuberosity (Fig. 2.41). When the infraspinatus tendon is torn, it is typically in combination with a tear of the supraspinatus tendon, allowing the humeral head to subluxate superiorly underneath the acromion process (Fig. 2.42). Partial-thickness tears are more common than full-thickness tears, and partial-thickness tears involving the articular surface of the cuff are more common than those involving the bursal side. Rotator cuff tears are much more common among older patients.

On radiographs, superior subluxation of the humeral head with loss of the normal radiographic space between the inferior aspect of the acromion process and the superior aspect of the humeral head is indicative of rotator cuff tear or atrophy. When the inferior surface of the acromion has remodeled to accommodate the humeral head, it is an indication that the supraspinatus and infraspinatus tendons are massively torn and retracted. These findings are often incidentally made on chest radiographs of elderly patients (Fig. 2.43).

On conventional arthrography, contrast medium or contrast medium and air are injected into the shoulder capsule. A full-thickness rotator cuff tear is indicated by leakage of contrast medium or air through the tear into the subdeltoid-subacromial bursa. The size of the tear is often difficult to establish using this technique. Partial tears involving the articular surface may be sometimes demonstrated on air contrast arthrography but generally not with single contrast arthrography. Arthrography may be combined with CT or MRI for greater accuracy.

On MRI, the shoulder should be examined in axial, oblique coronal, and oblique sagittal planes. The normal rotator cuff tendons have generally low signal on all

More than 90% of rotator cuff tears present with chronic symptoms.

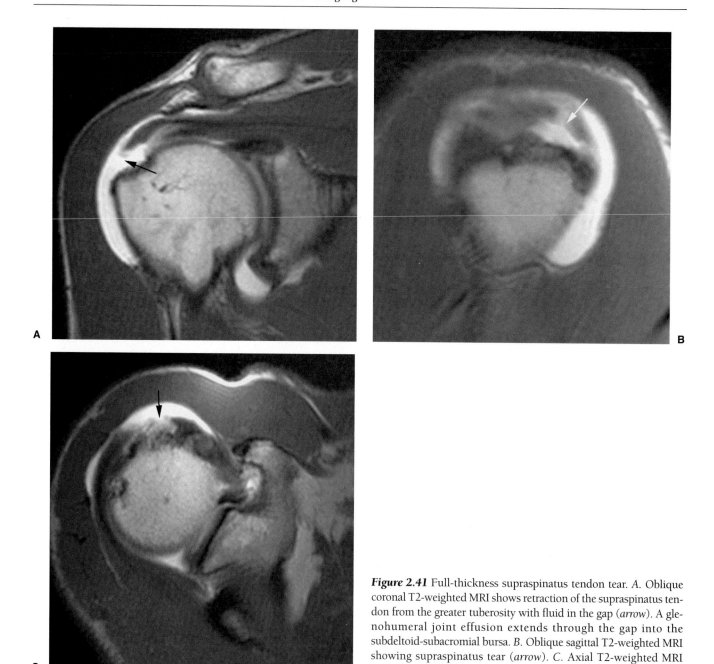

Figure 2.41 Full-thickness supraspinatus tendon tear. *A.* Oblique coronal T2-weighted MRI shows retraction of the supraspinatus tendon from the greater tuberosity with fluid in the gap (*arrow*). A glenohumeral joint effusion extends through the gap into the subdeltoid-subacromial bursa. *B.* Oblique sagittal T2-weighted MRI showing supraspinatus tear (*arrow*). *C.* Axial T2-weighted MRI showing supraspinatus tear (*arrow*).

On MRI, normal rotator cuff tendons have low signal on all sequences, similar to tendons in other parts of the body.

sequences, similar to that of tendons in other parts of the body. Many normal supraspinatus tendons have gray zones within the substance of the tendon that may reflect imaging artifact (magic angle phenomenon) or anatomic variation. Rotator cuff tears on MRI may be confidently recognized if there is a discontinuity of the tendon, retraction of the involved muscle belly, and fluid interposed between the fragments of the tendon. If a full-thickness tear does not involve the entire width of the tendon, and the gap is filled with granulation tissue rather than fluid, one may only see increased signal in the tendon without retraction of the muscle belly. Secondary signs of rotator cuff tears include fluid in the subdeltoid-subacromial bursa, fluid in the subcoracoid bursa, fluid in the glenohumeral joint, loss of the peribursal fat plane around the subdeltoid-subacromial bursa, and muscle atrophy. None of the secondary signs is diagnostic of a tear when occurring in isolation.

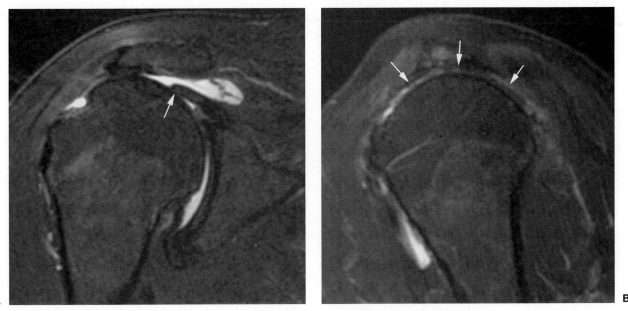

A   B

Figure 2.42 Full-thickness tears of the supraspinatus and infraspinatus tendons. *A*. Oblique coronal T2-weighted fat-suppressed MRI shows retraction of the supraspinatus tendon (*arrow*) and superior subluxation of the humeral head. *B*. Oblique sagittal T2-weighted fat-suppressed MRI shows absence of the supraspinatus and infraspinatus tendons (*arrows*) due to retraction.

Partial-thickness tears of the rotator cuff are evident as focal regions of high signal on T2-weighted images. Secondary signs of rotator cuff tear may be present. MRI is less accurate in identifying partial-thickness tears of the rotator cuff than full-thickness tears. The various appearances of rotator cuff tears on oblique coronal and oblique sagittal MRI may be likened to different hairstyles (Fig. 2.44).

Rotator cuff tendinopathy is evident on MRI as thickening of the tendon with increased signal on T2-weighted images. Tendinopathy is commonly found in the supraspinatus tendon (Fig. 2.45) and may progress to partial or complete tear.

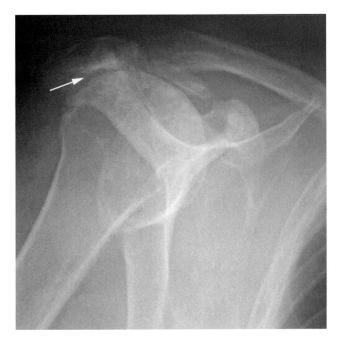

Figure 2.43 Chronic right rotator cuff tear seen on radiograph, with direct apposition of the acromion with the humeral head (*arrow*).

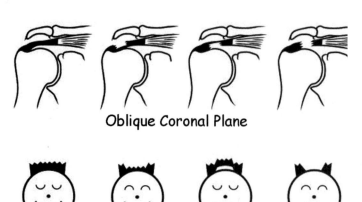

Oblique Coronal Plane

Oblique Sagittal Plane

Figure 2.44 Diagram of appearance of normal supraspinatus and partial and complete tears of the supraspinatus tendon on oblique coronal and oblique sagittal planes.

Tears of the subscapularis tendon are uncommon, and tears of the teres minor tendon are even less common. Isolated tears of the subscapularis tendon may occur with anterior dislocation (Fig. 2.46). Dislocations of the long head of the biceps tendon from the bicipital groove of the proximal humerus may accompany a subscapularis tendon tear, and sometimes the long head of the biceps tendon may dislocate into the glenohumeral joint.

Rotator cuff tears are repaired surgically if conservative methods do not improve symptoms. Imaging after a surgical repair can be difficult because of imaging artifacts from the surgery and the variable correlation between imaging findings of recurrent tear and patient symptoms.

SUBACROMIAL IMPINGEMENT

Subacromial impingement syndrome of the shoulder refers to trapping of the rotator cuff between the top of the humerus and the undersurface of the coracoacromial arch. The

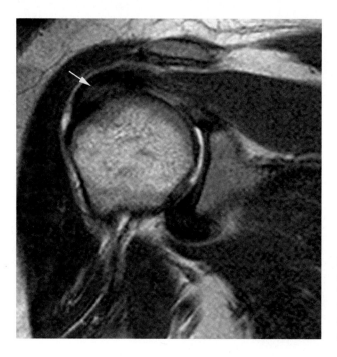

Figure 2.45 Rotator cuff tendinopathy. Oblique coronal T2-weighted MRI shows high signal (*arrow*) and thickening of the supraspinatus tendon, without discontinuity.

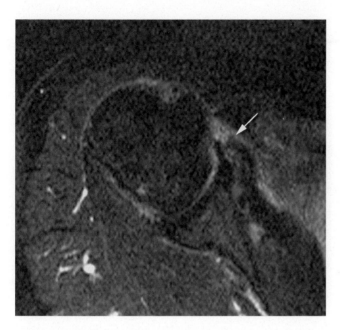

Figure 2.46 Subscapularis tendon avulsion (*arrow*).

coracoid process, the coracoacromial ligament, and the acromion process form the coracoacromial arch. A downward-projecting bony excrescence or degenerative hypertrophy of the acromioclavicular joint is commonly associated with impingement syndrome (Fig. 2.47). However, impingement syndrome is considered to be a clinical rather than a radiologic diagnosis. Other conditions that may impinge on the rotator cuff include congenital, developmental, or acquired variations in the size and shape of structures around the coracoacromial arch, including the acromion (Fig. 2.48) and the coracoid. Other types of shoulder impingement include posterior superior glenoid impingement and subcoracoid impingement.

Shoulder impingement syndrome is considered to be a clinical rather than a radiologic diagnosis.

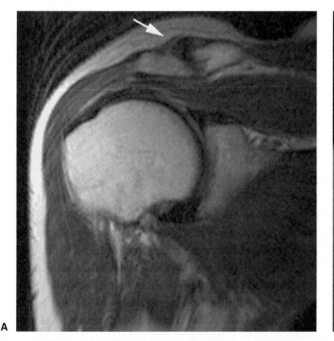

A

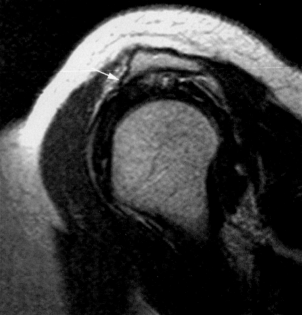

B

Figure 2.47 Rotator cuff impingement. *A.* Oblique coronal T1-weighted MRI shows osteoarthritis of the acromioclavicular joint with hypertrophy (*arrow*) and mass effect on the supraspinatus muscle. *B.* Oblique sagittal T1-weighted MRI shows anterior hooking (*arrow*) of the acromion process.

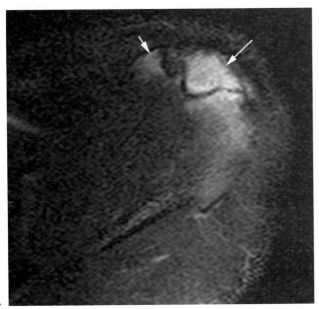
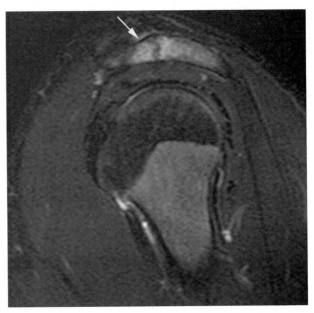

Figure 2.48 Symptomatic os acromiale. *A.* Axial T2-weighted with fat suppression MR image shows high signal in the os acromiale (*long arrow*) and distal clavicle (*short arrow*). *B.* Oblique sagittal T2-weighted with fat suppression MR image shows high signal in the os acromiale (*arrow*), which indents on the supraspinatus muscle.

GLENOID LABRUM AND GLENOHUMERAL LIGAMENTS

Injuries of the labrum and associated capsular structures are often related to sports activities. Most occur in one of two locations: the anterior-inferior labrum or the superior labrum (Table 2.3). A detachment of the anterior-inferior labrum during avulsion of the inferior glenohumeral ligament results in anterior shoulder instability. The superior

> Injury of the anterior-inferior labrum may be associated with anterior shoulder instability.

Table 2.3: Injuries of the Glenoid Labrum

Name	Salient Feature
SLAP lesion	Superior labrum anterior-to-posterior tear.
Bankart lesion	Detachment of the anterior-inferior labrum and inferior glenohumeral ligament from the glenoid process. The tear is between the labrum and the bone.
Perthes lesion	Incomplete avulsion of the anterior-inferior labrum with intact scapular periosteum. The labrum is displaced minimally or not at all.
ALPSA lesion	Anterior labroligamentous periosteal sleeve avulsion. The tear of the anterior-inferior labroligamentous is between the bone and the periosteum.
POLPSA lesion	Posterior labroligamentous periosteal sleeve avulsion.
GLAD lesion	Glenolabral articular disruption.
OCD	Osteochondritis dissecans or osteochondral defect of the glenoid has high incidence of associated labral tear.
GLOM	Glenoid labrum ovoid mass is the appearance of a labral tear.
Bennett lesion	Extra-articular posterior ossification associated with posterior labral injury and undersurface rotator cuff damage.
HAGL lesion	Humeral avulsion of the inferior glenohumeral ligament.
BHAGL lesion	Bony humeral avulsion of the inferior glenohumeral ligament.
FAIGHL	Floating anterior-inferior glenohumeral ligament. HAGL lesion with an associated labral tear.

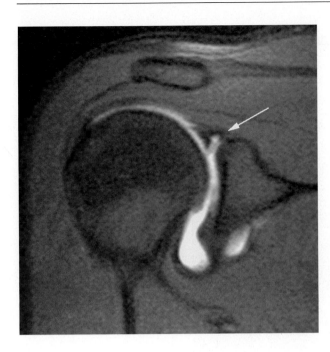

Figure 2.49 Superior labrum anterior-to-posterior tear. Oblique coronal T2-weighted with fat suppression MR arthrographic image shows globular high signal (*arrow*) within the superior labrum.

labral anterior to posterior tear, in which the labral-capsular-bicipital tendon complex is detached from the superior aspect of the glenoid process by traction on the long head of the biceps tendon during sudden arm abduction, does not result in instability (Fig. 2.49). A detachment of the anterior-inferior labrum by tension on the inferior glenohumeral ligament is a Bankart lesion, with its variants the Perthes lesion and the ALPSA lesion (anterior labroligamentous periosteal sleeve avulsion lesion) (Fig. 2.50). Labral and capsular injuries are shown best by MR arthrography or CT arthrography. Normal variants in the anterosuperior aspect of the glenoid may mimic labral pathology (Table 2.4). These variants include the sublabral sulcus (Fig. 2.51), the sublabral foramen (Fig. 2.52), and the Buford complex (Fig. 2.53).

Posterior labral tears at the attachment of the posterior cord of the inferior glenohumeral ligament may be associated with paralabral cysts (Fig. 2.54). These cysts are thought to arise from chronic leakage of synovial fluid through the tear into the periartic-

Posterior labral tears may be associated with paralabral cysts.

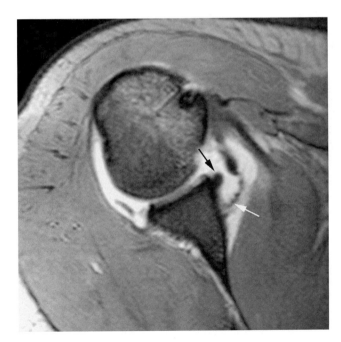

Figure 2.50 Anterior labroligamentous periosteal sleeve avulsion lesion. Axial gradient-echo MR image shows displacement of the anterior labrum (*black arrow*) and stripping of the periosteum anteriorly (*white arrow*).

Table 2.4: Anterosuperior Labral Variants of the Shoulder

Sublabral recess or sulcus	Potential space or recess between superior labrum and glenoid
Sublabral foramen or hole	Hole located anterior to glenoid providing communication of glenohumeral joint with subscapular recess
Buford complex	Cord-like or thickened middle glenohumeral ligament with absent or diminutive anterosuperior labrum

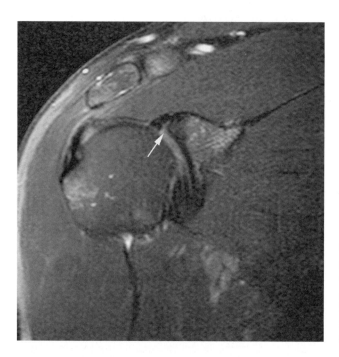

Figure 2.51 Sublabral sulcus. Oblique coronal T2-weighted with fat suppression MR image shows high signal (*arrow*) between the superior labrum and the glenoid, curving medially toward the glenoid.

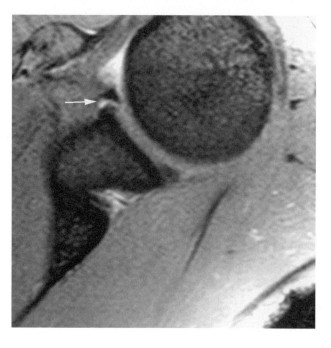

Figure 2.52 Sublabral foramen. Axial gradient-echo MR image shows high signal (*arrow*) between the anterosuperior labrum and the glenoid.

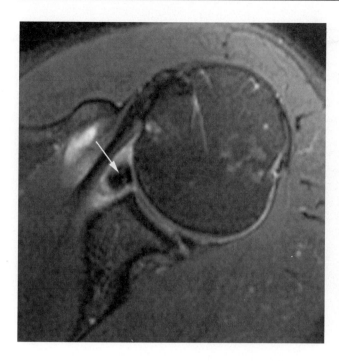

Figure 2.53 Buford complex. Axial gradient-echo MR image shows a thickened middle glenohumeral ligament (*arrow*) and an absent anterosuperior labrum.

ular soft tissues, perhaps with a one-way valve effect. The presence of such cysts is associated with a posterior labral tear in the majority of cases, although an actual communication between the cyst and the joint is often difficult to demonstrate. When large, such cysts may cause entrapment neuropathy of the suprascapular nerve in the suprascapular notch or spinoglenoid notch (Fig. 2.55), resulting in denervation atrophy changes in the supraspinatus muscle or supraspinatus and infraspinatus muscles, respectively. Early denervation atrophy may be recognized on MRI as a slight increase in muscle signal on T2-weighted images. Cysts are not generally associated with labral tears at other locations, because it is only posteriorly where the joint capsule is immediately apposed to the labrum. Posterior labral tears are commonly found in association with the Bennett lesion (Fig. 2.56), ossification adjacent to posteroinferior aspect of the glenoid rim. Bennett lesions are

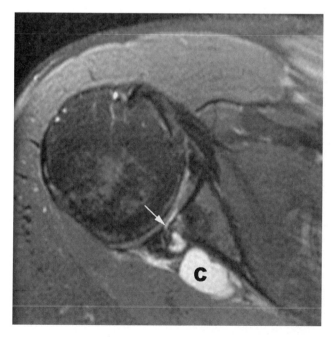

Figure 2.54 Posterior labral tear plus cyst. Axial gradient-echo MR image shows a paralabral cyst (C) associated with a posterior labral tear (*arrow*).

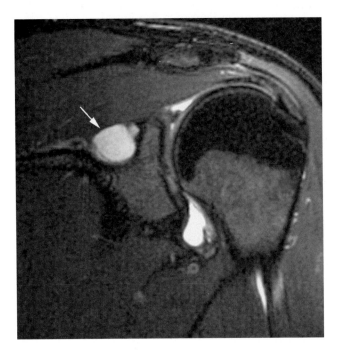

Figure 2.55 Paralabral cyst causing entrapment neuropathy. Oblique coronal T2-weighted fat-suppressed MRI shows a cyst (*arrow*) in the suprascapular notch.

found commonly in throwing athletes and usually have associated posterior undersurface rotator cuff damage.

Avulsions of the inferior glenohumeral ligament from the humeral attachment may also occur. These injuries are called *HAGL* (humeral avulsion of the inferior glenohumeral ligament) injuries when the ligament itself is torn (Fig. 2.57) or *BHAGL* (bony humeral avulsion of the inferior glenohumeral ligament) injuries when there is an associated bony fragment from the humerus (Fig. 2.58). HAGL lesions may occur anteriorly or posteriorly (Fig. 2.59), with or without bony avulsion, and with or without associated labral tear. When there is an associated labral tear with a HAGL, the lesion is called *floating anterior* (Fig. 2.60) or *posterior-inferior glenohumeral ligament*. The majority of patients with HAGL lesions have associated injuries. The most common associated injuries are labral tears, Hill-Sachs lesions, and rotator cuff tears.

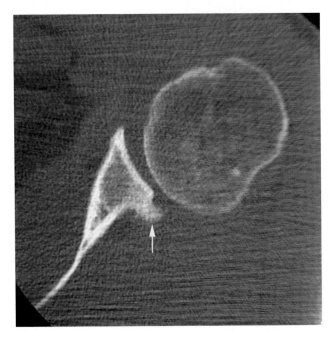

Figure 2.56 Bennett lesion. Axial CT image in bone window shows slight posterior subluxation of the humeral head, narrowing of the glenohumeral joint space posteriorly, and ossification in posteroinferior aspect of the glenoid rim (*arrow*).

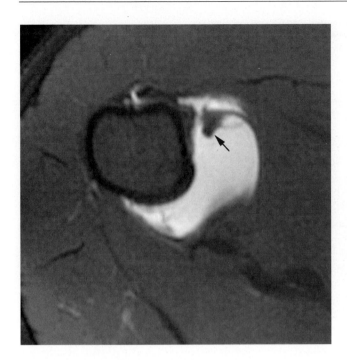

Figure 2.57 Humeral avulsion of the inferior glenohumeral ligament lesion. Axial T1-weighted MR arthrographic image shows detachment of the anterior band of the inferior glenohumeral ligament (*arrow*) with extravasation of joint fluid across the torn humeral attachment.

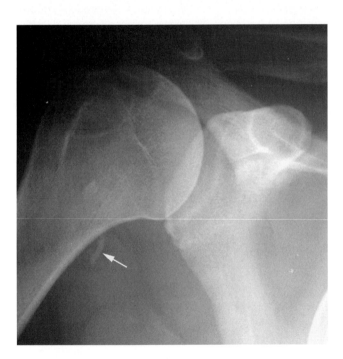

Figure 2.58 Bony humeral avulsion of the inferior glenohumeral ligament lesion. AP radiograph of the right shoulder shows a curvilinear fleck of bone (*arrow*) just medial to the proximal humerus.

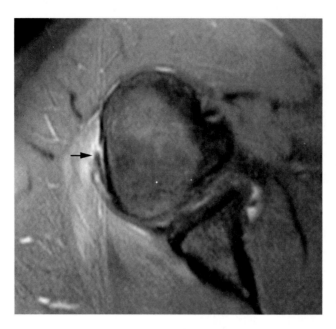

Figure 2.59 Posterior humeral avulsion of the inferior glenohumeral ligament lesion. Axial T2-weighted MR image with fat suppression shows that the posterior band of the inferior glenohumeral ligament (*arrow*) is avulsed from the proximal humerus with extravasation of joint fluid across the torn humeral attachment.

GLAD is a nondisplaced superficial anteroinferior labral tear associated with an adjacent chondral injury (Fig. 2.61). The mechanism of injury is forced adduction to the shoulder from an abducted and external rotated position. It has many similarities to osteochondral defect of the glenoid fossa (Fig. 2.62). History of dislocation, instability on physical examination, mechanism of injury, and radiologic findings distinguish osteochondral defect of the glenoid from the GLAD lesion.

CLAVICLE

Fractures of the clavicle usually occur in the middle third, medial to the coracoclavicular ligaments. The sternocleidomastoid muscle displaces the proximal fragment superiorly,

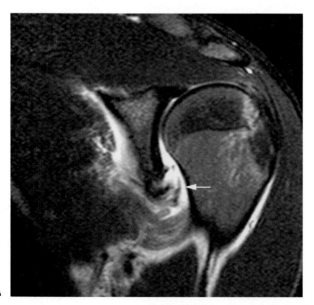
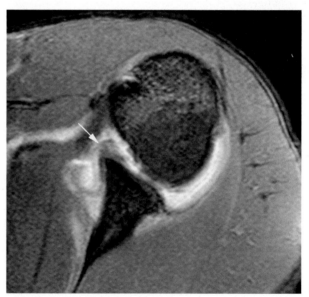

A   B

Figure 2.60 Floating anterior-inferior glenohumeral ligament. *A.* Oblique coronal T2-weighted MR image shows a J-shaped anterior band of the inferior glenohumeral ligament with extravasation of joint fluid across the torn humeral attachment (*arrow*). *B.* Axial gradient-echo MR image shows a glenoid labrum ovoid mass (*arrow*) consistent with anterior labral tear.

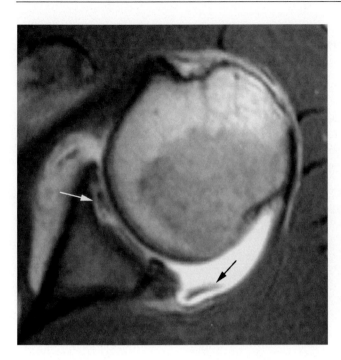

Figure 2.61 Glenolabral articular disruption lesion. Axial T1-weighted MR arthrographic image shows a chondral flap tear (*white arrow*) and a loose body within the glenohumeral joint (*black arrow*).

and the shoulder, acting through the coracoclavicular ligament, displaces the distal fragment inferiorly. With immobilization, healing is usually prompt. Clavicular fractures distal to the coracoclavicular ligaments may be complicated by tears of the coracoclavicular ligaments or avulsion of the coracoid process.

Acromioclavicular injuries (Table 2.5) involve the disruption of the acromioclavicular and coracoclavicular ligaments (shoulder separation). The inferior surfaces of the acromion process and the distal clavicle are normally at the same level on AP radiographs. In a type I injury, the acromioclavicular ligaments are stretched but not disrupted, and radiographs are normal or show a slight increase in the joint space. When the acromioclavicular ligaments are completely torn (type II), the distal clavicle subluxates superiorly (Fig. 2.63). If the coracoclavicular ligaments are also torn (type III), the clavicle dislocates, and the space between clavicle and coracoid process widens.

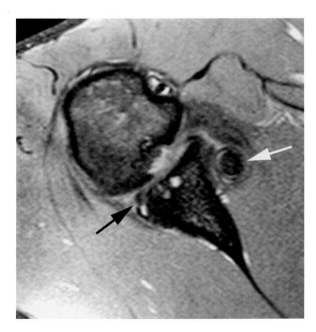

Figure 2.62 Osteochondral defect of glenoid. Axial gradient-echo MR image shows a multiloculated cyst (*black arrow*) in posterior aspect of the glenoid and a loose body (*white arrow*) anterior to the glenoid.

Table 2.5: *Common Types of Acromioclavicular Separations*

Type	Injury	Radiographic Findings
I	Stretched acromioclavicular ligament	Normal or slight increase in joint space with weight bearing
II	Ruptured acromioclavicular ligament	Superior subluxation of distal clavicle
III	Ruptured acromioclavicular and cora-coclavicular ligaments	Clavicle dislocation and widening of coracoclavicular space

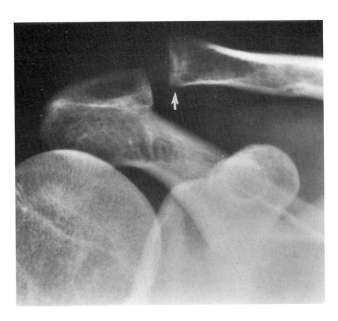

Figure 2.63 Acromioclavicular subluxation (type II) (*arrow*).

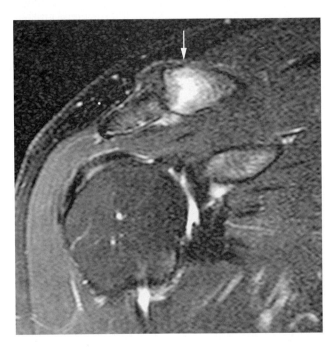

Figure 2.64 Posttraumatic osteolysis. Oblique coronal T2-weighted MR image shows high signal intensity in the distal clavicle (*arrow*) with periarticular soft tissue swelling.

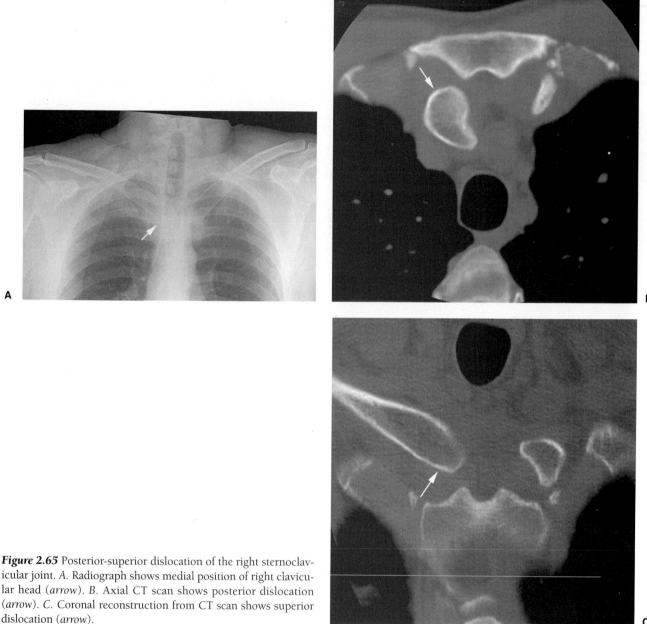

Figure 2.65 Posterior-superior dislocation of the right sternoclavicular joint. *A.* Radiograph shows medial position of right clavicular head (*arrow*). *B.* Axial CT scan shows posterior dislocation (*arrow*). *C.* Coronal reconstruction from CT scan shows superior dislocation (*arrow*).

Other types of acromioclavicular injuries are rare. Approximately 6% of patients who have had a previous acromioclavicular separation subsequently develop posttraumatic osteolysis, which can also be seen in athletes, particularly weight lifters (Fig. 2.64). Besides trauma, the differential diagnosis of osteolysis about the acromioclavicular joint includes hyperparathyroidism, rheumatoid arthritis, infection, collagen vascular disorders, spinal cord injury, and idiopathic causes.

Dislocations of the sternoclavicular joint are usually sustained in high-speed motor vehicle collisions. Although radiographs may demonstrate superior dislocation (Fig. 2.65), CT is often helpful and may be required to demonstrate a posterior dislocation. Anterior dislocations of the sternoclavicular joint are more common than posterior dislocations, but posterior dislocations of the sternoclavicular joint have more serious complications.

The inferior surfaces of the acromion process and the distal clavicle are normally at the same level on AP radiographs.

SOURCES AND READINGS

Barton N, ed. *Fractures of the hand and wrist.* Edinburgh: Churchill–Livingstone, 1988.

Bonsell S, Pearsall AW, Heitman RJ, et al. The relationship of age, gender, and degenerative changes observed on radiographs of the shoulder in asymptomatic individuals. *J Bone Joint Surg Br* 2000;82B:1135–1139.

Browner BD, Levine AM, Jupiter JB, et al., eds. *Skeletal trauma: fractures, dislocations, ligamentous injuries,* 2nd ed. Philadelphia: WB Saunders, 1998.

Bucholz RW, Heckman JD, eds. *Rockwood and Green's fractures in adults,* 5th ed. Philadelphia: Lippincott Williams & Wilkins, 2001.

Cerezal L, Abascal F, Canga A, et al. Usefulness of gadolinium-enhanced MR imaging in the evaluation of the vascularity of scaphoid nonunions. *AJR Am J Roentgenol* 2000;174:141–149.

De Maeseneer M, Jaovisidha S, Jacobson JA, et al. The Bennett lesion of the shoulder. *J Comput Assist Tomogr* 1998;22:31–34.

De Maeseneer M, Van Roy F, Lenchik L, et al. CT and MR arthrography of the normal and pathologic anterosuperior labrum and labral-bicipital complex. *Radiographics* 2000;20:S67–S81.

Feipel V, Rooze M. The capsular ligaments of the wrist: morphology, morphometry and clinical applications. *Surg Radiol Anat* 1999;21:175–180.

Firooznia H, Golimbu CN, Rafii M, et al. *MRI and CT of the musculoskeletal system.* St. Louis: CV Mosby, 1992.

Gilula LA, ed. *The traumatized hand and wrist: radiographic and anatomic correlation.* Philadelphia: WB Saunders, 1998.

Hilbrook TL, Grazier K, Kelsey JL, et al. *The frequency of occurrence, impact, and cost of selected musculoskeletal conditions in the United States.* Chicago: American Academy of Orthopedic Surgeons, 1984.

Hobby JL, Tom BD, Bearcroft PW, et al. Magnetic resonance imaging of the wrist: diagnostic performance statistics. *Clin Radiol* 2001;56:50–57.

Hunter TB, Peltier LF, Lund PJ. Radiologic history exhibit. Musculoskeletal eponyms: who are those guys? *Radiographics* 2000;20(3):819–836.

Lichtman DM, Alexander AH. *The wrist and its disorders,* 2nd ed. Philadelphia: WB Saunders, 1997.

May DA, Disler DG, Jones EA, et al. Abnormal signal intensity in skeletal muscle at MR imaging: patterns, pearls, and pitfalls. *Radiographics* 2000;20:S295–S315.

Mayfield JK. Patterns of injury to carpal ligaments. A spectrum. *Clin Orthop* 1984;187:36–42.

Morrey BF, ed. *The elbow and its disorders,* 3rd ed. Philadelphia: WB Saunders, 2000.

Palmer WE, Castlowitz PL, Chew FS. MR arthrography of the shoulder: normal intraarticular structures and common abnormalities. *AJR Am J Roentgenol* 1995;164:141–146.

Rafii M, Minkoff J. Advanced arthrography of the shoulder with CT and MR imaging. *Radiol Clin North Am* 1998;36:609–633.

Resnick D. *Diagnosis of bone and joint disorders,* 4th ed. Philadelphia: WB Saunders, 2002.

Rockwood CA Jr, Matsen FA, eds. *The shoulder,* 2nd ed. Philadelphia: WB Saunders, 1998.

Rogers LF. *Radiology of skeletal trauma,* 3rd ed. New York: Churchill-Livingstone, 2002.

Sanders TG, Tirman PF, Linares R, et al. The glenolabral articular disruption lesion: MR arthrography with arthroscopic correlation. *AJR Am J Roentgenol* 1999;172:171–175.

Stoller DW. *Magnetic resonance imaging in orthopaedics and sports medicine,* 2nd ed. Philadelphia: Lippincott-Raven, 1997.

Taleisnik J. Ligaments of the carpus. In: Razemon JP, Fisk GR, eds. *The wrist.* Edinburgh: Churchill-Livingstone, 1988:17–26.

Tang JB, Ryu J, Omokawa S, et al. Wrist kinetics after scapholunate dissociation: the effect of scapholunate interosseous ligament injury and persistent scapholunate gaps. *J Orthopaed Res* 2002;20:215–221.

Theumann N, Favarger N, Schnyder P, et al. Wrist ligament injuries: value of post-arthrography computed tomography. *Skeletal Radiol* 2001;30:88–93.

Tuite MJ, Cirillo RL, De Smet AA, et al. Superior labrum anterior-posterior (SLAP) tears: evaluation of three MR signs on T2-weighted images. *Radiology* 2000;215:841–845.

Wischer TK, Bredella MA, Genant HK, et al. Perthes lesion (a variant of the Bankart lesion): MR imaging and MR arthrographic findings with surgical correlation. *AJR Am J Roentgenol* 2002;178:233–237.

Yu YS, Dardani M, Fischer RA. MR observations of posttraumatic osteolysis of the distal clavicle after traumatic separation of the acromioclavicular joint. *J Comput Assist Tomogr* 2000;24:159–164.

Yu YS, Greenway G, Resnick D. Osteochondral defect of the glenoid fossa: cross-sectional imaging features. *Radiology* 1998;206:35–40.

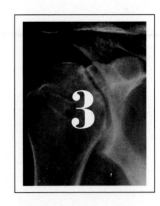

3

TRAUMA IN ADULTS: SPINE, THORACIC CAGE, AND PELVIS

This chapter describes the radiology of common injuries to the spine, thoracic cage, and pelvis in adults.

GENERAL PRINCIPLES

Injuries to the spine often occur in the setting of severe trauma. Approximately 45% of spine injuries are sustained in motor vehicle collisions, 20% in falls, 15% in recreational or sports-related accidents, 15% from intentional acts of violence, and 5% from other causes (Table 3.1). There is a 4:1 male predominance. Although spinal cord injuries often accompany spine trauma, neurologic damage is not an invariable concomitant (Table 3.2). Precautions against causing or worsening a neurologic injury should be scrupulously observed at all levels of care. Because spine injuries may be clinically occult, initial radiographs should be made expeditiously with the patient immobilized. If radiographs are equivocal, CT with thin slices (1- to 2-mm slice thickness in the cervical region, 3 mm elsewhere) is usually definitive; reconstructions in sagittal and coronal projections may be helpful. Abnormality of the spinal cord itself—mechanical transection, contusion, edema, or hemorrhage—can be imaged directly by MRI.

The vertebral bodies and intervertebral discs usually bear compressive loads, and the posterior elements and associated ligaments usually bear distractive (tensile) loads. The three-column concept is used widely to assess fracture stability (Fig. 3.1). The anterior column consists of the anterior part of the vertebral bodies, the anterior part of the intervertebral discs, and the anterior longitudinal ligament. The middle column consists of the posterior annulus of the intervertebral disc, the posterior wall of the vertebral body, and the posterior longitudinal ligament. The posterior column consists of the posterior elements, the facet joints, and the posterior ligament complex. An injury that disrupts the

Spine injuries are four times as common in men as in women.

Table 3.1: Causes of Spine Injuries

Causes	Frequency (%)
Motor vehicle collisions	45
Falls	20
Recreational or sports-related accidents	15
Intentional acts of violence	15
Other causes	5

Table 3.2: Neurologic Damage in Spine Trauma

Level of Injury	Patients with Neurologic Damage (%)
Cervical spine	39
Thoracic spine	10
Thoracolumbar junction (T11-L1)	4
Lumbar spine	3
Overall	14

Adapted from Riggins RS, Kraus JF. The risk of neurologic damage with fractures of the vertebrae. *J Trauma* 1977;126–133.

Flexion is the most common mechanism of spine injury.

middle and at least one other column is considered unstable. Most injuries can be described by the mechanisms of flexion, extension, shearing, and rotation (Table 3.3 and Fig. 3.2). These mechanisms may be combined with axial compression or axial distraction (tension). Flexion is by far the most common mechanism of injury and may occur throughout the spine. Flexion injuries result in compression of the anterior column and distraction of the posterior column. They have the radiologic features of vertebral body fractures and narrowing of the disc space anteriorly and widening of the interspinous space posteriorly. Severe injuries may disrupt the middle column, resulting in anterolisthesis and dislocated facets. Extension injuries are common only in the cervical region. They result from distraction of the anterior column and compression of the posterior column. They have the radiologic features of avulsion fractures of the anterior aspect of the vertebral end plate and widening of the disc space anteriorly and fractures of the neural arch posteriorly. Severe injuries may disrupt the middle column, resulting in retrolisthesis. Shearing injuries are common in the thoracic and lumbar regions and result from disruption of ligaments. Lateral distraction, lateral dislocation, avulsion fractures of the vertebral

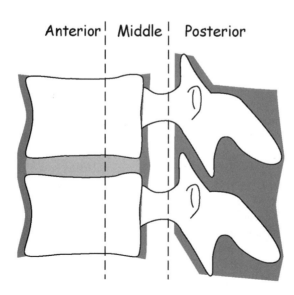

Figure 3.1 Diagram of the three-column concept.

Mechanism	Key Radiologic Features
Flexion	Vertebral body fracture
	Narrow disc space
	Wide interspinous space
	Facet dislocation
	Anterolisthesis
Extension	End-plate avulsion fracture
	Wide disc space
	Neural arch fracture
	Retrolisthesis
Shearing	Lateral distraction
	Lateral dislocation
	End-plate avulsion fracture
	Transverse process fracture
Rotation	Rotational misalignment
	Dislocation
	End-plate avulsion fracture
	Facet or pillar fracture

Table 3.3: Radiologic Features of Vertebral Injuries

Adapted from Daffner RH, Deeb ZL, Rothfus WE. "Fingerprints" of vertebral trauma—a unifying concept based on mechanisms. *Skeletal Radiol* 1985;15:518–525.

end plates, and transverse process fractures may be seen. Rotational injuries may occur throughout the spine and may be evident by rotational misalignment, dislocation, avulsion fractures of the vertebral end plates, and facet or pillar fractures. Axial compression may result in compression injuries in all three columns, whereas axial distraction may result in tension injuries.

A pragmatic approach to spine radiographs addresses technical film quality, alignment, soft tissue swelling, and fractures. Assessment of technical film quality is important

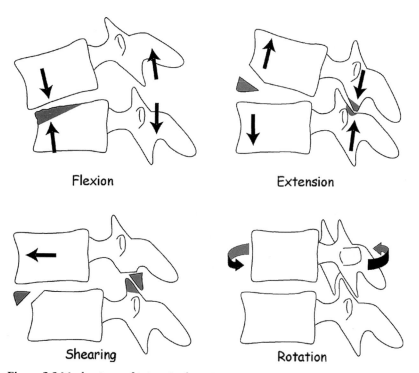

Flexion Extension

Shearing Rotation

Figure 3.2 Mechanisms of injury in the spine.

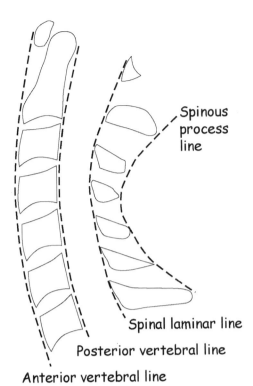

Figure 3.3 Useful lines and curves in the cervical region.

so that the interpreter is aware of which portions of the spine are adequately imaged and which are not. The most problematic area is the cervicothoracic junction, in which routine films often fail to show C7 and T1 adequately. In this circumstance, a "swimmer's" view should be obtained. Another common technical error is obtaining the lateral view with the spine rotated or tilted. The normal alignment of the spine is lordotic in the cervical region, kyphotic in the thoracic region, and lordotic in the lumbar region. Arcs drawn along any of the bony margins of the vertebrae on any view should be straight or curve smoothly. The most useful arcs in the cervical region on the lateral view are along the anterior margin of the bodies (anterior vertebral line), along the posterior margin of the bodies (posterior vertebral line), and along the posterior margin of the spinal canal (anterior margin of the spinous processes or spinal laminar line) (Fig. 3.3). The paraspinal soft tissues may be seen in the cervical region anteriorly and in the thoracic region laterally. As a general guideline, above the esophagus, the prevertebral soft tissues should measure 5 mm or less; at the level of the upper esophagus, (usually C6), they should measure 22 mm or less. In the thoracic region, the lateral soft tissues should follow the bony margins closely; they are more prom-

Table 3.4: Anatomic Distribution of Traumatic Spine Injuries[a]	
Region	*Frequency (%)*
Upper cervical (C1-C2)	13
Lower cervical (C3-T1)	53
Upper thoracic (T2-T10)	10
Thoracolumbar (T11-L2)	23
Lower lumbar (L3-L5)	1

[a]Based on 621 spine fractures, excluding isolated fractures of the spinous or transverse processes.
Adapted from Daffner RH, Deeb ZL, Rothfus WE. "Fingerprints" of vertebral trauma—a unifying concept based on mechanisms. *Skeletal Radiol* 1985;15:518–525.

inent in the presence of osteophytes. Discontinuity of any cortical margin on any view may indicate a fracture.

Because of differences in anatomy, biomechanics, and exposure to loading, spine trauma is considered in four regions: upper cervical (C1-C2), lower cervical (C3-T1), upper thoracic (T2-T10), and thoracolumbar (T11-L5). Spinal column injuries are most common in the lower cervical spine and in the thoracolumbar region (Table 3.4). A significant minority of patients have fractures at multiple noncontiguous levels. The most dangerous of these situations is a C2 fracture combined with a C7-T1 injury.

UPPER CERVICAL SPINE (C1-C2)

The cervical spine occupies a vulnerable position as the mobile linkage between the head and the thorax. The internal stresses on the spine and the injuries that result depend primarily on the positions of the head, spine, and body at the time of injury, and the sequence, direction, magnitude, and rate of loading. When structural failure occurs, it is most often restricted to a single intervertebral or vertebral level, but as many as 10% of patients with upper cervical spine injuries also have lower cervical spine injuries. In clinical practice, two types of events account for most cervical spine injuries: (a) axial loading on the head that is transmitted into the spine, and (b) acceleration or deceleration of the head and body relative to each other. Axial loading occurs when the moving head strikes a stationary object and may be combined with loading in flexion or extension. Acceleration and deceleration loading may occur because of the substantial difference in mass between the head and body. Forward or backward translation of the head relative to the body during acceleration or deceleration results in complex, changing forces on the cervical spine. In addition to the hyperflexion or hyperextension loading that occurs when the cervical spine reaches its limit of mobility, there are additional distractive forces in the axial direction. The predominant mode of loading is tensile in either flexion or extension. The injuries that occur depend on how the spine is loaded as well as individual variations in mechanics and anatomy.

> Upper and lower cervical spine injuries may occur simultaneously.

Fractures of the ring of C1 are sustained during axial loading. An axial load applied to the top of the head with the cervical spine in neutral position spreads apart the ring of C1 between the sloped articular surfaces of the occiput and C2. This results in multiple, displaced fractures of C1 (Jefferson fracture). More commonly, the axial load is applied obliquely, or the cervical spine does not remain straight, and the fractures of the ring of C1 are more posterior or lateral (Fig. 3.4). Neurologic damage is often absent because the spinal canal is relatively capacious at this level, and the fragments are displaced away from the cord. These injuries should be evident on radiographs, but CT is often helpful.

In traumatic spondylolisthesis of C2 (hangman's fracture), there are bilateral pars interarticularis fractures with forward subluxation of C2 over C3. The *pars interarticularis* is the bridge of bone that occupies the position in the articular mass between the superior and inferior articular facets. An individual subjected to judicial hanging drops feet first through a trap door with a rope secured around the neck and the hangman's knot located under the chin. When he or she reaches the end of the rope, the upper cervical spine is pulled violently into hyperextension and simultaneously subjected to massive distractive forces from the downward inertia of the body. The ligaments of the anterior column tear at the C2-C3 level, and the posterior elements are fractured at the pars interarticularis. Similar fractures of the C2 posterior elements may also occur when an axial load (compressive rather than distractive) is applied with the neck hyperextended (Figs. 3.5 and 3.6). This may occur in a motor vehicle collision in which the passenger slides forward and strikes the forehead, forcing the neck into hyperextension.

In young adults, most fractures of the odontoid process of C2 (dens) occur transversely across the base, probably as a result of hyperextension or hyperflexion. The fracture is accompanied by ligament tears at the same level separating the odontoid process and C1

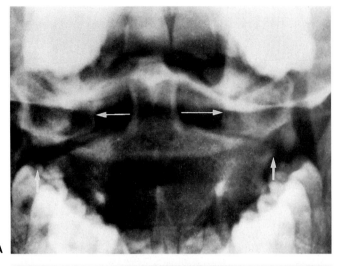

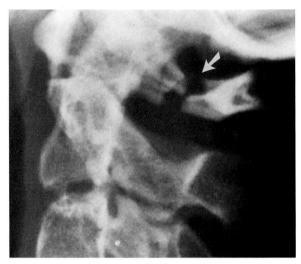

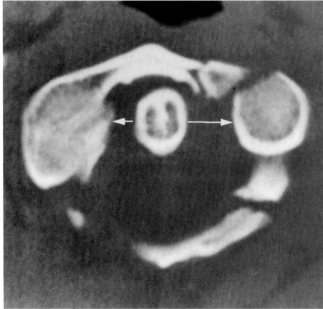

Figure 3.4 Axial compression fracture of C1 suffered in a diving accident. *A.* Open-mouth AP radiograph of the odontoid shows separation of the ring of C1 (*arrows*). *B.* Lateral radiograph shows soft tissue swelling and displaced fractures of the posterior arch (*arrow*). *C.* CT scan shows comminuted fractures involving the left lateral and the posterior portions of the ring of C1. The fragments have displaced asymmetrically from the odontoid process (*arrows*).

from the remainder of C2 as a single, mechanically unstable unit (Fig. 3.7). The odontoid is composed primarily of cortical bone, so that this fracture heals less well than fractures through portions of the vertebrae that are primarily cancellous.

In elderly adults, the most common odontoid fracture is through the base of the dens with extension into the body of C2 (Figs. 3.8 and 3.9). When the fracture is caused by flexion, a tension fracture begins at the posterior base of the dens and propagates anteriorly and inferiorly into the body of C2, where compression and impaction occur, resulting in an anteriorly angulated dens. When the fracture is caused by extension, a tension fracture begins at the anterior base of the dens and propagates posteriorly where compression and impaction occur, resulting in a posteriorly angulated dens.

Fractures of the dens can be classified according to Anderson and d'Alonzo (Table 3.5). A type I fracture involves the tip of the dens and is rare. A type II fracture extends transversely across the base of the dens and is the most common type. A type III fracture involves the body of C2.

An odontoid fracture that has progressed to atrophic nonunion is called an *os odontoideum* (Fig. 3.10). As with nonunions elsewhere, the margins of the fracture line become corticated; a fibrous union or a pseudoarthrosis may be present. Although some authorities argue that the os odontoideum is a developmental variant in which the odontoid process does

Type II odontoid fractures are common in young adults. Type III odontoid fractures are common in elderly adults.

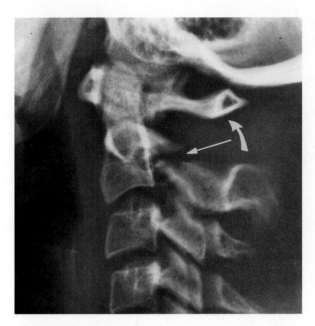

Figure 3.5 Traumatic spondylolisthesis (hangman's fracture) in a traffic collision victim. Horizontal fractures through the pars interarticularis (*long arrow*) allow C2 to incline forward, splaying the posterior elements (*curved arrow*).

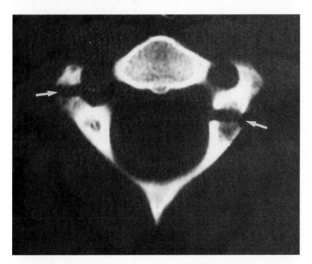

Figure 3.6 CT scan of C2 hangman's fracture (*arrows*).

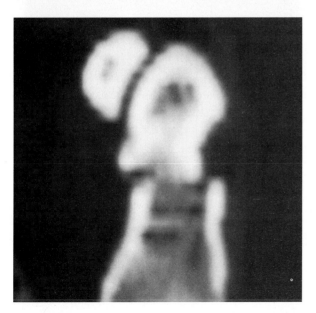

Figure 3.7 Odontoid fracture (type II) shown on sagittal CT reconstruction.

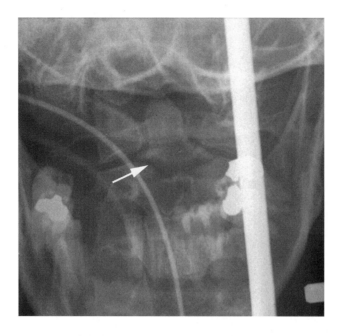

Figure 3.8 Odontoid fracture (type III) (*arrow*) shown on open-mouth AP radiograph.

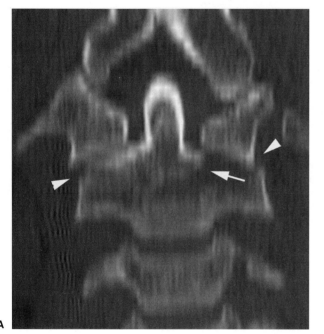

A

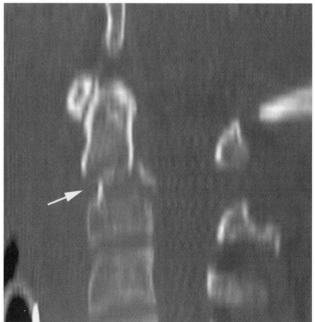

B

Figure 3.9 Odontoid fracture (type III) (*arrows*) shown on coronal (*A*) and sagittal (*B*) CT reconstructions. Note the subluxation of C1 relative to C2 (*arrowheads*).

Table 3.5: Anderson and d'Alonzo Classification of Fractures of the Dens

Type I	Avulsion fracture of the tip of the odontoid process	4%
Type II	Transverse fracture through the base of the dens at its junction with the body	64%
Type III	Fracture through the body of C2	15%

Adapted from Anderson LD, d'Alonzo RT. Fractures of the odontoid process of the axis. *J Bone Joint Surg Am* 1974;56:1663–1674.

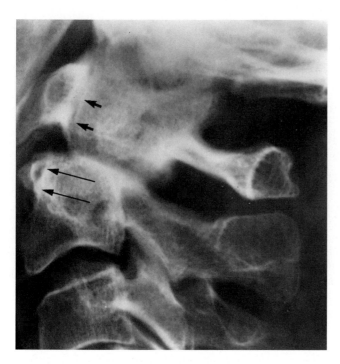

Figure 3.10 Nonunion of odontoid fracture. Lateral radiograph shows posterior subluxation of C1 over C2 allowed by a nonunited odontoid fracture. The anterior margins of the odontoid process (*short arrows*) and the body of C2 (*long arrows*) are misaligned. Instability was evident on flexion and extension radiographs (not shown).

not fuse to the body of C2, the site of the synchondrosis between the odontoid process and the body of C2 is not located here. Because of present or potential mechanical instability, surgical fusion of C1 and C2 is the common method of management. A fracture of the base of the odontoid process, through the substance of the body of C2 rather than through the odontoid process itself, also represents a mechanically unstable fracture. Because the fracture is through cancellous bone, healing is usually prompt, and nonunion is unlikely. These fractures are much less common than fractures through the odontoid process. Odontoid fractures are the most common cervical spine fractures in patients older than 70 years of age.

Isolated fractures of the anterior-inferior margin of the body of C2 are the most common type of hyperextension teardrop fracture (Fig. 3.11), so called because the mechanism

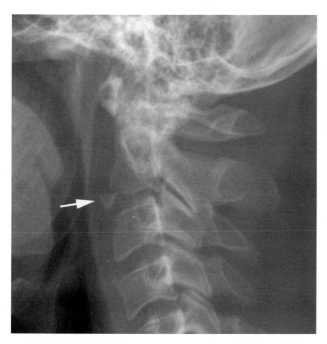

Figure 3.11 C2 hyperextension teardrop fracture (*arrow*) with displacement on radiograph.

of injury is hyperextension, and the fracture fragment resembles a teardrop. The hyperextension teardrop fracture represents an avulsion fracture with tension mediated through the anterior longitudinal ligament. The hyperextension teardrop fracture occurs less commonly at C3—and even less commonly at other levels—but may be associated with a hangman's fracture.

Dislocations of the occiput over C1 or of C1 over C2 require severe ligament disruption and are rare and usually fatal. Subluxation at the C1-C2 level requires disruption of the transverse ligament of C1 that maintains the normal anatomic position of the odontoid process. Nontraumatic laxity of the transverse ligament is associated with Down syndrome, rheumatoid arthritis, and mucopolysaccharidosis.

LOWER CERVICAL SPINE (C3-T1)

In the lower cervical spine, the most common levels of injury are C5 and C6.

Axial loading of the head occurs in events such as a fall from a height in which the individual lands on the head or a motor vehicle collision in which he or she is thrown forward and strikes the head. The attitude of the cervical spine and the location and direction of impact relative to the spine determine the stresses that result. Moderately severe axial loading with the cervical spine in neutral position causes vertebral body failure with central depression of the subjacent superior end plate, most often at C5. With massive axial loads, the intervertebral disc herniates through the end plate of the subjacent vertebral body and causes the body to explode from within, dispersing the fragments (burst fracture). Retropulsed fragments frequently damage the spinal cord. If the neck is flexed or if the location and direction of impact force the neck into flexion, the cervical spine is distracted posteriorly and compressed anteriorly. If the forces are relatively small, the injury may consist of a posterior ligament sprain (hyperflexion sprain) and possibly a compression fracture of the vertebral body. Disruption of the posterior ligament complex may be evident on radiographs as a focal kyphosis localized to the level of the sprain, often with subluxation of the facet joints and fanning of the spinous processes (Figs. 3.12 and 3.13). The abnormalities are accentuated with flexion and reduced with extension. The anterior compression fracture may be evident as loss of height, buckling of the anterior cortex, disruption of the end plate, and wedging of the disc space. Because the middle column is intact, this injury tends to be stable. Prevertebral soft tissue swelling tends to be minimal and focal, reflecting the integ-

Prevertebral soft tissue swelling tends to be minimal when the anterior longitudinal ligament is intact.

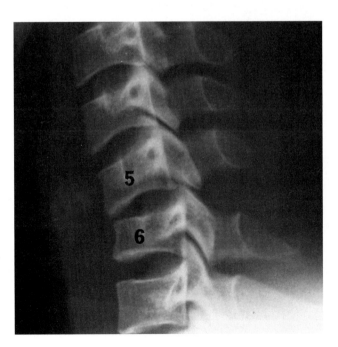

Figure 3.12 Posterior ligament tear between C5 and C6 without fracture (hyperflexion sprain).

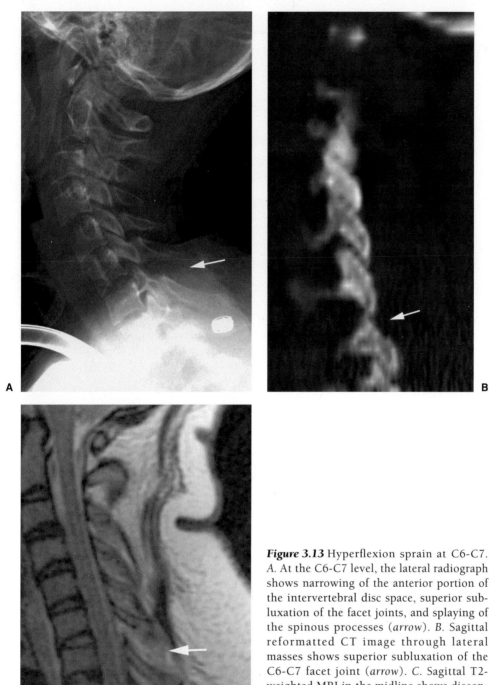

Figure 3.13 Hyperflexion sprain at C6-C7. A. At the C6-C7 level, the lateral radiograph shows narrowing of the anterior portion of the intervertebral disc space, superior subluxation of the facet joints, and splaying of the spinous processes (*arrow*). B. Sagittal reformatted CT image through lateral masses shows superior subluxation of the C6-C7 facet joint (*arrow*). C. Sagittal T2-weighted MRI in the midline shows discontinuity of the nuchal ligament at C6-C7 with splaying of the spinous processes (*arrow*) and narrowing of the anterior portion of the intervertebral disc space.

rity of the anterior longitudinal ligament. If the direction of force is slightly to one side, the injuries may be eccentric. Delayed or failed ligament healing is a common complication.

If axial compression with hyperflexion is caused by large forces, a fracture-dislocation may result (hyperflexion teardrop injury). This grievous injury is usually accompanied by quadriplegia from contusion of the anterior portion of the spinal cord. Massive posterior distractive forces disrupt the posterior ligament complex and dislocate the facet joints. The anterior and middle columns are disrupted with tears of the longitudinal ligaments and the

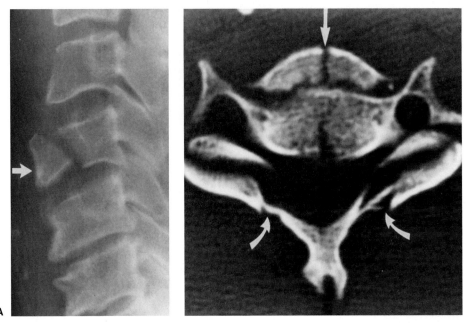

A   B

Figure 3.14 Hyperflexion teardrop fracture at C4. *A.* Lateral radiograph shows the teardrop fragment (*arrow*) and anterior soft tissue swelling. The major portion of the C4 vertebra is displaced posteriorly, although the teardrop fragment remains attached to the top of C5. *B.* CT scan through the C4 level shows a sagittal split of the body (*arrow*) and fractures of the laminae (*curved arrows*).

intervertebral disc. A triangular fragment (teardrop fragment) is sheared off the anterior-inferior corner of the dislocating vertebral body. The result is complete disruption of the cervical spine, with the superior portion displaced posteriorly and angulated anteriorly. The injury is recognized radiographically by focal kyphosis, posterior dislocation, distraction of the posterior elements, and the teardrop fragment of the anterior-inferior corner of the superior body (Figs. 3.14 and 3.15). Diffuse, marked anterior prevertebral soft tissue swelling is always present.

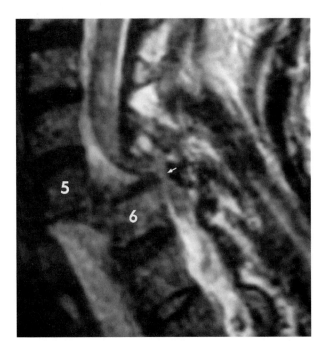

Figure 3.15 Hyperflexion fracture-dislocation at C5-C6. Sagittal T2-weighted MRI shows transection of the spinal cord (*arrow*).

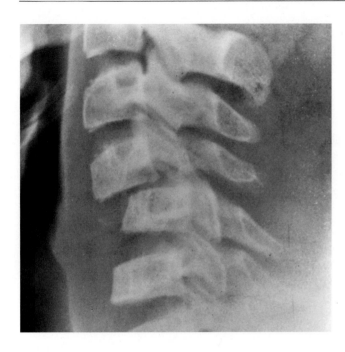

Figure 3.16 Bilateral facet dislocation at C4-C5. Approximately 50% of the body of C4 is displaced anterior to C5. Gross prespinal soft tissue swelling is present.

The major injury vector in bilateral facet dislocation is hyperflexion of large magnitude without axial compression. Bilateral facet dislocation is a tension injury that propagates from posterior to anterior. Complete disruption of the ligaments and forward displacement of one involved vertebra over another allow the inferior articular facets of the suprajacent vertebra to dislocate into the intervertebral foramen. The superior vertebra is anteriorly displaced by approximately 50% of the width of its body (Fig. 3.16). Sometimes the facets are subluxated (perched) but not dislocated. There may be accompanying fractures of the articular processes of the subjacent vertebra. The spine is unstable.

Axial loading with hyperextension places the anterior column under tension and the posterior column under compression. Structures of the spine fail in sequence, depending on the magnitude of the loading: tear of the anterior longitudinal ligament, disruption of the intervertebral disc, and tear of the posterior longitudinal ligament. A tension fracture of the vertebral body rather than disc disruption may occur; if the fracture involves only the anterior-inferior corner, a triangular (teardrop) fragment is present (hyperextension teardrop fracture). Compression fractures of the posterior elements are common, including fractures of the lamina and lateral masses. One or both facet joints may become dislocated. If only ligaments are disrupted and the spine relocates on the rebound, radiographs may show a nearly normally aligned spine without fracture in an acutely quadriplegic patient (hyperextension sprain) (Fig. 3.17). Marked prespinal soft tissue swelling should be present.

Large forces causing hyperextension and distraction, as might occur with a massive blow to the face or forehead, result in an injury similar to hyperextension with axial compression. The injury consists of tension injuries of the anterior and middle columns with transient posterior dislocation. Sometimes the disruption includes a tension fracture of the vertebral body, occasionally isolating a triangular fragment. Compressive injury to the posterior column is absent. Some degree of acute cervical cord syndrome is present, even though the cervical vertebrae on the lateral view may appear normally aligned after spontaneous reduction of the dislocation.

Unilateral facet dislocation occurs with hyperflexion, lateral bending, and rotation. Axial rotation and lateral bending are normally coupled in the middle and lower cervical spine because of the angle of the facet joints. With lateral bending, the facet joint on the concave side of the bend is compressed and essentially fixed; the contralateral articular mass rides forward and up and dislocates into the intervertebral foramen. The superior portion of the inferior facet is frequently fractured, presumably from impaction. Unilateral

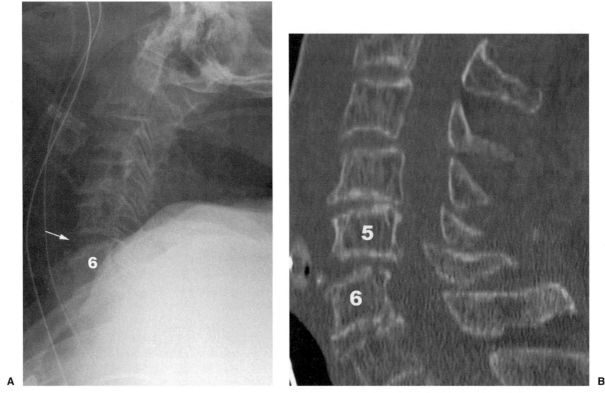

Figure 3.17 Hyperextension injury at C5-C6. *A.* Lateral radiograph shows anterior widening of intervertebral space at C5-C6 (*arrow*). *B.* Sagittal reformatted CT scan shows retrolisthesis.

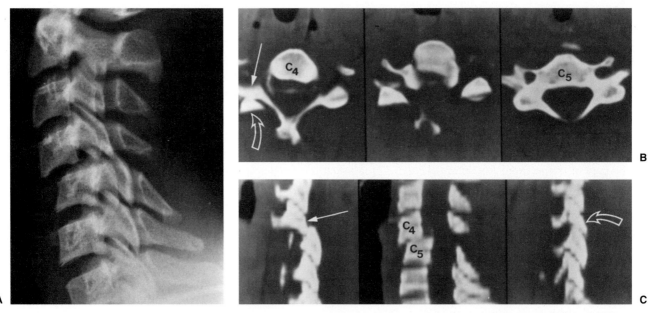

Figure 3.18 Unilateral facet dislocation at C4-C5. *A.* Lateral radiograph shows forward subluxation of C4. *B.* Three consecutive axial CT slices show the C4 vertebra on the left and the C5 vertebra on the right. C4 is rotated clockwise relative to C5. The right inferior articular process of C4 (*arrow*) is anterior to the right superior articular process of C5 (*curved arrow*). *C.* Sagittal reconstructions of the axial CT scan show the dislocated facet (*arrow*) on the patient's right side at C4-C5 but not on the patient's left (*curved arrow*).

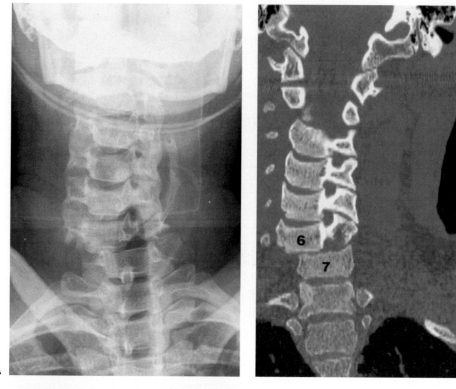

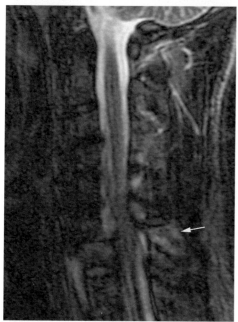

Figure 3.19 Lateral cervical spine fracture-dislocation. *A.* AP radiograph shows lateral fracture-dislocation at C6-C7. *B.* Coronal reformatted CT scan shows lateral translation of C6 over C7 with rotatory displacement. *C.* Sagittal T2-weighted MRI shows abnormal high signal (*arrow*) between the spinous processes of C6 and C7, indicative of ligamentous disruption. Spinal cord contusion is also present.

facet dislocation is recognized by forward subluxation and rotary misalignment (Fig. 3.18). The ligaments are disrupted on the side of the dislocation.

Lateral fracture-dislocations of the cervical spine are very uncommon (Fig. 3.19). In this circumstance, the lateral radiograph may be misleading in demonstrating normal or nearly normal alignment. Secondary sign, such as soft tissue swelling, should be present, and a cervical spinal cord injury may be clinically apparent. The mechanism of injury is likely to be lateral shearing.

Whiplash injuries occur in motor vehicle collisions when the individual's car is struck from behind, accelerating the body forward relative to the head. After the head

Lateral fracture-dislocations of the cervical spine are very uncommon.

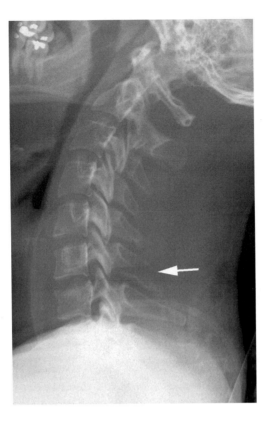

Figure 3.20 Clay shoveler's fracture at C6 (*arrow*).

bounces off the back of the car seat, the neck rebounds into flexion. The usual whiplash injury is a strain of the paravertebral and other neck muscles, often the *longus colli* group. In more severe injuries, the anterior longitudinal ligament and the anterior attachment of the intervertebral disc may be sprained. Bony fractures and dislocations are distinctly uncommon. Properly positioned headrests may prevent these injuries.

A clay shoveler's fracture is a horizontal tension fracture of a spinous process, most often C7 and less commonly C6 or T1 (Fig. 3.20). Workers digging drainage ditches in southwestern Australia in 1933 sustained these fractures when clay stuck to their shovels as they tried to throw the clay, suddenly increasing the stress on the neck musculature and its insertions. Similar injuries are sustained in motor vehicle collisions.

UPPER THORACIC REGION (T2-T10)

Traumatic fractures of the thoracic spine are uncommon.

The thoracic spine is supported by the rib cage and therefore is not very mobile. Fractures are uncommon and require major trauma. Acute traumatic compression fractures are most common at the T6-T7 levels. Most are anterior wedge fractures; the rest are lateral wedge fractures. Patients complain of localized pain and may have increased kyphosis. On imaging, paraspinal swelling, disruption of the cortical surface, and loss of height are present. Severe trauma may cause burst fractures, but these are much more common in the thoracolumbar region (discussed later in this chapter).

Although the upper thoracic spine is protected from bending forces by the rib cage, it is nonetheless vulnerable to torsional or shearing forces. Fracture-dislocations are severe injuries that are probably the result of torsional or shearing forces, presumably combined with hyperflexion or axial compression (Fig. 3.21). The posterior ligaments are torn, there is fracture or dislocation of the facet joints, and the vertebral body may have a rotary shear fracture just below the subjacent end plate. Horizontal shear-

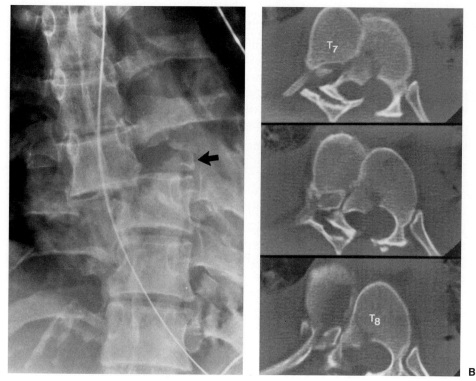

Figure 3.21 Thoracic fracture-dislocation. *A.* AP radiograph shows T7-T8 fracture dislocation with lateral translation of T7. An avulsed fragment of T7 remains attached to T8 (*arrow*). *B.* CT scan shows disruption of the posterior elements at both levels.

ing forces may be sustained in a direct blow that translates the upper portion of the spine over the lower portion at the level of injury. Typically, the blow is from behind and causes an anterior fracture-dislocation. The posterior column usually sustains traumatic spondylolisthesis with ligament tears, and the anterior and middle columns may have shear fractures of the vertebral body or soft tissue injuries of the intervertebral disc (Fig. 3.22). There is a high incidence of spinal cord injury; 60% to 70% of

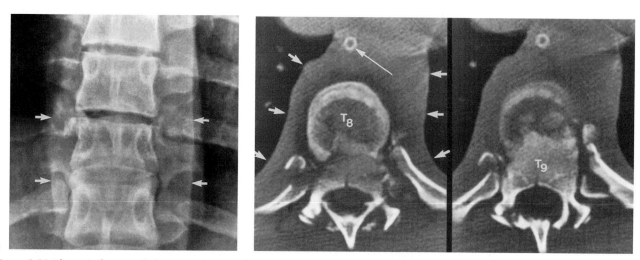

Figure 3.22 Thoracic fracture-dislocation. *A.* AP radiograph shows widening of the paraspinal line on both sides (*arrows*) with slight flattening of T9. *B.* CT scan shows forward translation of T8 over T9 with comminuted fractures that include the posterior elements. Paraspinal hematoma (*short arrows*) has displaced the esophagus and nasogastric tube (*long arrow*).

patients with thoracic fracture-dislocation have a neurologic deficit. Thoracic fracture-dislocations are often reduced or partially reduced when patients are placed on backboards for extrication or transport. A massive injury may then be present with only subtle signs on the obligatory AP radiograph of the chest. Misalignment of the spinous processes, misalignment of the lateral margins of the vertebral bodies, focal angulation, widening of the interspinous distance, and paraspinal hematoma should be carefully sought. Sometimes, the paraspinal hematoma dissects into the mediastinum and over the apex of the left lung, simulating transection of the thoracic aorta. The presence of any of these findings necessitates further investigation, usually by CT.

THORACOLUMBAR REGION (T11-L5)

The thoracolumbar junction is vulnerable to hyperflexion injuries.

Most injuries to the thoracolumbar region occur at the thoracolumbar junction (T11-L2), where the greatest degree of mobility is present. This region is particularly vulnerable to hyperflexion injuries. During hyperflexion, compression fractures with anterior wedging of the vertebral body may be sustained, but the tensile loads are not great enough to disrupt the posterior ligaments (Fig. 3.23). Pure axial loading of the spine causes axial compression fractures that appear indistinguishable from hyperflexion injuries. With moderate loading, a simple compression fracture of the superior end plate is typical. If the loads are asymmetric, the fractures may be eccentric. Lateral bending may cause tension fractures of the transverse processes. With massive loading, a burst fracture may occur (Fig. 3.24), with involvement of the posterior elements and possible injury to the spinal cord. Simple compression fractures are stable because the middle and posterior columns remain intact; they may be treated with a brace or body cast. Burst fractures involving anterior and middle columns may require internal fixation.

Seat belt injuries are sustained in hyperflexion when the body is thrown forward against a restraining lap belt during sudden deceleration. Unlike the usual flexion injury, in which the axis of rotation is through the vertebral body, the axis of rotation in seat belt injuries is at the anterior abdominal wall. Tensile forces disrupt the spine from pos-

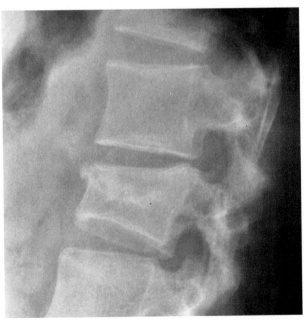
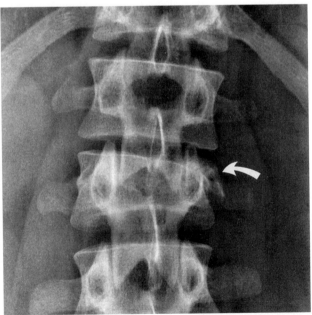

A

B

Figure 3.23 Compression fracture of L2. *A.* Lateral radiograph shows wedging of the L2 body at the superior end plate. *B.* AP radiograph shows greater loss of height on the left (*arrow*).

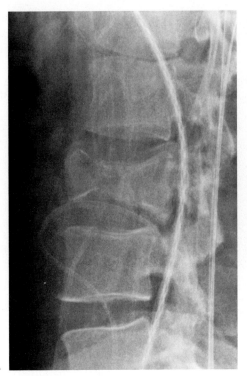
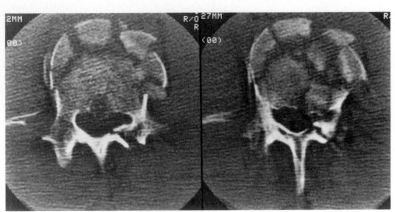

A   B

Figure 3.24 Lumbar burst fracture. *A.* Lateral radiograph shows L3 vertebral body flattened and spread apart. *B.* Axial CT shows comminution with centrifugal displacement of fragments. The fractures include the posterior elements. The spinal canal is compromised.

terior to anterior, usually at the L2 or L3 level. The resulting injury may consist of a tension fracture that extends horizontally through the vertebral body and neural arch (Chance fracture), intervertebral ligament disruption, or a combination of both (Fig. 3.25). A shoulder harness or air bag may prevent these injuries. Fractures or dislocations are uncommon at L3 or L4 and are rare at L5. Injuries to L3-L5 are seen most often in patients with multiple trauma.

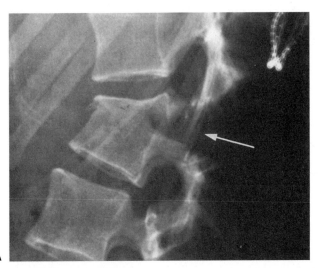
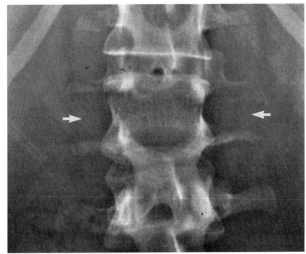

A   B

Figure 3.25 Tension fracture of the entire L2 vertebra in a motor vehicle collision victim (Chance fracture). *A.* Lateral view shows sharp kyphotic angulation at the fracture level. The fractures extend through the vertebra from the posterior elements (*arrow*) to the body. *B.* AP radiograph shows the fractures through the body, posterior elements, and transverse processes (*arrows*).

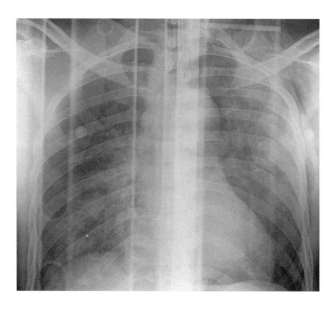

Figure 3.26 Multiple left rib fractures sustained in a high-speed automobile crash.

THORACIC CAGE

Blunt chest trauma sustained in motor vehicle collisions may crush the bony thorax on direct impact. Pulmonary contusion, pneumothorax, myocardial contusion, diaphragmatic rupture, and abdominal injuries may result. The sudden deceleration that accompanies direct impact may cause transection of the thoracic aorta.

    Rib fractures may occur from direct blows or crush injuries (Fig. 3.26). Oblique views of the chest are often necessary to demonstrate fractures of the ribs because of their arcuate course. Rib fractures may be difficult to see initially but are more obvious later as they become displaced by constant respiratory motion. Knowing the sites of

Rib fractures are more obvious after they become displaced by respiratory motion.

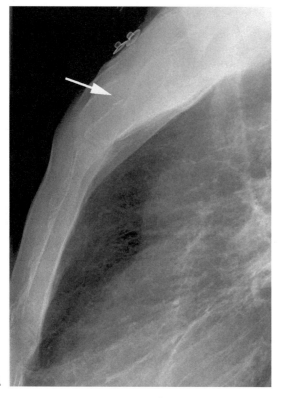

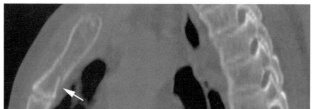

Figure 3.27 Manubrium fracture. *A.* Lateral radiograph and (*B*) sagittal reformatted CT show nondisplaced fracture (*arrows*) of the manubrium.

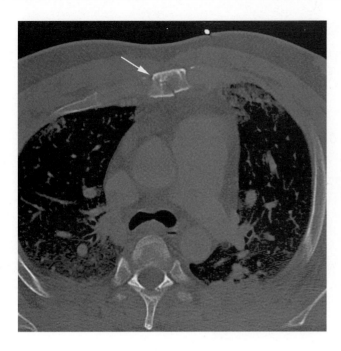

Figure 3.28 Sternal body fracture. Axial CT shows nondisplaced fracture (*arrow*) through the body of the sternum.

maximal pain and point tenderness is helpful. Rib fractures may be multiple, in which case they involve adjacent ribs in a linear array. A flail chest occurs when there are multiple rib fractures that isolate a segment of the chest wall and cause paradoxic motion with respiration. Complications and associated conditions include pulmonary contusion, pneumothorax, hemopneumothorax, hemothorax, tracheal or bronchial tear, and interstitial emphysema. Fractures of the first three ribs usually follow severe trauma. The most common rib fractures are of the posterior or lateral aspects of the fourth through ninth ribs. Fractures of the lower ribs may be associated with visceral injuries. A rib may fracture with violent coughing or sneezing, usually at the anterior aspect along the diaphragmatic insertion. Stress fractures may also occur at the insertions of the serratus anterior muscles (first through ninth ribs) or scalene muscles (first and second ribs). Rib fractures that occur without trauma or with minimal trauma raise suspicion for a pathologic fracture.

The sternum fractures only with severe trauma as might be sustained with direct impact on the chest, for example, hitting the steering wheel during a motor vehicle collision. Most sternal fractures are transverse through the body of the sternum or the sternomanubrial junction (Figs. 3.27 and 3.28). Hyperflexion of the thoracic cage is another mechanism of sternal fracture.

PELVIC RING

The pelvic ring comprises the sacrum and the two innominate bones. These three rigid components have resilient articulations where small degrees of motion are possible: the sacroiliac (SI) joints and the pubic symphysis. Thus, the pelvic ring is not a single rigid structure. Biomechanically, the sacrum can be considered the keystone of a femoral-sacral arch that supports the spine over the legs. The upper portion of the SI joint is a fibrous articulation with an extremely strong interosseous ligament; the lower portion of the SI joint is synovial and does not contribute mechanical strength to the joint. Anterior and posterior sets of SI ligaments attach the upper sacrum to the ilium, and sacrotuberous and sacrospinous ligaments attach the lower sacrum to the ischium. The functional stability of the pelvic ring depends on these ligaments. The pubic rami act as a stabilizing strut anteriorly, but their role is not crucial, provided that the posterior structures remain intact. Fractures of the pelvis can be divided into those that

Biomechanically, the pelvic ring is not a single rigid structure.

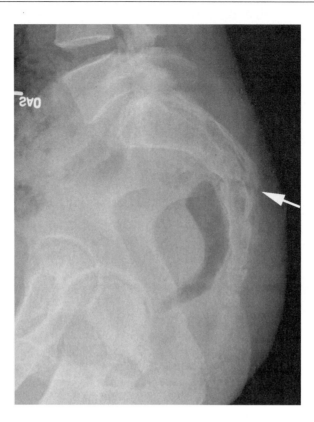

Figure 3.29 Fracture of the sacrum. Lateral radiograph shows a transverse fracture (*arrow*) through the sacrum at the S3 level.

do not disrupt the integrity of the weight-bearing femoral-sacral arch (stable fractures) and those that do (unstable fractures).

STABLE FRACTURES

Stable fractures account for approximately two-thirds of all pelvic fractures. These injuries include isolated fractures of the sacrum and pubic rami, avulsion fractures around the periphery of the pelvis, and simple acetabular fractures (see Chapter 4). Many stable fractures of the pelvis, especially isolated fractures around the obturator foramen, are sustained by elderly osteoporotic adults who fall. Although the bony margins of the obturator foramen form a rigid ring, the arrangement of its components is such that when the ring is loaded, one portion may be subjected to shearing forces, whereas another may be subjected to compressive forces. Bone resists shearing forces less well than compressive forces, so the bones may fail under shear but not under compression, leaving a single fracture of the ring. The most common pelvic fracture is an isolated fracture of an ischial ramus sustained in a fall. An isolated fracture of an iliac wing is called a *Duverney fracture*. It is frequently sustained in blunt trauma, such as motor vehicle crashes.

> The most common pelvic fracture is an isolated fracture of an ischial ramus.

Isolated fractures of the sacrum are caused by direct trauma or a fall. These fractures tend to be transversely oriented, below the level of the SI joints and anteriorly displaced or anteriorly angulated (Figs. 3.29 and 3.30). They are best demonstrated on the lateral radiograph or by CT images reformatted in the sagittal plane. Fractures of the sacrum that occur with pelvic ring fractures are typically vertical in orientation.

Stress fractures of the pubic rami may occur in runners. The clinical presentation is groin pain that is much worse with activity. As with stress fractures elsewhere, a radionuclide bone scan may be necessary to identify the injury.

UNSTABLE FRACTURES

Unstable fractures of the pelvic ring are the result of severe trauma, usually motor vehicle collisions involving either pedestrians or car occupants. Because these injuries are common

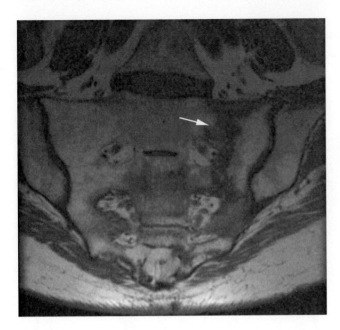

Figure 3.30 Fracture of the sacrum. Oblique coronal T1-weighted MRI shows dark signal (*arrow*) extending vertically along the left sacral ala, indicating the fracture line and adjacent hemorrhage and edema.

in the setting of multiple trauma, an AP radiograph of the pelvis should be part of the initial evaluation of all multiple trauma patients. Patients with pelvic fractures may have serious vascular injury, exsanguinate, and die. Because reduction and stabilization of pelvic fractures usually control bleeding, early discovery and evaluation of these injuries have significant practical importance for the orthopedist. Urologic injuries are commonly associated with severe pelvic fractures. Fractures that involve the vagina or rectum are open fractures and carry a grave risk of sepsis. Three distinct patterns of injury can be recognized (Table 3.6 and Fig. 3.31).

The most common mechanism of unstable pelvic ring injury is lateral compression. Lateral compression may occur when a pedestrian or a vehicle occupant is struck from the side. The pelvis is crushed as the hemipelvis on the side of impact is rotated inward by the force, sustaining a shear fracture of the pubis and a compression fracture of the ipsilateral sacral ala; ligamentous injury is minimal (Fig. 3.32). With force of greater magnitude, continued inward rotation causes either disruption of the posterior SI ligaments or fracture of the ilium. The opposite hemipelvis may be rotated outward, opening that SI joint anteriorly. Central hip dislocation may be associated with lateral pelvic compression injuries (Fig. 3.33). The severity of the injury depends on the precise direction and magnitude of the forces.

An AP radiograph of the pelvis should be part of the initial evaluation of all multiple trauma patients.

Table 3.6: Pelvic Ring Fractures

Lateral compression (inward rotation of hemipelvis)	
Type I	Compression fracture of sacrum, pubic rami fractures
Type II	Rupture of posterior SI ligaments or fracture of iliac wing
Type III	Outward rotation of contralateral hemipelvis with disruption of SI joint anteriorly
Anteroposterior compression (outward rotation of hemipelvis)	
Type I	Diastasis of symphysis pubis
Type II	Anterior diastasis of SI joint
Type III	Posterolateral dislocation of SI joint
Vertical shear	(superior fracture dislocation of hemipelvis)

SI, sacroiliac.
Adapted from Young JWR, Burgess AR. *Radiologic management of pelvic ring fractures. Systematic radiographic diagnosis.* Baltimore: Urban & Schwarzenberg, 1987.

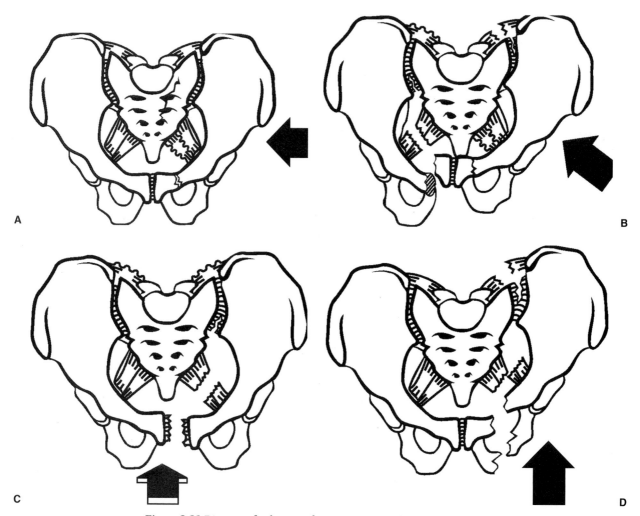

Figure 3.31 Diagram of pelvic ring fractures. *A.* Lateral compression (type I). Sacroiliac (SI) joint compression and pubic ramus fracture. The hemipelvis on the side of impact rotates inward. *B.* Lateral compression (type II). The SI joint is opened posteriorly as the hemipelvis continues to rotate inward. *C.* AP compression fracture (type II). Diastasis of the symphysis with opening of the SI joint anteriorly. *D.* Vertical fracture-dislocation of a hemipelvis.

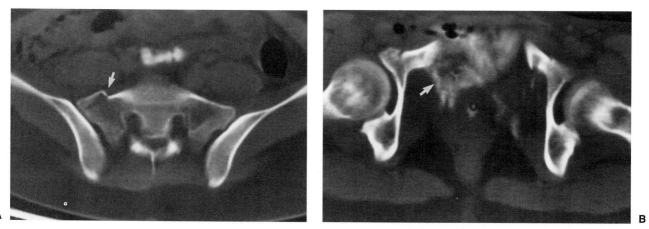

Figure 3.32 Lateral compression fracture (type I). *A.* CT scan shows a buckle fracture of the right sacral ala (*arrow*). *B.* CT slice at a lower level shows extravasated contrast (*arrow*) because of disruption of the urinary tract. Fractures of the pubic rami were present but not demonstrated at this anatomic level.

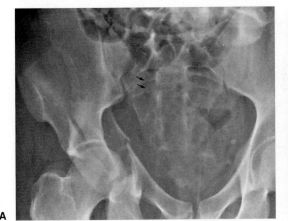

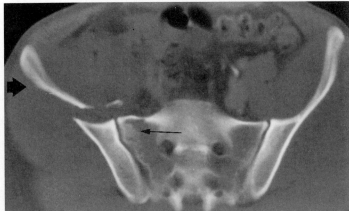

A

B

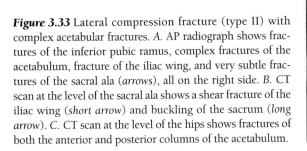

Figure 3.33 Lateral compression fracture (type II) with complex acetabular fractures. *A*. AP radiograph shows fractures of the inferior pubic ramus, complex fractures of the acetabulum, fracture of the iliac wing, and very subtle fractures of the sacral ala (*arrows*), all on the right side. *B*. CT scan at the level of the sacral ala shows a shear fracture of the iliac wing (*short arrow*) and buckling of the sacrum (*long arrow*). *C*. CT scan at the level of the hips shows fractures of both the anterior and posterior columns of the acetabulum.

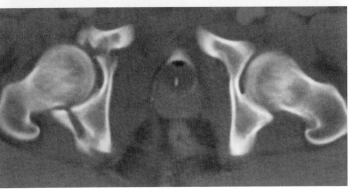

C

When force is applied anteriorly to the pelvis, the pelvis is flattened open. The anterior arch is first pulled apart and sustains a tension injury, usually a vertically oriented tension fracture of the pubic ramus or, less often, soft tissue disruption of the symphysis. If the force is of sufficient magnitude, one hemipelvis rotates outward, opening the pelvis like a book (Fig. 3.34). The sacrotuberous and sacrospinous ligaments are disrupted in turn and followed by the anterior, interosseous, and posterior SI ligaments. An even more severe injury is total SI joint disruption that leaves a floating, unsupported hemipelvis. AP compression fractures are associated with massive vascular damage and high mortality rates. A posterior column acetabular fracture may be an associated injury.

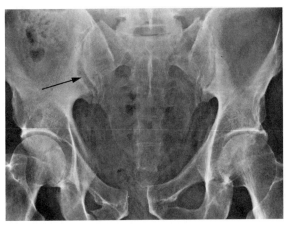

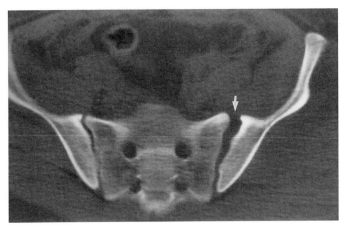

A

B

Figure 3.34 AP compression fracture (type II). *A*. The symphysis pubis is diastatic, and the right sacroiliac (SI) joint appears widened (*arrow*). Fractures of the right inferior pubic ramus are present. *B*. Another case of AP compression fracture (type II). CT scan shows the left SI joint has opened anteriorly (*arrow*).

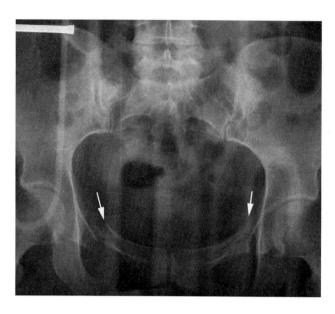

Figure 3.35 Straddle fractures of the pelvis, involving the right and left superior and inferior pubic rami (*arrows*).

A variant of the anterior compression fracture is the *straddle fracture*, which refers not to the mechanism of injury but to the morphology of the fractures. In this situation, there are bilateral vertical fractures of the superior and inferior pubic rami, with an intact pubis (Fig. 3.35).

Vertical shear forces typically occur in falls from a height onto an extended leg. The usual pattern of injury is a vertical fracture of the anterior ring and fracture-dislocation of the ipsilateral SI joint with vertical displacement (Malgaigne fracture) (Fig. 3.36). The vertical fractures of the anterior ring may be ipsilateral or contralateral to the SI joint lesion. Because there is total disruption of the posterior ligaments combined with anterior fractures, this relatively uncommon injury is grossly unstable. Occasionally, both SI joints are dislocated as the sacrum drops through the femoral-sacral arch.

Complex patterns of pelvic ring fractures occur with the application of forces from two or more directions, either together or sequentially. The most common combination is lateral compression and AP compression. The injuries have features of both types of injury.

One helpful clue in the analysis of pelvic ring fractures is the direction of displacement of the acetabulum. In lateral compression injuries, the acetabulum moves medially; in AP

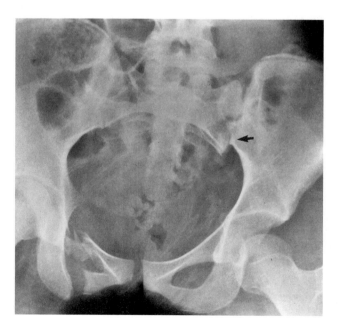

Figure 3.36 Vertical shear fracture in a 17-year-old patient. Vertical fractures of the right pubic rami are combined with superior dislocation of the left sacroiliac joint (*arrow*). The left hip is dislocated posteriorly.

compression, it moves laterally; and in vertical shear, it moves superiorly. The configuration of pubic rami fractures is another helpful clue. Pubic rami fractures oriented in the horizontal or coronal planes are sustained under lateral compression; fractures oriented in the vertical plane are sustained under AP compression or vertical shear.

SOURCES AND READINGS

Browner BD, Levine AM, Jupiter JB, et al., eds. *Skeletal trauma: fractures, dislocations, ligamentous injuries.* Philadelphia: WB Saunders, 1998.

Daffner RH, Brown RR, Goldberg AL. A new classification for cervical vertebral injuries: influence of CT. *Skeletal Radiol* 2000;29:125–132.

Daffner RH, Deeb ZL, Rothfus WE. "Fingerprints" of vertebral trauma—a unifying concept based on mechanisms. *Skeletal Radiol* 1985;15:518–525.

Dai LY, Yuan W, Ni B, et al. Os odontoideum: etiology, diagnosis, and management. *Surg Neurol* 2000;53:106–108.

Demetriades D, Charalambides K, Chahwan S, et al. Nonskeletal cervical spine injuries: epidemiology and diagnostic pitfalls. *J Trauma* 2000;48:724–727.

Fielding JW, Hensinger RN, Hawkins RJ. Os odontoideum. *J Bone Joint Surg [Am]* 1980;62A:376–383.

Gehweiler JA, Becker RF, Osborne RL. *Radiology of vertebral trauma.* Philadelphia: WB Saunders, 1997.

Goldberg W, Mueller C, Panacek E, et al. Distribution and patterns of blunt traumatic cervical spine injury. *Ann Emerg Med* 2001;38:17–21.

Hadley MN. Os odontoideum. *Neurosurgery* 2002;50:S148–S155.

Harris JH, Mirvis SE. *The radiology of acute cervical spine trauma,* 3rd ed. Philadelphia: Lippincott Williams & Wilkins, 1996.

Harris MB, Kronlage SC, Carboni PA, et al. Evaluation of the cervical spine in the polytrauma patient. *Spine* 2000;25:2884–2891.

Herkowitz HN, Rothman RH, eds. *The spine,* 4th ed. Philadelphia: WB Saunders, 1999.

Holmes JF, Miller PQ, Panacek EA, et al. Epidemiology of thoracolumbar spine injury in blunt trauma. *Acad Emerg Med* 2001;8:866–872.

Kaiser JA, Holland BA. Imaging of the cervical spine. *Spine* 1998;23:2701–2712.

Kerslake RW, Jaspan T, Worthington BS. Magnetic-resonance imaging of spinal trauma. *Br J Radiol* 1991;64:386–402.

Lowery DW, Wald MM, Browne BJ, et al. Epidemiology of cervical spine injury victims. *Ann Emerg Med* 2001;38:12–16.

Rapado A. General management of vertebral fractures. *Bone* 1996;18:191S–196S.

Resnick D. *Diagnosis of bone and joint disorders,* 4th ed. Philadelphia: WB Saunders, 2002.

Riggins RS, Kraus JF. The risk of neurologic damage with fractures of the vertebrae. *J Trauma* 1977;17:126–133.

Rogers LF. *Radiology of skeletal trauma,* 3rd ed. New York, Churchill-Livingstone, 2002.

Ryan MD, Henderson JJ. The epidemiology of fractures and fracture-dislocations of the cervical spine. *Injury* 1992;23:38–40.

Shaffrey CI, Shaffrey ME, Whitehill R, et al. Surgical treatment of thoracolumbar fractures. *Neurosurg Clin N Am* 1997;8:519–540.

Stahlman GC, Hanley EN. Surgical management of spinal fractures: guidelines for evaluation, patient selection, and surgical timing. *Neurosurg Q* 1999;9:73–86.

Tile M, Kellam J, Helfet DL, eds. *Fractures of the pelvis and acetabulum,* 3rd ed. Philadelphia: Lippincott Williams & Wilkins, 2002.

Veras LM, Pedraza-Gutierrez S, Castellanos J, et al. Vertebral artery occlusion after acute cervical spine trauma. *Spine* 2000;25:1171–1177.

Wasnich RD. Vertebral fracture epidemiology. *Bone* 1996;18:79S–183S.

White AA, Panjabi MM. *Clinical biomechanics of the spine,* 2nd ed. Philadelphia: Lippincott Williams & Wilkins, 1990.

TRAUMA IN ADULTS: LOWER EXTREMITY

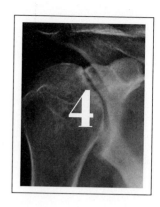

4

This chapter describes the radiology of many common injuries to the lower extremities in adults.

HIP

ACETABULAR FRACTURES

The acetabulum is nestled at the confluence of the ilium, pubis, and ischium under an arch formed by two columns: the iliopubic (anterior) and ilioischial (posterior). The posterior column, the thicker of the two, includes the major portion of the acetabular roof. The *acetabular roof*, or dome, is the articular and weight-bearing surface of the hip socket and includes portions of both columns. The quadrilateral plate forms the medial wall of the acetabulum and does not bear weight. The anterior column forms the iliopectineal line on AP radiographs; the posterior column forms the ilioischial line. Each column has a wall and a rim (Fig. 4.1). Acetabular fractures result from indirect forces transmitted through the femoral head, most often in high-energy motor vehicle collisions or falls. Approximately 20% of pelvic ring fractures in adults involve the acetabulum. The morphology of the fracture depends on the position of the femur at the moment of impact, the magnitude and direction of the force, and the strength of the bone. Acetabular fractures can be simple or complex (Table 4.1). Complex fractures can be described as combinations of fractures of the anterior and posterior columns, the anterior and posterior rims, and the acetabular roof. A transverse fracture separates the innominate bone into a superior iliac fragment and an inferior ilioischial fragment, and a T-shaped fracture combines a transverse fracture with a vertical separation of the anterior and posterior columns. The most common fracture of the acetabulum is a simple fracture of the posterior rim (Fig. 4.2), often associated with posterior hip dislocation (discussed in the next section). The other common fractures are simple

Approximately 20% of pelvic ring fractures in adults involve the acetabulum.

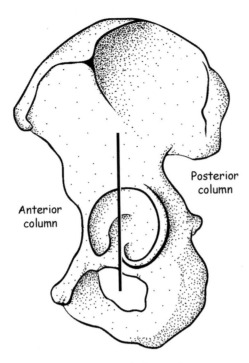

Lateral Aspect   *Figure 4.1* Columns of the acetabulum.

transverse fractures and complex fractures that involve the posterior column (Fig. 4.3). With complex fractures, the orthopedist is often most concerned about whether both anterior and posterior columns are involved or separated from each other, the severity of acetabular dome involvement, and the concomitant presence of pelvic ring injuries, especially ipsilateral iliac wing fractures or sacroiliac joint disruption. Acetabular fractures can be diagnosed by radiographs of the pelvis in AP and 45-degree oblique projections (Judet views) that show the anterior and posterior columns. CT is often necessary for full delineation of the sites of fracture and configuration of the fragments (Fig. 4.4).

HIP DISLOCATION

Eighty-five percent to 90% of hip dislocations are posterior.

Hip dislocations result from severe trauma such as motor vehicle collisions. Posterior dislocations with or without acetabular fractures (Fig. 4.5) account for 85% to 90% of cases. The mechanism of posterior dislocation is a blow along the axis of the femoral shaft with the hip flexed (as in hitting the dashboard with the knee in a motor vehicle collision). The posterior wall or column of the acetabulum is often fractured, and the femoral shaft or knee may also be injured. Sciatic nerve injury, sometimes transient, is present in approximately 10% of cases. Anterior dislocations may occur in motor vehicle collisions or falls from

Table 4.1: Acetabular Fractures	
Simple	Anterior rim
	Posterior rim
	Anterior column
	Posterior column
	Transverse
Complex	Combination of two or more simple fractures

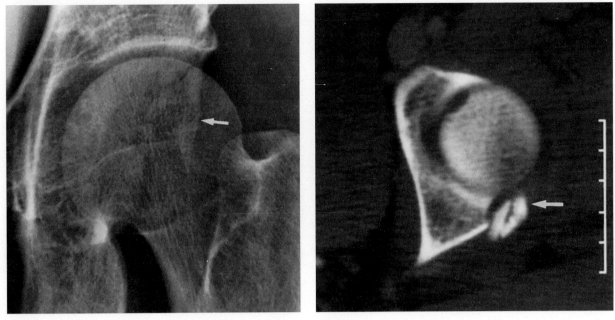

A   B

Figure 4.2 Posterior rim acetabular fracture. *A.* AP radiograph shows posterior rim fragment over-lapped by femoral head (*arrow*). *B.* CT shows the comminuted rim fragment (*arrow*).

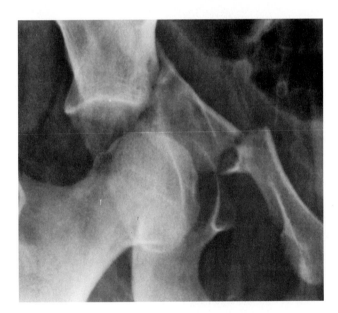

Figure 4.3 Complex acetabular fracture involving both columns.

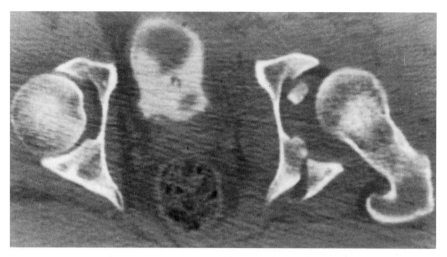

Figure 4.4 Posterior fracture dislocation of the left hip. Fractures of the rim and wall of the posterior column of the acetabulum are present. Because of the intra-articular fragment, the dislocation is not reducible.

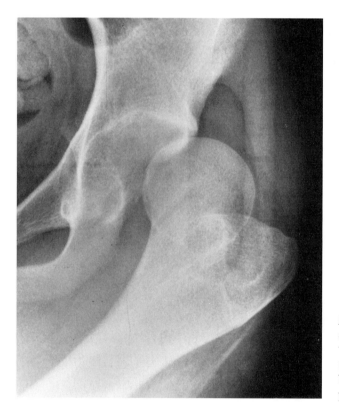

Figure 4.5 Posterior dislocation of the left hip without fracture. The femoral shaft is adducted. (The outline of a handhold of the backboard used to transport the patient overlies the femoral head.)

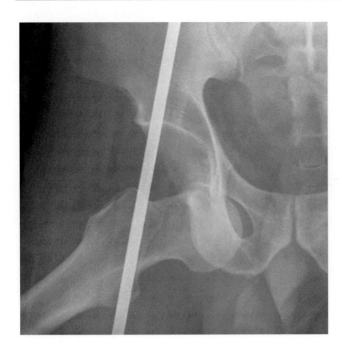

Figure 4.6 Anterior dislocation of the left hip. The femoral head lies anterior to the obturator ring. The femoral shaft is abducted.

heights when the hip is abducted (Fig. 4.6). CT can identify intra-articular fragments and confirm relocation of the hip after reduction. Complications of hip dislocation include avascular necrosis of the femoral head, transient or permanent sciatic nerve palsy, myositis ossificans, and posttraumatic degenerative joint disease. Associated fractures of the femoral head occur occasionally (Fig. 4.7).

ACETABULAR LABRUM

Patients with acetabular labral abnormalities may present with intractable, mechanical hip pain or snapping hip syndrome. The *acetabular labrum* is a fibrocartilaginous structure that is apposed to the bony acetabular rim. Similar to the glenoid labrum, it serves to deepen the hip socket. The labrum covers the anterior, superior, and posterior portions of the ace-

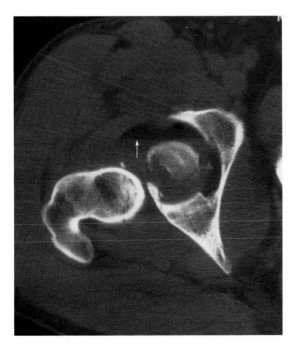

Figure 4.7 Posterior fracture-dislocation of the femoral head with a fragment remaining in the acetabulum. A fat-fluid level and gas bubble are present in the joint (*arrow*).

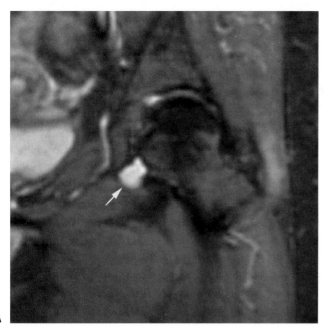
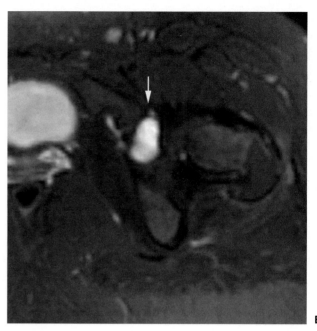

A   B

Figure 4.8 Tear of the anterior acetabular labrum. *A.* Coronal T2-weighted MRI with fat suppression shows a small cyst (*arrow*) at the anterior-inferior margin of the labrum. *B.* Axial T2-weighted MRI with fat suppression shows the tear (*arrow*) filled with fluid that is tracking into the cyst.

Abnormalities of the acetabular labrum are best identified with MR arthrography.

tabular rim; the deficient inferior portion is connected by a transverse ligament and is the site of insertion of the ligamentum teres. The labrum has a triangular cross section and normally has uniformly dark signal on T1-weighted, PD, and T2-weighted MR images, similar to the glenoid labrum or the menisci of the knee. Abnormalities of the labrum can be identified noninvasively with MRI or MR arthrography. As with the glenoid labrum, there is considerable variability in the appearance of the acetabular labrum, but tears can be identified by discontinuities in the fibrocartilage that are filled with fluid or contrast, in the case of MR arthrography. Disruptions of the peripheral attachment of the labrum to the bony acetabulum may also occur. The presence of a paralabral cyst is highly associated with labral tear (Fig. 4.8).

PROXIMAL FEMUR

Ninety-nine percent of fractures of the proximal femur in patients older than 50 years are caused by simple falls.

Fractures of the proximal femur are common only in the elderly because of osteoporosis (see Chapter 15); more than 95% of these fractures occur in patients older than 50 years, and the incidence is increasing as the population ages. The eventual mortality rate associated with hip fractures approaches 20%, and many survivors lose their independence of movement. Ninety-nine percent of fractures of the proximal femur are caused by simple falls. Even osteoporotic femurs are resistant to the compressive and tensile forces that occur during normal weight bearing, but there is great vulnerability to torsional or shearing stress. The roles of preexisting insufficiency microfractures in osteoporotic bone and decreased muscle tone as they relate to proximal femur fractures are unclear. Patients present with a painful, shortened, externally rotated limb that is unable to bear weight. Femoral fractures in persons younger than 40 years result from high-energy trauma and usually have associated injuries. Fractures of the proximal femur can be classified as intracapsular in 37% of cases, intertrochanteric in 49%, and subtrochanteric in 14%. Women sustain three to six times as many intracapsular fractures as men, but the incidence of intertrochanteric fractures is equal between the sexes. The initial evaluation in a suspected fracture should begin with radiographs. If a fracture is not identified and there is high clinical suspicion of a fracture, MRI should be obtained. If MRI is not available, CT or radionuclide bone scan should be used, although they are slightly less accurate than MRI. In the elderly population, fractures may not show radionuclide uptake until several days after the injury. A patient who was ambulatory before the fall but is unable to bear weight afterward should be presumed to have a fracture until proved otherwise.

> If radiographs are negative or equivocal and there is high clinical suspicion of fracture, MRI should be obtained.

INTRACAPSULAR FRACTURES

The capsule of the hip joint encloses the head and most of the neck of the femur, extending from the acetabulum to the intertrochanteric line anteriorly and to the mid-neck posteriorly. Most femoral neck fractures are intracapsular and therefore heal less rapidly (synovial fluid lyses clot) than intertrochanteric and subtrochanteric fractures. In addition, the vascular supply to the head is largely disrupted. Subcapital femoral neck fractures extend transversely across the neck, just below the femoral head. Intracapsular fractures can be classified as either nondisplaced (Fig. 4.9) or displaced (Fig. 4.10). Fractures through the base of the neck are similar to two-part intertrochanteric fractures in mechanism and treatment (discussed in the next section). The greater the displacement, the greater the likelihood of subsequent femoral head osteonecrosis. With displaced fractures, the incidence of osteonecrosis and nonunion is approximately 25%. Patients with impacted fractures are usually ambulatory with an antalgic limp and pain that is referred to the groin or the medial knee. Nondisplaced fractures have no inherent stability and may displace with continued ambulation. Femoral neck fractures heal by endosteal callus formation. Nondisplaced fractures are usually fixed with multiple pins placed in parallel; displaced fractures may be reduced and fixed with a variety of methods, including multiple pins, a telescoping hip screw, or some combination thereof. When the risk of femoral head osteonecrosis is high or the quality of trabecular bone is too poor for internal fixation, femoral endoprosthesis or total hip replacement may be used as primary treatment.

> Displaced femoral neck fractures have an incidence of osteonecrosis and nonunion of approximately 25%.

INTERTROCHANTERIC FRACTURES

The major fracture line of intertrochanteric fractures extends diagonally from superolateral (greater trochanter) to inferomedial (lesser trochanter). Most intertrochanteric fractures are comminuted, with the greater and lesser trochanters sometimes present as separate fragments (Fig. 4.11). In describing these fractures, the major fragments and the fracture

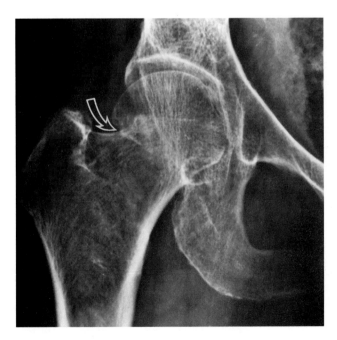

Figure 4.9 Impacted subcapital femoral neck fracture in an elderly woman (*arrow*).

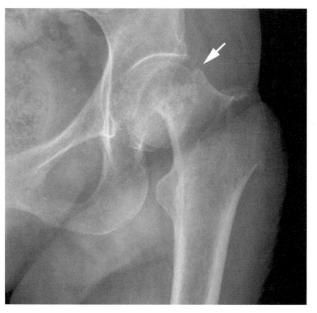
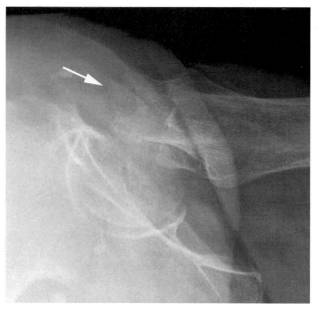

A   B

Figure 4.10 Displaced subcapital femoral neck fracture (*arrows*). *A.* AP radiograph. *B.* True lateral radiograph.

lines should be enumerated in relation to the trochanters, the neck, and the shaft. The degree of displacement and comminution and the presence or absence of subtrochanteric extension along the femoral shaft affect the orthopedic treatment plan and prognosis. Open reduction and internal fixation with a dynamic hip screw are usual. Unlike intracapsular femoral neck fractures, these injuries tend to heal promptly and without complication. The incidence of avascular necrosis of the femoral head is approximately 1%. Incomplete intertrochanteric fractures may occur in elderly adults as a result of falls. Radiographs in this circumstance may be normal, but MRI will demonstrate the fracture (Fig. 4.12). Isolated fractures of the greater trochanter occur in elderly adults as a result of direct trauma sustained in falls. Isolated fractures of the lesser trochanter in adults are pathologic and usually indicate an underlying osseous metastasis (see Chapter 10).

Incomplete intertrochanteric fractures may occur in elderly adults as a result of falls.

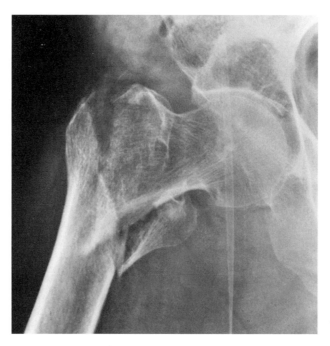

Figure 4.11 Four-part intertrochanteric fracture with the greater and lesser trochanters as separate fragments.

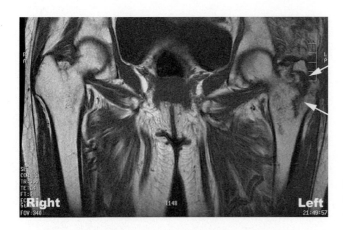

Figure 4.12 Incomplete intertrochanteric fracture (*arrows*) on coronal T1-weighted MRI.

SUBTROCHANTERIC FRACTURES

Subtrochanteric fractures in the elderly may represent extensions of intertrochanteric fractures into the shaft. In other age groups, subtrochanteric fractures are sustained in high-energy trauma such as motor vehicle collisions. The opposing pull of the gluteal and iliopsoas muscles and the thigh adductor muscles distracts and angulates the major fracture fragments. The cantilevered configuration of the femoral shaft and neck creates large stresses on the medial femoral cortex that complicate orthopedic management. A possibility of pathologic fracture must be considered in subtrochanteric fractures that occur in the absence of significant trauma.

SHAFT AND DISTAL FEMUR

Fractures of the femoral shaft occur typically in young adults as a result of major blunt force trauma, such as motor vehicle crashes. Because the femur is the largest and strongest bone in the human body and is protected by the largest and strongest muscle groups, considerable force is necessary to fracture it. Blood loss of two or more units typically accompanies an acute femoral shaft fracture. When the femoral shaft fractures with minimal trauma in an adult, an underlying pathologic lesion should be sought. Femoral fractures can also occur when there is advanced bony demineralization (Fig. 4.13). Insufficiency fractures in the elderly with osteoporosis may only be identified with MRI.

The femur is the largest and strongest bone in the human body.

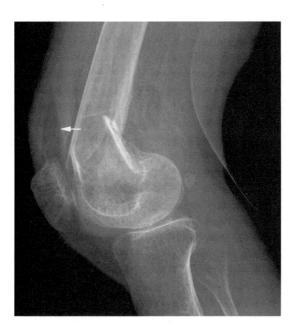

Figure 4.13 Osteoporotic supracondylar femur fracture. Lateral radiograph shows fat-fluid level (*arrow*).

KNEE

INTERNAL DERANGEMENT

As the knee extends, the tibia rotates externally in synchrony; as the knee flexes, the tibia rotates internally. Torque on the tibia helps control the position of the femur, making the knee an efficient screw joint that is stable in any position along the entire range of motion. The cruciate ligaments and menisci guide the tibia in this helicoid motion along the medial femoral condyle. The lateral condyle acts as a pivot. Motion at the proximal tibial fibular joint accommodates the rotation of the tibia. If tibial rotation is prevented during flexion or extension of the knee, the cruciate ligaments and menisci are placed under exceptional loads and may tear from tensile or shearing forces. Rotatory instability results, commonly leading to recurrent and chronic posttraumatic symptoms. Torn meniscal fragments can interfere with motion, causing locking, and may erode the articular cartilage, developing into early degenerative joint disease. Bone bruises within the tibia and femur, which are seen on MRI, can suggest commonly associated injuries.

Acute traumatic meniscal tears usually occur in young people when the meniscus is compressed between the femoral condyles and tibial plateaus during crush and twisting injuries. In older individuals, degenerative meniscal tears are thought to result from multiple subacute traumatic episodes that lead to chondrocyte death, increased mucinous ground substance (myxoid degeneration), and loss of mechanical integrity. The workup for internal derangement of the knee is dominated by MRI and arthroscopy. On MRI, the normal menisci and ligaments are visualized as low-signal structures. Meniscal tears are evident as high-signal regions on T1 or PD sequences that involve an articular margin (Figs. 4.14 and 4.15). Gross distortions of meniscal shape or intrameniscal fluid collections indicate meniscal tears with displaced fragments (Fig. 4.16). Fluid collections adjacent to the menisci are also associated with meniscal tears (Fig. 4.17).

Injury of the collateral ligaments may be imaged directly with MRI. Partial tears are thickened and edematous and may contain hemorrhage (Fig. 4.18); complete tears are discontinuous. An old tear of the medial collateral ligament may ossify, an appearance known as *Pellegrini-Stieda disease* (Fig. 4.19). A *Stieda fracture* is an avulsion injury from the medial femoral condyle at the origin of the tibial collateral ligament.

Because the anterior cruciate ligament (ACL) is active throughout the knee's range of motion, the ACL can be injured by a variety of noncontact, deceleration, hyperextension, twisting, and pivoting mechanisms. The ACL is the most frequently injured knee ligament and is

> Acute traumatic meniscal tears usually occur in young people when the meniscus is compressed between the femoral condyles and tibial plateaus during crush and twisting injuries. In older individuals, degenerative meniscal tears are thought to result from multiple subacute injuries.

> The ACL is the most frequently injured knee ligament.

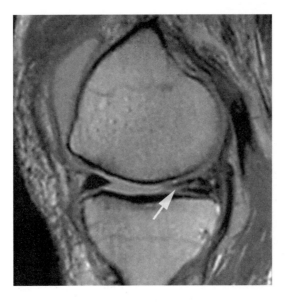

Figure 4.14 Sagittal PD-weighted MRI shows oblique tear (*arrow*) of the posterior horn of the medial meniscus extending into the inferior articulating surface.

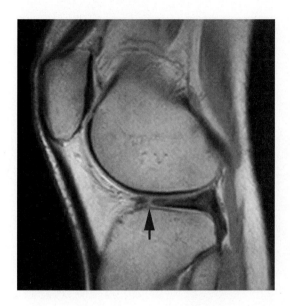

Figure 4.15 Sagittal PD-weighted MRI shows vertical tear (*arrow*) in anterior horn of lateral meniscus.

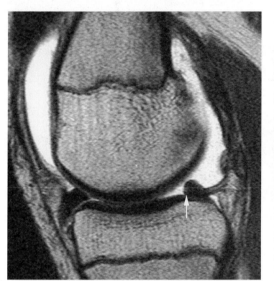

A

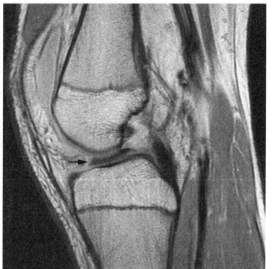

B

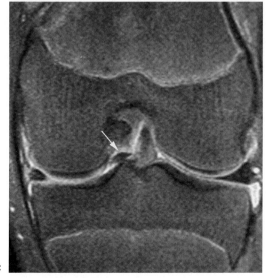

C

Figure 4.16 Bucket-handle tear of the medial meniscus. *A.* Sagittal T2-weighted MRI through the medial compartment shows a displaced tear of the posterior horn of the medial meniscus with a small peripheral stump (*arrow*). *B.* Sagittal PD MRI through the middle of the knee shows a displaced meniscal fragment (*arrow*). *C.* Coronal T2-weighted MRI shows the displaced meniscal fragment (*arrow*) adjacent to the anterior cruciate ligament.

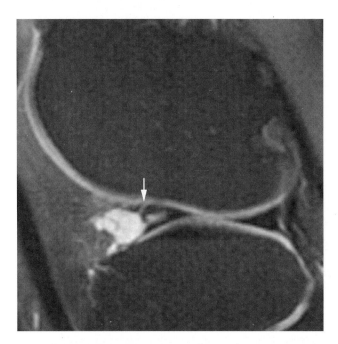

Figure 4.17 Lateral meniscus tear with meniscal cyst. Sagittal T2-weighted MRI with fat suppression shows horizontal tear in anterior horn of lateral meniscus associated with a meniscal cyst (*arrow*).

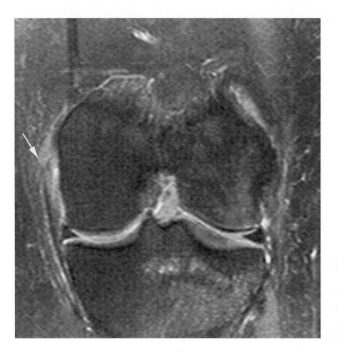

Figure 4.18 Medial collateral ligament (MCL) tear. Coronal inversion recovery MRI shows a grade III sprain of the femoral origin of the MCL (*arrow*) with surrounding high signal.

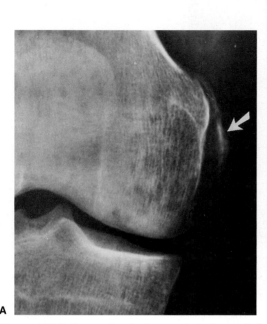
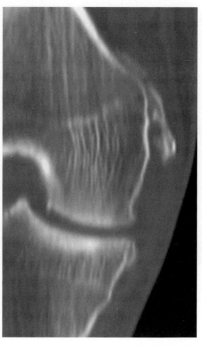

A   B

Figure 4.19 Pellegrini-Stieda disease. *A.* Radiograph shows ossification of the medial collateral ligament (MCL) (*arrow*), indicative of previous MCL tear. *B.* Coronal CT-reformatted image shows ossification.

commonly associated with medial meniscal tears, capsular tears, and transchondral impaction fractures (Fig. 4.20). Occasionally, loading of the ACL results in an avulsion fracture of its insertion at the medial tibial spine (Fig. 4.21). An avulsion fracture at the margin of the lateral tibial plateau where the knee capsule attaches (Segond fracture) is indicative of severe internal

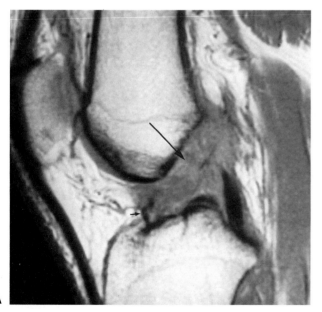
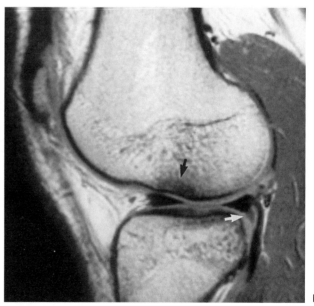

A   B

Figure 4.20 Anterior cruciate ligament (ACL) tear. *A.* Sagittal PD-weighted MRI through the intercondylar notch of the femur shows abnormal signal in the normal location of the ACL (*long arrow*). A curled fragment of the ACL is seen anteriorly (*short arrow*). *B.* Image through the lateral compartment shows femoral condylar bone bruise (*black arrow*) and posterior displacement of the posterior horn of the lateral meniscus (*white arrow*).

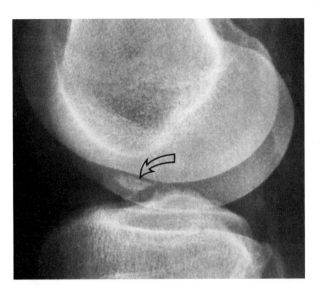

Figure 4.21 Avulsion of the medial tibial spine (*arrow*).

Up to 50% of PCL sprains are isolated and are sustained in a dashboard injury or a severe fall on a flexed knee.

derangement, including ACL tear (Fig. 4.22). Posterior cruciate ligament (PCL) sprains are 10% as common as ACL sprains. As many as 50% of PCL sprains are isolated and sustained in a dashboard injury or a severe fall on a flexed knee (Fig. 4.23). The remaining PCL sprains have complex mechanisms of injury and are associated with injuries of the ACL, medial collateral ligament (reverse Segond fracture), medial meniscus, or other structures. ACL and PCL injuries are associated with injuries to the posterolateral complex (popliteus tendon, arcuate ligament complex, lateral collareral ligament) (Fig. 4.24). Chronic knee instability can result if the posterolateral complex is not repaired within 3 weeks of the injury.

Trabecular microfractures (also called *bone bruises*) are caused by impaction trauma and are seen on MRI as regions of localized edema with intact overlying articular cartilage and subcortical bone. The specific pattern of bone bruises may suggest the mechanism of injury and associated injuries: Bruises of the anterior aspect of lateral femoral condyle and posterolateral

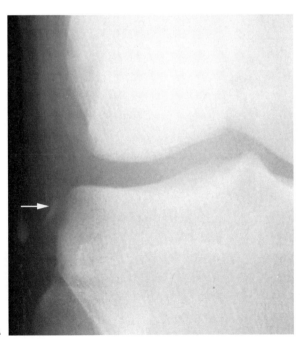

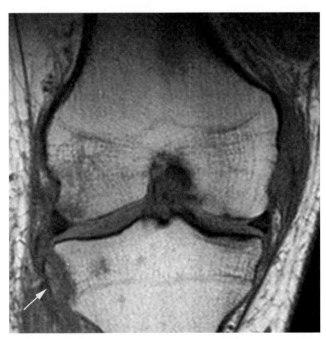

A   B

Figure 4.22 Segond fracture with tear. *A.* Radiograph shows a small bone fragment (*arrow*) adjacent to the lateral tibial plateau. *B.* Coronal T1-weighted MRI shows a laterally displaced bone fragment (*arrow*). The anterior cruciate ligament and medial collateral ligament were torn.

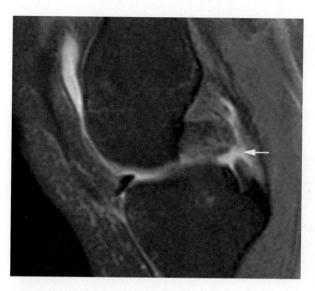

Figure 4.23 Posterior cruciate ligament tear. Sagittal T2-weighted fat-suppressed MRI shows the tear with fluid in the gap (*arrow*).

tibial plateau are associated with pivot shift injury (ACL rupture, medial meniscal tear, and lateral meniscal tear); bruises of the anterior aspect of the tibial tubercle are associated with a dashboard injury (PCL rupture); bruises of the medial aspect of the anterior tibia and anterior aspect of medial femoral condyle are associated with hyperextension injury (ACL and PCL ruptures); bruises of the lateral aspect of lateral femoral condyle and medial aspect of medial femoral condyle are associated with a clipping injury (ACL rupture, MCL rupture, and medial meniscal tear); and bruises of the inferomedial aspect of the patella and anterior aspect of lateral femoral condyle are associated with lateral patellar dislocation (osteochondral fracture of patella and medial patellofemoral ligament rupture).

The knee may dislocate in any direction—anterior, posterior, lateral, medial, or rotary—but many dislocations relocate spontaneously. In most cases, both the ACL and the PCL are torn, with or without tears of one or both collateral ligaments (Fig. 4.25). In cases of knee dislocation in which the cruciate ligaments remain intact, there are typically avulsion fractures of their attachments to the tibia. Angiography is important to exclude injury to the popliteal artery and vein. Damage to the peroneal nerve can be permanent.

> The knee can dislocate in any direction.

EXTENSOR MECHANISM

The extensor mechanism of the knee is composed of the quadriceps muscles and tendons, the patella, and theinfrapatellar tendon. The *patella* is a large sesamoid bone. The quadri-

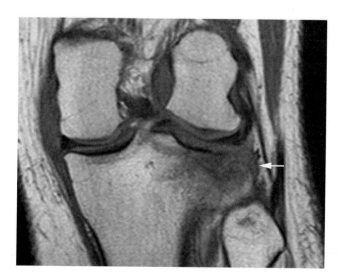

Figure 4.24 Posterolateral complex injury. Coronal PD MRI shows impacted fracture (*arrow*) in posterolateral tibial plateau and edema in proximal fibular head. An anterior cruciate ligament tear was also present.

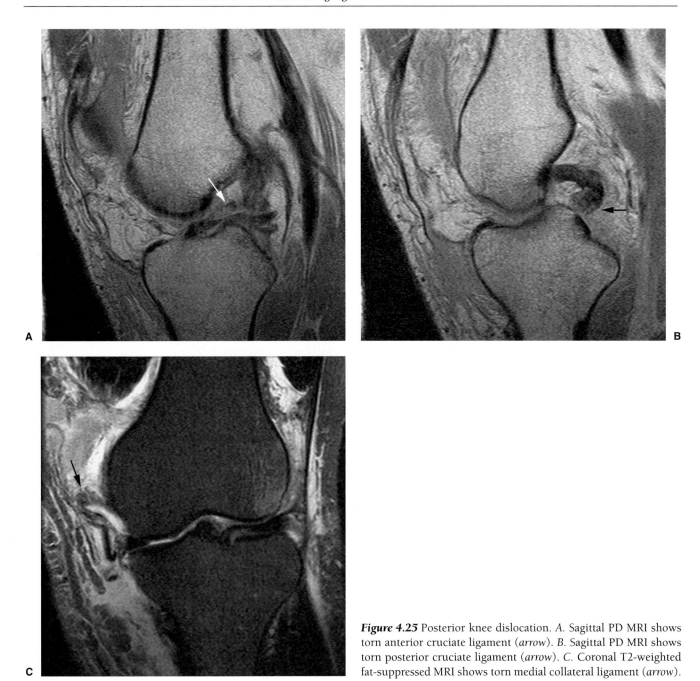

Figure 4.25 Posterior knee dislocation. *A.* Sagittal PD MRI shows torn anterior cruciate ligament (*arrow*). *B.* Sagittal PD MRI shows torn posterior cruciate ligament (*arrow*). *C.* Coronal T2-weighted fat-suppressed MRI shows torn medial collateral ligament (*arrow*).

ceps and infrapatellar tendons are continuous with each other across the patella; the medial and lateral retinacula are tendinous extensions that pass beside the patella.

Injuries to the extensor mechanism may result from forced flexion during strong quadriceps contraction. With complete disruption of the extensor mechanism, voluntary knee extension is lost; a partial disruption results in weakness of extension. In the adult, the extensor tendons are thinnest where they pass over the patella. Tear of the tendon coupled with a fracture of the patella from tensile loading results in a transverse patellar fracture with the fragments distracted by the quadriceps muscle (Fig. 4.26). Hemarthrosis in the knee capsule is invariably present. The quadriceps and infrapatellar tendons are also subject to injury. Quadriceps tears usually occur at the musculotendinous junction in patients older than 50 years who have degenerative changes in their tendons. Quadriceps injuries are best demonstrated by MRI (Fig. 4.27). Infrapatellar tendon tears are seen most often in young adult athletes. In complete tears, superior retraction of the patella by unop-

With complete disruption of the extensor mechanism, voluntary knee extension is lost.

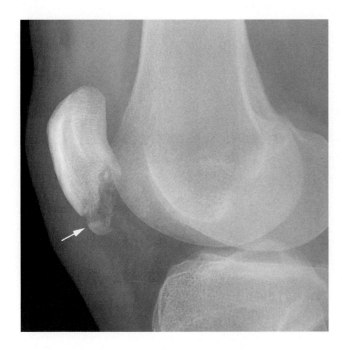

Figure 4.26 Avulsion fracture of interior pole of patella (*arrow*).

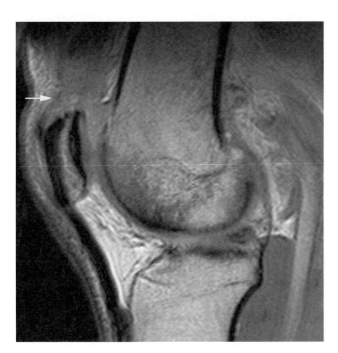

Figure 4.27 Quadriceps tendon tear. Sagittal PD MRI shows discontinuity of the tendon (*arrow*) at the superior pole of the patella.

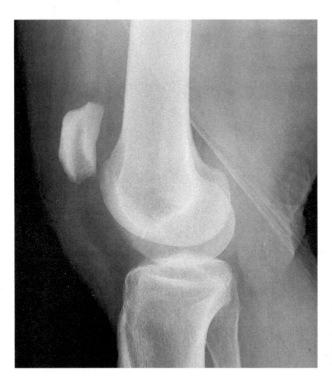

Figure 4.28 Infrapatellar tendon sprain (grade III). Proximal retraction of the patella by the quadriceps muscles. Note high position of patella (patella alta).

posed pull of the quadriceps results in a high-riding patella (patella alta) (Fig. 4.28). Partial tears of the infrapatellar tendon are seen as increased T2-weighted signal within the tendon on MRI (Fig. 4.29).

Stellate fractures of the patella may be caused by a direct blow. The extensor mechanism remains intact, and the fragments are not distracted (Fig. 4.30). Osteochondral fractures of the patella may occur secondary to patellar dislocation. Most patellar dislocations are lateral and result from direct trauma. The lateral margin of the patellofemoral groove may be fractured as the patella dislocates (Fig. 4.31). For the patella to dislocate laterally, there must be either a tear of the medial retinaculum (Fig. 4.32) or a fracture at the medial patellofemoral ligament attachment.

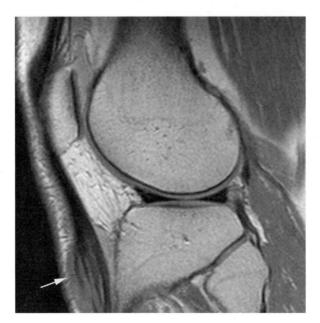

Figure 4.29 Infrapatellar tendon sprain (grade II). Sagittal PD MRI shows partial tear of the infrapatellar tendon (*arrow*) at its insertion on the anterior tibial tubercle. The patella has not retracted proximally because the tear is incomplete.

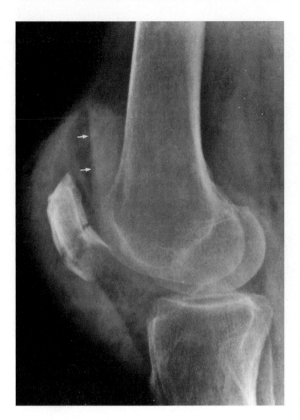

Figure 4.30 Minimally displaced comminuted patellar fracture from direct trauma. Lateral radiograph with horizontal x-ray beam demonstrates a fat-fluid level (*arrows*) indicative of intra-articular fracture.

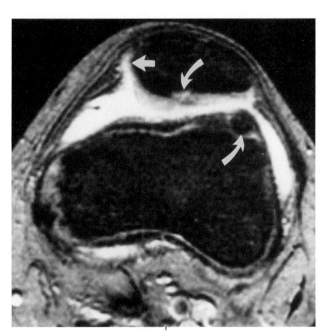

Figure 4.31 Axial T2-weighted MRI shows reduced lateral patellar dislocation with medial retinacular separation (*short arrow*) and osteochondral injuries of the patella and lateral patellofemoral groove (*curved arrows*).

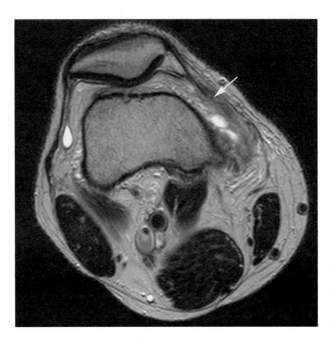

Figure 4.32 Medial retinaculum tear postpatellar dislocation. Axial T2-weighted fast spin echo MRI of the knee shows tear of medial retinaculum (*arrow*).

TIBIA

TIBIAL PLATEAU

Most tibial plateau fractures are sustained in motor vehicle collisions, but fractures of the tibial plateau may also occur in older individuals during twisting falls (Figs. 4.33 and 4.34). Isolated lateral tibial plateau fractures are the most common (55% to 70%); the rest involve the medial plateau alone or both plateaux. These injuries consist of compression fractures of the subchondral cancellous bone with depressions of the articular surface, vertical splits (shear fractures) of the joint margin, or a combination of depression and vertical split. A knee effusion is invariably present. Conventional tomography can establish the depth of the

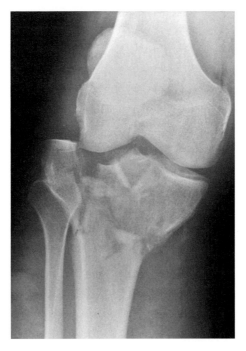

Figure 4.33 Severely comminuted lateral tibial plateau fracture.

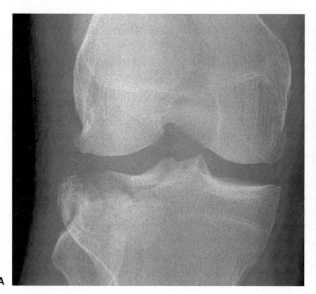 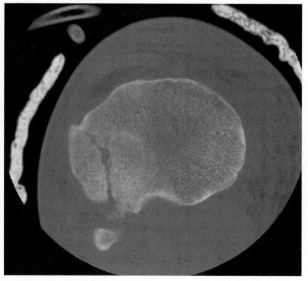

Figure 4.34 Lateral tibial plateau fracture. *A.* Radiograph. *B.* Axial CT.

depression and the number and location of depressed fragments; CT with coronal and sagittal reconstructions serves the same purpose. Associated injuries include lateral meniscal tears (50% of cases), lateral femoral condylar fractures, cruciate ligament tears, and fibular head fractures. These injuries may be treated surgically, depending on the amount of depression and displacement. Posttraumatic degenerative joint disease occurs in 20% of cases.

Posttraumatic degenerative joint disease follows a tibial plateau fracture in 20% of cases.

TIBIAL SHAFT

Transverse and segmental tibial shaft fractures commonly occur in high-energy motor vehicle collisions, particularly in pedestrians and motorcyclists. Because the soft tissues covering the tibia anteriorly are thin, many of these fractures are open. The complications of infection and osteonecrosis of large cortical fragments are common. Even if uncomplicated, these high-energy fractures tend to heal slowly and may take as long as 2 years to unite completely. The combination of transverse fractures of the femoral shaft and tibial shaft isolates the knee joint and is called a *floating knee*. Twisting injuries may result in spiral fractures of the tibia.

Many fractures of the tibial shaft are open.

ANKLE

The leg articulates with the foot at the talus. The *talus* is a hard, slippery bone with much of its surface covered by articular cartilage. Because the talus has no direct muscular control, its movements follow the push and pull of adjacent bones and ligaments. The talus is maintained in the ankle mortise (tibiofibular socket) by geometric fit and with ligaments. The articular surfaces of the ankle mortise are the tibial plafond superiorly and the medial (tibial) and lateral (fibular) malleoli on either side. The mortise is wider anteriorly than posteriorly. The posterior lip of the tibia is designated the *posterior malleolus*. At the distal tibiofibular syndesmosis, anterior and posterior tibiofibular ligaments bind the fibula to the tibia. The tibial and fibular shafts are also joined along their length by an interosseous membrane. The lateral malleolus is attached to the foot by anterior and posterior talofibular ligaments and a calcaneofibular ligament. The medial malleolus has a superficial deltoid ligament that inserts on the talus, calcaneus, and navicular and a deep deltoid ligament that inserts on the talus. The mortise, ligaments, and calcaneus form a ring in the coronal plane with the talus in the center (Fig. 4.35).

Most ankle injuries are sustained by indirect loading when the leg angulates or rotates around a malpositioned and stationary foot. Forced movement of the talus breaks open the

The *talus* is a hard, slippery bone with no direct muscular control.

Most ankle injuries are sustained by indirect loading.

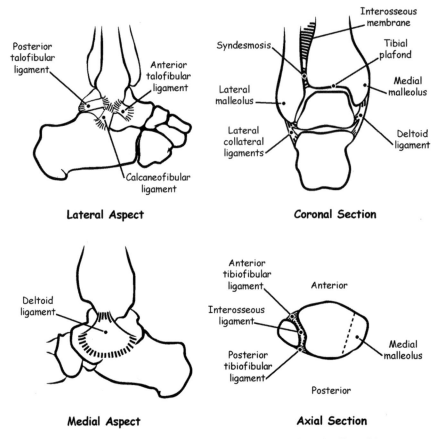

Figure 4.35 Ligaments of the ankle. Lateral aspect shows the lateral collateral ligaments. Medial aspect shows the deltoid ligament. Coronal section shows how the structures of the ankle joint form a ring with the talus in the center. Axial section shows how the distal fibula is attached to the tibia by the syndesmosis.

mortise. Most ankle injuries are reduced or partially reduced by the time they are radiographed, so the direction and magnitude of loading must be inferred from the pattern of injury. There are several classifications of ankle injuries in wide usage (Table 4.2), the most useful of which is the AO-Weber classification (Table 4.3), and ankle injuries may also be

Table 4.2: Classifications of Ankle Injuries[a]

Initial Side of Injury	Inferior Extent of Characteristic Fibular Fracture (If Present)	Lauge-Hansen	AO-Weber[b]	Simplified[c]	Over-Simplified[d]
Lateral	Below syndesmosis, transverse avulsion fracture	Supination-adduction	A	Adduction (Inversion)	Adduction
	At syndesmosis, oblique	Supination–external rotation	B	External rotation	External rotation/abduction
	Anteroinferior to posterosuperior				
Medial	Above syndesmosis, oblique anterosuperior to posteroinferior	Pronation–external rotation	C	Abduction (Eversion)	—
	Above syndesmosis, oblique inferomedial to superolateral	Pronation-abduction	—	—	—
Central	Incidental to tibial pilon fracture	Pronation-dorsiflexion	—	Axial compression	Axial compression

[a]Each classification system has two or more stages of severity, which are not listed.
[b]AO-Weber classification is only for malleolar fractures; other classifications include sprains.
[c]Adapted from Kelikian H, Kelikian AS. *Disorders of the ankle.* Philadelphia: Saunders, 1985.
[d]Adapted from Rockwood CA Jr, Green DP, Bucholz RW, eds. *Rockwood and Green's fractures in adults,* 3rd ed. Philadelphia: Lippincott, 1991.

Table 4.3: AO-Weber Classification of Ankle Fractures

Type	Defining Characteristic	Associated Injuries
A	Lateral malleolar fracture below the level of the ankle joint space.	The syndesmosis and the deltoid ligament remain intact, but there may be an associated oblique fracture of the medial malleolus.
B	Oblique fracture of the lateral malleolus through the syndesmosis.	Deltoid ligament tear or transverse fracture of the medial malleolus. May also have an associated posterior malleolar fracture.
C	Fracture of the fibula above the syndesmosis.	Rupture of the syndesmosis. Deltoid ligament tear or transverse medial malleolar fracture. May also have an associated posterior malleolar fracture.

described by the location and morphology of the fractures. Mixed patterns of injury occur, and some fractures defy classification. The practical simplified classification of indirect ankle injuries favored here has four mechanisms: adduction, external rotation, abduction, and axial compression.

Adduction or inversion of the foot is inward rotation along the foot's long axis. With forcible inversion, the lateral malleolus and its ligaments are loaded. The first injury is a sprain of the anterior talofibular ligament, which may be followed by a sprain of the calcaneofibular ligament. The appearance on radiographs is lateral soft tissue swelling; the talus may be tilted but will not be displaced. This lateral ankle sprain is the most common ankle injury in adults (Fig. 4.36). Less commonly, a tension fracture of the lateral malleolus occurs rather than a ligamentous sprain. With continued loading, the talus impinges against the medial malleolus and moves medially, causing an oblique or vertical shear fracture of the medial malleolus as the talus subluxates.

External rotation of the foot loads the anterior portion of the lateral malleolus and the posterior portion of the medial malleolus as the talus moves within the mortise like a lever.

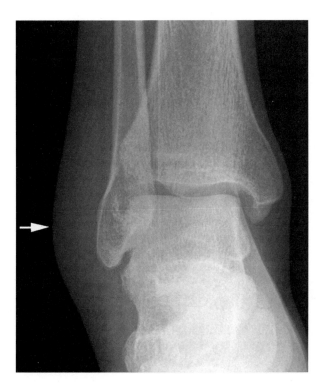

Figure 4.36 Lateral ankle sprain as demonstrated by soft tissue swelling (*arrow*) without fracture on the AP radiograph.

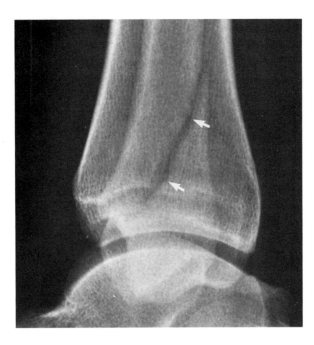

Figure 4.37 Lateral radiograph shows external rotation injury of the ankle with oblique fibular fracture (*arrows*).

The first injury is disruption of the anterior tibiofibular ligament of the syndesmosis. Loading then transfers to the lateral malleolus, resulting in a short oblique fracture that runs antero-inferior to posterosuperior (Fig. 4.37). With continued loading, the talus displaces the lateral malleolar fragment, causing the posterior malleolus to be avulsed by the strong posterior tibiofibular ligaments; the lateral and posterior malleoli remain attached to the talus and each other. Finally, with loss of the lateral and posterior supports of the ankle, the medial side is loaded as the talus dislocates laterally and posteriorly, and either the medial malleolus fractures or the deltoid ligament tears (Fig. 4.38). In an isolated lateral malleolar external rotation injury, the talus is subluxated; in a trimalleolar injury, it may be completely dislocated. If the

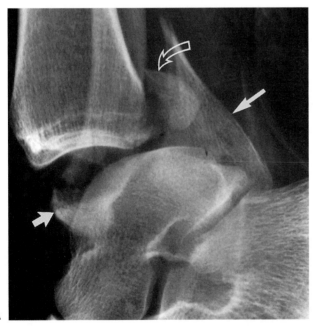
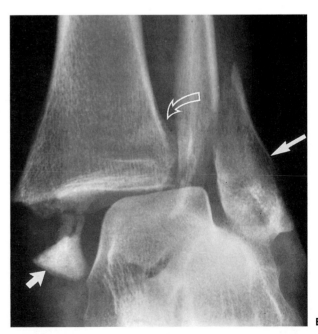

Figure 4.38 External rotation fracture-dislocation of the ankle. *A,B.* Lateral and AP radiographs show displaced fractures of the medial malleolus (*short arrows*), lateral malleolus (*long arrows*), and posterior malleolus (*curved arrows*), with lateral and posterior subluxation of the talus.

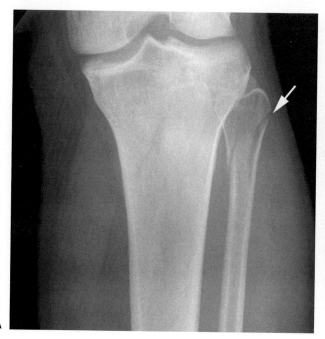 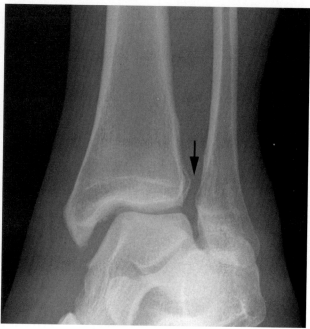

Figure 4.39 *A.* Maisonneuve fracture (*arrow*) of the proximal fibula. *B.* Associated abduction of the lateral malleolus and tear of the syndesmosis (*arrow*).

posterior malleolar fragment includes 25% or more of the articular surface, an associated component of axial compression can be inferred. Sometimes, CT is necessary to establish the proportion of articular surface involvement. The most common ankle fracture in adults is an isolated lateral malleolar fracture from external rotation.

Abduction or eversion of the foot relative to the ankle causes a tension fracture of the medial malleolus more often than a tear of the deltoid ligament. With continued loading in abduction, the talus impinges against the lateral malleolus and displaces it laterally, disrupting the syndesmotic ligaments or avulsing their bony attachments. As the talus dislocates laterally, taking the fibula with it, the interosseous ligament tears until the fibular shaft fractures. The fibular fracture may occur anywhere along the shaft and typically runs inferomedial to superolateral. A proximal fracture of the fibula may be missed on routine films of the ankle.

Three fracture eponyms may be encountered in clinical consultation. The *Maisonneuve fracture* is an abduction injury in which the fibular fracture is quite proximal (Fig. 4.39). The *Tillaux fracture* is an abduction injury with an avulsion fracture of the anterior tibial tubercle by the anterior tibiofibular ligament (Fig. 4.40). The *Wagstaffe-LeFort fracture* is an avulsion fracture of the anterior medial portion of the distal fibula by the anterior tibiofibular ligament.

Ankle injuries usually require anatomic restoration of the mortise; otherwise, excessive motion and instability lead to early degenerative joint disease. Simple ankle sprains are treated conservatively with casting and bracing. Most heal over a period of several weeks, but a few have chronic pain and recurrent instability. MRI in this circumstance may reveal a chronic anterior talofibular ligament tear (Fig. 4.41) or other pathology. If satisfactory restoration of the mortise is not achieved by closed means, open reduction and internal fixation are performed. Displacements of 1 to 2 mm are acceptable for the medial joint space; displacements of 3 to 4 mm are acceptable for the posterior malleolus. Medial malleolar fractures are usually fixed by lag screws. Lateral malleolar fractures may be fixed by various methods such as cortical plates, screws, pins, or combinations of these appliances.

Axial compression (vertical loading) fractures (also called *pilon fractures*) are sustained in falls from a height or in automobile collisions in which the talus is driven into the tibial plafond. These injuries are characterized by severe distal tibial shaft comminution,

To prevent posttraumatic osteoarthritis, ankle injuries typically require anatomic restoration of the mortise.

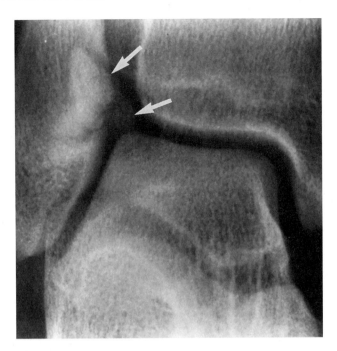

Figure 4.40 Avulsion fracture (*arrows*) of lateral aspect of tibia (Tillaux fracture).

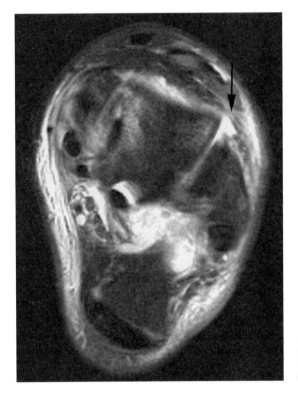

Figure 4.41 Chronic anterior talofibular ligament tear (*arrow*) on axial T2-weighted fat-suppressed MRI.

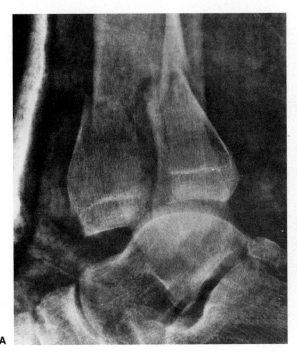

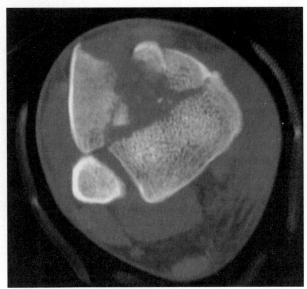

A

B

Figure 4.42 *A.* Intra-articular axial compression fracture of the distal tibia (pilon fracture) seen on lateral radiograph through plaster cast. *B.* Pilon fracture shown by CT at level of distal tibia.

intra-articular fractures through the tibial plafond, and talar fractures (Fig. 4.42). Malleolar fractures and ligamentous disruption may coexist, indicating some combination of axial compression with adduction, external rotation, or abduction.

ACHILLES TENDON INJURIES

Achilles tendon tears and tendonitis generally occur during athletic activity in middle-aged men. Conditions that predispose the tendon to injury include rheumatoid arthritis, systemic lupus erythematosus, diabetes mellitus, and gout. The normal Achilles tendon is a tapered structure with uniformly dark signal on all sequences. In cross section, it has a shape like the letter *C* that is concave toward the tibia. Complete tendon tears are evident on MRI as discontinuities with high signal on T1- and T2-weighted images (Figs. 4.43 and 4.44). Partial tears are evident as thickening of the tendon with longitudinal bands of increased signal on T1- and T2-weighted MRI. Because the Achilles tendon does not have a tendon sheath, frank fluid around the tendon is not seen. However, soft tissue edema in the soft tissues surrounding the tendon may be seen after an acute tear.

The Achilles tendon does not have a tendon sheath.

TIBIALIS POSTERIOR TENDON INJURIES

Tibialis posterior tendon injuries are frequently chronic, classically presenting in mature women as a unilateral flatfoot deformity. The normal tibialis posterior tendon traverses the ankle posterior and inferior to the medial malleolus and then turns anteriorly along the sole of the foot to insert at the tuberosity of the navicular bone, with multiple fibrous slips at the plantar aspects of the navicular and medial cuneiform bones. The tibialis posterior provides dynamic support for the medial longitudinal arch of the foot, and ruptures of it are therefore associated with acquired, unilateral flatfoot deformity, often without a history of trauma. On lateral weight-bearing radiographs, loss of the longitudinal arch may be evident. On MRI, tears of the tibialis posterior are seen most frequently at or within a few centimeters of its navicular insertion, distal to the medial malleolus. The tendon will be thickened and have increased signal on T1- and T2-

Tibialis posterior tendon injuries are usually chronic.

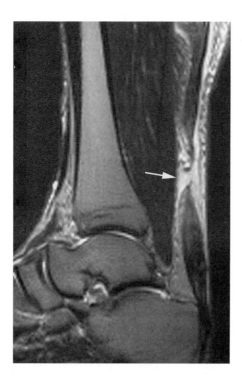

Figure 4.43 Achilles tendon tear. Sagittal T2-weighted MRI of the ankle shows discontinuity of the fibers of the Achilles tendon several centimeters above the calcaneal tuberosity, consistent with a complete tear (*arrow*).

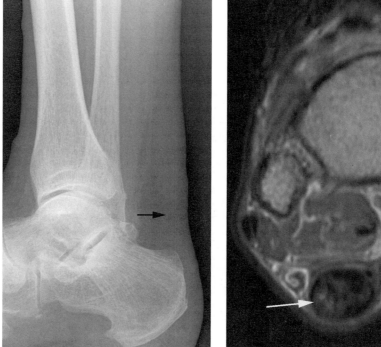

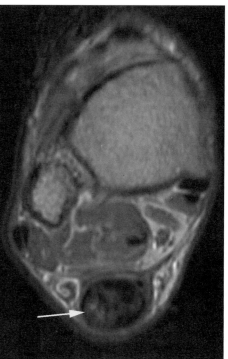

Figure 4.44 Achilles tendon tendinopathy. *A.* Lateral radiograph of ankle shows thickening of Achilles tendon (*arrow*). *B.* Axial T2-weighted MRI of the same ankle shows an abnormally round contour of the distal Achilles tendon with hyperintense T2 signal interspersed throughout its fibers (*arrow*).

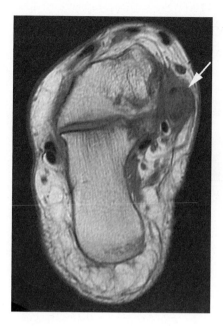

Figure 4.45 Tibialis posterior tendon tear. Axial PD MRI shows tear within the tibialis posterior tendon with inflammation surrounding the ligament (*arrow*).

weighted MRI, with loss of continuity, surrounding edema, and fluid in the tendon sheath (Fig. 4.45). Similar MRI findings without loss of continuity may indicate tendonitis of the tibialis posterior.

TIBIALIS ANTERIOR TENDON INJURIES

Tibialis anterior tendon injuries are most commonly seen in patients whose athletic activities involve forced plantar flexion and ankle eversion; the superficial location of the tendon also leaves it vulnerable to lacerations (Fig. 4.46).

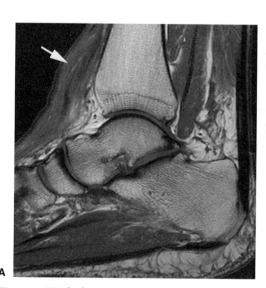
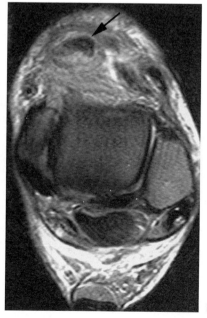

A   B

Figure 4.46 Tibialis anterior tendon tear and tendinopathy. *A.* Sagittal T1-weighted MRI of the ankle shows abnormal thickening and signal hypointensity within the partially torn tibialis anterior tendon (*arrow*). *B.* Axial T2-weighted fat-saturated fast spin echo MRI of the ankle shows abnormal thickening of and signal hyperintensity within the tibialis anterior tendon, consistent with a hypertrophic partial tear (*arrow*).

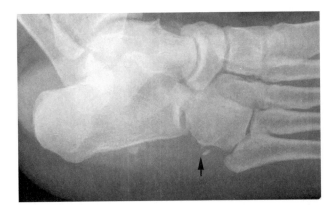

Figure 4.47 Fractured os peroneum (*arrow*) associated with peroneus longus tear.

PERONEAL TENDON INJURIES

Peroneal tendon injuries are usually acute.

Peroneal tendon injuries usually occur in acute injury. An os peroneum, if present, may be fractured (Fig. 4.47) or may migrate proximally with the retracting tendon. Tears of the peroneus brevis typically occur at the level of the lateral malleolus as it makes its turn anteriorly from behind the malleolus. Longitudinal splits are more common than transverse tears (Fig. 4.48). Tears of the peroneus longus may accompany injuries of the peroneus brevis but are less common and generally do not occur in isolation.

POSTERIOR ANKLE IMPINGEMENT SYNDROME

Posterior ankle impingement syndrome is a common cause of ankle impingements and results from trauma or overuse. Patients have symptoms of pain, stiffness, tenderness, and soft tissue swelling at the posterior ankle. In the presence of an os trigonum (accessory ossicle resulting from unfused ossification center of posterior talar process), extreme plantar flexion in activities such as ballet may cause compression and entrapment of the posterior ankle soft tissues, including the flexor hallucis longus tendon between the posterior lip of the tibia and the calcaneus. There is edema surrounding and often involving the os trigonum as well as flexor hallucis longus tenosynovitis (Fig. 4.49). MRI and radionuclide bone

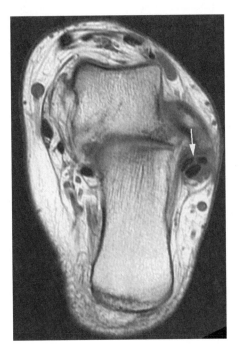

Figure 4.48 Longitudinal tear of the peroneus brevis tendon. Axial T1-weighted MRI of the ankle shows an abnormal split morphology of the peroneus brevis tendon with low signal in the surrounding tendon sheath (*arrow*).

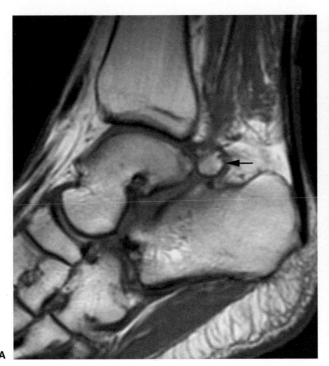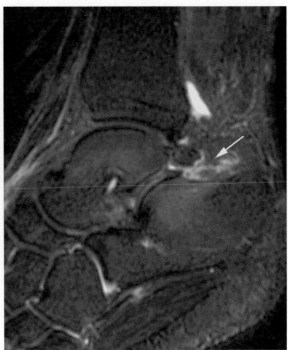

Figure 4.49 Posterior ankle impingement syndrome. *A.* Sagittal T1-weighted MRI shows a large os trigonum (*arrow*). *B.* Sagittal T2-weighted fat-suppressed MRI shows tenosynovitis of flexor hallucis longus and bone marrow edema (*arrow*) in os trigonum and calcaneus.

scan can be used for diagnosis. The condition may also be called *os trigonum syndrome*, although impingement may occur without the presence of an os trigonum.

FOOT

TALUS

Lateral osteochondral fractures of the talus may occur when forced inversion shears the lateral edge of the talar dome against the fibula (Fig. 4.50). The less common medial osteochondral fracture may follow impaction of the talus against the tibia. Clinical presentation may be nonspecific ankle pain. The terms *osteochondral defect* and *osteochondritis dissecans* are often applied to osteochondral fractures of the talar dome. Osteochondral defects may require CT or MRI for demonstration. Associated osteochondral injuries of the fibula or tibial plafond may be found (Fig. 4.51). The severity of osteochondral defects ranges from a cartilage injury (stage 1), to an attached osteochondral fragment (stage 2), to a detached but nondisplaced fragment (stage 3), and, finally, to a displaced fragment (stage 4). Osteonecrosis of attached and detached fragments is common. If displaced, the fragment becomes a loose body within the joint capsule.

Hyperdorsiflexion of the foot may produce a vertical fracture of the talus through the talar neck. In more severe cases, the fracture displaces, and the subtalar joint subluxates or dislocates (Fig. 4.52). In very severe cases, the subtalar and ankle joints are both dislocated. Because the vascular supply of the talus passes from distal to proximal, osteonecrosis of the proximal fragment may occur, suggested by the acute osteoporosis that accompanies fracture healing. Stress fractures of the talus are unusual, but their typical location is vertically through the neck.

A fracture of the lateral tubercle of the posterior process of the talus is called a *Sheperd fracture.*

A displaced osteochondral fragment may become a loose body within the ankle joint.

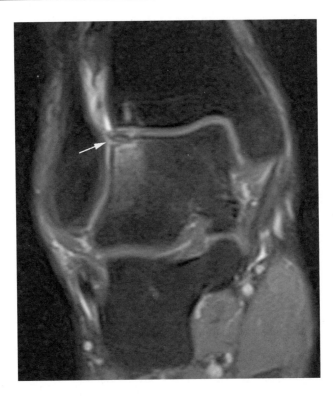

Figure 4.50 Osteochondral defect of the talar dome. Coronal fat-saturated PD-weighted MRI of the ankle shows a small osteochondral defect in the lateral talar dome. The central fragment is detached and partially displaced from the dome of the talus (*arrow*), and there is surrounding fluid. Subchondral bone marrow edema is also seen in lateral aspect of tibial plafond.

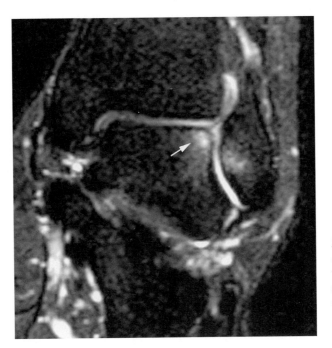

Figure 4.51 Osteochondral defect of the talar dome. Coronal T2-weighted with fat suppression shows a cartilage injury with subchondral bone marrow edema (*arrow*) in lateral talar dome and distal fibula.

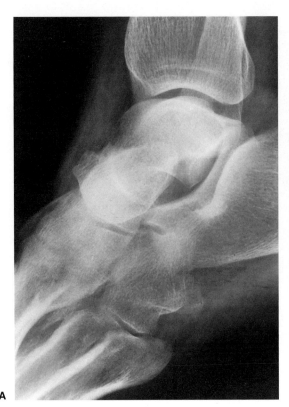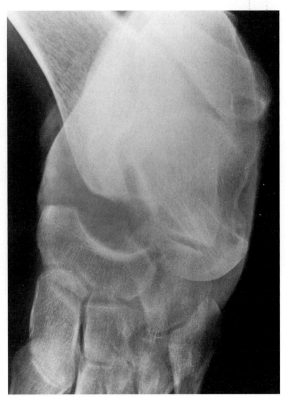

A   B

Figure 4.52 *A,B.* Subtalar foot dislocation. The talus remains within the ankle mortise, but the rest of the foot has dislocated as a unit through the subtalar and talonavicular joint.

CALCANEUS

Intra-articular calcaneal fractures are caused by axial loading in falls from a height in which the heel sustains the initial impact. Such calcaneal fractures are bilateral in 10% of cases and, because of the common mechanism of loading, may be associated with compression or burst fractures of the thoracolumbar spine and other fractures of the lower extremities. Although the loading that occurs during these injuries may be rapid and massive, resulting in gross comminution, there is a consistent pattern of injury. The calcaneus, along with the cuboid and fifth metatarsal, forms a weight-bearing longitudinal arch on the lateral side of the foot that supports the talus and structures above. With excessive axial loading, the arch consistently breaks in the center at the tarsal sinus, where the lateral process of the talus descends like an ax. The sustentaculum tali breaks off as a separate fragment, and the arch collapses. With continued loading, the talus may depress the posterior calcaneal facet into the substance of the body of the calcaneus, which in turn may explode into a multitude of tiny fragments (joint depression type) (Fig. 4.53). Alternatively, the posterior facet and superior portion of the body may shear off horizontally as the talus is driven downward (tongue type) (Fig. 4.54). Intra-articular calcaneal fractures are usually obvious on plain films because of flattening of the normal bony longitudinal arch and the presence of many fragments. The soft tissues are often extensively injured in calcaneal fractures. Occasionally, if the fractures are impacted and not displaced, a decrease in Böhler's angle is a helpful radiographic sign. The long-term prognosis is poor: The sequelae of residual widening of the heel and posttraumatic subtalar degenerative joint disease are commonplace.

The most common of the extra-articular calcaneal fractures—those not involving the subtalar joint—is an avulsion fracture of the anterior process. This fracture occurs where the bifurcate ligament links the calcaneus to the cuboid and navicular. These injuries may occur with inversion of the foot and are easily overlooked when the ankle is examined.

Calcaneal fractures sustained in falls from a height are bilateral in 10% of cases.

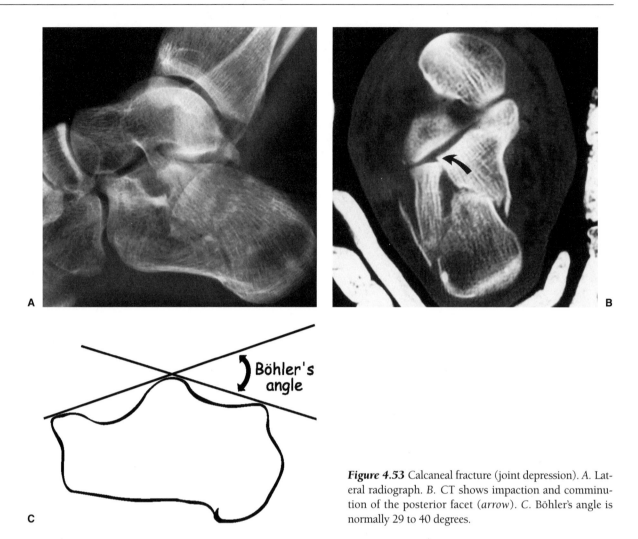

Figure 4.53 Calcaneal fracture (joint depression). *A.* Lateral radiograph. *B.* CT shows impaction and comminution of the posterior facet (*arrow*). *C.* Böhler's angle is normally 29 to 40 degrees.

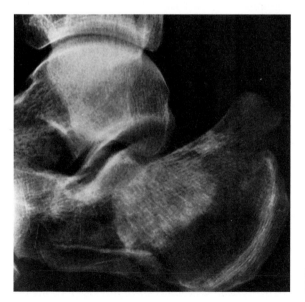

Figure 4.54 Comminuted intra-articular calcaneal fracture (tongue type).

Stress fractures of the calcaneus typically occur through the tuberosity. The fracture plane is perpendicular to the stress-bearing trabeculae.

MIDFOOT AND FOREFOOT

Fracture-dislocation of the midfoot (Chopart fracture-dislocation) may occur through the talonavicular and calcaneo-cuboid articulations during incidents such as motorcycle crashes.

Dislocation of the forefoot (Lisfranc fracture-dislocation) may occur after a variety of traumas, including falls, longitudinal compression with hyperflexion, and rotary loading. In most cases, multiple metatarsals are dislocated in the same direction (homolateral) laterally and dorsally; occasionally, the second through fifth metatarsals are dislocated laterally, and the first metatarsal is dislocated medially (divergent) (Fig. 4.55). A transverse fracture through the base of the second metatarsal and avulsion fractures of the proximal metatarsals or distal tarsals are frequently associated.

Avulsion fractures at the base of the fifth metatarsal, proximal to the metatarsal tuberosity, are caused by tensile loading transmitted through the lateral cord of the plantar aponeurosis during sudden inversion of the foot. As a tension injury, the fracture line is oriented transversely to the direction of applied force (Fig. 4.56). These fractures are intra-articular and occur commonly with ankle trauma. The fracture fragment includes the insertion of the peroneus brevis tendon.

Avulsion fractures at the base of the fifth metatarsal resemble ankle injuries in mechanism and presentation.

Fractures of the metatarsal shafts commonly occur with direct trauma. The distal shafts of the metatarsals are common locations for stress fractures, particularly those associated with running and marching. Stress fractures of the metatarsals may be radiographically occult at presentation and may require a radionuclide bone scan or MRI for demonstration (Fig. 4.57). With healing, the fractures become apparent as calcified callus becomes visible (Fig. 4.58). A fracture of the proximal shaft of the fifth metatarsal that is

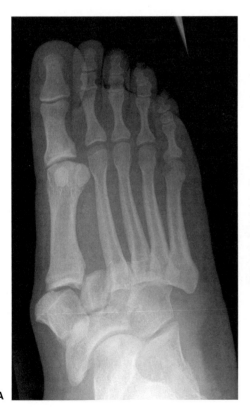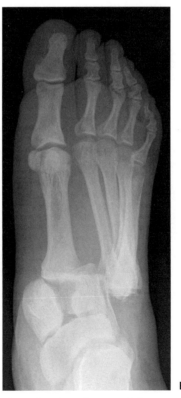

Figure 4.55 *A,B.* Radiographs of the foot show a homolateral Lisfranc fracture-dislocation at the tarsalmetatarsal joint with separation of the first and second cuneiforms.

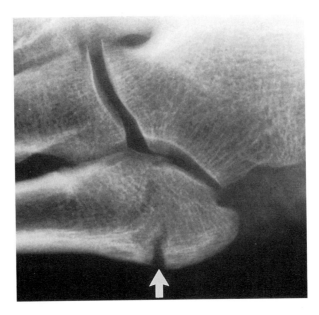

Figure 4.56 Avulsion fracture (*arrow*) of the fifth metatarsal base.

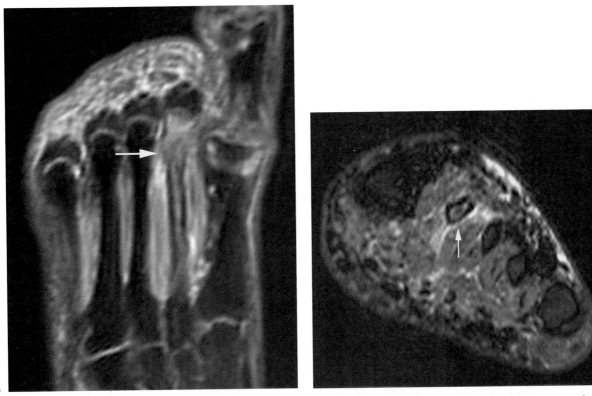

Figure 4.57 Stress fracture metatarsal. Axial (*A*) and coronal (*B*) T2-weighted fat-suppressed MRIs of the foot show high signal at the neck of the second metatarsal (*arrows*). There is edema within the marrow space and in the surrounding soft tissues.

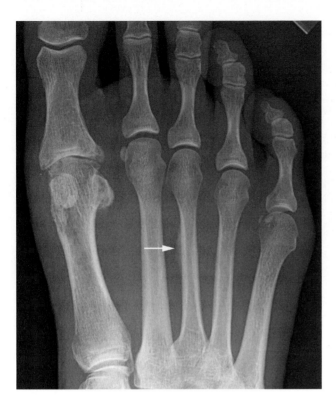

Figure 4.58 Healing stress fracture of the third metatarsal (*arrow*) in a patient who had recent podiatric surgery.

extra-articular and distal to the metatarsal tuberosity may be known by the eponym *Jones fracture* (Fig. 4.59). Jones fractures are typically stress fractures and require treatment different from that of avulsion fractures of the fifth metatarsal base.

Stubbed toe injuries generally load the affected digits axially, resulting in oblique fractures of the phalangeal shafts. Alternatively, comminuted fractures at the ends of the phalanges may occur. These usually have an inverted Y shape. Direct trauma to the toes from dropped objects and misadventures with wheeled or motorized conveyances are common.

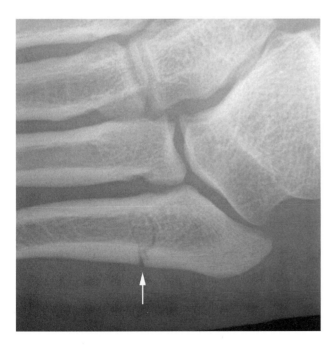

Figure 4.59 Extra-articular fracture of the proximal fifth metatarsal (Jones fracture) (*arrow*).

SOURCES AND READINGS

Aharonoff GB, Dennis MG, Elshinawy A, et al. Circumstances of falls causing hip fractures in the elderly. *Clin Orthop* 1998;348:10–14.

Berquist TH. *MRI of the musculoskeletal system*, 4th ed. Philadelphia: Lippincott Williams & Wilkins, 2001.

Berquist TH, ed. *Radiology of the foot and ankle*, 2nd ed. Philadelphia: Lippincott Williams & Wilkins, 2000.

Bray TJ. Femoral neck fracture fixation. Clinical decision making. *Clin Orthop* 1997;339:20–31.

Browner BD, Levine AM, Jupiter JB, et al., eds. *Skeletal trauma: fractures, dislocations, ligamentous injuries*, 2nd ed. Philadelphia: WB Saunders, 1998.

Bucholz RW, Heckman JD, eds. *Rockwood and Green's fractures in adults*, 5th ed. Philadelphia: Lippincott Williams & Wilkins, 2001.

Crim JR, Cracchiolo A, Hall RL. *Imaging of the foot and ankle*. Philadelphia: Lippincott–Raven, 1996.

De Laet CE, Pols HA. Fractures in the elderly: epidemiology and demography. *Best Pract Res Clin Endocrinol Metab* 2000;14:171–179.

Dennison E, Cooper C. Epidemiology of osteoporotic fractures. *Horm Res* 2000;54[Suppl]:58–63.

Escobedo EM, Mills WJ, Hunter JC. The "reverse" Segond fracture: association with a tear of the posterior cruciate ligament and medial meniscus. *AJR Am J Roentgenol* 2002;178:979–983.

Firooznia H, Golimbu CN, Rafii M, et al. *MRI and CT of the musculoskeletal system*. St. Louis: Mosby, 1992.

Kaplan P, Dussault R, Helms CA, et al. *Musculoskeletal MRI*. Philadelphia: WB Saunders, 2001.

Kelikian H, Kelikian AS. *Disorders of the ankle*. Philadelphia: WB Saunders, 1998.

Lofman O, Berglund K, Larsson L, et al. Changes in hip fracture epidemiology: redistribution between ages, genders and fracture types. *Osteoporosis Int* 2002;13:18–25.

Michelson JD, Myers A, Jinnah R, et al. Epidemiology of hip fractures among the elderly. Risk factors for fracture type. *Clin Orthop* 1995;311:129–135.

Pavlov H, Torg J. *The running athlete. Roentgenograms and remedies*. Chicago: Yearbook, 1987.

Petersilge CA. Chronic adult hip pain: MR arthrography of the hip. *Radiographics* 2000;20:S43–S52.

Plancher KD, Donshik JD. Femoral neck and ipsilateral neck and shaft fractures in the young adult. *Orthop Clin North Am* 1997;28:447–459.

Robinson CM, Court-Brown CM, McQueen MM, et al. Hip fractures in adults younger than 50 years of age. Epidemiology and results. *Clin Orthop* 1995;312:238–246.

Robinson P, White LM, Salonen D, et al. Anteromedial impingement of the ankle: using MR arthrography to assess the anteromedial recess. *AJR Am J Roentgenol* 2002;178:601–604.

Rogers LF. *Radiology of skeletal trauma*, 3rd ed. New York: Churchill Livingstone, 2002.

Siliski JM, ed. *Traumatic disorders of the knee*. New York: Springer-Verlag New York, 1994.

Stoller DW. *Magnetic resonance imaging in orthopaedics and sports medicine*, 2nd ed. Philadelphia: Lippincott–Raven Publishers, 1997.

Taylor DC, Erpelding JM, Whitman CS, et al. Treatment of comminuted subtrochanteric femoral fractures in a young population with a reconstruction nail. *Mil Med* 1996;161:735–738.

Tile M, Kellam J, Helfet DL, eds. *Fractures of the pelvis and acetabulum*, 3rd ed. Philadelphia: Lippincott Williams & Wilkins, 2002.

Verettas DA, Galanis B, Kazakos K, et al. Fractures of the proximal part of the femur in patients under 50 years of age. *Injury* 2002;33:41–45.

TRAUMA IN CHILDREN

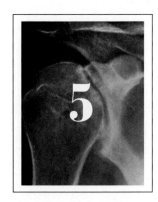

Fractures in children are not the same as fractures in adults because of differences in anatomy, biomechanics, and exposure to trauma.

EPIDEMIOLOGY OF CHILDREN'S FRACTURES

The incidence, type, and age distribution of children's fractures vary across countries and regions because of cultural and environmental differences. Fractures in children are first seen at childbirth, from birth trauma. They become more prevalent with walking (and falling) in toddlers and peak in incidence in girls at approximately 11 years of age and in boys at approximately 14 years of age. By 16 years of age, 42% of boys and 27% of girls will have sustained at least one fracture. In the United States, most fractures in children are the result of playing accidents and sports-related injuries. Fractures are more common in boys than girls by a ratio of nearly 2:1. The upper extremity is fractured more commonly than the lower extremity, and the left upper extremity is fractured more frequently than the right.

After the first year of life, trauma is the leading cause of death in children, accounting for 50% of all deaths in children between 1 and 14 years of age. As with fractures, boys are at greater risk of dying from trauma than girls. Most trauma deaths in children are the result of head injuries.

Fractures in children peak in incidence in girls at approximately 11 years of age and in boys at approximately 14 years of age. Boys have twice as many fractures as girls. After the first year of life, trauma is the leading cause of death in children.

BIOMECHANICS OF CHILDREN'S FRACTURES

The immature, growing skeleton has cartilaginous growth plates, cartilaginous epiphyses, and a thick, strong periosteum. Immature bone is more porous than adult bone and functions less as a single mechanical unit and more as an aggregate of smaller units. Children's bone is less stiff and more malleable (ductile) than adult bone. Fracture lines do not propagate as far, and a loaded bone is more likely to bend and deform than to break and splinter. There are five general types of children's fractures: buckle fractures, plastic deformation, greenstick fractures, complete fractures, and growth plate fractures.

Cortical bone in children can fail under compressive as well as tensile loading. Failure of bone under compressive loading results in a buckle fracture. *Buckle fractures* (also called

Immature bone functions less as a single mechanical unit and more as an aggregate of smaller units.

Failure of bone under compressive loading results in a buckle fracture.

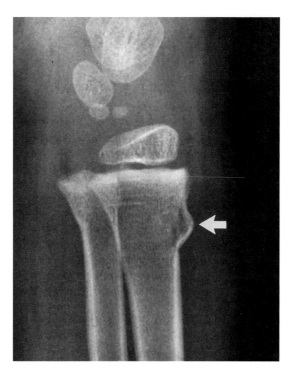

Figure 5.1 Buckle fracture of the distal radial metaphysis (*arrow*).

torus fractures) are incomplete impaction fractures in which the cortex around all or part of the circumference of the bone is buckled (Fig. 5.1). They occur at the metaphysis, where the porosity of the bone is greatest, and are most common in preschool-aged children. On radiographs, buckle fractures can be recognized by a focal, angular protrusion of the cortex with a modest angulation of the shaft and overlying soft tissue swelling.

With angular loading, elastic and then plastic bowing occurs (Fig. 5.2). Traumatic plastic bowing results in a permanent bend caused by a series of microscopic shear frac-

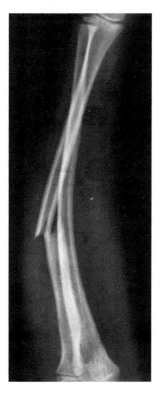

Figure 5.2 Plastic bowing deformity of the ulna and a complete fracture of the radius.

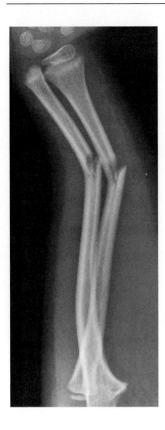

Figure 5.3 Greenstick fractures of the forearm.

tures on the concave aspect without gross disruption of the cortex or trabeculae. Elastic recoil allows a bent bone to recover part of its normal shape. Plastic bowing is most often seen at the ulna, in association with fractures of the radius, and at the fibula, in association with fractures of the tibia. On radiographs, plastic bowing may be recognized by an abnormal bend in the affected bone.

Traumatic plastic bowing results in a permanent bend.

When a bone is angulated beyond the limits of bowing, the convex side fails in tension, and the concave side bends, resulting in an angulated, incomplete transverse fracture. Such a fracture is called a *greenstick fracture* (Fig. 5.3). Elastic recoil usually decreases the degree of angulation; muscle pull may increase it. The periosteum is intact on the concave side of the bend but not on the convex side, leaving a periosteal hinge. Greenstick fractures are seen most often in children of elementary school age. The only anatomic sites where greenstick fractures are common are the shafts of the radius and ulna. On radiographs, greenstick fractures may be recognized by the bowing deformity of the affected bone with a transverse fracture extending through the cortex on the convex side of the bow.

Muscle pull may increase the angulation of a fracture.

The displacement of complete fractures depends on whether the periosteum is torn. A periosteal hinge usually is present on one side, allowing angulation but not much displacement. Children's fractures are rarely comminuted. As with adult bones, the direction of loading determines the configuration of the fracture line.

An intact periosteum may prevent a complete fracture from becoming displaced.

GROWTH PLATE INJURIES

The cartilage of the growth plate absorbs and dissipates some of the energy of loading, reducing the likelihood of a fracture. The growth plate is attached to the metaphysis internally by the interdigitation of bone with the zone of calcified cartilage and externally by the periosteum. The growth plate is relatively weak compared with the capsule and ligaments of adjacent joints, and mechanisms of injury that tend to result in ligamentous joint injuries in adults typically result in growth plate fractures in children. The growth plate is particularly vulnerable to injury when loaded in torsion or shear but is relatively resistant to

Mechanisms of injury that tend to result in ligamentous joint injuries in adults typically result in growth plate fractures in children.

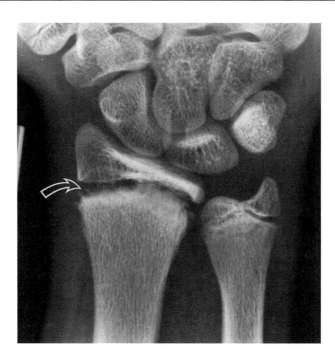

Figure 5.4 Healing distal radius growth plate fracture (Salter type I) with widening and irregularity of the zone of provisional calcification (*arrow*).

tension and compression. When the epiphysis is separated from the metaphysis, the plane of separation through the growth plate is in the zone of cartilage transformation between the calcified and uncalcified layers of cartilage, leaving the germinal cell layers with the epiphysis and the calcified cartilage with the metaphysis. Displacement does not occur unless the periosteum is also torn.

The growth plate obtains its blood supply from the epiphysis.

The production of growing cartilage may not be interrupted by a fracture if the blood supply to the separated epiphysis remains intact. After a fracture, the growth plate becomes wider until the normal zone of cartilage transformation is reestablished and the plate returns to normal (Fig. 5.4). The healing process is much more rapid than that of a fracture through bone and may leave no scar.

Injuries to the growth plate represent approximately one-third of skeletal injuries in children. The most common sites of growth plate fractures are the wrist and ankle. Growth plate fractures are more common in boys than in girls. The peak incidence in boys is at 14 years of age, but the peak incidence in girls is at 11 and 12 years of age. The difference can

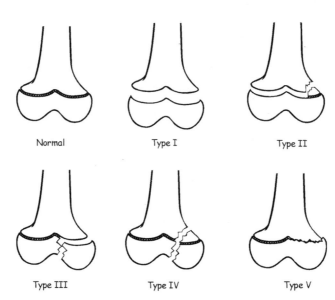

Figure 5.5 Salter-Harris classification of fractures of the growth plate.

Table 5.1: Relative Frequency of Types of Growth Plate Fractures

Salter Type	Frequency (%)
I	6
II	75
III	8
IV	10
V	1

Adapted from Rogers LF. The radiography of epiphyseal injuries. *Radiology* 1970;96:289–299.

Table 5.2: Most Common Sites of Salter Type I Fractures

Location	Frequency (%)
Distal fibula (lateral malleolus of ankle)	25
Distal radius	21
Phalanges (fingers)	17
Distal humerus	6
Others	31

Adapted from Peterson HA. Physeal and apophyseal injuries. In: Rockwood CA, Wilkins KE, Beaty JH, eds. *Fractures in children*, 4th ed. Philadelphia: Lippincott, 1996:103–165.

be accounted for by the differences in the rate of skeletal maturation between boys and girls. Sometimes, a normal growth plate may be mistaken for a fracture. Keats and Smith's *Atlas of Normal Developmental Roentgen Anatomy* is a handy reference for reviewing the radiologic appearance of the skeleton at various ages; in some circumstances, it may be necessary to radiograph the contralateral body part for comparison.

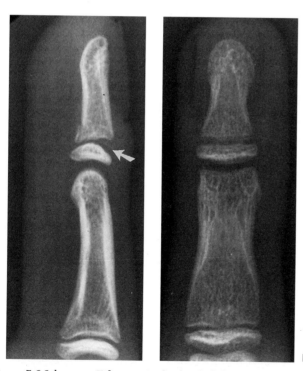

A   B

Figure 5.6 Salter type II fracture in the distal phalanx. *A.* The fracture passes through the growth plate (*arrow*) and includes a small piece of the metaphysis. *B.* The fracture is barely visible on the PA view.

Table 5.3: Most Common Sites of Salter Type II Fractures

Location	Frequency (%)
Phalanges (fingers)	48
Distal radius	16
Distal tibia	9
Distal fibula	6
Phalanges (toes)	6
Others	15

Adapted from Peterson HA. Physeal and apophyseal injuries. In: Rockwood CA, Wilkins KE, Beaty JH, eds. *Fractures in children*, 4th ed. Philadelphia: Lippincott, 1996:103–165.

Salter and Harris described five types of growth plate fractures (Fig. 5.5). Their classification should be used in describing fractures of the growth plate. The most common type of growth plate fracture is a Salter type II fracture (Table 5.1). There are many other systems of classifying growth plate injuries of varying complexity, but the Salter-Harris system is universally understood.

A Salter type I fracture extends through the growth plate without involving bone. This type is usually caused by shearing, torsion, or avulsion. Because Salter type I fractures do not displace unless the periosteum is torn, they may be difficult to demonstrate radiologically without stress views. The most common sites of Salter type I fractures are the lateral malleolus of the ankle and the distal radius (Table 5.2).

In Salter type II fractures, the plane of the fracture passes through much of the growth plate but includes a piece of metaphyseal bone on one side (Fig. 5.6). The periosteum is intact on the side with the metaphyseal fragment but torn on the opposite side. The most common sites of Salter type II fractures are the phalanges of the fingers and the distal radius (Table 5.3).

Salter type III fractures include a piece of the epiphysis and are intra-articular. Salter type III fractures are most common when the growth plate is partially closed, so they tend to occur in teenagers. Most Salter type III fractures are avulsion fractures that occur at sites of ligamentous or tendinous attachment. The most common sites of Salter type III fractures

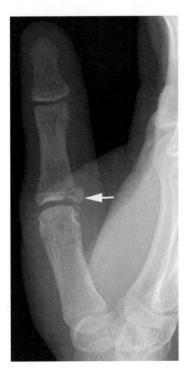

Figure 5.7 Radiograph of the thumb shows a Salter type III fracture (*arrow*) at the base of the proximal phalanx of the thumb (gamekeeper's fracture).

Table 5.4: Most Common Sites of Salter Type III Fractures

Location	Frequency (%)
Phalanges (fingers)	40
Distal tibia	25
Distal ulna	9
Phalanges (toes)	8
Metacarpal	7
Others	11

Adapted from Peterson HA. Physeal and apophyseal injuries. In: Rockwood CA, Wilkins KE, Beaty JH, eds. *Fractures in children*, 4th ed. Philadelphia: Lippincott, 1996:103–165.

are the phalanges of the fingers and thumb (Fig. 5.7) and the medial malleolus of the ankle (Table 5.4).

Salter type IV fractures involve both metaphysis and epiphysis and are intra-articular. The most common sites of Salter type IV fractures are the lateral condyle of the elbow and the medial malleolus of the ankle (Fig. 5.8). Because displacement of the fracture fragment is likely to result in premature closure of the growth plate (Table 5.5), Salter type IV fractures have a worse prognosis than Salter type I or II fractures. Open reduction and internal fixation may be required for treatment of these fractures.

A Salter type V injury is a crush injury of the growth plate from axial loading. These injuries are exceedingly rare and are absent from many large series of growth plate fractures, raising doubts about their existence. Almost by definition, these injuries may not be recognized until the cessation of growth is noticed (Fig. 5.9).

The growth plate is surrounded by a perichondrial ring that appears to regulate its diameter. Displacement of the perichondrial ring allows growth away from the plate laterally, resulting in a posttraumatic osteochondroma (see Chapter 9). Removal of a segment of the ring, for example, by a lawn mower blade injury, permits a bony bridge (physeal bar) to develop across the growth plate, tethering it and leading to angular deformity as growth proceeds (Fig. 5.10).

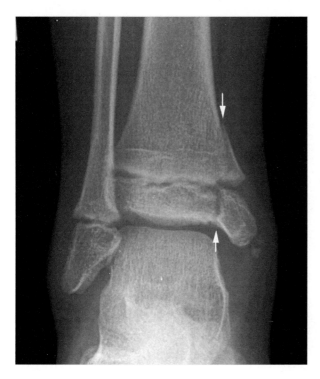

Figure 5.8 Salter type IV fracture of distal tibial growth plate. Fracture lines (*arrows*) extend through the epiphysis, physis, and metaphysis at the medial aspect of the ankle.

Table 5.5: Most Common Sites of Salter Type IV Fractures

Location	Frequency (%)
Distal humerus	34
Distal tibia	31
Phalanges (fingers)	19
Phalanges (toes)	6
Others	10

Adapted from Peterson HA. Physeal and apophyseal injuries. In: Rockwood CA, Wilkins KE, Beaty JH, eds. *Fractures in children*, 4th ed. Philadelphia: Lippincott, 1996:103–165.

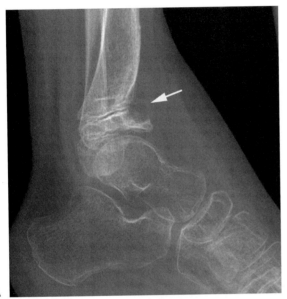

A

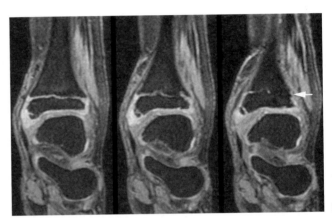

B

Figure 5.9 Salter type V fracture of the distal tibial growth plate. *A.* Lateral ankle radiograph 1 year after injury shows a growth deformity (*arrow*). *B.* Coronal PD fat-suppressed MRI shows the prematurely closed portion of the growth plate (*arrow*).

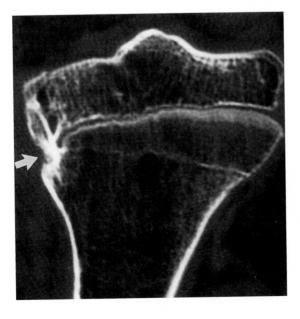

Figure 5.10 Coronal CT of proximal tibia shows physeal bar (*arrow*) caused by a boat propeller injury of the proximal tibial growth plate. Asymmetric growth with angular deformity has resulted.

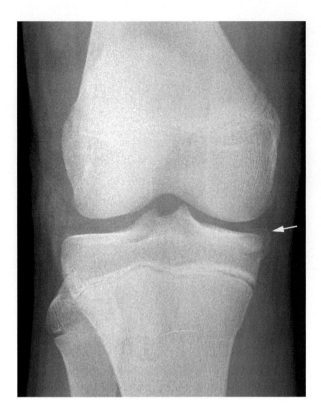

Figure 5.11 Tibial epiphyseal fracture (*arrow*).

Fractures of the epiphysis in children without involvement of the growth plate may occur as osteochondral fractures or avulsion fractures (Fig. 5.11). When the fractures involve only cartilage, they may be unrecognized. These injuries were not included in the original Salter-Harris classification.

    Apophyses are bony prominences that typically accept traction from an attached tendon or muscle, and fractures involving apophyses are almost always avulsion fractures. Fractures of the apophyses are Salter type I or type III injuries. There are several specific sites where apophyseal avulsion fractures are likely to occur (Table 5.6).

Fractures of the epiphysis in children without involvement of the growth plate may occur.

Table 5.6: Common Sites of Apophyseal Avulsion Fractures in Children
Upper extremity
Coracoid
Medial epicondyle
Olecranon
Ulnar coronoid
Pelvis
Iliac crest
Anterior-superior iliac spine
Anterior-inferior iliac spine
Periacetabular rim
Ischial tuberosity
Lower extremity
Femoral greater trochanter
Femoral lesser trochanter
Anterior tibial tubercle
Calcaneal apophysis

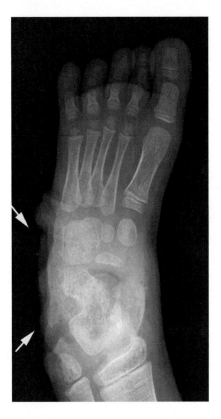

Figure 5.12 Lawn mower accident in a child with open fractures (*arrows*) of the lateral foot.

OPEN FRACTURES

Open fractures in children are typically the result of accidents, many of which are preventable (Fig. 5.12). Open fractures account for approximately 3% of fractures in children. On radiographs, open fractures may be recognized by the presence of gas within the fracture site, a soft tissue wound extending to the fracture site, protrusion of bone through the soft tissues, missing fragments of bone, or penetration of foreign bodies to the bone.

FRACTURE HEALING AND TREATMENT

Fracture healing in children is rapid (Table 5.7). The younger the child and the greater the remaining growth potential of the fractured bone, the faster and more complete are the healing

Table 5.7: Radiographic Timetable of Fracture Healing in Children

	Time after Fracture to Initial Observation	
Radiographic Finding	Typical	Range
Resolution of soft tissue swelling	4–10 d	2–21 d
Periosteal new bone	10–14 d	4–21 d
Loss of fracture-line definition	14–21 d	10–21 d
Soft callus	14–21 d	10–21 d
Hard callus	21–42 d	14–90 d
Remodeling	1 yr	3 mo to physeal closure

Adapted from Kleinman PK. *Diagnostic imaging of child abuse,* 2nd ed. St. Louis: Mosby–Year Book Inc., 1998.

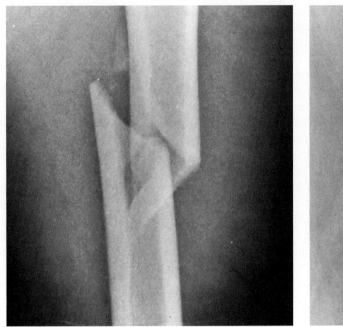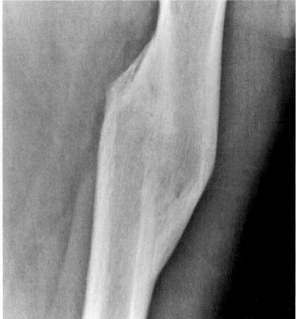

A B

Figure 5.13 Healing spiral femoral shaft fracture. *A*. Acute fracture. *B*. Follow-up after 8 weeks.

and remodeling. Fracture remodeling is a process of bone resorption and periosteal deposition. Fracture remodeling can round off protruding edges by bone resorption and fill in concavities by periosteal new bone. However, varus, valgus, and rotary misalignments do not improve by this process (Fig. 5.13). As growth proceeds and the bone enlarges, asymmetric activity at the growth plate and at the periosteum may tend to correct angular misalignment. Hyperemia from fracture healing may lead to overgrowth, so that a reduction may be left intentionally shorter than anatomic in anticipation of overgrowth. Nonunion of children's fractures is rare unless the fractures are intra-articular. Most fractures in children are treated by closed means, but open reduction and internal fixation by pins, wires, plates, screws, and rods are sometimes necessary.

> Hyperemia from fracture healing may lead to overgrowth of the limb.

SOFT TISSUE INJURIES

Bruises and contusions are common in children and usually are inconsequential. Bruises around the head and neck or chest and abdomen may suggest more severe underlying injuries of the central nervous system or viscera, respectively. Unexplained multiple bruises of different ages may suggest child abuse. Because a child's bones and growth plates are usually weaker than the tendons and ligaments, strains and sprains in children are uncommon until adolescence, when adult patterns of injury begin to emerge as the growth plates close.

> Unexplained multiple bruises of different ages may suggest child abuse.

HAND AND FOREARM

Fractures of the hand account for approximately 20% of all fractures of the extremities in children. The most common fractures in the hand are crush injuries of the distal phalanx and growth plate fractures of the proximal phalanx. The index and little fingers are the most likely to be fractured.

Distal phalanges are most commonly injured by closing doors and falling objects. These are generally extra-articular fractures that do not involve the growth plate and may have a transverse, longitudinal, or comminuted morphology. Forced flexion may result in fractures of the distal phalanx that involve the growth plate. Because the extensor tendon inserts at the epiphysis of the distal phalanx, and the flexor digitorum profundus tendon inserts along the metaphysis, these fractures may become angulated or displaced and assume a fixed position in flexion (mallet finger equivalent). These mallet finger–equivalent injuries may represent Salter type I or II fractures with displacement or angulation at the fracture site or Salter type III or IV fractures with retraction of the fragment by the extensor tendon and unopposed flexion by the flexor digitorum profundus.

In young children, proximal phalangeal fractures are typically Salter type I or II fractures (Fig. 5.7). In adolescents, Salter type III fractures occur with avulsion of a portion of the articular surface by an attached tendon or ligament. Such fractures occur commonly at the thumb and are the children's equivalent of a gamekeeper's fracture. Salter type III avulsion fractures may also occur at other phalanges of the fingers.

The most common metacarpal fracture in children is the *boxer's fracture*, a volarly angulated fracture of the fifth (or sometimes fourth) metacarpal neck.

Fractures and dislocations involving the carpal bones are rare in children. A fracture of the scaphoid is the most common of these rare injuries. Similar to the fractures in adults, fractures across the scaphoid waist may lead to osteonecrosis of the proximal pole. Ligamentous injuries of the wrist in children are rarer than fractures of the carpal bones.

Fractures of the distal radius account for approximately 23% of all fractures of the extremities in children, making it the most common site of children's fractures. These injuries are most commonly sustained in falls onto an outstretched, dorsiflexed hand. The severity of the fracture depends on the energy involved in the fall, ranging from gravity falls from standing height, to falls in which the body has significant momentum (e.g., in roller skating), to falls from a great height. Simple buckle fractures are common in preschool-aged children with simple gravity falls (Fig. 5.1). Buckle fractures are usually located 2 to 3 cm proximal to the growth plate. Complete fractures are seen in higher-energy injuries. When displaced, the fragments are most often displaced dorsally, resulting in a bayonet deformity. The distal radius is the most common location for growth plate fractures in children. These are most often Salter type I or II fractures (Fig. 5.14), and the epiphysis may be displaced.

Fractures of the shafts of the radius and ulna may be impacted, greenstick (Fig. 5.3), or complete (Fig. 5.15). Rotational deformity is usually present and evident as angulated fractures of both bones at different levels. Because the radius has a normal bowing curve

> Fractures and dislocations involving the carpal bones are rare in children.

> The distal radius is the most common site of children's fractures.

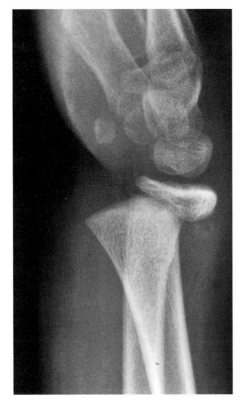

Figure 5.14 Displaced Salter type II fracture of the distal radius.

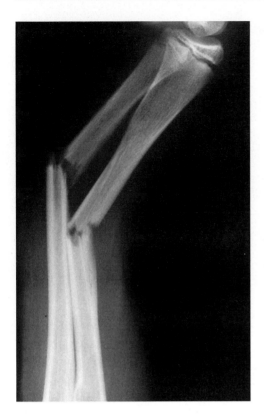

Figure 5.15 Complete fractures of the forearm.

and a pear-shaped cross section, interruption of the smooth curve of the radius or an apparent change in shaft diameter across the fracture site indicates radial malrotation. The bicipital tuberosity may serve as a guide to the rotation of the proximal radius. The position of the proximal fragments in complete fractures depends on the direction of muscle pull.

ELBOW

Fractures of the bones around the elbow account for approximately 12% of all fractures of the extremities in children, making it the third most common location for fractures after the distal radius and the hand.

In children, 60% of elbow fractures are supracondylar fractures, 15% are lateral condylar fractures, and 10% are medial epicondylar avulsion fractures (Table 5.8). Fractures may occur in combinations or in association with elbow dislocation. Isolated fractures of the proximal ulna, olecranon, or coronoid processes are rare. It is important to know the order and timing of the appearance of the ossification centers in the elbow (Table 5.9).

The anterior humeral line, the radiocapitellar line, and the fat pad sign are radiographic clues to the presence of an elbow fracture (Fig. 5.16). The anterior humeral line is a line drawn down the anterior humeral cortex on a true lateral radiograph; it should pass

Isolated fractures of the proximal ulna, olecranon, or coronoid processes are rare in children.

Table 5.8: Common Elbow Injuries in Children

Supracondylar fracture
Lateral condylar fracture
Medial epicondylar avulsion fracture
Radial neck fracture
Pulled elbow (nursemaid's elbow)
Dislocation with medial epicondylar fracture

Table 5.9: Order and Age of Appearance of Ossification Centers at the Elbow

Ossification Center	Boys	Girls
Capitellum	6 wk–8 mo	1–6 mo
Head of radius	46–60 mo	33–66 mo
Medial/internal epicondyle	57–84 mo	27–61 mo
Trochlea	8–9 yr	7–9 yr
Olecranon	9–11 yr	8–11 yr
Lateral/external epicondyle	12–14 yr	12–14 yr

Adapted from Girdany BR, Golden R. Centers of ossification of the skeleton. *AJR Am J Roentgenol* 1952;68:922–924.

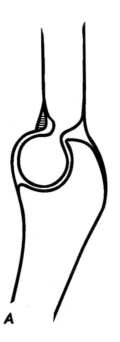
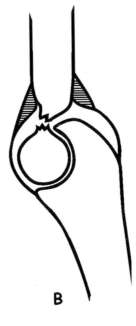

Figure 5.16 Diagram of supracondylar fracture mechanism (hyperextension of the elbow). *A.* Elbow before the fracture. *B.* After the fracture, the capsule distends with blood, making visible the anterior and posterior fat pads.

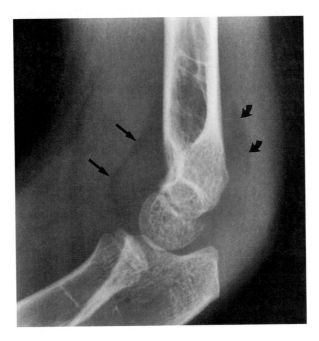

Figure 5.17 Supracondylar children's fracture with anterior (*straight arrows*) and posterior (*curved arrows*) fat pad signs and slight posterior angulation of the capitellum.

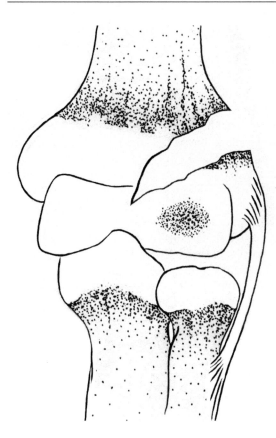

Figure 5.18 Diagram of lateral condylar fracture. If the fracture extends completely through the epiphysis, the fragment may displace.

through the middle third of the capitellum. The radiocapitellar line is drawn through the proximal radial shaft; it should intersect the capitellum on every radiographic projection. The elbow has anterior and posterior fat pads that abut the joint capsule. The posterior fat pad is usually not seen because it lies in the intercondylar depression. The anterior fat pad is typically visible, extending obliquely toward the forearm. Elbow joint distention from any cause will displace both the anterior and posterior fat pads, making them visible. After trauma, the capsule is distended with blood. More than 90% of children and adolescents

More than 90% of children and adolescents with a posterior fat pad sign have a demonstrable fracture.

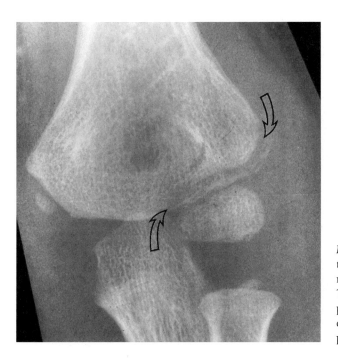

Figure 5.19 Lateral condylar fracture. The fracture through the metaphysis is indicated by arrows. The fracture crosses the growth plate and continues through the cartilaginous portion of the epiphysis (Salter type IV).

with a posterior fat pad sign have a demonstrable fracture. Absence of the fat pad sign in children virtually excludes an intra-articular fracture unless the injury is so severe that there is disruption of the elbow joint capsule.

The age of peak incidence of supracondylar fractures is 5 to 8 years of age, and they are rare after 15 years of age. Supracondylar fractures of the elbow occur with hyperextension, usually in a fall. The fracture extends transversely across the distal humerus through the coronoid and olecranon fossae, above the level of the condyles. The distal fragment is angulated posteriorly, so that the anterior humeral line passes anterior to the capitellum. A posterior fat pad sign is almost always present (Fig. 5.17). The fracture is usually complete, but greenstick fractures, torus fractures, and plastic bowing are possible. The typical treatment is closed reduction with casting.

Lateral condylar fractures are most common between 4 and 10 years of age. These are usually Salter type IV injuries sustained during a fall on an outstretched hand. In most cases, the fracture line begins in the metaphysis, extends across the growth plate, and, if complete, exits through the cartilaginous portion of the epiphysis (Fig. 5.18). Because the fracture usually extends through the cartilaginous portion of the growth plate, it may resemble a Salter type II fracture (Fig. 5.19). An incomplete fracture leaves a distal cartilaginous hinge. A minority of lateral condylar fractures involves the ossified portion of the epiphysis. A posterior fat pad sign is almost always present. The extensors of the forearm originate from the lateral condyle and may distract the distal fragment. Displaced fractures are treated with open reduction and internal fixation.

The medial epicondylar ossification center appears at approximately 5 years of age. It is the site of insertion of the common tendon of the flexor pronator muscle group and can be avulsed by muscular contraction. This often results in a displaced fracture (Fig. 5.20). Dislocation of the elbow also separates the medial epicondyle from the distal humerus by stress applied through the medial ulnar collateral ligament. The medial epicondylar fragment may then become entrapped in the elbow joint as it opens with valgus stress. Medial epicondylar injuries are usually seen between 5 and 15 years of age; after the medial epicondyle fuses in late adolescence, this injury no longer occurs.

Radial neck fractures are not as common in children as in adults because of the greater vulnerability of other structures in the growing elbow. The radial neck may be fractured by indirect forces applied across the humerus during a fall on an outstretched arm with the elbow extended. The injury is usually a Salter type II separation of the radial head (proxi-

Lateral condylar fractures are usually Salter type IV injuries.

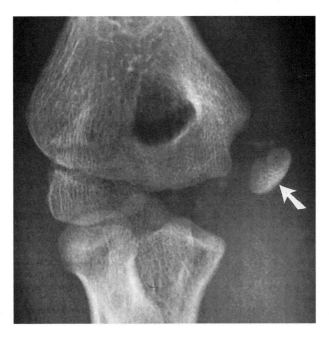

Figure 5.20 Medial epicondyle avulsion (*arrow*) in a 9-year-old boy (Salter type I).

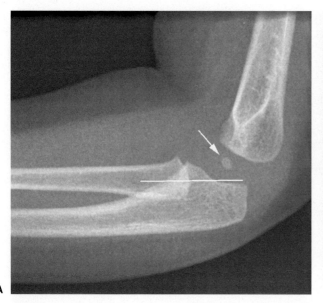
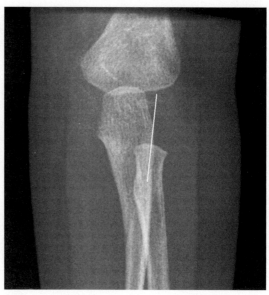

Figure 5.21 Small child with pulled elbow. *A,B.* Lateral and AP radiographs show that the radiocapitellar line (*white lines*) does not intersect the middle of the ossification center (*arrow*) of the capitellum.

mal epiphysis) that may be accompanied by impaction of the lateral metaphysis and lateral angulation of the distal shaft.

Pulled elbow (nursemaid's elbow) is a common injury in ambulatory preschoolers. Longitudinal traction on the pronated hand or wrist as an adult pulls a young child along may dislocate the radial head and tear the attachment of the annular ligament to the radial head. The annular ligament binds the radial head to the ulna and is weakly attached until 5 years of age. The ligament may slip over the radial articular surface, preventing relocation of the radial head. The child may complain of pain and refuse to move the arm. Supination of the slightly flexed elbow during positioning for radiographs often reduces the ligament, resulting in normal radiographs. If the elbow has not been reduced, subluxation of the radial head relative to the capitellum is indicative of the injury (Fig. 5.21). In the normally located elbow, a line drawn through the proximal radial shaft should intersect the ossification center of the epiphysis of the capitellum on all views.

SHOULDER AND HUMERUS

Injuries of the proximal humerus are mostly Salter type II fractures that occur in adolescents. In children younger than 5 years of age, Salter type I fractures usually occur. Hyperextension of the glenohumeral joint during a fall from a height is a common mechanism. The growth plate fracture leaves the humeral head normally located, but the humeral shaft angulates posteriorly and medially (Fig. 5.22). Treatment is usually sling or traction. The adult injury of anterior shoulder dislocation is seen only after the proximal humeral epiphysis has closed.

Scapular fractures in children are rare and are usually the result of severe direct violence such as motor vehicle collisions or child abuse.

Fractures of the clavicle account for approximately 6% of all fractures of the extremities in children. Most clavicle fractures are fractures of the middle portion of the shaft. The medial fragment is pulled cephalad by the sternocleidomastoid muscle, while the distal fragment is pulled caudad by the pectoralis minor muscle. Midshaft fractures may be complete or greenstick, but both unite quickly and remodel completely (Fig. 5.23). Because of the double curve of the normal clavicle, multiple views may be required to demonstrate the fracture. Rarely, injuries can occur at the medial or lateral ends of the

The adult injury of anterior shoulder dislocation is seen only after the proximal humeral epiphysis has closed.

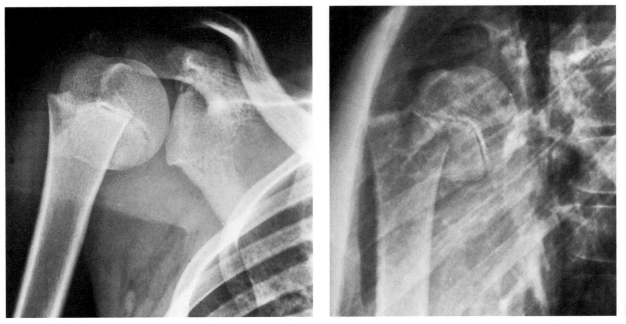

Figure 5.22 Salter type II fracture of the humerus in an 11-year-old boy. *A.* AP radiograph shows proximal humeral fracture. *B.* Transthoracic lateral radiograph of humerus shows the fracture is displaced and angulated.

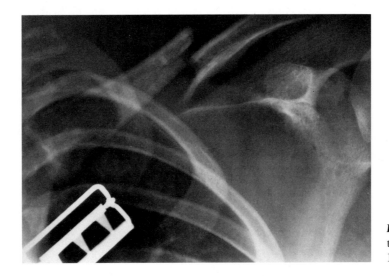

Figure 5.23 Acute fracture of the clavicle in a 14-year-old boy.

clavicle. At the medial end, an epiphyseal separation may occur and mimic a sternocla-vicular dislocation. These injuries occur between 18 and 25 years of age, when the medial clavicular ossification center is present. At the lateral end, the distal tip may be fractured by a backward blow. If the periosteum becomes stripped from the clavicular shaft, the radiographic appearance may suggest acromioclavicular dislocation, but true acromio-clavicular dislocation is rare in children.

SPINE

ACUTE TRAUMA

Cervical spine injuries in children are rare, accounting for less than 1% of all fractures in children. Most involve C1 or C2 and are sustained in motor vehicle collisions, as pedestrian or passenger, or in falls from a height. Weak neck musculature and relatively large head size predispose the upper cervical spine to injuries from acceleration-deceleration or axial distraction. The most common injuries are odontoid fractures and C1-C2 fracture-disloca-tions. Growth plates in children may make the interpretation of radiographs confusing. Growth plates have smooth, regular, sclerotic margins and are found in predictable loca-tions (Fig. 5.24). The vertebral ring apophyses appear in adolescence and persist into young adulthood. Fracture lines are irregular, without sclerosis, and often in unpredictable locations. Forward glide of one vertebral body over the next by up to 3 mm is normal but may mimic subluxation, particularly at the C2-C3 level (Fig. 5.25). The retropharyngeal soft tissues may appear thickened as a result of the child's crying. The neck may normally appear lordotic, neutral, or kyphotic, depending on positioning and the presence or absence of muscle spasm. After 8 to 10 years of age, the spine reaches mature proportions, and the adult pattern of injuries emerges.

Thoracolumbar fractures from acute trauma in children are even less common than cervical spine fractures. Because children's bones are more elastic and ductile, relatively greater amounts of loading can be sustained as the force is dissipated over more levels than

Cervical spine injuries in children are rare, with most involving C1 or C2.

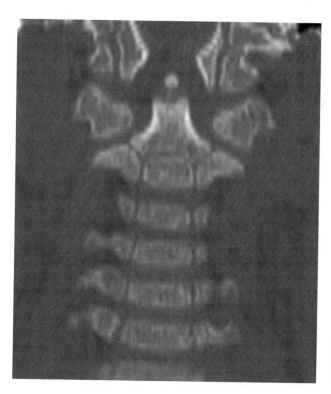

Figure 5.24 Coronal CT recon-struction of the cervical spine of a 2-year-old patient, showing nor-mal ossification centers.

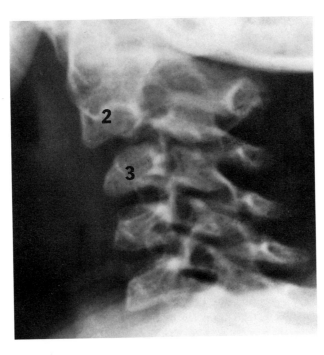

Figure 5.25 Normal cervical spine in a 6 year old with forward glide (pseudosubluxation) at C2-C3.

in adults. When injuries do occur, however, they may be at multiple levels and catastrophic. Spinal cord injury without radiographic abnormality may occur. Avulsion fractures of the spinous processes in infants are highly specific to child abuse (discussed later in this chapter).

SPONDYLOLYSIS AND SPONDYLOLISTHESIS

Spondylolysis refers to discontinuity of the pars interarticularis. Usually seen at the L4 or L5 level, this lesion is a stress fracture of the pars interarticularis caused by axial loads. Predisposing congenital and developmental factors are likely, and many patients with spondylolysis also have various minor deficiencies of the posterior elements such as dysraphic or malformed lamina. Spondylolysis is very rare in young children, has an increasing incidence that coincides with the adolescent growth spurt, and has a prevalence of 5% in the general population. Only a small fraction of children and adolescents with spondylolysis appear to develop symptoms before adulthood. Symptoms may be initiated or aggravated by strenuous activities involving the spine such as football, gymnastics, wrestling, rowing, tennis, baseball pitching, and hockey. The neurologic examination is usually normal. Spondylolysis can be demonstrated on radiographs (Fig. 5.26) and is seen best on lateral or oblique views as a radiolucent discontinuity in the pars interarticularis (the part of the posterior elements that connects the superior and inferior articular facets of a vertebra). On the oblique view, the posterior elements have an appearance that has been likened to a "Scottie dog." When spondylolysis is present, the "Scottie dog" appears to be wearing a radiolucent collar. Radionuclide bone scan may show a stress reaction (hot spot) in the absence of a demonstrable fracture, but a fracture is usually evident later. Nonunion is the common outcome. CT and MRI can demonstrate spondylolysis but should be reserved for problem solving or surgical planning.

The incidence of spondylolysis is highest during the adolescent growth spurt.

Spondylolisthesis, anterior subluxation of the vertebral body, is a common sequela. The severity of spondylolisthesis can be graded from 1 to 4 by dividing the end plate of the lower vertebra into four equal parts on the lateral projection. If the posterior margin of the upper vertebral body has slipped forward up to one-fourth of the AP length of the end plate of the lower vertebra, it is grade 1 spondylolisthesis; a slip of between one-fourth and one-half is grade 2, and so forth. Complete anterior dislocation is considered to be grade 5.

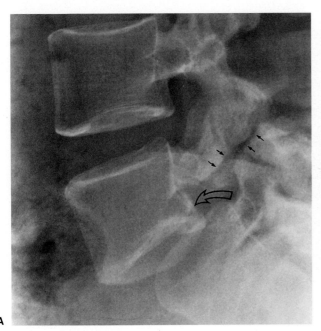 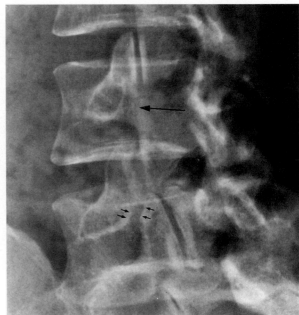

A   B

Figure 5.26 Spondylolysis with spondylolisthesis. *A.* Lateral radiograph shows spondylolysis at L5 (*small arrows*) with grade 2 spondylolisthesis (*large arrow*). *B.* Oblique radiograph shows the bony defect at the pars interarticularis with sclerotic margins (*small arrows*). The pars interarticularis at L4 is normal (*long arrow*).

PELVIS AND PROXIMAL FEMUR

Fractures of the lower extremity in children occur much less frequently than fractures of the upper extremity.

The majority of fractures of the pelvis in children do not interrupt the continuity of the pelvic ring. Avulsion fractures of the apophyses typically occur with sports-related activities. The most common sites of pelvic apophyseal avulsion fractures are the ischial tuberosity (the origin of the hamstring muscles) (Fig. 5.27) and the anterior superior iliac spine (the origin of the sartorius muscle).

Fractures of the pelvic ring in children are caused by severe trauma, such as when a child pedestrian is struck by a car. The likelihood of concomitant injuries, especially of the thorax and head, is high. Depending on the child's age, the hip, trochanters, shaft, or condyles of the femur are at the level of the bumper. A preponderance of left-sided injuries occurs in the United States because a child running across a street is more likely to be hit by a car in the near lane,

The majority of fractures of the pelvis in children do not interrupt the continuity of the pelvic ring.

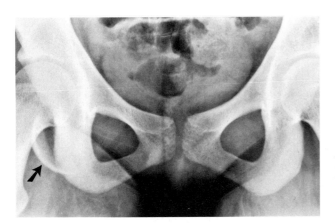

Figure 5.27 Avulsion of the right ischial apophysis (*arrow*) by the hamstrings in a 15-year-old girl who performed a side-split maneuver on the trampoline (Salter type I).

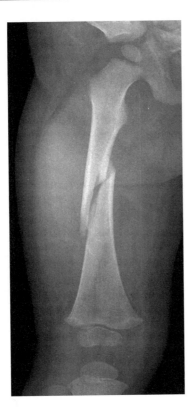

Figure 5.28 Boy who is 21 months old with spiral fracture of the femur suspicious for child abuse.

whose driver has less time to react than a driver of a car in the far lane. In Great Britain and other countries where drivers stay on the left side of the road, there is a preponderance of right-sided injuries.

Hip dislocations are more common than fractures, probably because of the soft cartilaginous structure of the acetabulum in young children. When hip fractures do occur, they may be complicated by osteonecrosis of the femoral head and malunion.

Fractures of the femoral shaft in children younger than 4 years of age are commonly the result of child abuse (Fig. 5.28). In older children, high-energy trauma, such as that sustained in motor vehicle crashes, is required to fracture the femur. Because of muscle pull, fractures of the femoral shaft tend to be shortened and displaced, with the distal fragment angulated posteriorly. Because femoral shaft fractures tend to heal with overgrowth, reduction with overriding is a common orthopedic practice (Fig. 5.13).

KNEE

Knee injuries in children differ from knee injuries in adults because of the relative strength of the ligaments and the thick, energy-absorbing articular and growth cartilages.

The most common intra-articular fracture is an avulsion of the anterior tibial spine by the anterior cruciate ligament. In an adult, the ligament would probably tear. The size of the ossified fragment may be large or small, but the cartilaginous portion is always larger. The fracture may be complete and displaced, incomplete and undisplaced, or hinged posteriorly. A bloody effusion is consistently present.

Internal derangements of the knee in children are less common than in adults.

Internal derangements of the knee in children are less common than in adults. Internal derangements are unusual in young children, and the incidence increases with age as the skeleton gains strength relative to the soft tissue structures of the knee, and there is increased exposure to knee trauma.

Meniscal tears in children and adolescents may be repaired primarily if they extend through the vascularized periphery of the meniscus. The normal meniscus receives its blood supply from its peripheral attachment to the joint capsule.

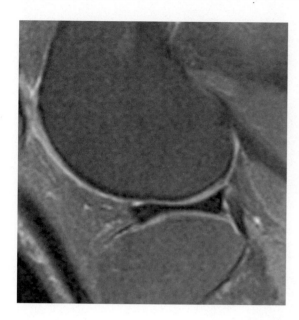

Figure 5.29 Discoid lateral meniscus with biconcave shape on sagittal PD fat-suppressed MRI.

Discoid meniscus is a developmental variant in which the meniscus is shaped like a biconcave disc rather than the letter *C* (Fig. 5.29). The extension of meniscal cartilage into the joint makes it susceptible to degeneration and tears, and a significant proportion of adolescents with meniscal tears have a discoid meniscus. Chronic irritation of the discoid meniscus is thought to cause it to thicken and, in some cases, become slab-like, shaped like a hockey puck with parallel superior and inferior surfaces. Patients typically present with snapping or chronic pain. Discoid meniscus is much more common in the lateral compartment. On MRI, a discoid meniscus can be recognized by the presence of a sheet of fibrocartilage connecting the anterior and posterior horns on sagittal images. An intact discoid meniscus should have a transverse dimension of at least 12 mm on coronal images, and the bow-tie configuration should be seen on three or more consecutive 4-mm-thick slices on sagittal images.

Osteochondral fractures may accompany lateral dislocation of the patella, with a fragment shearing off the lateral femoral condyle or off the medial facet of the patella (Fig. 5.30).

MRI is the recommended method for identifying osteochondral fracture fragments.

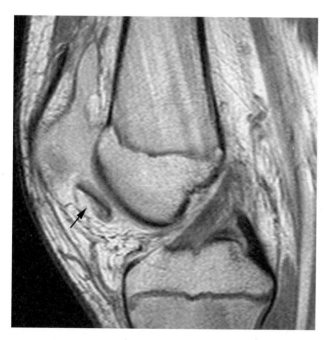

Figure 5.30 Patellar dislocation with osteochondral fragment (*arrow*) shown on sagittal PD MRI.

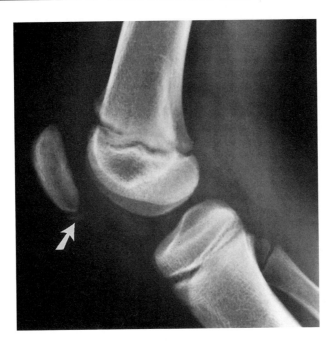

Figure 5.31 Avulsion fracture of the inferior pole of the patella (*arrow*) in a 6-year-old boy. On physical examination, acute tenderness was localized to the site of fracture.

Direct trauma to the medial femoral condyle, as might occur with a fall on stairs, may also result in an osteochondral fracture. A flexion-rotation injury of the knee may also cause an osteochondral fracture involving the medial or lateral femoral condyle. On radiographs, the fragments may be difficult to identify. MRI is the recommended method for identifying such fragments and has the added advantage of displaying the condition of the other structures of the knee.

Fractures of the patella are uncommon in children. Most are sleeve fractures in which tensile loading through the quadriceps mechanism distracts the patella (Fig. 5.31). The inferior fragment typically consists of a large sleeve of cartilage—including the inferior, medial, lateral, and articular surfaces—and sometimes a sliver of the ossification center. As healing occurs, this displaced ossification center enlarges and eventually fuses with the main ossification center. These intra-articular fractures have an associated knee effusion. Fractures of the patella must be distinguished from developmental variants, particularly a patella with multiple ossification centers (multipartite patella). Accessory ossification centers have rounded contours and sclerotic margins and typically occur in the superior lateral quadrant of the patella.

TIBIAL SHAFT

The tibia is the most frequently fractured bone of the lower extremity in children.

The tibia is the most frequently fractured bone of the lower extremity in children. Fractures of the tibial shaft are more common than fractures of the medial malleolus and are seen more frequently in younger children. Approximately one-third of tibial shaft fractures have an accompanying fracture of the fibula. Pedestrian-automobile collisions are common with children, but because of their shorter stature, they tend to sustain fractures of the hip and femur rather than the lower leg.

TODDLER'S FRACTURES

Toddler's fractures may be exceedingly subtle on radiographs.

Isolated spiral or oblique fractures of the tibial shaft are common injuries in ambulatory preschoolers (toddler's fracture) (Fig. 5.32). The fibula is usually intact. These injuries result from falls with torsion of the foot, and the traumatic episode is often innocuous or not witnessed. These fractures may be exceedingly subtle on radiographs because the low

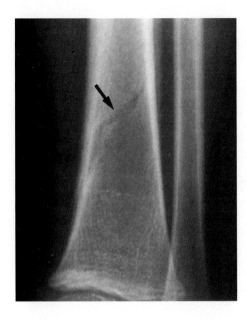

Figure 5.32 Toddler's fracture of the distal tibial shaft (*arrow*) in a 2 year old.

energy that produces the fractures is insufficient to displace it. The clinical presentation is failure to bear weight, limping, or simply the appearance of pain when bearing weight. Follow-up examinations show periosteal new bone, indicative of healing. Fractures from a similar mechanism occur less frequently in the femur or metatarsals. Toddler's fractures must be distinguished from inflicted trauma in the battered child (discussed later in this chapter). Tibial shaft fractures from inflicted trauma are often caused by high-energy direct trauma. The clinical history and physical examination in inflicted trauma are often inconsistent with the radiologic findings.

ANKLE

The ankle ligaments in children are stronger than the growth plates and the bone. The ankle mortise usually remains intact, with the injuries occurring proximally in the growth plates of the tibia and fibula. The most common fractures are Salter type II fractures of the distal tibia and Salter type I or II fractures of the lateral malleolus (Fig. 5.33).

The ankle mortise usually remains intact in injuries of the ankle in children.

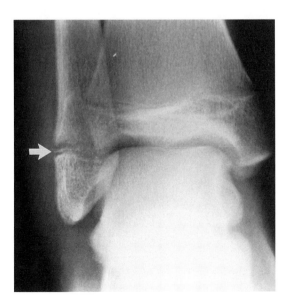

Figure 5.33 Salter type II fracture of the lateral malleolus (*arrow*). Note the soft tissue swelling.

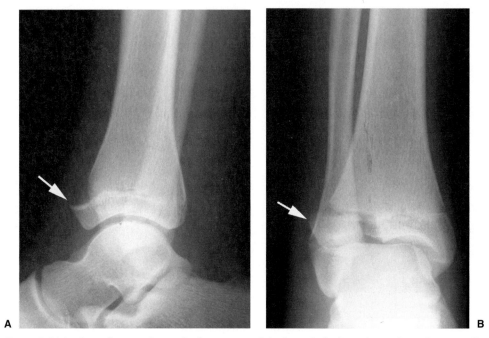

Figure 5.34 Avulsion fracture (*arrows*) of a portion of the lateral tibial epiphysis through a partially closed growth plate (juvenile Tillaux fracture, Salter type III) in a 15-year-old boy. *A.* Lateral radiograph. *B.* AP radiograph.

Gross displacement and angulation may accompany the distal tibial fracture. The lateral malleolar fracture is seen as soft tissue swelling and sometimes as widening of the fibular growth plate.

As the epiphyses begin to close, two unusual fractures may occur in the ankle through the partially fused growth plates. The juvenile Tillaux fracture is an avulsion of a portion of the lateral tibial epiphysis after closure of the medial portion of the tibial growth plate. This avulsion occurs instead of rupture of the syndesmosis or fracture of the lateral malleolus (Fig. 5.34). The fragment may be anterior or posterior depending on whether the ante-

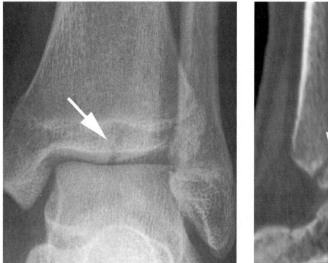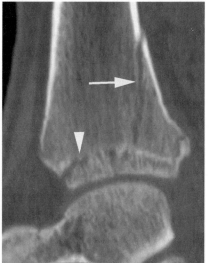

Figure 5.35 Triplane fracture. *A.* AP radiograph shows a fracture (*arrow*) in the sagittal plane through the distal tibial epiphysis. *B.* Sagittal reformatted CT image shows a fracture in the axial plane (*arrowhead*) through the partially opened physis connecting with a fracture through the metaphysis in the coronal plane (*arrow*). (*continued*)

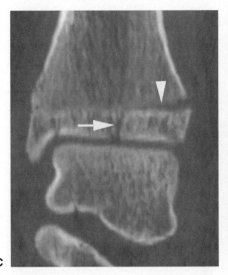 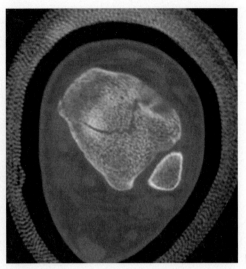

Figure 5.35 *(continued) C.* Coronal reformatted CT image shows a fracture in the sagittal plane (*arrow*) through the distal tibial epiphysis and a fracture in the axial plane (*arrowhead*) through the physis. *D.* Axial CT image through the distal tibial epiphysis shows fractures in the coronal and sagittal planes.

rior or posterior portion of the syndesmosis was under tension. The tibial triplane fracture also occurs in the distal tibia when the growth plate is partially fused. This is a Salter type IV fracture that extends in the coronal plane through the tibial metaphysis, in the axial plane through the growth plate, and in the sagittal plane through the epiphysis (Fig. 5.35).

SPORTS-RELATED INJURIES

American football and wrestling have by far the highest injury rates among school sports. Swimming and tennis have the lowest, and soccer and gymnastics are in between. Fractures and acute soft tissue injuries may occur during play or practice from discrete incidents of trauma. These are more likely to occur in contact sports if the participants are mismatched in size and ability. Chronic overuse injuries similar to those suffered by adults have become common in children who participate in organized single-sport athletics such as gymnastics and hockey. Children are also at risk for injuries peculiar to the growing skeleton, and repetitive loading of growing bones may lead to mechanical adaptation and growth aberration.

Stress fractures are common in the proximal tibia at the junction of the proximal and middle thirds (Fig. 5.36). Stress fractures often follow a change in the training regimen. Stress fractures may involve the growth plates or synchondroses such as those of the pelvis (Fig. 5.37). Children at particular risk for such injuries are usually participants in activities in which repetitive shearing forces are applied to growth plates or synchondroses (Table 5.10).

Avulsion fractures of apophyses by inserting tendons are most common about the pelvis but may also involve the knee, elbow, and shoulder. Avulsion fractures of apophyses and epiphyses at tendinous insertions are Salter type I injuries if the growth plates are open and Salter type III injuries if the growth plates are partially closed. These fractures are distracted because of excessive muscle pull. The most common sites of avulsion fractures are the fingers, around the pelvis, the lesser trochanter, the medial epicondyle, and the anterior tibial tubercle.

Osgood-Schlatter disease of the knee is thought to be a stress injury of the tibial apophyseal growth plate at the insertion of the infrapatellar tendon. The clinical presentation of Osgood-Schlatter disease is painful prominence of the tibial tubercle in an adolescent

Sports-related injuries in contact sports are more likely to occur if the participants are mismatched in size and ability.

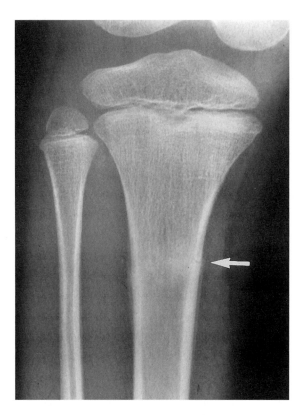

Figure 5.36 Stress fracture (*arrow*) of the tibia in a 7-year-old boy with healing.

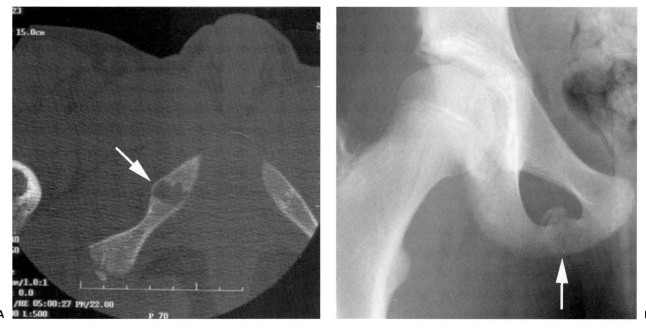

Figure 5.37 Ischial stress fracture in a 14-year-old boy participating in kickboxing. *A.* Axial CT scan shows a stress fracture (*arrow*) in the right ischium. *B.* Radiograph shows healing fracture (*arrow*) after 3 weeks of rest.

Table 5.10: Common Sites of Stress Fractures in Children
More common sites
Proximal tibia
Metatarsals
Pars interarticularis
Medial epicondyle
Less common sites
Proximal humerus
Distal radius
Ulna
Vertebral end plate
Femoral neck
Femoral shaft
Fibular shaft
Calcaneus
Adapted from Staheli LT. *Fundamentals of pediatric orthopedics*. Philadelphia: Lippincott–Raven, 1998.

(11 to 15 years of age) who participates in jumping sports such as basketball. Symptoms may be prolonged and intermittent but always cease when the growth plate closes. Stress fractures of the anterior tibial apophysis may also occur potentially resulting in avulsion of the apophysis by the infrapatellar tendon.

A stress injury of the inferior pole of the patella carries the eponym Sinding-Larsen-Johansson disease. In this condition, there is repetitive incomplete avulsion trauma to the inferior pole of the patella mediated through tension on the infrapatellar ligament.

THE BATTERED CHILD

The battered child has horrified and fascinated the medical profession since 1946 when Caffey, a pediatric radiologist, published his findings of a series of six infants with chronic subdural hematomas and unrecognized skeletal trauma. He suggested inflicted trauma as the cause for both. Described initially by physicians as a medical syndrome with predictable implications in terms of treatment, prognosis, and prevention, the concept of child abuse has expanded to include broad psychological, cultural, social, and legal implications. A contemporary concept of the physical abuse of children categorizes it as one permutation in a "world of abnormal rearing." Children who are raised in such a world do not complete the tasks of childhood; they are not taught many of the basic skills necessary for successful social interaction because their parents or caretakers themselves lack these skills. Inadequacies in behavior and parenting can be passed down through successive generations: Except for the rare psychotic individual, child abusers have had abnormal rearing, and many were battered as children. There is no broadly accepted, precise definition of child abuse. Some of these children are physically abused; others may be sexually molested, neglected, or unloved. This section is concerned with physical abuse inflicted in the home by a parent or caretaker.

Approximately 10% of children reported to governmental agencies as abused have radiologic evidence of injury. Approximately 10% of children younger than 5 years of age who are seen in hospital emergency departments for trauma have child abuse as the cause. Intentional trauma is one of the leading causes of death in infancy and childhood. Because the acts of violence are nearly always multiple, any physician with reasonable suspicion of child abuse has a duty to prompt further formal investigation. Moreover, failure to do so may expose the physician to criminal, civil, or professional liability. The standard for the radiologist is to report findings and suspicions to the referring physician. The referring physician is in a better position to correlate the radiologic findings with history and phys-

The battered child syndrome was first described by a radiologist.

Approximately 10% of children younger than 5 years of age who are seen in hospital emergency departments for trauma have child abuse as the cause.

Table 5.11: Skeletal Injuries in Child Abuse
High specificity
Classic metaphyseal lesions
Rib fractures, especially posterior
Scapular fractures
Spinous process fractures
Sternal fractures
Moderate specificity
Multiple fractures, especially bilateral
Fractures of different ages
Epiphyseal separations
Vertebral body fractures and subluxations
Digital fractures
Complex skull fractures
Low specificity
Subperiosteal new bone formation
Clavicular fractures
Long bone shaft fractures
Linear skull fractures

Adapted from Kleinman PK. *Diagnostic imaging of child abuse*, 2nd ed. St. Louis: Mosby–Year Book, 1998.

ical examination. However, if the radiologic findings are highly specific and the referring physician fails to report, the obligation for reporting then falls to the radiologist. Statutes requiring the reporting of suspected cases of child abuse are in place throughout the United States and Canada.

The radiologist can suggest, support, or even establish the diagnosis of child abuse. Radiologic findings may range from suggestive to virtually pathognomonic (Table 5.11); normal radiographs do not exclude the possibility, however. Abused children often present with misleading histories and complaints, and an absent, inconsistent, or implausible history of injury raises the suspicion of abuse. In this circumstance, the radiologic report may become a key medicolegal document.

> The skeletal survey is the usual screening examination for evidence of abuse.

The skeletal survey is the usual screening examination for evidence of abuse. In children 2 years of age or younger, a full skeletal survey with the best technique available for bone detail is required. A single view of the entire baby, including skull, trunk, and extremities (babygram), is almost never adequate or satisfactory. The skull, trunk, and extremities should all be examined and are best radiographed separately. In children older than 2 years of age, radiologic findings are limited to those in whom there is a history or physical evidence of inflicted trauma; in these, radiologic screening can be limited to the specific areas of suspicion. In a few imaging departments, the radionuclide bone scan is used for screening. Compared to the skeletal survey, the bone scan has higher sensitivity but greater cost and lower specificity. A high level of technical and interpretive expertise is required to perform high-quality bone scans in young children. Many use the bone scan only when there is a high level of suspicion but a normal skeletal survey.

The most common fractures seen in child abuse are spiral fractures of the femur and tibia, fractures of the clavicle, and simple linear fractures of the skull outside the occiput. These fractures are not specific to child abuse and may also occur with accidental trauma. Child abuse is likely when injuries are discovered that are more extensive or more severe than the history given for the trauma; when the injuries are of different ages, indicating prior episodes of trauma; or when there is fracture without adequate explanation.

Some skeletal injuries are highly specific to child abuse regardless of the clinical circumstance. Patterns of fractures that are specific to child abuse are caused by indirect torsional, acceleration, and deceleration forces generated when an infant is gripped around the thorax or by the extremities and shaken violently. Massive forces develop as the head

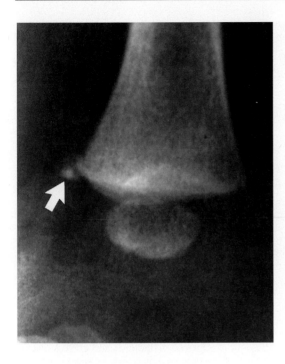

Figure 5.38 Distal femur of a 6-month-old girl shows a corner fracture (*arrow*).

and extremities flail about. Torsional and tractional forces are applied as an infant is twisted or pulled by an extremity. The radiologic alterations from such forces are found in infants and young children.

In the long bones of the extremities, radiologic-pathologic studies have shown the fundamental lesion to be a series of microfractures occurring in a plane through the immature metaphyseal primary spongiosa, which is the zone of growing bone where delicate trabeculae are first apposed to central calcified cores. The fracture fragment consists of a thin plate of bone, calcified cartilage, the growth plate, and the attached epiphysis. This fracture is recognized as a transverse subepiphyseal lucency with an adjacent linear density abutting the growth plate. If the fragment is tipped or viewed obliquely, it has a bucket-handle appearance. If the periphery is thicker than the central portion, it has a corner fracture appearance (Figs. 5.38 through 5.40). These metaphyseal lesions are injuries highly spe-

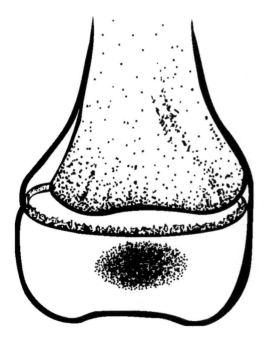

Figure 5.39 Diagram of the metaphyseal lesion that is pathognomonic of child abuse. The fracture plane extends through the metaphysis just beneath the growth plate. Because the bone plate is often very thin, it may only be visible in areas of overlap or after the start of healing.

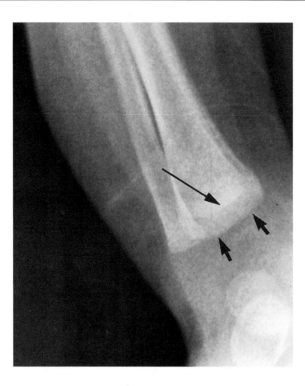

Figure 5.40 Healing metaphyseal fracture in a 1-month-old boy. The original extent of ossification is indicated by the long arrow; the extent of the new bone made by the fractured and displaced metaphysis and growth plate is indicated by the short arrows.

cific for intentional injury and differ from the usual Salter types of growth plate fractures, in which the fracture plane is between the calcified and uncalcified zones of cartilage. Shaking may also separate a long bone from its periosteal envelope, leading to subperiosteal hemorrhage and periosteal elevation. Once the periosteum begins to make new reactive bone, its displaced position becomes evident (Fig. 5.41).

In the head, violent shaking produces rapid rotational accelerations and decelerations of the brain within the skull. Disruption of the bridging veins between the cortical surface and the dural sinuses results in subdural hematoma, often interhemispheric. Subarachnoid

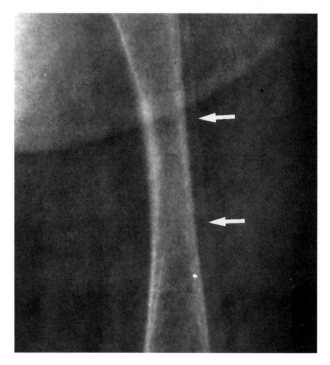

Figure 5.41 Postmortem radiograph of the femur of a 5-month-old girl shows periosteal elevation from subperiosteal hemorrhage with early reactive bone (*arrows*).

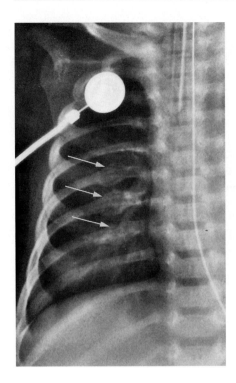

Figure 5.42 Posterior rib fractures (*arrows*) in a 5-week-old boy with advanced callus formation indicating that the fractures are at least 14 days old.

hemorrhage may also occur, but not epidural hemorrhage. If the child's head strikes a wall or other solid object while he or she is being shaken, skull fractures may occur in the occipital or posterior parietal regions. Accidental intracranial trauma is so rare in early childhood that virtually all serious intracranial injuries in infants have been intentionally inflicted. In the absence of an adequate history of massive trauma, skull fractures that are depressed, complex, or associated with dural tear are probably caused by abuse. The incidence of skull fractures in infants after accidental falls is no higher than 2%; these fractures are generally narrow, linear, and uncomplicated. Head injuries may be acutely life threatening; in survivors, posttraumatic long-term developmental effects such as mental retardation and learning

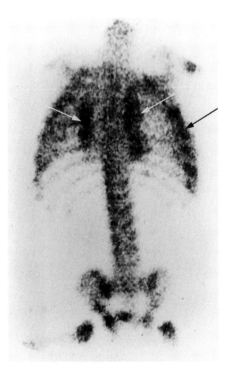

Figure 5.43 Bone scan of a 1-month-old girl shows three separate sets of rib fractures (*arrows*). The two sets of posterior rib fractures (*white arrows*) are virtually pathognomonic for child abuse.

disabilities are common. Fractures are best detected by plain films, and intracranial injuries are best demonstrated by MRI. Facial fractures are unusual in child abuse.

Rib fractures may result from AP compression of the rib cage when a child is grabbed around the trunk and shaken. This compression causes fractures of the inside cortex of the posterior portions of the ribs and the outside cortex of the lateral portions at multiple contiguous levels (Figs. 5.42 and 5.43). Rib fractures at these sites also may occur in motor vehicle collisions, but not as a result of falls or attempted cardiopulmonary resuscitation.

It may become critical to establish the age of a fracture by radiologic appearance in relation to the historical timing of the trauma. Dating fractures by roentgenography is imprecise. In general, a fracture with definite but slight periosteal new bone may be as recent as 4 to 7 days old. Unless immobilized or internally fixed, a fracture that is 20 days old will almost always have well-defined periosteal new bone and soft callus. A fracture with a large amount of periosteal new bone or callus is more than 14 days old. Long-bone fractures in infants heal with widespread periosteal new bone formation.

The radiologic differential diagnosis of extremity fractures in child abuse is limited.

Dating fractures by radiographs is imprecise.

SOURCES AND READINGS

Berson L, Davidson RS, Dormans JP, et al. Growth disturbances after distal tibial physeal fractures. *Foot Ankle Int* 2000;21:54–58.

Caffey J. Multiple fractures in the long bones of children suffering from chronic subdural hematoma. *AJR Am J Roentgenol* 1946;56:163–173.

Carey J, Spence L, Blickman H, et al. MRI of pediatric growth plate injury: correlation with plain film radiographs and clinical outcome. *Skeletal Radiol* 1998;27:250–255.

Futami T, Foster BK, Morris LL, et al. Magnetic resonance imaging of growth plate injuries: the efficacy and indications for surgical procedures. *Arch Orthop Traum Surg* 2000;120:390–396.

Green NE, Lampert R, Swiontkowski MF, eds. *Skeletal trauma in children*, 2nd ed. Philadelphia: WB Saunders, 1998.

Helfer RE, Kempe RS, eds. *The battered child*, 4th ed. Chicago: University of Chicago Press, 1987.

John SD. Trends in pediatric emergency imaging. *Radiol Clin North Am* 1999;37:995–1034.

Kao SC, Smith WL. Skeletal injuries in the pediatric patient. *Radiol Clin North Am* 1997;35:727–746.

Keats TE, Smith TH. *An atlas of normal developmental roentgen anatomy*, 7th ed. Chicago: Year Book, 2002.

Kleinman PK. *Diagnostic imaging of child abuse*. St. Louis: Mosby–Year Book, 1998.

Loder RT, Kuhns LR, Swinford AE. The use of helical computed tomographic scan to assess bony physeal bridges. *J Pediatr Orthop* 1997;17(3):356–359.

Lohman M, Kivisaari A, Vehmas T, et al. MRI in the assessment of growth arrest. *Pediatr Radiol* 2002;32:41–45.

Noerdlinger MA, Cole PA, Lifrak JT. Proximal tibial physis fractures and the use of noninvasive studies in detecting vascular injury: a case report and literature review. *Am J Orthop* 2000;29(11):891–895.

Ogden JA. Injury to the growth mechanisms of the immature skeleton. *Skeletal Radiol* 1981;6:237–253.

Perron AD, Miller MD, Brady WJ. Orthopedic pitfalls in the ED: pediatric growth plate injuries. *Am J Emerg Med* 2002;20:50–54.

Peterson CA, Peterson HA. Analysis of the incidence of injuries to the epiphyseal growth plate. *J Trauma* 1972;12:275–281.

Rang M. *Children's fractures*, 2nd ed. Philadelphia: JB Lippincott Co, 1983.

Reynolds R. Pediatric spinal injury. *Curr Opin Pediatr* 2000;12:67–71.

Rhemrev SJ, Ekkelkamp S, Sleeboom C. Epiphyseal fractures of the proximal tibia. *Injury* 2000;31:131–134.

Rogers LF. The radiography of epiphyseal injuries. *Radiology* 1970;96:289–299.

Rogers LF. *Radiology of skeletal trauma*, 3rd ed. New York: Churchill Livingstone, 2002.

Salter RB, Harris WR. Injuries involving the epiphyseal plate. *J Bone Joint Surg Am* 1963;45A:587–622.

Scoles PV. *Pediatric orthopedics in clinical practice*, 2nd ed. Chicago: Year Book, 1988.

Shin AY, Moran ME, Wenger DR. Intramalleolar triplane fractures of the distal tibial epiphysis. *J Pediatr Orthop* 1997;17(3):352–355.

Swift DM, McBride L. Chronic subdural hematoma in children. *Neurosurg Clin N Am* 2000;11:439–446.

Wilkins KE. The incidence of fractures in children. In: Rockwood CA, Wilkins KE, Beaty JH, eds. *Fractures in children*, 4th ed. Philadelphia: Lippincott, 1996.

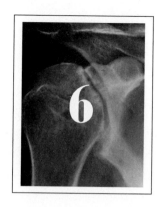

IMAGING OF FRACTURE TREATMENT AND HEALING

The seriousness of an injury is not always related to the radiographic severity of the fracture. The patient's general state of health, associated injuries and conditions, degree of soft tissue injury, and consistency of underlying bone can have a vast influence on outcome. For example, a minimally displaced, closed femur fracture in a frail, osteoporotic woman is often life threatening, whereas a comminuted, displaced femoral fracture in an otherwise healthy child probably is not. In choosing the mode of fracture treatment, considerations other than the location and morphology of the fracture are crucial.

FRACTURE HEALING

The natural history of an uncomplicated long-bone fracture is union through the formation of callus. This *secondary fracture healing* occurs in three stages: an inflammatory stage, a reparative stage, and a remodeling stage (Table 6.1 and Fig. 6.1). Immediately after the fracture, hematoma and devitalization of soft tissues and bone at the fracture site provoke an acute, intense inflammatory reaction. On radiographs, soft tissue swelling and sharp fracture lines are present. By 10 to 14 days after injury, the fracture lines may have become more readily visible because of bone resorption. Acute regional osteoporosis of the involved extremity, caused by the hyperemia that accompanies inflammation, is usual (Fig. 6.2). As the hematoma organizes into granulation tissue capable of osteogenesis, the reparative phase begins. External periosteal callus is formed in the subperiosteal regions adjacent to the fracture. Fibrous tissue, cartilage, and immature bone form within the mass of granulation tissue around the fracture. This mass, called *primary* or *soft callus*, is fusiform

Secondary fracture healing occurs through the formation of fracture callus.

Acute regional osteoporosis is caused by the hyperemia that accompanies fracture healing.

Table 6.1: Stages of Fracture Healing

Stage	Time Frame	Tissue at Fracture Site
Inflammatory	Days to weeks	Hematoma and granulation tissue
Reparative	Weeks to months	Callus
Remodeling	Months to years	Remodeling bone

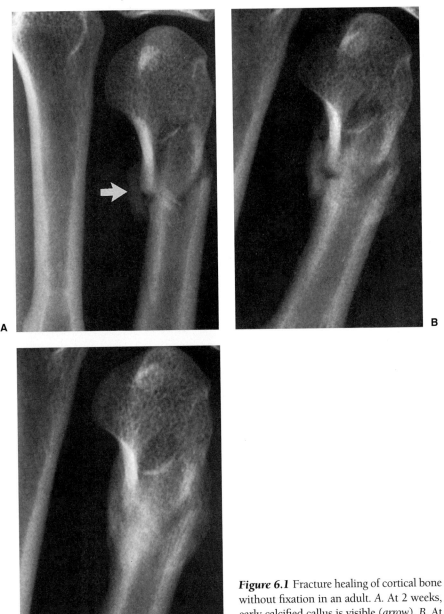

Figure 6.1 Fracture healing of cortical bone without fixation in an adult. *A.* At 2 weeks, early calcified callus is visible (*arrow*). *B.* At 6 weeks, more callus is visible, and the fracture lines are becoming obscured. *C.* At 13 weeks, the fracture has almost completely healed.

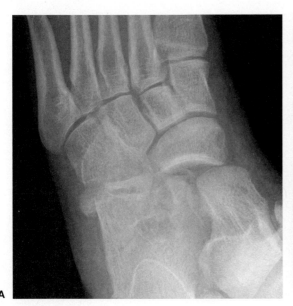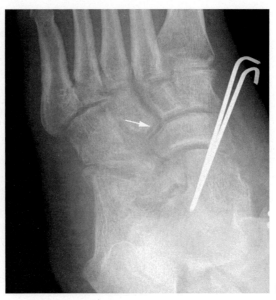

A   B

Figure 6.2 Acute osteoporosis accompanying fracture healing. *A.* Oblique radiograph of the foot at the time of presentation shows fracture dislocations of the Chopart and subtalar joints. *B.* Radiograph 6 weeks later shows subchondral bone resorption (*arrow*) indicating acute osteoporosis.

in shape and bridges the fracture gap. In the proper environment of ample blood supply and limited motion and stress, the primary callus forms bone. Ossification in primary callus may be seen on radiographs as early as 10 days after injury in children and 2 weeks in adults. Because external callus expands the diameter of the bone at the site of fracture healing, often by a factor of two or three, mechanical stability (clinical union) is generally achieved within 6 to 12 weeks. Radiographs should show abundant, well-defined callus bridging the fracture site, with fracture lines becoming fuzzy. Bone repair continues with the formation of intramedullary callus and the eventual remodeling of woven bone to lamellar bone along lines of stress. Remodeling of callus may take place over a period of months to years (Fig. 6.3). In time, there may be scant radiographic indication of the pre-

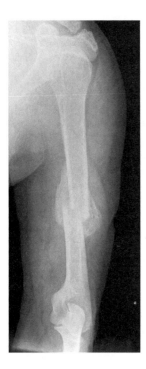

Figure 6.3 Remodeling fracture callus at the humeral shaft (3 months).

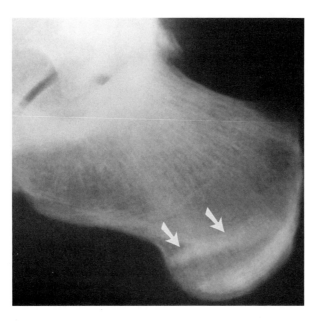

Figure 6.4 Sclerosis (*arrows*) indicates healing fracture in the cancellous bone of the calcaneus.

Endosteal healing may be evident radiographically as increasing and then decreasing sclerosis at the fracture site.

vious fracture. In contrast, fractures of cancellous bone, particularly if impacted, tend to form internal callus rather than external callus as they heal. Healing in a fracture that is wholly confined to cancellous trabeculae may be evident radiographically only as increasing and then decreasing sclerosis at the fracture site (Fig. 6.4).

Injuries of the soft tissues heal through the process of localized necrosis, inflammation, and repair. Ligament and tendon injuries heal with a bridging scar if the ends are not too far distracted. The scar may eventually remodel along lines of stress. Cartilage heals through a different process because of the lack of vascularization. Localized necrosis occurs, but there is no inflammatory phase. Superficial injuries that do not extend to the bone marrow heal by migration of cells from the synovial fluid or from elsewhere in the cartilage. In injuries that extend to the bone marrow, an initial blood clot is replaced by granulation tissue. The resulting fibrous scar undergoes progressive hyalinization and chondrification to become fibrocartilage.

CLOSED FRACTURE TREATMENT

The vast majority of fractures are treated closed—that is, without open surgery. The fractures and soft tissues are reduced, and the fracture is stabilized but not completely immobilized. Muscle activity, joint motion, and load transmission promote external callus formation. The two common methods of closed fracture treatment are casts and traction.

Muscle activity, joint motion, and load transmission promote the formation of external callus.

Casts can be used to reduce and control fractures with angular deformity through three-point fixation. The cast is shaped so that it pushes at the apex of the fracture and at the opposite ends of the bone, tending to keep it straight. Slow-setting plaster of Paris (Fig. 6.5) is applied while reduction maneuvers are performed. Casts are typically applied over a stockinette and a layer of padding so that a radiolucent zone is present between the limb and the cast on radiographs. A second layer of cast material can be applied to provide strength and durability. Plaster casts are often covered with a layer of fiberglass for durability and may be replaced completely by fiberglass as the fracture begins to heal and the patient regains the use of the limb (Fig. 6.6). Fiberglass casts can be made into more functional braces through the addition of hinges where the cast crosses a joint. Some fractures of the thoracic and lumbar spine are treated with casts or braces that envelop the torso and stabilize the spine by compressing the soft tissues of the abdomen. The position and alignment of reduced fractures of the limbs can be maintained in a similar manner. The shape and relative rigidity of the cast use the patient's own soft tissues to turn the cast into a fluid-filled cylinder that resists swelling and deformation. Stable fractures, when subjected to

Plaster casts are often covered with a layer of fiberglass for durability.

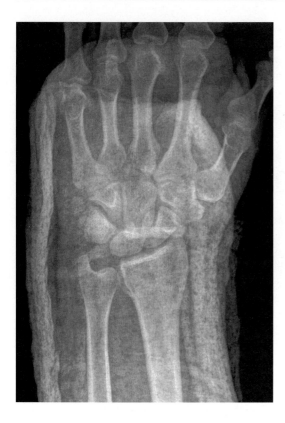

Figure 6.5 Plaster cast applied to distal radius fracture.

normal stresses, maintain their reduction. External supports such as casts, splints, or braces are load-sharing devices that restrict motion after a stable fracture has been reduced. Traction can be applied and maintained in a variety of ways. Skin traction, in which the limb is gripped with adhesive bandages and connected to a system of hanging weights, is

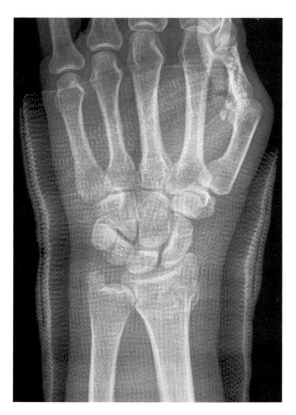

Figure 6.6 Fiberglass cast applied to distal radius fracture.

seldom used except for femoral fractures in small children. Skeletal traction is applied by placing pins into the extremity distal to the fracture and connecting the pins to weights. Dynamic traction allows the physiologic motion that is generally beneficial to the formation of periosteal callus. Traction on fractures of the clavicle and proximal humerus can be applied with a figure-of-eight harness or a long-arm cast, respectively. The upper limb itself becomes the hanging weight, and the direction of traction depends on the point of suspension along the cast. Some fractures of the cervical spine are treated with a halo brace that functions on the same principle but works against gravity by stretching the neck.

OPEN REDUCTION AND INTERNAL FIXATION

Open reduction and internal fixation (osteosynthesis) requires surgical exposure of the fracture. The fracture is reduced, the soft tissues are repaired, and the fragments are fixed with hardware. If a bone undergoes plastic deformation before fracturing, the fracture fragments may not fit back together because of the distortion in shape that preceded the fracture. Fracture fixation hardware does not substitute for the native bony structure; rather, it provides temporary mechanical stability while the natural healing process occurs. The stability that comes with internal fixation is crucial to rapid restoration of mobility and function; many patients cannot tolerate bed rest and prolonged hospitalization. Fixation devices include screws, plates, rods, pins, nails, and wires. Many fixation devices can be inserted percutaneously under fluoroscopic guidance or through minimal incisions. A second operation is necessary to remove many types of hardware after the fractures have healed.

Internal fixation that holds bone fragments together rigidly promotes direct bony union (primary fracture healing). New intracortical haversian systems drill across the fracture site, leaving cores of new bone. Fracture callus is minimal or absent as the osteocytes remodel the fracture away (Fig. 6.7). On radiographs, primary fracture healing is seen as a

Fracture fixation hardware provides temporary mechanical stability for bone healing to occur.

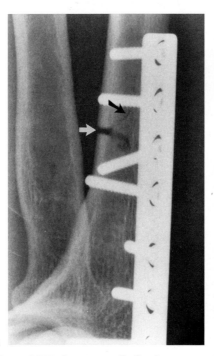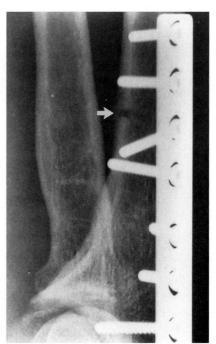

A   B

Figure 6.7 Healing internally fixed transverse fracture of the ulna with posterior butterfly fragment. *A.* Immediate postoperative film shows that a cortical plate has fixed the fragments of the transverse portion of the fracture with 1- to 2-mm distraction (*white arrow*), while the oblique fractures are compressed (*black arrow*). *B.* After 7 weeks, endosteal callus bridges the transverse fracture (*arrow*), and the oblique fractures have remodeled and disappeared.

gradual disappearance of the fracture line. A gap between fragments or excessive motion at the fracture site interferes with the migration of osteocytes across the fracture plane, and the fracture heals through the formation of periosteal and endosteal callus. Secondary fracture healing occurs more slowly in fractures with internal fixation because restriction of motion interferes with formation of callus.

Internal fixation devices are designed to function on the biomechanical principles of static or dynamic interfragmentary compression, bridging, or splintage. In static compression, a metal implant holds the fracture fragments together under compression. In dynamic compression, the implant transforms physiologic loading into compression at the fracture site. There is direct bony union in both types of compression. Internal fixation bridges a fracture site when it is secured to uninjured bone on either side of the fracture. Physiologic loads are transferred from the bone on one side of the fracture to the bone on the other side. If the fragments are not directly apposed and there is motion between them, periosteal and endosteal callus fills the gaps between the bones. Length and alignment are maintained while the bones heal. Internal fixation devices that function as internal splints allow motion at the fracture site and promote periosteal callus while maintaining reduction.

> Callus is minimal or absent in internally fixed fractures.

SCREWS

Orthopedic screws are available in a variety of sizes and shapes, often for use in specific circumstances (Fig. 6.8). The parts of a screw are the head, shaft, thread, and tip. Most

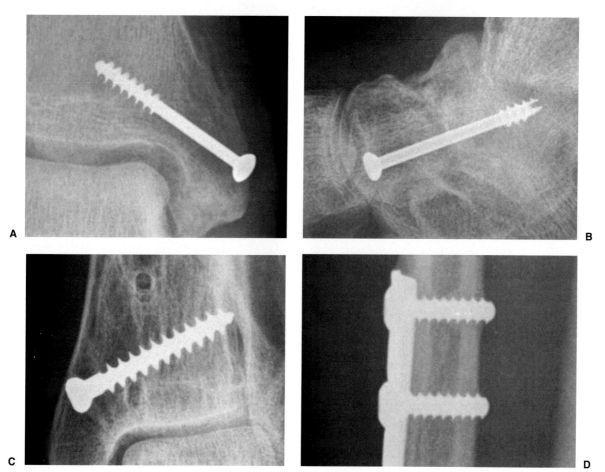

Figure 6.8 Common types of orthopedic screws. *A.* Compression or lag screw. *B.* Cannulated screw. *C.* Machine screw with cancellous threads. *D.* Machine screws with cortical threads.

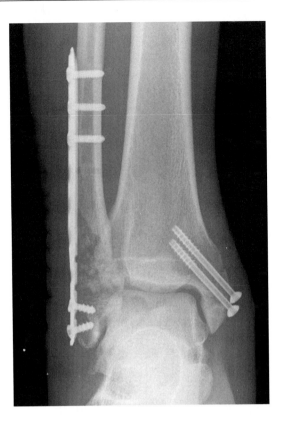

Figure 6.9 Ankle fracture with internal fixation. Two lag screws with cancellous threads fix the medial malleolus. The contoured cortical plate is fixed to the fibular shaft by three screws with cortical threads and to the lateral malleolus by two cannulated cancellous screws.

types of screws have a head socketed to receive a hexagonal shaft driver and a threaded shank. The heads have a hemispheric undersurface that allows contact even when the screw is inclined. Screws used for cancellous bone have a wider thread diameter relative to the core shank diameter and a deeper thread pitch (larger distance between threads) than screws used for cortical bone (Fig. 6.9). Most screws are inserted into drill holes. These holes may be tapped or threaded to receive a screw, or the screw may be self-tapping and cut its own threads as it is driven into the hole. Cannulated screws are hollow in the center. These allow the placement of screws over a guide wire, improving the ability of the orthopedist to place screws accurately without the need for supplementary clamp fixation of the site. Some cannulated screws are self-drilling and self-tapping and can be percutaneously inserted over a guide wire. Screws are made of metal, commonly stainless steel or titanium alloy. There has been considerable research and development in the field of bioabsorbable screws and other nonmetallic orthopedic implants for fracture fixation. The initial bioabsorbable hardware had problems with failure and bone resorption. The current bioabsorbable technology is more reliable and is gaining more widespread use despite its high cost. These implants may be difficult to recognize on radiographs (Fig. 6.10).

Bioabsorbable implants may be difficult to recognize on radiographs.

When screws are used to secure bony fragments to each other, they are called *interfragmentary screws*. Interfragmentary screws work biomechanically by converting torque applied to the screw into axial tension between the bone fragments. When screws are used to secure cortical plates or other hardware to bone, they are called *position screws* or *neutralization screws*.

Headless screws are used where the presence of a head may interfere with motion or cause soft tissue irritation. Headless screws may be inserted below the surface of the bone, which is desirable in osteochondral fractures and intra-articular fractures. Screws with heads may also be inserted flush with the bone surface by countersinking or drilling a larger hole for the head to drop into as the screw is driven.

Compression screws, also called *lag screws*, are threaded only at the distal portion of the shank. This type of screw compresses two objects together (bone against bone or

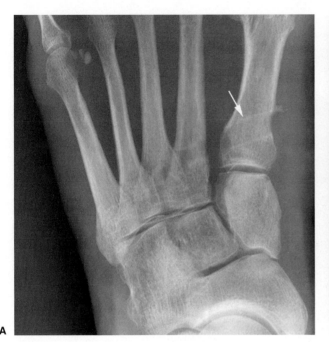
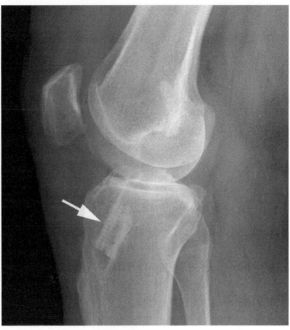

A   B

Figure 6.10 Bioabsorbable screws (different patients). *A.* Radiograph of the foot shows lucency indicating a drill hole for a bioabsorbable screw fixing first and second metatarsals (*arrow*). *B.* Radiograph of the knee shows a bioabsorbable screw (*arrow*) fixing an anterior cruciate ligament repair.

bone against another fixation device). The object into which the screw is threaded is pulled against the object through which the screw is passed. Maximal compression is obtained when the screw is oriented perpendicular to the fracture plane. A fully threaded screw fixes objects together without compressing them because the threads force them to maintain their relative positions. Screws that are fully threaded along their shanks may also be used in compression if the drill hole near the head (the glide hole) is drilled to a

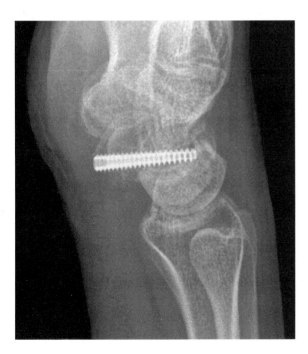

Figure 6.11 Headless, tapered, variable thread pitch compression screw fixing scaphoid waist fracture.

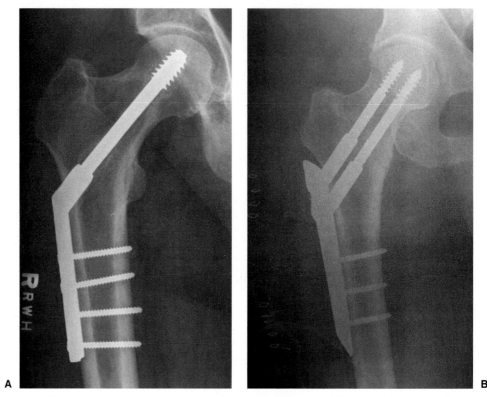

A   **B**

Figure 6.12 Fixation for intertrochanteric fractures. *A.* Telescoping (dynamic) hip screw fixing an intertrochanteric fracture. *B.* Percutaneous compression plate fixing an intertrochanteric fracture. Note the small size of the skin incisions as indicated by the skin staples.

size that the threads pass through freely. Subsequent extraction of screws is easier if they are fully threaded.

The *Accutrak screw* is a headless, fully threaded, cannulated screw with a tapered profile and a variable thread pitch (Fig. 6.11). The thread pitch is wider at one end of the screw, so that each turn of the screw compresses fragments together because of the difference in thread pitch. These screws are commonly used for internal fixation of intra-articular fractures of small bones such as the scaphoid. Were it not for the cost, they could be exceedingly useful in cabinetmaking.

Dynamic hip screws (telescoping hip screw, sliding hip screw, Richards screw) (Fig. 6.12) and dynamic condylar screws with side-plates are designed for dynamic compression of fractures of the proximal and distal femur, respectively. The screw fits into a sleeve in the side-plate into which it can slide or telescope. In an intertrochanteric hip fracture, for example, the screw extends through the femoral neck into the head, and the side-plate is fixed to the lateral cortex of the proximal shaft. With weight bearing, the unthreaded shank of the screw slides into the sleeve at the end of the side-plate, compressing the fracture fragments together. A smaller set screw that is threaded into the near end of the large-diameter sliding screw can be used to apply static compression to the fracture site at the time of surgery.

WIRES AND CABLES

Kirschner wires (K-wires) are used to fix cancellous bone in situations in which a screw might also be suitable. They are introduced percutaneously, and their purchase in bone is exclusively by friction (Fig. 6.13), which makes them easier to pull out than screws. The

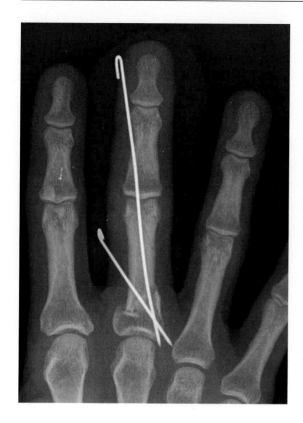

Figure 6.13 K-wire fixation. Radiograph of hand shows two K-wires fixing a fracture of the proximal phalanx of the middle finger.

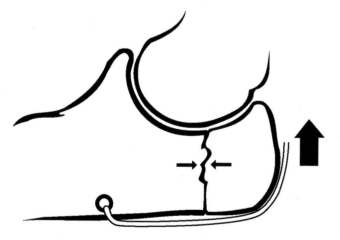

Figure 6.14 Biomechanical concept of tension band fixation. The band acts as a hinge, transforming tension on the olecranon into interfragmentary compression.

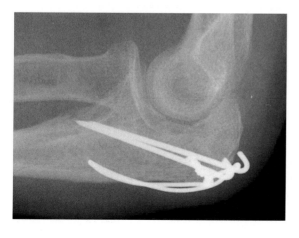

Figure 6.15 Tension band fixing olecranon fracture. The tension band passes through a hole drilled in the posterior ulnar cortex and hooks over the head of the K-wires. (Courtesy of Catherine C. Roberts, MD.)

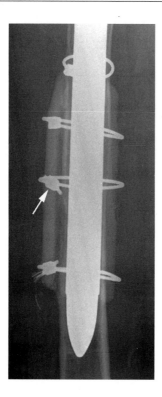

Figure 6.16 High-tension braided cable used for cerclage at the femoral shaft. The ends of the cable are secured by a crimp (*arrow*).

One end of percutaneously introduced K-wires is typically left protruding through the skin.

end of the wire is typically left protruding from the skin so that the wires can be extracted when the fracture heals.

A tension band transforms tensile stress into interfragmentary compression (Fig. 6.14). Tension bands are commonly used where asymmetric muscle tension tends to distract fragments. The tension band is usually a wire loop or figure-of-eight that is placed across the fracture site along the line of tensile force. When the muscle contracts, the tension band acts like a hinge to compress the fracture fragments together. For example, a transverse fracture of the olecranon process could be fixed by a tension band along the posterior aspect of the triceps mechanism. With contraction of the triceps muscles, the tension band functions as a hinge and converts the distractive force along the posterior aspect of the olecranon to compressive force on the opposite side (Fig. 6.15). Tension bands are also commonly used to fix transverse fractures of the patella.

Cerclage wires encircle the shaft of a bone and can be used to hold fragments to the shaft. They are usually placed in combination with intramedullary (IM) rods or cortical plates. Wires are made of stainless steel and cobalt chrome alloy and are commonly in the form of monofilament wires or high-tension braided cables with multiple filaments attached with a crimp (Fig. 6.16).

CORTICAL PLATES

Cortical plates placed on the periosteal surface are secured to bone by position screws and should be considered internal splints for holding together structural defects and not load-bearing members. Compression across the fracture components is critical to protect the plate from failure. Plates function through the biomechanical principles of static compression, dynamic compression, buttressing, and neutralization. Static compression can be maintained by a plate when it is applied while the fracture site is being compressed during surgery (Fig. 6.17). Compression can also be applied through specially designed screw holes and eccentrically placed screws. Small plates may be used

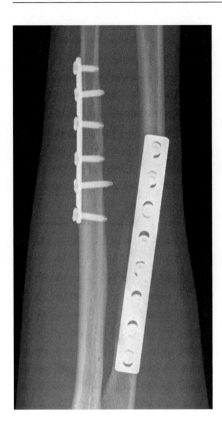

Figure 6.17 Cortical plates (dynamic compression plates) fixing fractures of the distal radial and ulnar shafts. Note the eccentric screw placement in the oval holes of the plate.

to fix small fragments. When placed on a bone with asymmetric muscle pull such as the femur, a plate placed with initial static compression may subsequently function with dynamic compression through the tension band principle when weight bearing resumes. Plates can also be contoured to fit the particular shape of the bone to which they are applied (Fig. 6.18), either at the time of manufacture or at the time of surgery. Buttress plates are broader on one end than the other and may be used to fix meta-

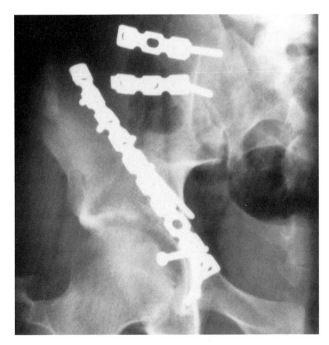

Figure 6.18 Malleable cortical plates fixing pelvic fractures.

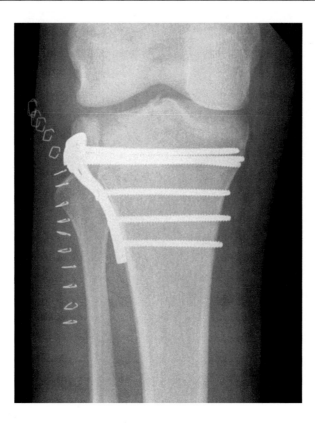

Figure 6.19 Buttress plate fixating proximal metaphyseal fracture of the tibia.

Neutralization plates counter the stresses on an internally fixed fracture but generally do not provide interfragmentary compression.

physeal fractures of long bones such as the distal radius or the proximal tibia (Fig. 6.19). A buttress plate used dynamically transforms shearing stress directed along the longitudinal axis of the bone into compressive force across the fracture plane. Neutralization plates counter the stresses on an internally fixed fracture but are not intended to

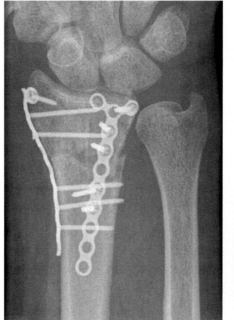

A

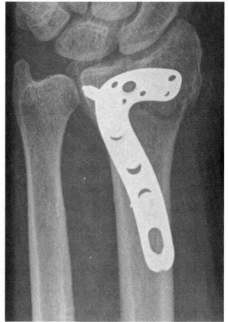

B

Figure 6.20 Specialized cortical plates for distal radius fixation. *A.* Small cortical plates and screws fixing a comminuted intra-articular fracture. *B.* Contoured low-profile cortical plate fixing a comminuted intra-articular fracture.

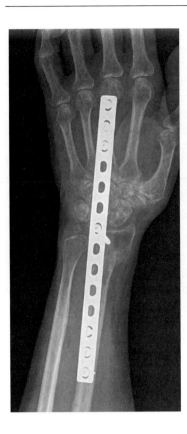

Figure 6.21 Cortical plate used as a bridge for comminuted intra-articular fractures of the distal radius and ulna.

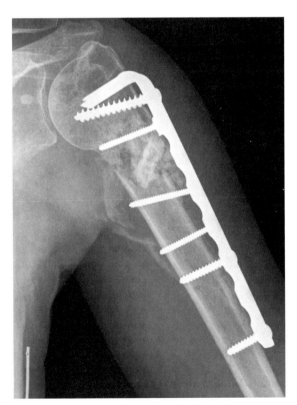

Figure 6.22 Blade plate traversing a comminuted proximal humerus fracture.

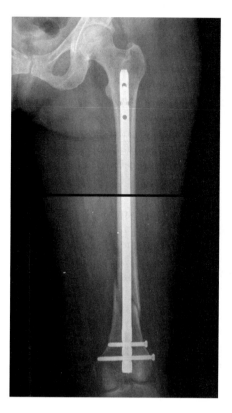

Figure 6.26 Retrograde intramedullary rod fixing an oblique fracture of the distal femoral shaft with locking screws.

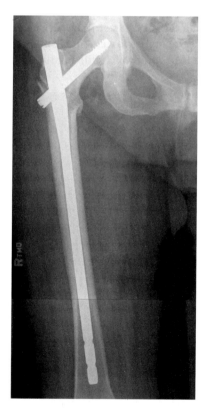

Figure 6.27 Gamma nail fixation of a subtrochanteric femur fracture.

provide interfragmentary compression. When neutralization plates are used to maintain length and position, one or more interfragmentary screws are also used to hold the fracture fragments together. The interfragmentary screws are generally oriented perpendicular to the fracture plane for maximum compression. Interfragmentary screws may also pass through one of the holes in the neutralization plate.

Recent developments in plate technology have emphasized low-profile designs for specific anatomic sites and specific types of fractures. An example is at the distal radius, a common site of fracture, where cortical plates have become much smaller and specific plates are available for various subtypes of fractures (Fig. 6.20). Cortical plates can be used for bridging a comminuted distal radius fracture (Fig. 6.21). In this circumstance, the bridge extends from the radial shaft, across the fracture site and the carpal bones, to the third metacarpal.

A blade plate is a cortical plate with an angled blade that is inserted sideways into the end of a bone while the plate is affixed to the cortex of the shaft with position screws. Blade plates are used at sites like the proximal femur, the distal femur, and the proximal humerus (Fig. 6.22), where normal muscle pull would tend to destabilize a simple plate. Blade plates have been replaced in many circumstances by telescoping screws with side-plates and by specialized IM rods.

RODS AND NAILS

An IM rod is an internal splint that promotes fracture healing through callus formation.

IM rods or nails are used to treat long-bone fractures. In closed nailing, the rod is inserted into one end of the fractured bone and passed across the fracture site under fluoroscopic guidance. In open nailing, the rod is passed across the fracture site under direct surgical visualization. The medullary space is usually reamed so that it can accommodate the rod, destroying the endosteal blood supply but depositing finely morselized bone and marrow elements at the fracture site; this osseous autograft enhances fracture healing. The endosteal blood supply reconstitutes in approximately

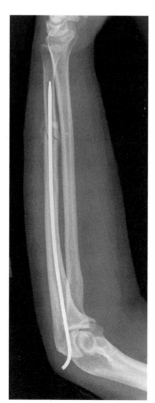

Figure 6.23 Small intramedullary rod for fixation of an ulnar shaft fracture.

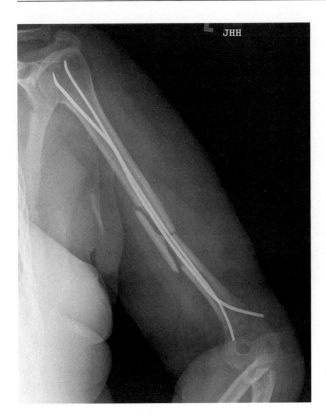

Figure 6.24 Humeral shaft fracture fixed by two Enders rods inserted retrograde through the condyles.

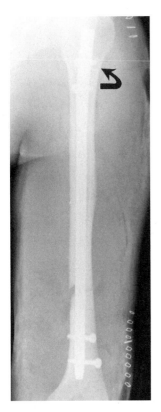

Figure 6.25 Humeral shaft fracture fixed by proximally (*arrow*) and distally locked intramedullary rod.

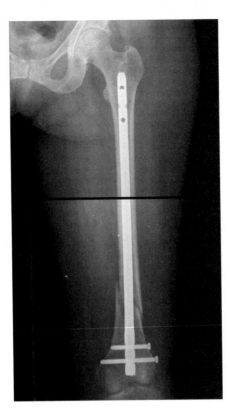

Figure 6.26 Retrograde intramedullary rod fixing an oblique fracture of the distal femoral shaft with locking screws.

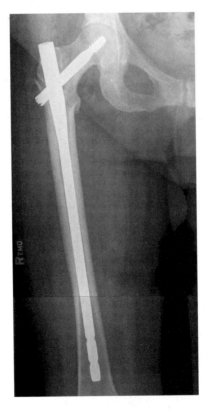

Figure 6.27 Gamma nail fixation of a subtrochanteric femur fracture.

3 weeks. The periosteal blood supply is preserved. An IM rod typically functions as a load-sharing device or an internal splint. Small, flexible IM rods can be placed into small non–weight-bearing bones (Fig. 6.23). Larger bones may require multiple IM rods for fixation and strength (Fig. 6.24). If the rod is locked on both ends by cross-screws (Fig. 6.25), it ceases to function as a load-sharing device and becomes a load-bearing device. When the limb is loaded, the stresses are transferred from the bone to one end of the rod by the cross-screws, travel along the length of the rod past the fracture site, and finally are dispersed by the cross-screws at the other end, thus preventing load on the fracture site. Locking also allows control and reduction of rotary displacement. As periosteal callus is formed and the fracture begins to stabilize, one set of locking screws may be removed, allowing load sharing by the healing bone. This technique of removing the locking screws from the longer fragment is called *dynamization.*

Rods may be inserted across a fracture site in an antegrade fashion or a retrograde fashion (Fig. 6.26). The direction of insertion can be identified on radiographs by the locations of the blunt and tapered ends, with the tapered end pointing in the direction of insertion and the blunt end located at the site of insertion.

New designs in IM rods have resulted in rods intended for fractures of specific bones, including the humerus, radius, ulna, femur, and tibia. These rods take into account the biomechanical requirements of each site as well as the unique anatomy and the technical demands of the various operative sites. For example, the gamma nail is designed specifically for subtrochanteric femur fractures (Fig. 6.27).

EXTERNAL FIXATION

External fixation allows a fractured limb to be reduced or stabilized by the manipulation of externally projecting pins or wires secured to the limb on both sides of the fracture

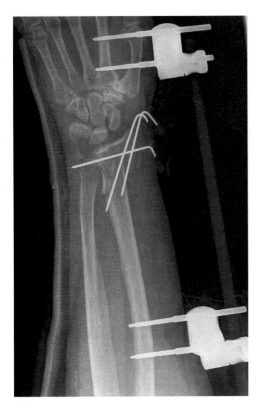

Figure 6.28 Comminuted intra-articular fractures of the distal radius and ulna. The distal radius fragments have been fixed by K-wires. The entire wrist has been stabilized by a pin-rod external fixator.

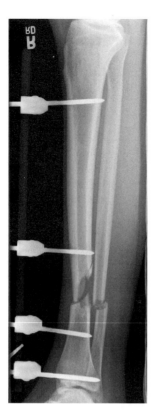

Figure 6.29 Distal tibial fractures stabilized with pin-rod external fixator. The rod is radiolucent carbon fiber.

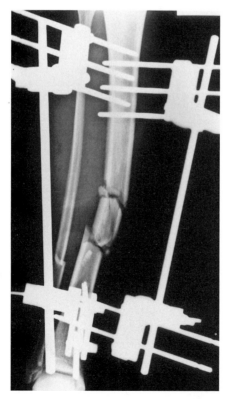

Figure 6.30 Segmental tibial shaft fracture stabilized with pin-rod external fixation in two planes.

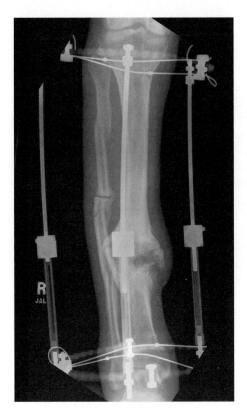

Figure 6.31 Ilizarov external fixator for treatment of nonunion.

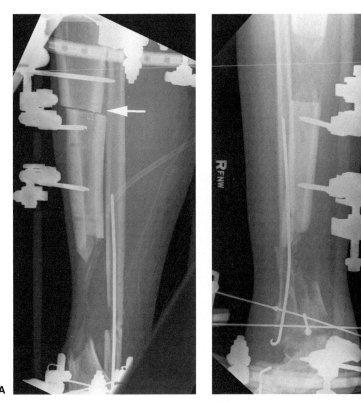

A   B

Figure 6.32 Hybrid pin-rod and ring external fixation for bone transport after loss of a segment of bone during an open tibial fracture. *A.* Lateral radiograph 1 month after trauma shows the large proximal gap in the tibial shaft, the ring fixator, and a proximal osteotomy (*arrow*). *B.* Lateral radiograph at 6 months shows further transport of the middle fragment.

Externally fixed fractures unite by secondary bone healing.

site. Surgical trauma to the fracture site is avoided. The fixation is more rigid and allows earlier mobility than closed methods. The fractures unite by secondary bone healing. External fixation is favored for types II and III open fractures, in which distraction of the limb is appropriate and rapid surgical stabilization is necessary. The two major types of external fixators are pins attached to rods (pin fixators) and wires stretched on circular frames that are attached to rods (ring fixators). Pin fixators are secured to bone with pins that are introduced surgically or percutaneously (Figs. 6.28 and 6.29). Different fixator configurations can be tailored to the specific fracture site and morphology. Many fractures require external fixation in two planes for stability (Fig. 6.30). Pin fixators can be applied rapidly in emergent situations and are used often for pelvic fractures in which early reduction and fixation can realign the soft tissues and avert life-threatening hemorrhage. Ring fixators (Ilizarov fixators) are secured to bone through a pair of crossed, unthreaded, transfixion wires that are stretched on a circular frame. These circular frames are attached to longitudinal connecting rods. The fragments are reduced by adjusting the position of the rings relative to each other. A nonunion may be addressed by compression to induce healing followed by distraction to restore length (Fig. 6.31). A fragment of bone can be transported axially by successive adjustments of the rings along the longitudinal rods on the order of 1 mm per day (Fig. 6.32). Modular systems of external fixation allow the surgeon to fit hybrid frames to complex, complicated fractures using both pins and rings.

SOFT TISSUE HEALING AND REPAIR

Healing tendons and ligaments remodel along lines of stress.

Tendon and ligament healing occurs in phases. Initially, the wound fills with blood, inflammatory products, and fibrin. Proliferating granulation tissue then fills the gap, and over a period of weeks to months, fibroblasts and collagen fibers begin to unite the injured ends. The healing tissue then remodels and matures as the fibroblasts and collagen fibers become oriented along the lines of stress, a process that may continue over

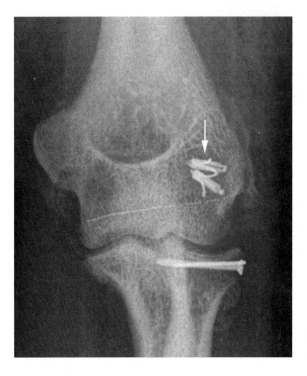

Figure 6.33 Soft tissue anchors in the distal humerus (*arrow*).

many months. Direct repair of tendons and ligaments is generally performed by suturing the injured ends together. When a soft tissue structure has been avulsed from a bony attachment, it may be reattached using a variety of devices, including sutures, wires, screws, pins, and soft tissue anchors. When screws are used, washers are generally placed between the screw head and the soft tissues to increase the surface area apposed to the bone and to decrease trauma caused by the screw itself. Soft tissue anchors are small devices that are embedded into the bone and have loops through which sutures may be passed (Fig. 6.33). Soft tissue anchors are available in a variety of sizes, shapes, and materials, including plastic, metal, and bioabsorbable materials. With healing, the biomechanical integrity of the soft tissue attachment is reestablished, and the fixation device is no longer needed.

GRAFTS AND IMPLANTS

Soft tissue grafts and bone grafts are commonly used to reconstruct severe open fractures, particularly where significant fragments of bone have been ejected from the limb at the time of trauma or débrided at the time of initial treatment (Fig. 6.34). Bone grafts used for trauma reconstruction are typically small pieces of cortico-cancellous bone rather than massive allografts. Large defects in cortical bone are generally reconstructed by bone transport rather than grafting.

Structural biomaterials as substitutes for bone is an active area of research in orthopedics. Materials that may soon gain widespread use in the United States include genetically engineered bone growth factors, bioabsorbable hardware, and metallic implants with bone-like mechanical and physical properties.

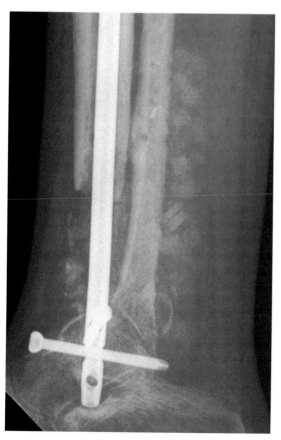

Figure 6.34 Bone graft for open fracture of the ankle.

SPINE FIXATION

Because of the complex anatomy, the presence of the spinal cord and nerve roots, the small bones, and the large number of joints, fixation of the spinal column after trauma requires specialized hardware and techniques.

Stable injuries of the posterior column may require only fixation of the posterior elements at the levels involved. Many cervical spine injuries are treated with reduction and fusion of the posterior elements using wires and bone graft (Fig. 6.35). Posterior column injuries may also be treated with pedicle screws and rods, a process in which a series of pedicle screws inserted posteriorly are attached to contoured rods. Depending on the biomechanical stresses at the level of injury, multiple levels above and below the injury may be included in the stabilization procedure. Anterior column fractures such as compression fractures can be treated by internal fixation of the vertebral bodies above and below the level of injury with plates and screws and restoration of the height of the fractured vertebra using bone graft. The bone graft may be structural allograft or small cortico-cancellous chips and fragments, maintained in place by a wire fusion cage (Fig. 6.36).

Unstable injuries involving the anterior and posterior column generally require both anterior and posterior stabilization. The rods may be placed posterior to the spine and secured to the vertebral bodies by pedicle screws above and below the level of injury. Anterior stabilization can be performed with bone graft, hardware, or a combination (Fig. 6.37). At the time of surgery, the spinal canal is also decompressed.

Simple osteoporotic compression fractures may be treated by vertebroplasty. Vertebroplasty is a procedure in which methylmethacrylate cement is injected percutaneously under fluoroscopic guidance into the involved vertebral body (see Chapter 18). The injected cement is rendered radiodense by the addition of barium or other materials so that it can be observed during fluoroscopy and on subsequent radiographs (Fig. 6.38).

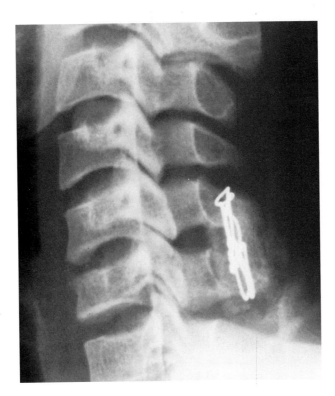

Figure 6.35 Posterior fusion of cervical spine (C5-C6) with bone graft and wires.

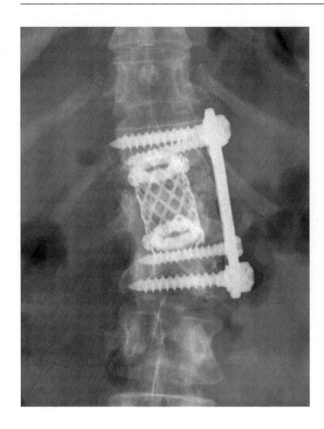

Figure 6.36 Healing T12 burst fracture. AP radiograph shows T12 corpectomy with bone graft and internal fixation. A fusion cage filled with bone graft has been inserted between T11 and L1.

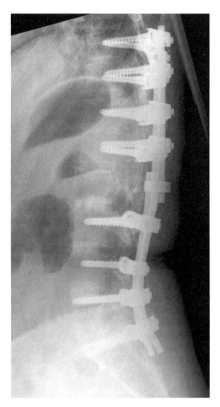

Figure 6.37 Combined anterior and posterior thoracloumbar spine fusion with anterior bone graft and posterior pedicle screws with rods.

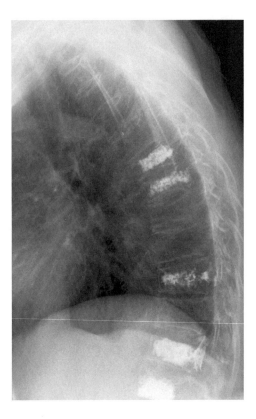

Figure 6.38 Multiple osteoporotic compression fractures after vertebroplasty. Lateral radiograph shows osteoporosis with multiple wedging deformities, five of which have been treated by vertebroplasty.

COMPLICATIONS

Complications of fractures may be immediate or delayed (Table 6.2).

FAILURE OF FRACTURE HEALING

Fracture healing is impaired or slow when the patient is elderly or in poor nutritional condition, when the local blood supply is poor, and when the fragments are displaced rather than apposed. Intracapsular fractures (within the joint capsule) heal slowly because the intracapsular part of the bone does not support periosteal callus formation, and synovial fluid lyses the blood clot. Necrotic bone fragments cannot participate in the healing process until they are revascularized. An extensive fracture heals more slowly than a limited one. A fracture through cortical bone heals more slowly than one through cancellous bone. A fracture with significant soft tissue damage heals more slowly than one with little soft tissue damage. An infected fracture will not heal.

Distraction of fragments or excessive motion between them may result in nonunion. Nonunion is an arrest of the healing process before there is bony union of the fragments. The bone ends become osteoporotic and atrophied or hypertrophic and sclerotic (Figs. 6.39 and 6.40). The space between the bony fragments usually contains dense fibrous tissue and sometimes may be clinically stable. Alternatively, a false joint lined with synovium and filled with synovial fluid (pseudoarthrosis) may form in the gap between nonunited fracture fragments (Fig. 6.41); this tends to occur when there has been excessive motion at the fracture site. Malunion occurs when the fracture fragments heal in poor position or alignment so that functional or cosmetic problems ensue. The presence of malunion is a clinical, not a radiologic, diagnosis. Other notable variations in fracture healing include delayed union, in which there is a longer-than-average healing process, and slow union, in which the healing process is protracted but progressive.

Failure of an internally fixed fracture to heal is usually caused by a gap between fragments or excessive motion at the fracture site. The result is failure or loosening of the fix-

Nonunion is an arrest of the healing process before there is bony union of the fragments.

Table 6.2: Fracture Complications

Immediate complications
  Shock
  Hemorrhage
  Thromboembolism
  Disseminated intravascular coagulopathy
  Fat embolism
  Gas gangrene
  Tetanus
  Osteonecrosis
  Posttraumatic reflex sympathetic dystrophy
  Compartment syndrome
  Osteomyelitis
Delayed complications
  Failure to heal
  Posttraumatic degenerative joint disease
  Posttraumatic chondrolysis
  Remote stress injuries
  Refracture
  Chronic pain and instability
  Myositis ossificans
  Failure or migration of implant
  Synostosis

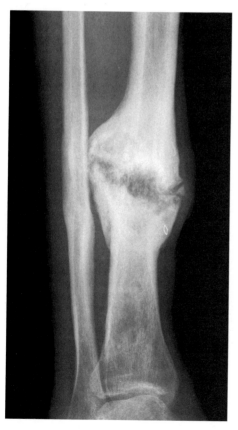

Figure 6.39 Hypertrophic nonunion of the tibial shaft.

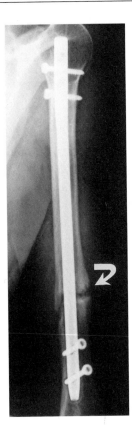

Figure 6.40 Humeral shaft fracture with nonunion (*arrow*). The ends of the fragments have developed cortex.

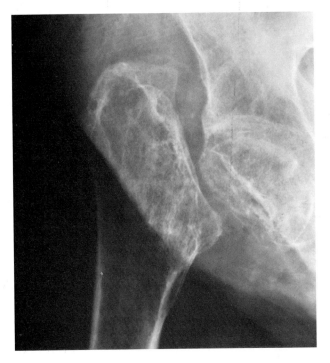

Figure 6.41 Nonunion of a femoral neck fracture with pseudoarthrosis. The femoral neck and distal head have been resorbed. The margins of bone adjacent to the fracture line are sclerotic and smooth.

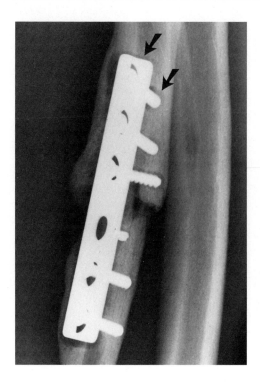

Figure 6.42 Cortical plate with loss of fixation and atrophic nonunion. The lucent zones (*arrows*) around the plate and each of the individual screws indicate bone resorption. The fracture lines are clearly visible, and no callus is present.

ation device. Loosening is evident on radiographs by the presence of a lucent zone around the device. This lucent zone corresponds to resorption of bone, indicating that the device no longer has a stable purchase (Fig. 6.42). There is often a thin zone of sclerosis at the metal–bone interface (Fig. 6.43). Hardware that shifts in position from examination to examination may indicate loosening (Fig. 6.44). Catastrophic loss of fixation with breakage of hardware may occur when there is too much biomechanical stress on the reconstructed part and there is progressive angulation or displacement (Figs. 6.45 and 6.46).

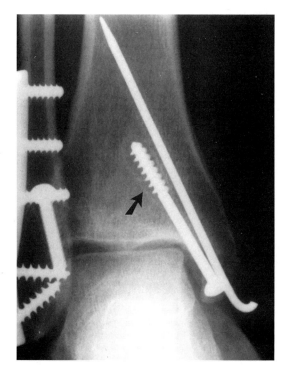

Figure 6.43 Loose compression screw and K-wire in healed medial malleolar fracture. A thin zone of sclerosis (*arrow*) demarcates the region of bone resorption around the hardware.

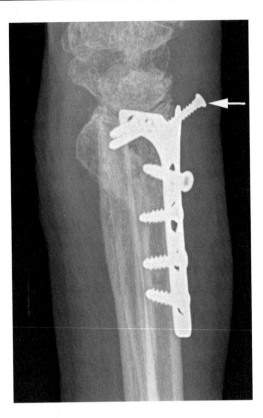

Figure 6.44 Loose screw protruding into soft tissues.

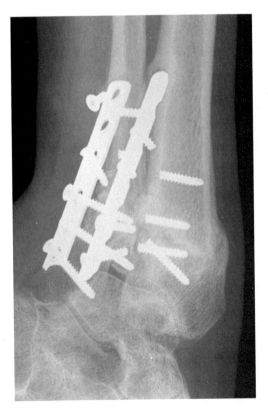

Figure 6.45 Fractured screws at the ankle.

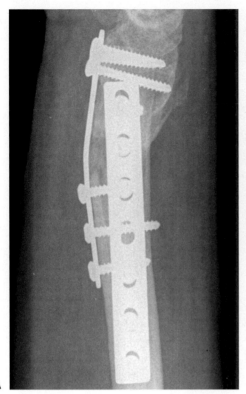
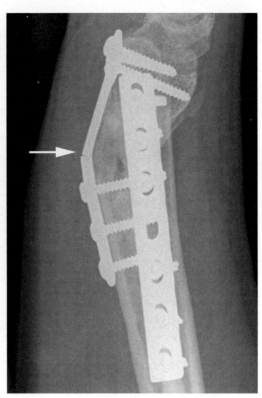

Figure 6.46 Fractured plate at a comminuted distal radius fracture. *A.* Lateral radiograph 6 weeks after internal fixation shows mild dorsal angulation and bending of the volar cortical plate. *B.* Lateral radiograph 12 weeks after internal fixation shows progression of angulation with fracture of plate (*arrow*).

OTHER COMPLICATIONS

Fat embolism is an acute complication that may occur when fatty marrow gains access to the venous system as a result of a fracture, usually of the long bones. Fat is liquid at body temperature and pours out of a fractured bone into the soft tissues, where it may enter the veins and travel to the lungs. Fat emboli appear to provoke a chemical pneumonitis rather than cause pulmonary infarction.

Avascular necrosis of bone may occur when the blood supply is compromised by the injury or by the fixation device. Normally, bones become osteoporotic in response to fracture healing. Avascular necrosis can be recognized on radiographs because necrotic, devascularized bone does not become osteoporotic (Fig. 6.47). Common sites of avascular necrosis after fracture include the femoral head, the proximal pole of the scaphoid, and the proximal pole of the talus. MRI may show osteonecrosis before radiographs.

Infection may occur as a complication of the primary injury or secondarily during treatment. Infection can be recognized radiographically as a nonhealing fracture with progressive bone loss, but the process may be far advanced before radiographic changes are noticeable (Fig. 6.48). External fixators are vulnerable to infection at the insertion sites of wires or pins through the skin into the bone (Fig. 6.49). Pin infections can be recognized by osteolysis at the site of insertion.

Untreated or unrecognized soft tissue injuries may result in chronic pain and instability, often with devastating disability. This is a particular problem in the wrist, knee, and shoulder. MRI and arthrography are the two radiologic modalities most useful for delineating injuries to ligaments and cartilage in these regions.

Posttraumatic reflex sympathetic dystrophy (complex regional pain syndrome, Sudeck atrophy) is a painful swelling of an extremity with rapid onset after an injury. The injury may be a fracture but is often minor. The site of swelling and pain is usually

Common sites of posttraumatic avascular necrosis include the femoral head, the proximal pole of the scaphoid, and the proximal pole of the talus.

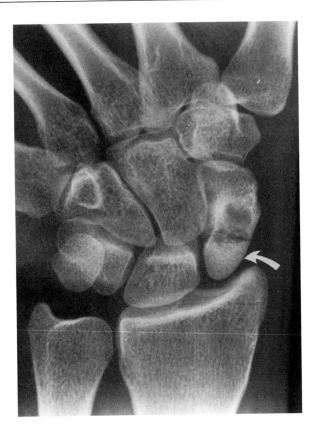

Figure 6.47 Scaphoid wrist fracture with nonunion and osteonecrosis. The proximal fragment is denser (*arrow*) than the other bones. Bone has been resorbed from the fracture site.

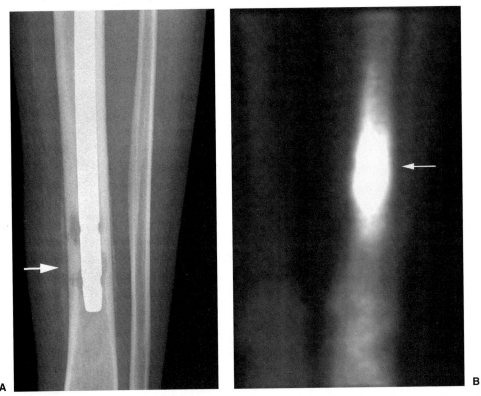

A

B

Figure 6.48 Infected intramedullary rod. *A.* Radiograph of the tibia shows lucencies (*arrow*) around the distal end of the rod. *B.* White cell scan shows intense accumulation of activity (*arrow*) corresponding to the same location.

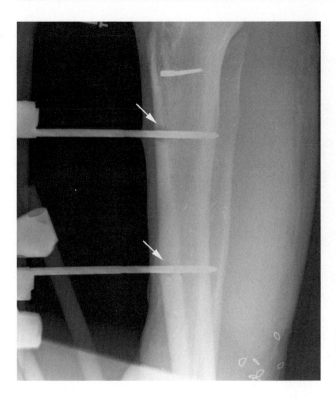

Figure 6.49 Infected pin-rod external fixator. Focal osteolysis (*arrows*) is present where the pins traverse the tibial cortex.

in the ipsilateral limb but remote from the site of trauma. The cause is thought to be neurovascular. Regional soft tissue swelling and acute osteoporosis are evident at onset (Fig. 6.50). Soft tissue atrophy may follow subsidence of the acute symptoms; the bone usually remains osteoporotic.

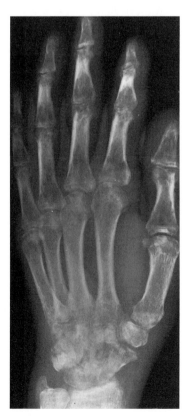

Figure 6.50 Posttraumatic reflex sympathetic dystrophy. Acute osteoporosis and painful soft tissue swelling of the entire hand occurred after a fracture of the ipsilateral scapula.

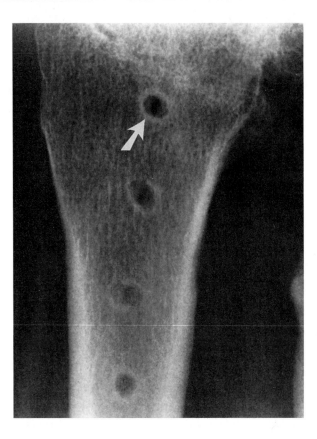

Figure 6.51 Healed screw holes in the distal radial metaphysis where a cortical plate was used for fixation. The margins of the holes have become corticated (*arrow*).

   Failure of implanted orthopedic devices may lead to poor healing or chronic pain. Some implant failures have led to multi million-dollar class-action lawsuits.
   Scars in bone may remain after removal of internal fixation devices. Small holes in the cortex from the removal of screws or pins do not fill in with bone but remodel by cortication of the edges (Fig. 6.51). During loading, stress tends to concentrate at irregularities in bone or at the sites of hardware. Subsequent fractures tend to begin at such "stress risers" (Fig. 6.52).

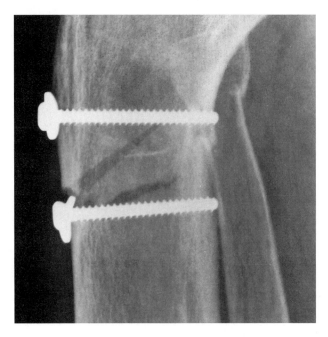

Figure 6.52 Tibial fracture line passes through screws from previous osteotomy.

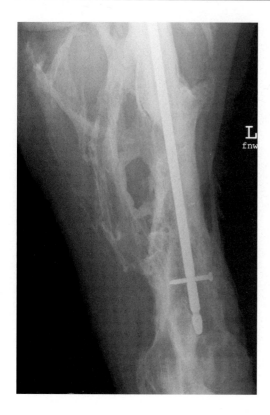

Figure 6.53 Posttraumatic myositis ossificans.

Altered stresses and biomechanics related to a fracture may result in remote complications such as stress injuries to contralateral limbs. A fracture with mechanical fixation in place may not remodel because the site is shielded from mechanical stress. An insufficiency fracture may follow the removal of the fixation device.

Posttraumatic degenerative joint disease may occur because of direct damage to the articular surfaces or the subchondral bone (see Chapter 13). Malunion and altered patterns of stress on joints adjacent to a fracture site may also lead to degenerative changes, particularly in weight-bearing joints. Posttraumatic chondrolysis is an articular complication in which there is rapid, generalized dissolution of the articular cartilage of the traumatized bones; the process is poorly understood.

Myositis ossificans is heterotopic ossification in the soft tissues. Posttraumatic myositis ossificans may follow soft tissue injury, resulting in mature bone formation at the site (Fig. 6.53). Although mechanical problems may ensue, the heterotopic bone will usually remodel and may ultimately be resorbed. Occasionally, myositis ossificans may be mistaken for sarcoma on MRI or other imaging, but clinical correlation and follow-up will clarify the issue.

COMPLICATIONS OF SPINE FIXATION

Complications of spine fixation include misplacement of pedicle screws (Fig. 6.54), nerve root injury, dural sac tear, infection, and loss of fixation (Fig. 6.55). CT with myelography is often the best method for imaging the spine after fixation, although MRI can be safely used. Artifacts on MRI from metallic implants may render a study difficult to interpret.

IMAGING AFTER TREATMENT

Standard radiographs are the usual method of imaging fracture healing. Early radiographs may be obtained to check the accuracy of the reduction and the appropriateness of fixation device placement. Subsequent films follow the healing process or investigate complications. The presence of hardware often requires nonstandard oblique views so that the frac-

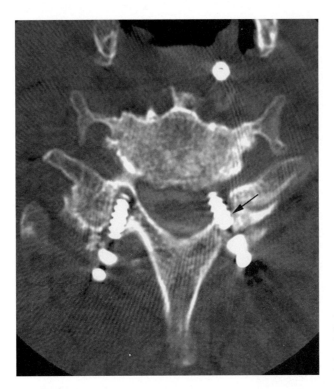

Figure 6.54 Misplaced pedicle screw. Axial CT image after myelography shows a pedicle screw (*arrow*) extending into spinal canal and neural foramen.

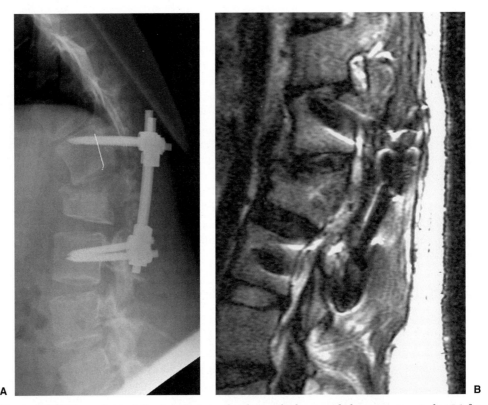

A   B

Figure 6.55 Failure of spinal fixation. *A.* Lateral radiograph shows pedicle screws inserted at L1 for posterior stabilization of superior end-plate compression fracture of L2 have shifted in position, allowing the spine to collapse into kyphosis. *B.* Sagittal T1-weighted MRI excludes nonmechanical causes of failure.

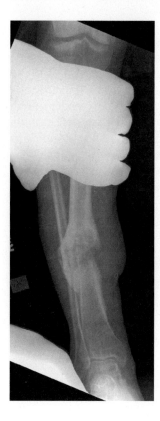

Figure 6.56 Fracture nonunion demonstrated by AP radiograph with valgus stress.

ture site is not obscured by the device. Sometimes, positioning under fluoroscopy may be helpful in projecting metal away from the bone, revealing the fractures. Stress radiographs may identify motion at a fracture site, indicating nonunion (Fig. 6.56). Additional constraints on positioning for radiographs may be imposed by external fixators, external supports, or traction devices.

Conventional tomography may help blur overlying bones and devices, improving the visibility of the fracture site, but this modality is no longer available in some radiology departments. CT can be helpful when the examination has been tailored to a specific situation (Fig. 6.57). Because many fractures are oriented transversely to the axis of the long

Multidetector CT with multiplanar reconstructions is the study of choice for imaging complicated fractures with hardware.

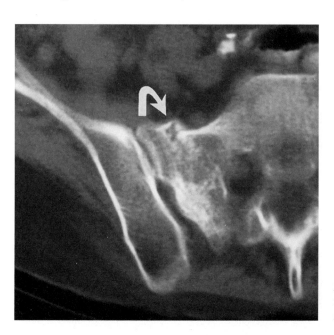

Figure 6.57 Healing impacted fracture of the right sacral wing shown by axial CT (*arrow*).

bones, the fractures are often in the same plane as the imaging, and structures smaller than 1 mm may be obscured by partial volume averaging. Metal implants cause artifacts on CT occasionally severe enough to obscure the fracture site. Fracture hardware and small implants such as metallic sutures or vascular clips may produce major artifacts on MRI that limit its usefulness after fractures. Even when nothing has been implanted, microscopic metal debris from drills and other instruments may produce artifacts that render a study useless. However, orthopedic hardware used for fracture fixation does not deflect in the magnetic fields used for MRI, and patients may be safely placed into these scanners for imaging anatomic regions somewhat remote from the implant. Radionuclide bone scans are occasionally helpful in demonstrating the presence of physiologic activity at a fracture site. Nuclear scans with labeled leukocytes or gallium as well as positron emission tomography may occasionally be helpful when there is a question of infection.

SOURCES AND READINGS

Behrens F. A primer of fixator devices and configurations. *Clin Orthop* 1989;241:5–14.

Boles CA, Daniel WW, Adams BD, et al. Hand and wrist. *Radiol Clin North Am* 1995;33:319–354.

Browner BD, Levine AM, Jupiter JB, et al., eds. *Skeletal trauma: fractures, dislocations, ligamentous injuries*, 2nd ed. Philadelphia: WB Saunders, 1998.

Bucholz RW, Heckman JD, eds. *Rockwood and Green's fractures in adults*, 5th ed. Philadelphia: Lippincott Williams & Wilkins, 2001.

Buckwalter JA, Einhorn TA, Simon SR. *Orthopaedic bioscience: biology and biomechanics of the musculoskeletal system*, 2nd ed. American Academy of Orthopaedic Surgeons, 2000.

Chew FS, Pappas CN. Fracture fixation hardware in the extremities. *Radiol Clin North Am* 1995;33:375–390.

Eustace S, Goldberg R, Williamson D, et al. MR imaging of soft tissues adjacent to orthopaedic hardware: techniques to minimize susceptibility artefact. *Clin Radiol* 1997;52:589–594.

Leibovic SJ. Internal fixation sets for use in the hand. A comparison of available instrumentation. *Hand Clin* 1997;13:531–540.

Pruefer D, Kalden P, Schreiber W, et al. In vitro investigation of prosthetic heart valves in magnetic resonance imaging: evaluation of potential hazards. *J Heart Valve Dis* 2001;10:410–414.

Rommens PM, Blum J, Runkel M. Retrograde nailing of humeral shaft fractures. *Clin Orthop* 1998;350:26–29.

Scalea TM, Boswell SA, Scott JD, et al. External fixation as a bridge to intramedullary nailing for patients with multiple injuries and with femur fractures: damage control orthopedics. *J Trauma* 2000;48:613–621.

Shellock FG, Morisoli S, Kanal E. MR procedures and biomedical implants, materials, and devices: 1993 update. *Radiology* 1993;189:587–599.

Slone RM, Heare MM, Van der Griend RA, et al. Orthopedic fixation devices. *Radiographics* 1991;11:823–847.

Slone RM, Slone RM, McEnery KW, et al. Fixation techniques and instrumentation used in the thoracic, lumbar, and lumbosacral spine. *Radiol Clin North Am* 1995;33:233–265.

Suh JS, Jeong EK, Shin KH, et al. Minimizing artifacts caused by metallic implants at MR imaging: experimental and clinical studies. *AJR Am J Roentgenol* 1998;171:1207–1213.

Tencer AF, Johnson KD. *Biomechanics in orthopedic trauma: bone fracture and fixation*. Philadelphia: JB Lippincott, 1994.

Uhthoff HK, ed. *Current concepts of external fixation of fractures*. New York: Springer-Verlag, 1982.

Watson MA, Mathias KJ, Maffulli N. External ring fixators: an overview. *Proc Inst Mech Eng* 2000;214:459–470.

Wyrsch B, Mencio GA, Green NE. Open reduction and internal fixation of pediatric forearm fractures. *J Pediatr Orthop* 1996;16:644–650.

Yang AP, Iannacone WM. External fixation for pelvic ring disruptions. *Orthop Clin North Am* 1997;28:331–344.

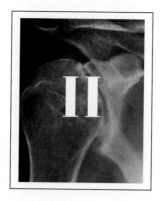

TUMORS

Approach to Bone Lesions

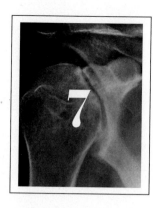

- Incidence
- Cardinal Principle
- Patient Factors
- Location of Lesion
- Rate of Growth
- Tissue Characterization
- Staging
- Treatment
- Metastases
- Sources and Readings

Incidence

Malignant primary musculoskeletal tumors represent less than 1% of all cancers. Approximately 2,500 new cases of primary bone malignancies and 6,400 new cases of primary connective tissue malignancies are reported annually in the United States. A malignant tumor located in bone is much more likely to be a metastasis or multiple myeloma than a primary sarcoma. The average practicing radiologist may see a new primary bone malignancy every few years; many clinicians never see one. Thus, it is often the radiologist who is the physician with the first and best opportunity to suggest the diagnosis and who may guide the initial evaluation and management. Because the prognosis of primary bone and soft tissue malignancies is often related to initial management, it is crucial for the radiologist to know both the clinical and the radiologic features of these lesions. As a general rule, patients in whom a primary malignant musculoskeletal tumor is suspected should be referred to a medical center with special expertise. Obtaining the biopsy should be the very last (not first) step in the diagnostic process and is best performed by a member of the multidisciplinary team that will provide the definitive care. A hasty attempt at biopsy that violates and contaminates otherwise unaffected tissue planes may compromise the definitive procedure and necessitate a more extensive operation with a worse prognosis.

Primary bone tumors are rare, but radiologists must be able to recognize them.

A situation that arises more frequently than the tumors themselves is the discovery of an incidental bone lesion for which a primary malignant bone tumor is a differential diagnostic possibility. It is more important for the radiologist to know with confidence which lesions are not aggressive tumors than to know which specific entity an aggressive bone tumor might be.

Cardinal Principle

The cardinal principle in the diagnosis of solitary bone lesions is that the radiologic appearance reflects the underlying pathology of the abnormal lesional tissue and its interplay with the host bone. The radiologic images are best understood when the underlying pathologic processes are also understood; this principle applies regardless of the particular imaging

The radiologic appearance of a lesion reflects the lesion's underlying pathology and its interplay with the host bone.

Table 7.1: Frequency of 8,591 Primary Malignant Bone Tumors in the Mayo Clinic Series

Type of Tumor	Frequency (%)
Myeloma	44
Osteosarcoma (including variants)	20
Chondrosarcoma (including variants)	12
Lymphoma	8
Ewing sarcoma	6
Chordoma	4
Fibrosarcoma/malignant fibrous histiocytoma	4
Hemangioendothelioma	1
Others	1

Adapted from Unni KK. *Dahlin's bone tumors. General aspects and data on 11,087 cases,* 5th ed. Philadelphia: Lippincott–Raven, 1996.

modality. Knowledge regarding the histogenesis and clinicopathologic classification of many lesions is controversial and in constant flux. However, a few pathologic entities account for the majority of these lesions (Table 7.1).

The standard radiologic approach addresses four issues: (a) patient factors, especially age; (b) location within the skeleton and within the involved bone; (c) rate of growth or aggressiveness; and (d) tissue characterization from specific features such as mineralization. Careful consideration of these factors may lead to a diagnostic conclusion that is almost certain. Often, however, the diagnosis can only be narrowed to several entities or may even be completely uncertain.

In many musculoskeletal lesions, the pathologic examination is not sufficient to provide a definitive diagnosis. In many cases, the radiologic appearance and clinical course of the lesion are equally important. Thus, if a lesion has specific radiologic features that narrow the differential diagnosis, the radiologist should be prepared to defend his or her diagnosis—even in the face of a contrary opinion from the pathologist.

PATIENT FACTORS

Most bone lesions tend to affect particular age groups. Therefore, knowing the patient's age is often valuable in distinguishing among lesions with similar radiologic features or lesions with nonspecific appearances (Table 7.2). Many lesions affect a broad age range. Most bone

Table 7.2: Most Frequently Encountered Types of Primary Malignant Bone Tumors at Various Ages[a]

0–9 yr	10–19 yr	20–29 yr	≥30 yr
Ewing sarcoma	Osteosarcoma	Osteosarcoma	Myeloma
Osteosarcoma	Ewing sarcoma	Chondrosarcoma	Chondrosarcoma
Primary lymphoma	Primary lymphoma	Ewing sarcoma	Osteosarcoma
		Primary lymphoma	Primary lymphoma
		MFH/fibrosarcoma	Chordoma
			MFH/fibrosarcoma

MFH, malignant fibrous histiocytoma.
[a]For each age range, the tumor types are listed in order of frequency and account for more than 90% of the primary tumors.
Adapted from Unni KK. *Dahlin's bone tumors. General aspects and data on 11,087 cases,* 5th ed. Philadelphia: Lippincott–Raven, 1996.

Table 7.3: Sex Predominance of Bone Lesions

	Male Predominance	Ratio[a]	No Predominance	Female Predominance	Ratio
Malignant	PNET	>2:1	Adamantinoma	Parosteal osteosarcoma	Slight
	Osteosarcoma, telangiectatic	Slight			
	Chondrosarcoma	2:1			
	Chordoma	2:1			
	Osteosarcoma, conventional	Slight			
	Ewing sarcoma	Slight			
	Myeloma	Slight			
	Lymphoma of bone	Slight			
	MFH of bone	Slight			
Benign	Simple cyst	3:1	Enchondroma	Giant cell tumor	Slight
	Osteoid osteoma	3:1	Fibrous dysplasia	Aneurysmal bone cyst	Slight
	Osteoblastoma	2:1		Hemangioma	Slight
	Osteochondroma	2:1			
	Periosteal chondroma	2:1			
	Chondroblastoma	2:1			
	Chondromyxoid fibroma	2:1			
	Fibrous cortical defect	2:1			
	Nonossifying fibroma	2:1			
	Eosinophilic granuloma	2:1			
	Desmoplastic fibroma	Slight			
	Intraosseous lipoma	Slight			
	Intraosseous ganglion	Slight			

MFH, malignant fibrous histiocytoma; PNET, primitive neuroectodermal tumor.
[a]Ratios are approximate and rounded.
Adapted from Unni KK. *Dahlin's bone tumors. General aspects and data on 11,087 cases*, 5th ed, Philadelphia: Lippincott–Raven, 1996; and Fechner RE, Mills SE. *Tumors of the bones and joints*. Washington DC: Armed Forces Institute of Pathology, 1993.

Table 7.4: Precursors of Malignancy in Bone

Precursor Condition	Comment
Enchondroma	Very low risk with solitary lesion; higher risk with multiple lesions
Osteochondroma	Very low risk with solitary lesion; higher risk with multiple lesions
Paget disease	Higher risk with more extensive, polyostotic disease
Radiation injury	Low risk with ≤7,000 rads
Osteomyelitis with chronic sinus tract	Long latency period (≥20 yr)
Bone infarct	Rare; ≥90% have multiple infarcts
Fibrous dysplasia	Case reports
Metallic implants	Case reports
Bone cysts	Case reports
Osteogenesis imperfecta	Case reports
Genetic predisposition	Association with mutant Rb gene and retinoblastoma
Synovial chondromatosis	Case reports
Giant cell tumor	Rare malignant recurrence after treatment
Osteoblastoma	Rare locally aggressive form that does not metastasize
Osteofibrous dysplasia	Coexistent with adamantinoma; possibly subsets of the same disease

Adapted from Dorfman HD, Milchgrub S. Bone. In: Henson DE, Albores-Saavedra J. *Pathology of incipient neoplasia*, 2nd ed. Philadelphia: Saunders, 1993.

Table 7.5: Typical Longitudinal Locations of Solitary Bone Lesions

Epiphysis	Metaphysis	Diametaphysis	Diaphysis
Chondroblastoma	Osteochondroma	Benign fibrous lesions	Ewing sarcoma
Eosinophilic granu- loma	Osteosarcoma	Malignant fibrous lesions	Myeloma
Giant cell tumor	Enchondroma	Chondromyxoid fibroma	Lymphoma
Subchondral cyst	Chondrosarcoma	Simple bone cyst	
Brodie abscess		Osteoid osteoma	
Clear cell chondro- sarcoma		Osteoblastoma	

Table 7.6: Typical Transverse Locations of Solitary Bone Lesions

Medullary Cavity	Cortex	Juxtacortical
Conventional osteosarcoma	Cortical osteoid osteoma	Osteochondroma
Medullary chondrosarcoma	Fibrous cortical defect	Periosteal chondroma
Ewing sarcoma	Adamantinoma	Parosteal osteosarcoma
Myeloma		Exostotic chondrosarcoma
Lymphoma		
Giant cell tumor		
Enchondroma		
Simple bone cyst		
Nonossifying fibroma		

lesions are more common in men (Table 7.3). A few precursor conditions increase the risk of developing a bone malignancy (Table 7.4).

LOCATION OF LESION

The location of a lesion within the skeleton and within the involved bone may have considerable differential diagnostic significance (Tables 7.5 and 7.6). The site of origin of a large, extensive lesion may be difficult to localize. Although there may be considerable variability in location, tumors of a given cell type seem to arise preferentially at sites where the homologous normal cells are most active.

RATE OF GROWTH

The rate of growth of a lesion is classified according to the type of bone destruction and the type of bone proliferation in response to the presence of the lesion.

Bone destruction occurs when normal bone tissue is replaced by lesional tissue. Bone destruction is described as *geographic* when it is confined to a focal area, forming a single hole in the bone (Fig. 7.1). The demarcation between the lesion and normal unaffected bone can be sharp or gradual. Bone destruction is described as *moth-eaten* when there are multiple medium-sized holes with irregular edges randomly distributed in the area of involvement (Fig. 7.2). It is described as *permeated* when the multiple holes are so small that the overall outline of the bone remains intact in the presence of extensive destruction (Fig. 7.3). In moth-eaten and permeated destruction, the transition between normal and abnormal bone is usually gradual.

Proliferative bone is a reaction to the lesion by the host bone. This reaction can be endosteal, within the bone, or periosteal, on the cortical surface. A sclerotic rim is a layer

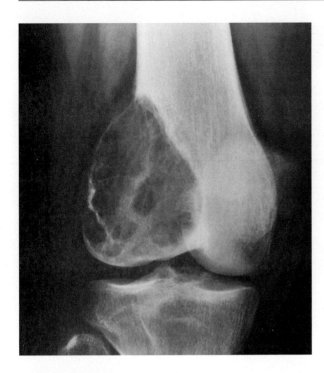

Figure 7.1 Geographic bone destruction in distal femur (giant cell tumor).

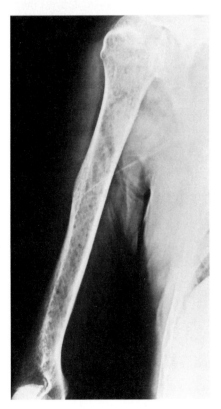

Figure 7.2 Moth-eaten bone destruction in humerus (multiple myeloma).

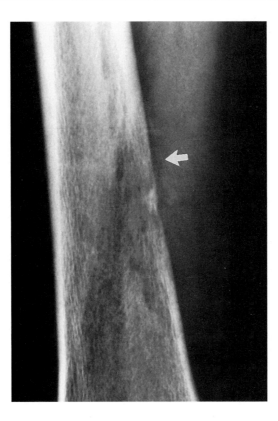

Figure 7.3 Permeated bone destruction in medial femoral cortex (*arrow*) (metastasis).

A sclerotic rim around a lesion indicates stable size or slow growth.

of dense endosteal reactive bone surrounding the lesion and separating it from normal adjacent bone (Fig. 7.4). A sclerotic rim implies that the growth rate of the lesion is slow enough for new bone to form around it and confine it. An expanded cortical shell is a layer of periosteal new bone that confines a lesion that has already destroyed the cortex and expanded beyond the original contour of the bone (Fig. 7.5). The periosteal new bone is formed as the endosteal surface of the cortex is destroyed; the faster the cortical destruction and expansion of the lesion, the thinner is the cortical shell. An expanded shell may have ridges or trabeculations on the endosteal surface, reflecting an uneven growth rate. Nodules of tumor have grown more rapidly beneath the thinner areas of bone and less rapidly where the trabeculations are located. True bony septations that divide a lesion into com-

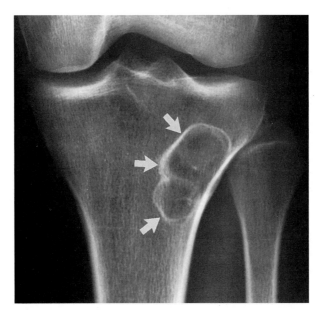

Figure 7.4 Sclerotic rim (*arrows*) around lesion in proximal tibia (nonossifying fibroma).

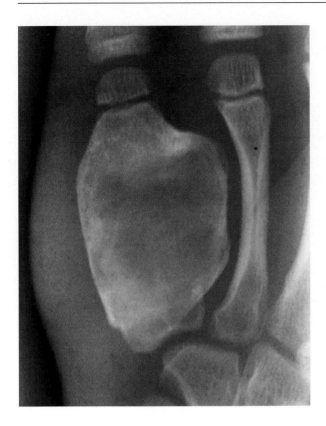

Figure 7.5 Expanded cortical shell in fifth metacarpal (osteoblastoma).

partments are rare. If a lesion expands so rapidly that the periosteal bone response cannot keep up, a shell will not be visible. Mottled sclerosis, scattered throughout cancellous bone adjacent to a lesion, suggests disorganized reactive bone formation in the presence of an aggressive, fast-growing lesion.

Cortical penetration by an intramedullary lesion is indicative of an aggressive process (Fig. 7.6) typically apparent by the presence of a soft tissue mass. Periosteal reaction may

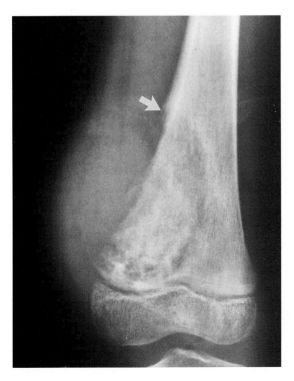

Figure 7.6 Cortical penetration with Codman triangle (*arrow*) in distal femur (osteosarcoma).

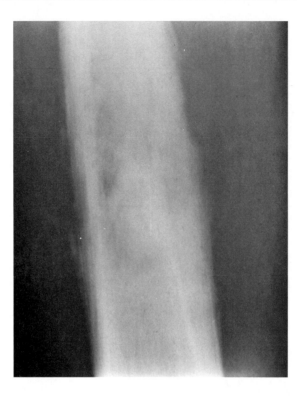

Figure 7.7 Layers of periosteal reaction with Codman triangle (osteosarcoma).

also indicate cortical penetration. Layers of periosteal reaction may be caused by cortical penetration of the lesion into the subperiosteal region (Fig. 7.7). A sunburst periosteal reaction or streaks of periosteal new bone indicate penetration with reactive bone-forming periosteum being carried along by an expanding lesion (Fig. 7.8). An interrupted layer of

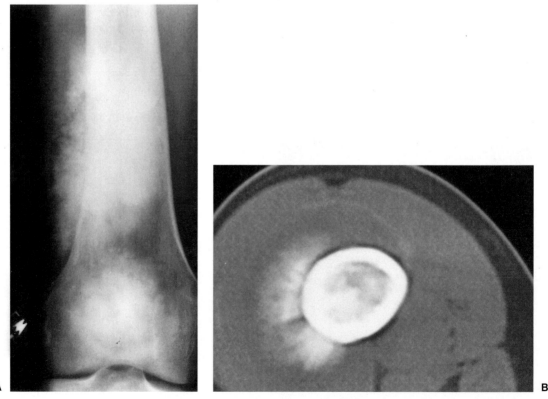

A   B

Figure 7.8 Sunburst periosteal reaction (osteosarcoma). *A.* AP radiograph. *B.* Axial CT scan.

Table 7.7: Radiologic Grading of Destructive Bone Lesions

AFIP System	Defining Characteristics	Simplified System
I-A	Geographic destruction; well-defined lucent destruction *with* sclerotic margin; cortex expanded ≤1 cm	Low grade; nonaggressive
I-B	Geographic destruction; well-defined lucent destruction *without* sclerotic margin or cortex expanded >1 cm	Medium grade; moderately aggressive
I-C	Geographic destruction; complete cortical penetration with ill-defined margin	
II	Geographic destruction combined with moth-eaten or permeated destruction; middle-sized holes in bone with irregular, poorly defined contours	High grade; very aggressive
III	Moth-eaten or permeated destruction only; numerous elongated slotted holes parallel to long axis	

AFIP, Armed Forces Institute of Pathology.
Adapted from Hudson TM. *Radiologic-pathologic correlation of musculoskeletal lesions.* Baltimore: Williams & Wilkins, 1987.

bone at the edge of a lesion that has expanded beyond the periosteum may be present, the so-called Codman triangle.

The rate of growth reflects the biologic aggressiveness of the lesion and can be assigned a radiologic grade. The grading system devised by Lodwick at the Armed Forces Institute of Pathology (AFIP) is commonly used (Table 7.7). Growth rate I-A is geographic destruction with a complete sclerotic margin and partial or no cortical destruction; the cortex may be expanded by up to 1 cm (Fig. 7.4). Growth rate I-B is geographic destruction with either no sclerotic rim or cortical expansion greater than 1 cm (Fig. 7.9). Growth rate I-C is geographic destruction with complete cortical penetration (Fig. 7.6). Growth rate II is geographic destruction combined with moth-eaten or permeated destruction, or both (Fig. 7.10). Growth rate III is moth-eaten destruction with or without permeated destruction only (Figs. 7.2 and 7.3). Higher-grade growth rates may have features of lower-grade growth rates, but not vice versa. Lesions with growth rate I-A are low grade and nonaggressive, lesions with growth rate I-B or I-C are medium grade and moderately aggressive, and lesions with growth rate II or III are high grade and very aggressive. It may

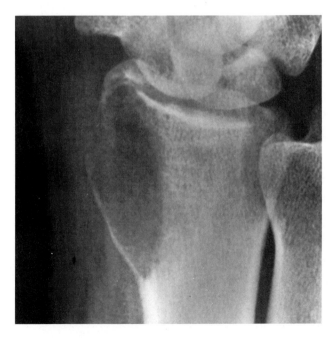

Figure 7.9 Geographic destruction with no sclerotic margin in distal radius (giant cell tumor).

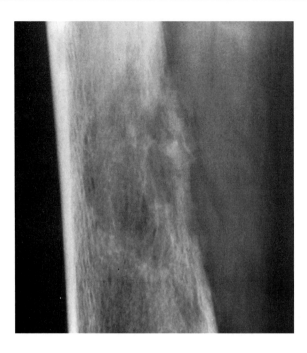

Figure 7.10 Geographic destruction combined with permeated destruction in distal femur (metastasis).

be difficult to distinguish growth rate I-B from I-C and growth rate II from III, but the distinction is not important clinically.

TISSUE CHARACTERIZATION

The pattern of matrix mineralization may indicate a specific tissue type.

Many primary musculoskeletal tumors form an intercellular matrix. The internal radiologic characteristics of tumors that form a matrix are determined by the relative proportions of cells and matrix and the composition and mineralization of the matrix. Types of tumor matrix include osteoid (osseous), chondroid (cartilaginous), myxoid (proteinaceous), fat (lipomatous), and fibrous (collagenous). Identifying the type of matrix often suggests a specific diagnosis (Table 7.8). The pattern of mineralization on radiographs, the attenuation on CT, and the signal on MRI may be helpful in identifying tumor matrix.

Dense homogeneous mineralization is typical of osteoid matrix, formed by benign and malignant bone-forming lesions (Fig. 7.11). Alternatively, osteoid matrix may have a ground-glass or intermediate pattern of matrix mineralization. Osteoid matrix is not always mineralized; therefore, the lack of densely mineralized matrix does not rule out the possibility of an osteoid-forming lesion. Nonmineralized osteoid matrix may have attenuation on CT similar to muscle and often has low signal on both T1- and T2-weighted MRI.

Calcified rings and arcs, dense punctate calcifications, and flocculent calcifications (small, loosely aggregated masses) are patterns of mineralization of chondroid matrix (Figs. 7.12 through 7.14), formed by benign and malignant cartilage-forming lesions. The

Table 7.8: Matrix Mineralization in Bone Tumors

	Osteoid Matrix	*Chondroid Matrix*	*Intermediate Matrix*
Benign	Osteoid osteoma	Enchondroma	Fibrous dysplasia
	Osteoblastoma	Osteochondroma	Osteoblastoma
	Bone island	Periosteal chondroma	
	Osteoma	Chondroblastoma	
		Chondromyxoid fibroma	
Malignant	Osteosarcoma	Chondrosarcoma	Osteosarcoma

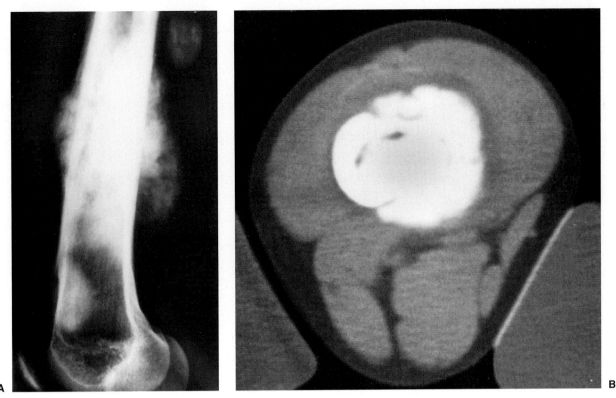

Figure 7.11 Mineralized osteoid matrix (osteosarcoma). *A.* Lateral radiograph. *B.* Axial CT scan.

rings-and-arcs configuration of mineralization corresponds to calcification and ossification around the periphery of cartilaginous lobules. Chondroid matrix that is not mineralized typically has attenuation on CT that is lower than muscle but greater than water. On MRI, chondroid matrix has low signal on T1-weighted images and high signal on T2-weighted images, similar to hyaline cartilage.

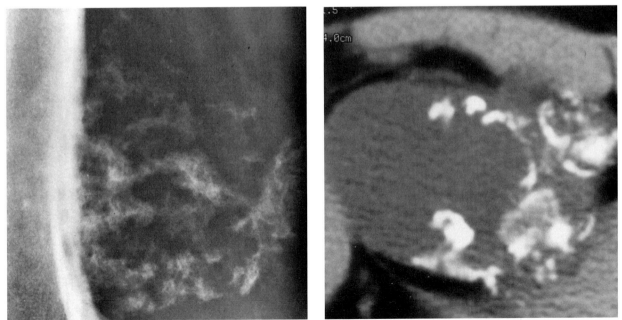

Figure 7.12 Rings-and-arcs cartilage matrix mineralization (chondrosarcoma). *A.* Lateral radiograph. *B.* Axial CT scan.

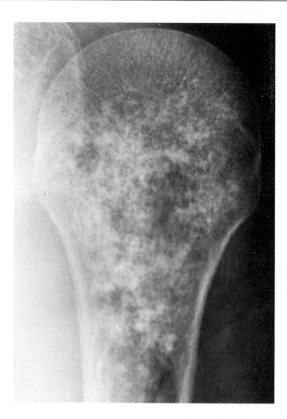

Figure 7.13 Flocculent cartilage matrix mineralization (enchondroma).

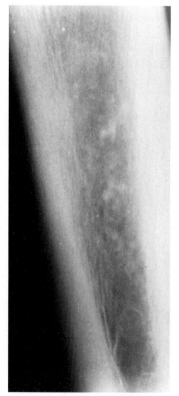

Figure 7.14 Punctate cartilage matrix mineralization (enchondroma).

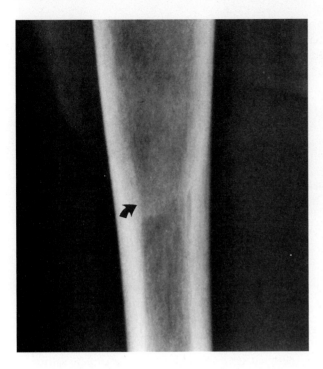

Figure 7.15 Intermediate mineralization (ground-glass appearance) of matrix (fibrous dysplasia) in the proximal femur (*arrow*).

Myxoid matrix may be formed by benign and malignant cartilage-forming tumors and by other benign and malignant mesenchymal tumors, including chordomas. Myxoid matrix generally does not mineralize and typically has attenuation on CT that is lower than muscle and greater than water. On MRI, myxoid matrix has high signal on T2-weighted images, presumably due to its high water content, and variable signal on T1-weighted images, presumably due to its variable protein content.

Lesions that form fibrous matrix range from densely cellular fibrous tissue to myxoid tissue, often within the same lesion. Fibrous matrix typically does not mineralize. On CT, fibrous matrix has variable, nonspecific attenuation, depending on its composition. On MRI, fibrous matrix has variable, nonspecific signal, also depending on its composition. Fibrous dysplasia characteristically has the intermediate pattern of mineralization (ground-glass appearance). However, this appearance results from the presence of dysplastic, microscopic bone spicules rather than mineralization of the fibrous matrix itself. On radiographs, the ground-glass appearance may be difficult to recognize: The lesion is more dense than the marrow space but less dense than the cortical bone (Figs. 7.5 and 7.15). CT is often helpful (Fig. 7.16). A lesion with no mineralization will have either

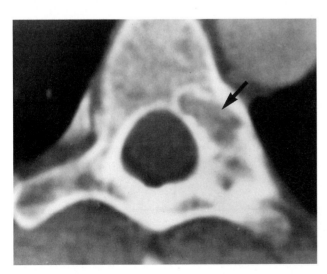

Figure 7.16 Intermediate matrix mineralization (ground-glass appearance) on CT (*arrow*) (fibrous dysplasia).

matrix that is not mineralized or no matrix at all. Lesions without matrix may be densely cellular (e.g., Ewing sarcoma, lymphoma, myeloma), or they may be acellular (e.g., bone cyst) (Figs. 7.1, 7.4, and 7.9). MRI may be diagnostic when a nonaggressive lesion can be demonstrated to be fluid filled and therefore cystic. A localized change in the character of tumor matrix from mineralized to nonmineralized may indicate a focus of higher-grade tumor cells.

STAGING

Staging requires full and exact anatomic delineation of the tumor tissue and its surrounding reactive tissue. This reactive tissue may contain micrometastases. The anatomic relationship of the lesion to all surrounding structures, anatomic compartments, and neurovascular bundles must be established. In addition to plain films, cross-sectional imaging is necessary. Although CT is much better than MRI for establishing a diagnosis, the two modalities are equal for evaluating the extent and anatomic setting of the tumor. Chest CT can exclude lung metastases; a radionuclide bone scan or whole-body MRI can exclude skeletal metastases.

> CT and MRI are equivalent for evaluating the extent and anatomic setting of the tumor.

The Musculoskeletal Tumor Society and the American Joint Committee for Cancer Staging and End Results Reporting have adopted the surgical staging system described in Table 7.9 for primary malignant musculoskeletal tumors. The staging system is based on a combination of the histologic grade (designated G_0 through G_2), the anatomic setting of the tumor itself (designated T_0 through T_2), and the presence or absence of metastases (designated M_0 or M_1). Benign lesions have three stages that are designated by Arabic numbers; malignant lesions have three stages designated by Roman numerals. Stage I lesions are low-grade malignancies, stage II lesions are high-grade malignancies, and stage III lesions are those with metastases, whether low or high grade. The additional letter designation of A or B reflects the anatomic setting. Stages I-A, II-A, and III-A are intracompartmental lesions in which the tumor is confined within a natural anatomic barrier to tumor growth such as cortical bone, articular cartilage, major fascial septa, or joint capsules. Stages I-B, II-B, and III-B are extracompartmental lesions, in which the lesion has expanded beyond the confines of a single anatomic compartment. At presentation, 30% of musculoskeletal sarcoma patients have stage I lesions (66% of these are stage I-A, and 33% are stage I-B), 60% have stage II lesions (10% of these are stage II-A, and 90% are stage II-B), and 10% have stage III lesions. As a general observation, benign lesions in stages 1 and 2

Table 7.9: Staging for Bone and Soft Tissue Tumors

Benign	Stage 1	Latent	G_0	T_0	M_0
	Stage 2	Active	G_0	T_0	M_0
	Stage 3	Aggressive	G_0	T_{1-2}	M_{0-1}
Malignant	Stage I	Low grade			
		A: Intracompartmental	G_1	T_1	M_0
		B: Extracompartmental	G_1	T_2	M_0
	Stage II	High grade			
		A: Intracompartmental	G_2	T_1	M_0
		B: Extracompartmental	G_2	T_2	M_0
	Stage III	Distant metastasis, low or high grade			
		A: Intracompartmental	G_{1-2}	T_1	M_1
		B: Extracompartmental	G_{1-2}	T_2	M_1

G, histologic grade; M, metastases; T, tumor setting.
Adapted from Enneking WF. *Clinical musculoskeletal pathology,* 3rd ed. Gainesville, FL: University of Florida Press, 1991.

are radiologically low grade or nonaggressive, stage 3 benign lesions and stage I malignant lesions are medium grade or moderately aggressive, and stage II or III malignant lesions are high grade or very aggressive.

TREATMENT

Treatment of musculoskeletal tumors is individualized. Benign lesions whose radiologic appearance and clinical presentation are typical often do not require a histologic diagnosis and may be ignored, followed, or treated according to symptoms and natural history. Most other benign lesions can be treated with curettage or simple excision. Aggressive or malignant lesions usually require both local and systemic therapy. Although lesions such as lymphoma and Ewing sarcoma are treated with radiation (Fig. 7.17), local therapy for most malignant or aggressive lesions is surgical (Fig. 7.18). The size of the surrounding cuff of tissue that is ideally excised with the lesion is usually related to the histologic grade of the tumor. Depending on the operation chosen and the site and extent of the tumor, amputations and local limb-sparing operations may leave behind gross tumor, macroscopic or microscopic residual tumor, or no residual tumor at all. A contaminated biopsy site can enlarge the scope of the operation required to achieve a particular biologic goal; the biopsy site is generally resected with the tumor. Newer regimens of neoadjuvant and adjuvant therapy—including radiation therapy, chemotherapy, and immunotherapy—are aimed at reducing tumor bulk before surgery and at eliminating residual (often microscopic) tumor and subclinical metastases after surgery. Major advances in the staging and treatment of primary bone and joint cancers have improved the 5-year survival rates for children younger than 15 years of age from 20% in 1960 to 1963 to 64% in 1986 to 1991. Primary bone sarcomas that have been resected segmentally are usually reconstructed with large

> A contaminated biopsy site can enlarge the scope of the operation required to achieve a particular biologic goal.

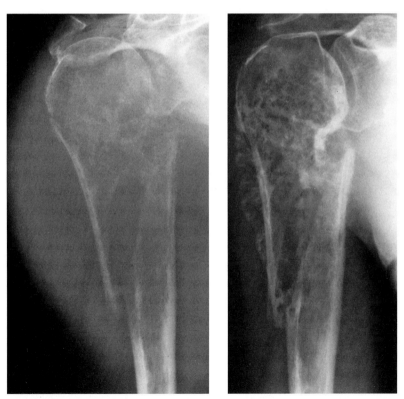

A   **B**

Figure 7.17 Ewing sarcoma in the proximal humerus with pathologic fracture. *A.* At presentation, there is permeated destruction and a large soft tissue mass. *B.* Ten months after radiation therapy, the mass has regressed, and reactive bone is present.

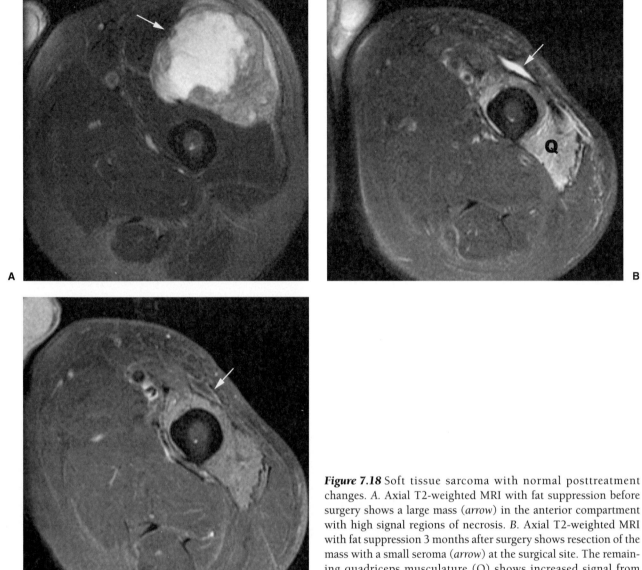

Figure 7.18 Soft tissue sarcoma with normal posttreatment changes. *A.* Axial T2-weighted MRI with fat suppression before surgery shows a large mass (*arrow*) in the anterior compartment with high signal regions of necrosis. *B.* Axial T2-weighted MRI with fat suppression 3 months after surgery shows resection of the mass with a small seroma (*arrow*) at the surgical site. The remaining quadriceps musculature (Q) shows increased signal from denervation atrophy. *C.* Axial T1-weighted MRI with fat suppression after gadolinium injection shows modest enhancement around the periphery of the seroma (*arrow*).

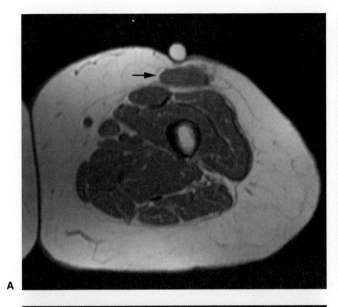

A

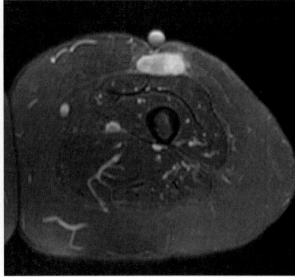

B

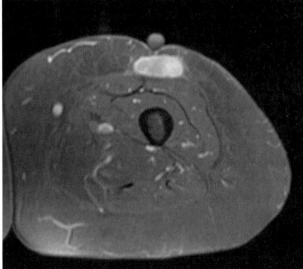

C

Figure 7.19 Recurrent soft tissue sarcoma. *A.* Axial T1-weighted MRI shows a lesion (*arrow*) with intermediate signal intensity in the anterior subcutaneous tissues of the proximal thigh. The marker has been placed on the incision scar from previous surgery. *B.* Axial T2-weighted MRI with fat suppression shows heterogeneous high signal within the lesion. *C.* Axial T1-weighted MRI with fat suppression after gadolinium injection shows heterogeneous enhancement in the lesion.

allografts. If a joint is included in the resection, the reconstruction may include a prosthesis or an arthrodesis. Involvement of major vessels is not necessarily a contraindication to limb-sparing resection if a vascular graft can be successfully placed. However, in some cases, an amputation is necessary. For benign disease in which intralesional excision is appropriate—for example, enchondroma or osteoblastoma—the resulting defect at the surgical site may be filled with material such as bone graft or methylmethacrylate cement. After the initiation of therapy, imaging may be used to monitor the response and to screen for complications or recurrences (Fig. 7.19).

METASTASES

Metastases to the lungs are common in patients with musculoskeletal sarcomas. The lung lesions typically have a cannonball morphology. The pulmonary metastases of matrix-forming bone tumors also form similar matrix. In many clinical circumstances, pulmonary metastases are aggressively pursued, even when multiple. Musculoskeletal malignancies also metastasize to other bones. The metastatic lesions generally resemble the primary lesions (Fig. 7.20).

Metastases to the lungs typically have a cannonball morphology.

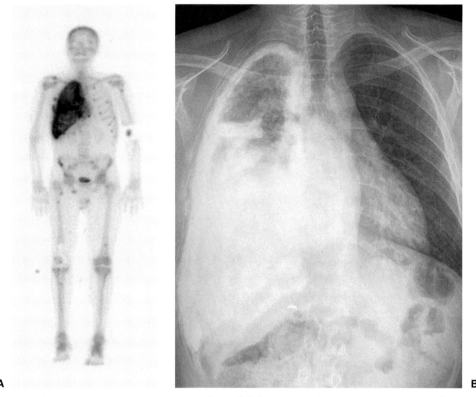

A   **B**

Figure 7.20 Metastatic osteosarcoma. *A.* Radionuclide bone scan shows intense activity in the right hemithorax. There are multiple small lesions scattered throughout the skeleton. The primary site of tumor at the right distal femur was reconstructed with a joint replacement and shows no abnormal activity. *B.* PA chest radiograph shows densely mineralized tumor filling the right hemithorax.

SOURCES AND READINGS

Anderson MW, Temple HT, Dussault RG, et al. Compartmental anatomy: relevance to staging and biopsy of musculoskeletal tumors. *AJR Am J Roentgenol* 1999;173:1663–1671.

Daldrup-Link HE, Franzius C, Link TM, et al. Whole-body MR imaging for detection of bone metastases in children and young adults: comparison with skeletal scintigraphy and FDG PET. *AJR Am J Roentgenol* 2001;177:229–236.

Dorfman HD, Milchgrub S. Bone. In: Henson DE, Albores-Saavedra J. *Pathology of incipient neoplasia*, 2nd ed. Philadelphia: WB Saunders, 1993:508–525.

Enneking WF. *Clinical musculoskeletal pathology*, 3rd ed. Gainesville, FL: University of Florida Press, 1991.

Fechner RE, Mills SE. *Tumors of the bones and joints*. Washington, DC: Armed Forces Institute of Pathology, 1993.

Ghelman B. Biopsies of the musculoskeletal system. *Radiol Clin North Am* 1998;36:567–580.

Heare TC, Enneking WF, Heare MM. Staging techniques and biopsy of bone tumors. *Orthop Clin North Am* 1989;20:273–285.

Hudson TM. *Radiologic-pathologic correlation of musculoskeletal lesions*. Baltimore: Williams & Wilkins, 1987.

Jemal A, Thomas A, Murray T, et al. Cancer statistics, 2002. *CA Cancer J Clin* 2002;52:23–47.

Lodwick GS. *Atlas of tumor radiology. The bones and joints*. Chicago: Year Book, 1971.

Lodwick GS, Wilson AJ, Farrell C, et al. Determining growth rates of focal lesions of bone from radiographs. *Radiology* 1980;134:577–583.

Lodwick GS, Wilson AJ, Farrell C, et al. Estimating rate of growth in bone lesions: observer performance and error. *Radiology* 1980;134:585–590.

Moser RP, Madewell JE. An approach to primary bone tumors. *Radiol Clin North Am* 1987;25:1049–1093.

Olson PN, Everson LI, Griffiths HJ. Staging of musculoskeletal tumors. *Radiol Clin North Am* 1994;32:151–162.

Parker SL, Tong T, Bolden S, et al. Cancer statistics, 1996. *CA Cancer J Clin* 1996;46:5–30.

Parkin DM. Global cancer statistics in the year 2000. *Lancet Oncol* 2001;2:533–543.

Peh WCG. The role of imaging in the staging of bone tumors. *Crit Rev Oncol Hematol* 1999;31:147–167.

Temple HT, Bashore CJ. Staging of bone neoplasms: an orthopedic oncologist's perspective. *Semin Musculoskelet Radiol* 2000;4(1):17–23.

Unni KK. *Dahlin's bone tumors. General aspects and data on 11,087 cases*, 5th ed. Philadelphia: Lippincott–Raven, 1996.

MALIGNANT AND AGGRESSIVE TUMORS

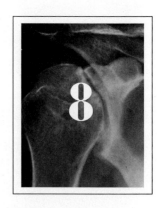

OSTEOSARCOMA

Osteosarcomas are malignant osteoid-producing sarcomas (Table 8.1). Although they are the most common of the primary bone sarcomas, there are fewer than 1,000 new cases per year in the United States. Eighty-five percent of cases occur at age 30 years or younger, but osteosarcomas may occur at any age. Most arise de novo, but in patients older than 40 years of age, as many as 15% to 20% of osteosarcomas are associated with Paget disease, therapeutic irradiation, or bone infarct.

Osteosarcoma is the most common primary bone sarcoma.

CONVENTIONAL OSTEOSARCOMA

Conventional (intramedullary) osteosarcoma is found within the cancellous portion of a long or flat bone. Aggressive growth within the medullary cavity leads to early cortical penetration and invasion of the soft tissues. The typical longitudinal location is the metaphysis; the typical transverse location is eccentric within the medullary cavity. An open growth plate can act as a barrier to tumor spread, sparing the epiphysis in the immature skeleton. The common locations are the distal femur (32% of cases), proximal tibia (15%), proximal femur and femoral shaft (9%), proximal humerus (8%), and ilium (7%). Note that nearly 50% of osteosarcomas occur around the knee.

Nearly 50% of osteosarcomas occur around the knee.

The typical clinical presentation is nonspecific: pain, swelling, and limited joint motion for a few weeks or months. Some patients present with pathologic fractures, especially those with rapidly growing, sparsely ossified tumors. An osteosarcoma may be overlooked in the presence of a healing pathologic fracture, but appreciation of the presence of bone destruction leads to the correct diagnosis. Fracture callus and osteosarcoma can be virtually indistinguishable histologically.

Most osteosarcomas are heavily or moderately ossified, with the dense blastic areas corresponding to mineralized osseous matrix made by the tumor and reactive medullary bone

Table 8.1: Classification of Osteosarcomas

Type	Frequency (%)
Intramedullary (central)	
High grade	75
Low grade	4–5
Parosteal (low grade)	6–9
Juxtacortical (high grade)	1–2
Intracortical	0.2
Extraskeletal	2–3
Multifocal	1–2
Osteosarcoma of jaw	6
Secondary	5–7

(Figs. 8.1 and 8.2). Lytic areas, when present, correspond to destruction and replacement of bone by tumor tissue containing scant or no ossification. Cortical penetration with a large soft tissue mass is common (Fig. 8.3). Confluent bone densities within a soft tissue mass correspond to mineralized matrix. Reactive periosteal new bone may have a linear, laminated, or perpendicular sunburst bone configuration, all of which are indicative of cortical penetration. Approximately 50% of osteosarcomas have features typical enough to allow a confident radiologic diagnosis. Approximately 25% of osteosarcomas are chondroblastic, with large amounts of chondroid matrix mixed with the osteoid, so that the appearance on imaging may resemble a chondroid or myxoid lesion. Approximately 25% of osteosarcomas are fibroblastic, with large amounts of fibrous matrix. Recurrent tumors resemble the primary. Any cloudlike, solid, dense bone formation within the medullary cavity, even in the absence of overt bone destruction and soft tissue extension, should suggest the possibility of an osteosarcoma.

> Approximately 50% of osteosarcomas have atypical radiologic features.

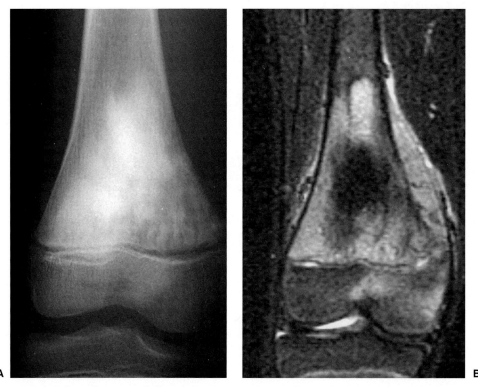

A   B

Figure 8.1 High-grade intramedullary osteosarcoma. *A.* AP radiograph shows sclerotic lesion in the distal femoral metaphysis. *B.* Coronal T2-weighted fat-suppressed MRI shows low signal in the mineralized portion of the tumor with high signal in nonmineralized portions, including a significant soft tissue component. There is extension into the epiphysis. (*continued*)

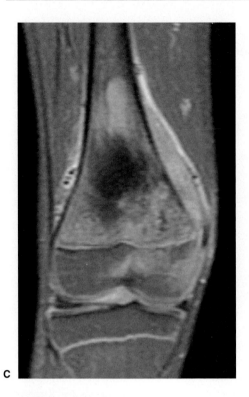

C

Figure 8.1 (*continued*) *C.* Coronal T1-weighted fat-suppressed MRI after gadolinium injection shows enhancement in the tumor.

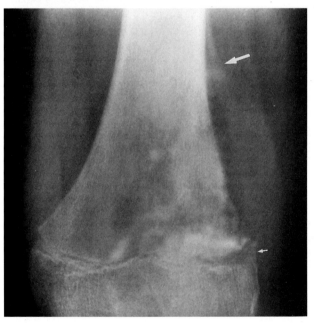

Figure 8.2 High-grade intramedullary osteosarcoma of distal femur. AP radiograph with Codman triangle (*large arrow*) and involvement of the growth plate (*small arrow*).

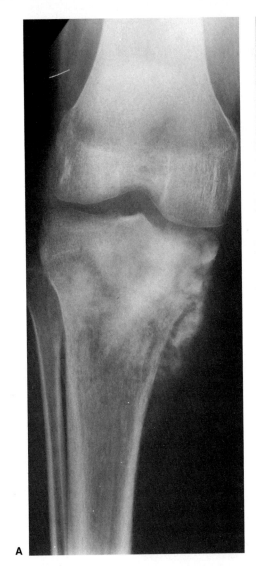

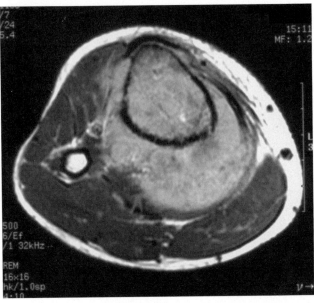

Figure 8.3 Osteosarcoma of the proximal tibia with associated soft tissue mass. *A.* AP radiograph shows a blastic lesion with soft tissue component. *B.* Axial T1-weighted MRI shows permeated destruction of the cortex with large soft tissue mass. The lesion enhanced after gadolinium injection.

Osteosarcoma metastasizes to the lung, where the deposits may form dense, mineralized osteoid, accumulate bone-scanning agents, cavitate, and cause pneumothorax. At presentation, 10% to 20% of patients have metastases, usually to the lungs. Occasionally, skip metastases occur in the medullary cavity of the host bone, sparing an interval of normal marrow between the primary tumor and the metastasis (Fig. 8.4). A metastasis may even skip across a joint.

Osteosarcomas are rapidly growing tumors with a median doubling time of 34 days. Local recurrences are usually apparent within the first year. The current treatment consists of neoadjuvant chemotherapy to reduce the tumor mass, aggressive resection of the tumor, adjuvant chemotherapy, and resection of pulmonary metastases. Segmental limb-sparing resections may improve function without necessarily compromising local control. The disease-free, overall 5-year survival rate of those without metastatic disease at presentation (up to stage II-B) approaches 80%.

OSTEOSARCOMA VARIANTS

Radiation-induced osteosarcomas have the radiologic appearance and biologic behavior of conventional high-grade intramedullary osteosarcomas (Fig. 8.5). Approximately 5% of osteosarcomas are postirradiation in etiology. Osteosarcoma is the most common type of postirradiation musculoskeletal sarcoma.

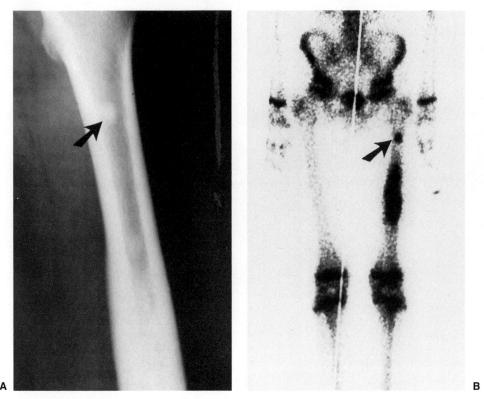

Figure 8.4 High-grade intramedullary osteosarcoma with skip metastasis. *A.* AP radiograph shows a long lesion in the middle third of the femoral shaft with dense, ossified matrix. The lesion gradually merges with normal bone. A satellite lesion with similar characteristics is present proximally (*arrow*). *B.* Bone scan shows accumulation of tracer in the primary and satellite (*arrow*) lesions.

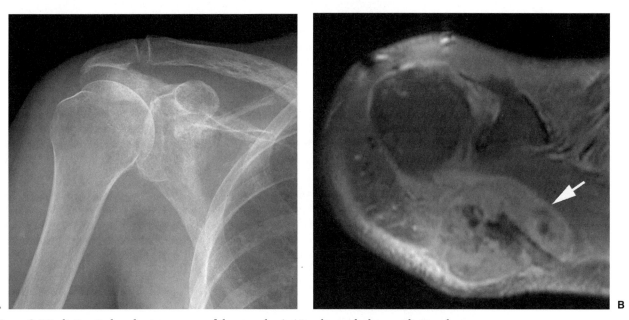

Figure 8.5 Radiation-induced osteosarcoma of the scapula. *A.* AP radiograph shows radiation change in the clavicle and scapula, with coarsened trabecular bone pattern. The humerus overlies a destructive lesion of the scapular spine. *B.* Axial T2-weighted fat-suppressed MRI shows heterogeneous high signal in a large scapular mass with soft tissue extension (*arrow*).

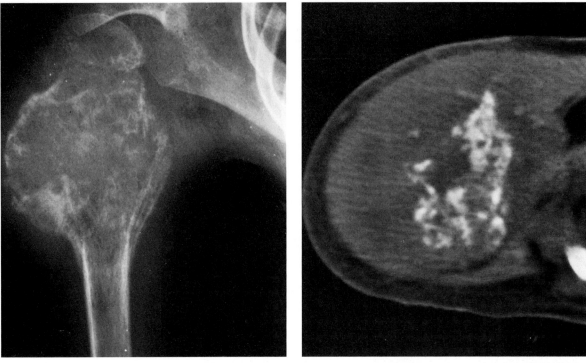

A   B

Figure 8.6 Telangiectatic osteosarcoma in the proximal humerus. *A.* Radiograph shows an expansile, destructive lesion in the proximal humerus with cortical penetration (blow-out). *B.* CT shows the circumferential cortical penetration and soft tissue extension with neoplastic and reactive ossification.

Telangiectatic osteosarcomas represent approximately 4% of all osteosarcomas and display distinctive pathologic features. The lesions are destructive and lytic, with large extraosseous masses incompletely surrounded by thin shells of bone (Fig. 8.6). They grow rapidly and elicit relatively little bone reaction. Pathologically, telangiectatic osteosarcomas are mostly cystic and vascular, containing little or no tumor matrix or other solid tumor tissue. Fluid-fluid levels may be demonstrated on CT or MRI. Telangiectatic osteosarcomas were previously thought to be more lethal but were subsequently shown to have the same prognosis as conventional osteosarcomas with neoadjuvant chemotherapy and wide resection.

Parosteal osteosarcomas represent 6% to 9% of osteosarcomas. This variety arises on the cortical surface and affects a slightly older age group, with most patients older than 20 years of age. Virtually all are found in the metaphysis of a long bone, especially the posterior surface of the distal femoral metaphysis (66% of cases). The presentation is nonspecific, often dull, aching pain or mechanical difficulties caused by the mass itself. The lesions are commonly diagnosed and treated incorrectly for years as atypical osteochondromas that somehow recur locally. Even with late diagnosis, the prognosis is often better than for conventional osteosarcoma. The radiographic appearance is a lobulated juxtacortical mass with densely ossified tumor tissue attached to the cortex, often by a stalk; variable amounts of lucent, nonossified tissue are usually present, making the lesion larger than apparent on plain radiographs (Figs. 8.7 and 8.8). CT or MRI can document tumor invasion of the medullary cavity by direct extension through the stalk.

Periosteal osteosarcomas are found in a periosteal location most commonly along the shaft of the femur or tibia. These osteosarcomas are generally chondroblastic and therefore not densely ossified (Fig. 8.9). They are predominantly radiolucent on radiographs and CT, with a lobulated morphology. A sunburst appearance is often present. On MRI, the bulk of the lesion typically has heterogeneous low signal on T1-weighted images and high signal on T2-weighted images. The age of onset is similar to conventional osteosarcomas, and periosteal osteosarcomas are of moderate histologic grade and biologic aggressiveness.

Other osteosarcoma variants with distinctive histologic or clinical features account for approximately 1% of all osteosarcomas. These include multifocal osteosarcoma (synchro-

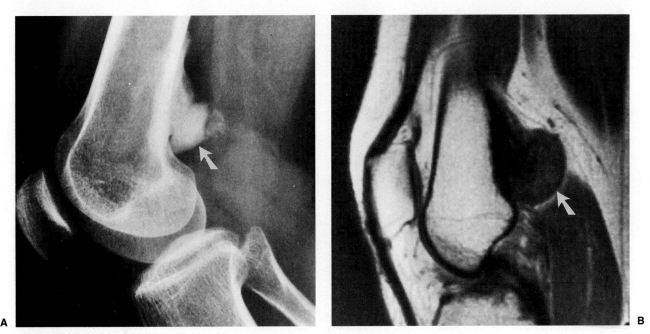

A

B

Figure 8.7 Parosteal osteosarcoma. *A.* Radiograph shows a homogeneously dense, lobulated mass (*arrow*) on a short broad stalk along the posteromedial cortex of the distal femoral metaphysis. *B.* Sagittal T1-weighted MRI shows a lobulated soft tissue mass (*arrow*). No invasion of the marrow cavity is present.

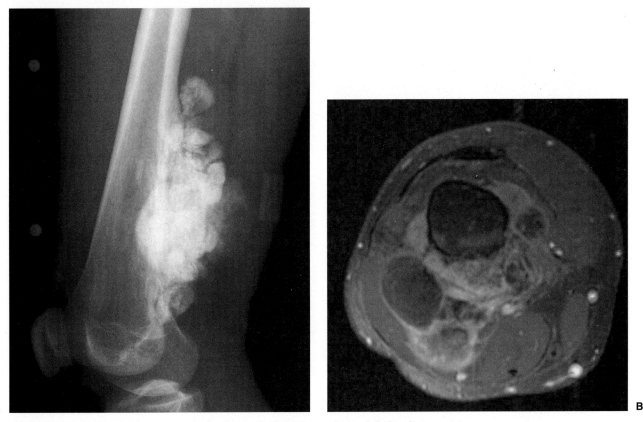

A

B

Figure 8.8 Parosteal osteosarcoma. *A.* Lateral radiograph shows large, dense, lobulated mass arising from the posterior cortex of the distal femur. *B.* Axial T1-weighted fat-suppressed MRI after gadolinium injection shows regions of enhancement. (*continued*)

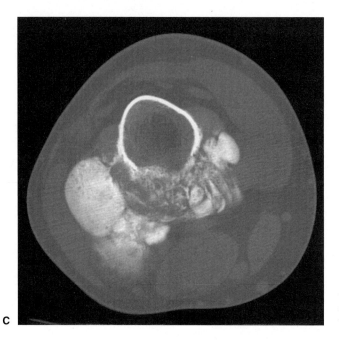

Figure 8.8 (*continued*) *C.* Axial CT scan shows variation in mineralization of the lesion.

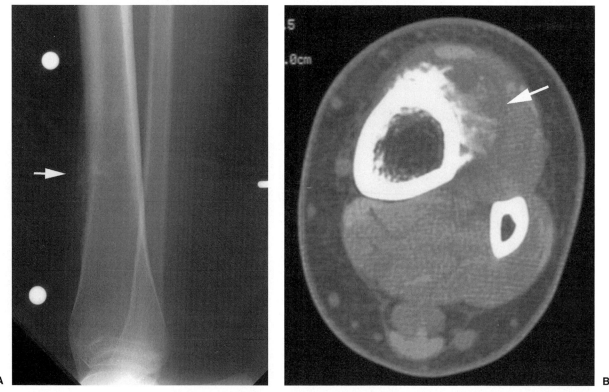

Figure 8.9 Periosteal osteosarcoma. *A.* Lateral radiograph shows a partially mineralized lesion arising from the tibial cortex (*arrow*). *B.* Axial CT scan shows lesion arising from tibial cortex with soft tissue mass (*arrow*). (*continued*)

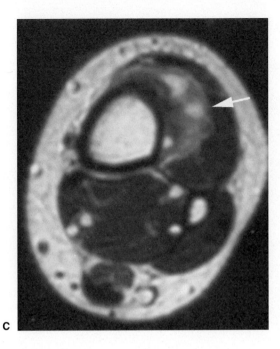

c

Figure 8.9 (continued) C. Axial T2-weighted MRI shows heterogeneous signal within the lesion (*arrow*).

nous and asynchronous types), small cell osteosarcoma (see the section Small Cell Osteosarcoma), intraosseous well-differentiated osteosarcoma, intracortical osteosarcoma, and high-grade surface osteosarcoma.

CHONDROSARCOMA

Chondrosarcomas are malignant cartilage-producing tumors that arise de novo or in preexisting cartilage lesions or rests. They present a wide variation in form and aggressiveness, and low-grade malignant lesions may be almost indistinguishable morphologically from benign cartilage-containing lesions. A limited focus of malignancy may be embedded in a much larger mass of clearly benign tissue. At the other end of this spectrum are high-grade, frankly malignant tumors that recur and spread by local extension or metastasis. Chondrosarcomas follow a slow clinical evolution; they tend to metastasize late in the clinical course, and patients rarely present with metastatic disease.

A small chondrosarcoma may arise within a larger, benign cartilaginous lesion.

MEDULLARY CHONDROSARCOMA

Medullary (central) chondrosarcomas are primary lesions that arise within cancellous bone or the medullary cavity. The most common locations are the pelvis (23% of cases), femur (22%), ribs (11%), and humerus (11%). The presenting symptom is deep pain lasting for months or years. If the tumor has breached the cortex, local swelling may be present. Presentation is over a wide age range, but most patients are between 35 and 70 years of age, and men are affected more frequently than women. The treatment is surgical. The incidence of metastasis and the prognosis are related to the histologic grade, with 10-year survival ranging from 28% for high-grade lesions to 85% for low-grade lesions. The radiographic appearance is osseous destruction with matrix mineralization characteristic of cartilage. A typical lesion would be a lucent area in the center of a long bone with endosteal scalloping, cortical thickening, and geographic margins. Often, the tumor contains the punctate or flocculent calcification and ring-shaped ossification characteristic of cartilage tissue (Figs. 8.10 through 8.13). The lucent appearance is a result of the replacement of normal bone by noncalcified cartilage. On CT, the nonmineralized regions have a myxoid appearance with attenuation in the range of 10 to 30 Hounsfield units (HU). On MRI, these regions have

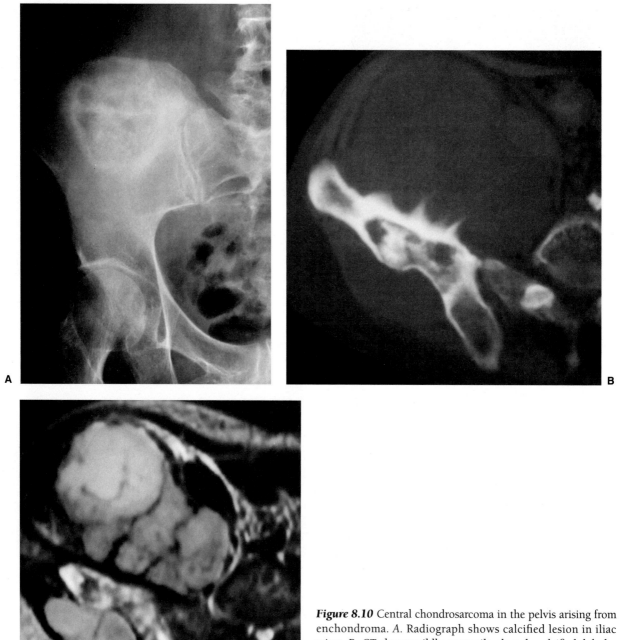

Figure 8.10 Central chondrosarcoma in the pelvis arising from enchondroma. *A.* Radiograph shows calcified lesion in iliac wing. *B.* CT shows mildly expansile, densely calcified, lobular intraosseous lesion (underlying enchondroma). There is a large soft tissue mass on both sides of the iliac wing with a sunburst periosteal reaction anteriorly. *C.* Axial T2-weighted MRI shows high signal in the nonmineralized portions of the intraosseous lesion and in the soft tissue mass.

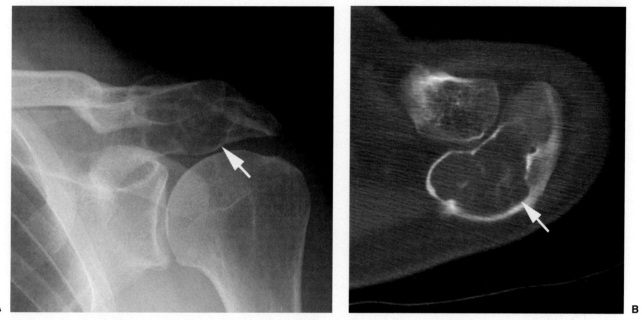

Figure 8.11 Low-grade chondrosarcoma of the scapula. *A.* AP radiograph shows a well-circumscribed, mildly expansile lesion in the acromion process (*arrow*) with cartilage-type calcifications. *B.* Axial CT scan demonstrates endosteal scalloping and chondroid matrix (*arrow*).

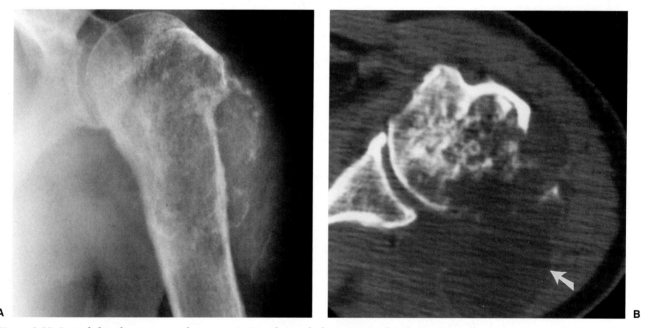

Figure 8.12 Central chondrosarcoma in humerus. *A.* AP radiograph shows geographic destruction, soft tissue mass, and rings-and-arcs calcifications. *B.* CT shows calcified intramedullary lesion with cortical penetration and low-attenuation posterior soft tissue mass (*arrow*).

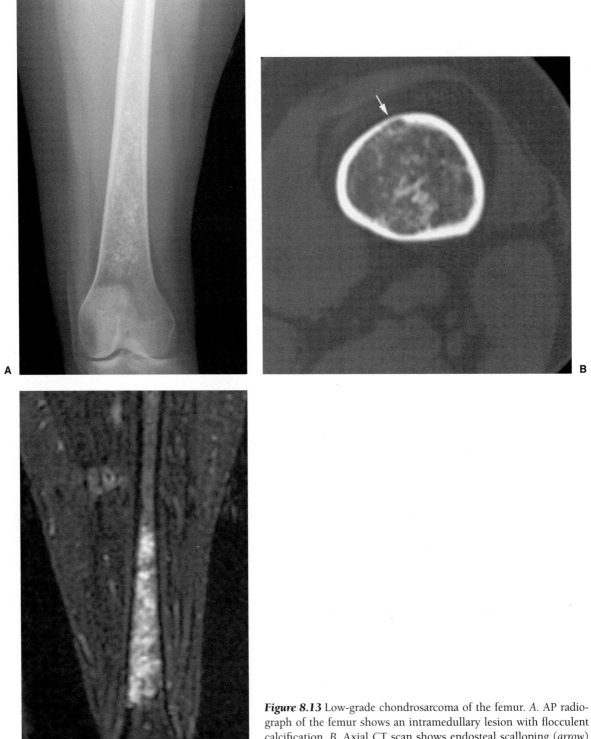

Figure 8.13 Low-grade chondrosarcoma of the femur. *A.* AP radiograph of the femur shows an intramedullary lesion with flocculent calcification. *B.* Axial CT scan shows endosteal scalloping (*arrow*) and mineralized matrix. There is no cortical penetration. *C.* Coronal STIR MRI shows high signal in a lobular morphology.

high signal on T2-weighted images and variable signal on TI-weighted images. A lobular growth pattern is often evident on CT or MRI. The bone scan shows increased tracer accumulation.

EXOSTOTIC CHONDROSARCOMA

Exostotic (peripheral) chondrosarcomas arise in the cartilage cap of a previously benign exostosis (osteochondroma) or from the surface of a bone involved by multiple heritable exostoses. They represent approximately 15% of chondrosarcomas. Men are affected twice as often as women. A wide age range is affected, but most patients are young adults. The tumors tend to be of low histologic grade and may be difficult to distinguish from the cartilaginous cap, but a nonmineralized soft tissue component larger than 1 cm should raise suspicion. If a lesion recurs, it tends to be of a higher histologic grade. The radiographic appearance is that of an exostosis with an attached mass of soft tissue density containing variable amounts of cartilaginous calcification (Fig. 8.14). CT and MRI reliably demonstrate nonmineralized cartilaginous matrix. Serial films may document destruction of ossified portions of the underlying exostosis. These lesions appear as areas of increased tracer uptake on bone scan, with the intensity of radionuclide accumulation roughly proportional to the combined amount of enchondral ossification, osteoblastic activity, and hyperemia in the tumor. The intensity of uptake does not reliably predict whether the lesion is benign or malignant.

Patients with multiple heritable exostoses are at risk for developing chondrosarcoma.

CHONDROSARCOMA VARIANTS

Dedifferentiated chondrosarcomas contain a limited focus of anaplastic sarcoma within a larger mass of typical low-grade chondrosarcoma. The clinical course is that of the higher-grade tumor, and the prognosis is grim. These account for approximately 11% of chondrosarcomas. Other chondrosarcoma variants with distinctive histologic or gross pathologic features comprise approximately 5% of all chondrosarcomas. These include clear cell chondrosarcoma, mesenchymal chondrosarcoma, and juxtacortical (parosteal or periosteal) chondrosarcoma.

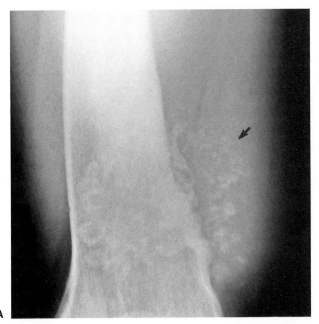 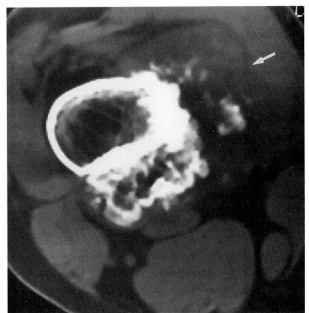

A B

Figure 8.14 Exostotic chondrosarcoma. *A.* AP radiograph of distal femur shows rings-and-arcs calcifications and lateral soft tissue mass (*arrow*). *B.* CT shows lobulated, low-attenuation soft tissue mass (*arrow*) and dense calcifications.

PRIMARY MARROW CELL TUMORS

MULTIPLE MYELOMA

Multiple myeloma is a malignant neoplasm of plasmacytes, the cells of the bone marrow that make immunoglobulins. The most common primary tumor arising in bone, multiple myeloma has an incidence in the United States of 14,600 per year. The age of onset is usually between 45 and 80 years. Although palliative treatments exist, the condition is uniformly fatal and without cure. Myeloma arises in the bone marrow and involves it diffusely. Bony abnormalities usually occur at multiple sites, including the vertebrae in 66% of patients, the ribs in 45%, the skull in 40%, the shoulder girdle in 40%, the pelvis in 30%, and the long bones in 25%. Myeloma lesions are sharply defined, purely lytic areas of bone destruction with no reactive bone formation. The pattern of destruction may be geographic, moth-eaten, or permeated; involvement may be so diffuse that the bones are simply osteopenic or even normal in radiographic appearance (Figs. 8.15 through 8.17). Pathologically, the marrow and bone have been replaced by myeloma tissue. Focal holes in the involved bones are filled with closely packed sheets of plasmacytes of varying maturity. The lesions may be expansile, penetrate the cortex, and form large extraosseous soft tissue masses. Pathologic fractures are common. The radionuclide bone scan is typically normal or may show areas of decreased uptake ("cold" spots). These cold spots represent destruction and replacement of bone by myeloma tissue without evocation of osteoblastic bone reaction. For this reason, the plain-film skeletal survey is the best method for disclosing sites of bone destruction. MRI shows the replacement of the normal marrow by myeloma tissue (Fig. 8.18).

Several differential points may help distinguish between multiple myeloma and osseous metastases (Table 8.2) in a patient with multiple destructive bone lesions. Myeloma tissue produces a number of osteoclast-stimulating factors that result in bone destruction that is cleanly marginated and purely lytic. Although metastases also produce osteoclast-stimulating factors, they tend to provoke reactive bone, frequently resulting in a more ragged and irregular appearance. Myeloma may involve the intervertebral discs and the mandible, but metastases rarely do so. Metastases often involve the vertebral pedicles, but myeloma rarely does so. A large soft tissue mass is more likely to be present with myeloma than with metastases. The bone scan is usually positive in the presence of bone metastases and often negative in myeloma.

Myeloma does not provoke reactive bone formation.

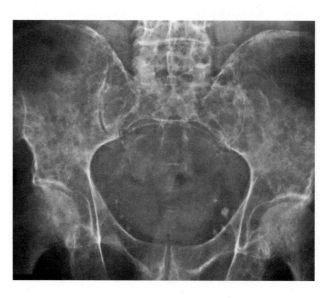

Figure 8.15 Multiple myeloma. Radiograph shows moth-eaten destruction.

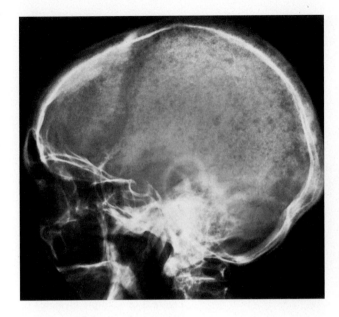

Figure 8.16 Multiple myeloma. Lateral skull radiograph shows moth-eaten destruction of the calvaria.

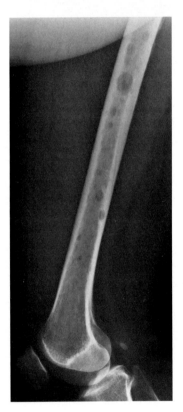

Figure 8.17 Multiple myeloma. Lateral femur radiograph shows multiple lytic lesions of varying size.

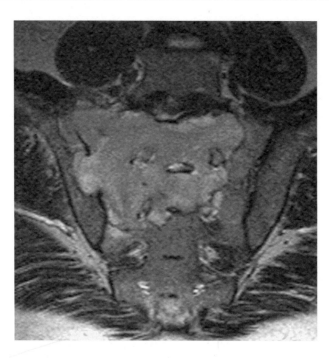

Figure 8.18 Multiple myeloma of the sacrum shown on a coronal T2-weighted MRI.

SOLITARY MYELOMA

Solitary myeloma (plasmacytoma) is myeloma that has a single focus of involvement. The findings from marrow aspiration may therefore be negative, and laboratory manifestations may be absent. Virtually all patients with solitary myeloma develop multiple myeloma, but 10 years or more may pass before the progression of disease becomes apparent. Solitary myeloma commonly presents as an expansile lesion in the spine, a rib, the pelvis, or the sacrum (Figs. 8.19 and 8.20).

PRIMARY LYMPHOMA

The radionuclide bone scan shows the extent of skeletal involvement in lymphoma.

Lymphoma presenting as a primary tumor of bone without concurrent regional lymph node or visceral involvement represents 5% of all extranodal (non-Hodgkin) lymphomas. Most are large cell lymphomas of B-cell origin and are histologically similar or identical to extranodal lymphomas arising at other sites. Lymphoma may develop at any age, but most patients are adults, and men are affected more frequently than women. The common presentation is localized pain, often with a mass, and minimal or absent systemic symptoms. Approximately 50% have symptoms for a year or longer before diagnosis. Most lesions have a diaphyseal location in a long bone, especially the femur or humerus, but other frequent sites of involvement include the clavicle, ribs, and pelvis. Ill-defined, permeated, or moth-eaten destruction of bone with little or no periosteal reaction is the usual radiographic appearance. This appearance reflects the insidious spread of tumor cells along the

Table 8.2: Distinguishing Features of Multiple Myeloma and Metastases

	Myeloma	*Metastases*
Margin	Cleanly marginated	Irregular, more ragged
Mandible	Yes	Rarely
Pedicle	Rarely	Yes
Disc space	Yes	Rarely
Soft tissue mass	More likely	Less likely
Bone scan	Negative	Positive

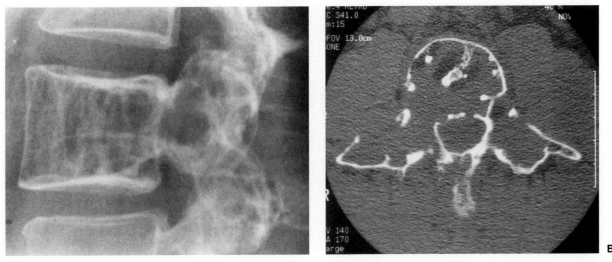

Figure 8.19 Plasmacytoma. *A.* Radiograph shows expansile, lytic lesion involving entire L2 vertebra. *B.* CT shows the extent of destruction.

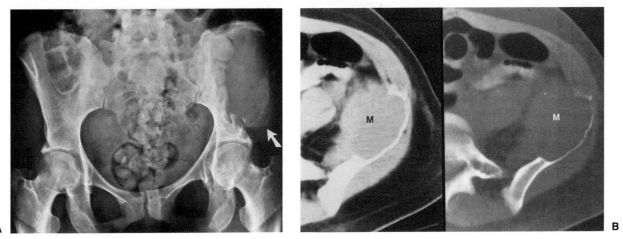

Figure 8.20 Plasmacytoma. *A.* AP radiograph of pelvis shows expansile, lytic lesion in left iliac wing (*arrow*). *B.* CT at soft tissue and bone windows shows destruction of anterior cortex with soft tissue mass (M).

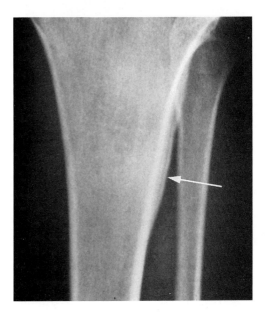

Figure 8.21 Lymphoma of the tibia. There is poorly defined medullary sclerosis and layered periosteal reaction (*arrow*).

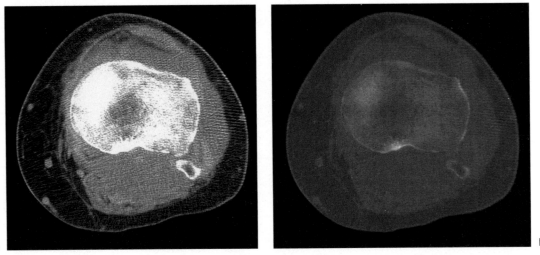

Figure 8.22 Lymphoma of the proximal tibia. *A.* Axial CT scan with soft tissue settings shows abnormal soft tissue surrounding the tibia. *B.* Axial CT scan with bone settings shows severe osteopenia.

marrow spaces and through the cortex by way of the haversian systems, growing through and enlarging them. The lesions may be extensive at presentation, often involving more than 50% of the affected bone. A large, nonmineralized soft tissue mass may be present when there is extensive cortical destruction. Mild to moderate bone reaction is seen in approximately 45% of lesions, consisting of a mottled sclerotic reaction within cancellous bone, new reactive periosteal bone, or both (Figs. 8.21 through 8.23). Sequestra were seen in 11% of the cases of primary lymphoma of bone. Lymphoma always shows increased isotope uptake on bone scan. CT and MRI are useful for demonstrating tumor extent, especially cortical penetration and extraosseous tumor. Primary lymphomas may also occur in muscle (Fig. 8.24). The treatment of lymphoma involves radiation therapy, adjuvant chemotherapy, and sometimes surgery. The prognosis is related to the cell type and pattern of

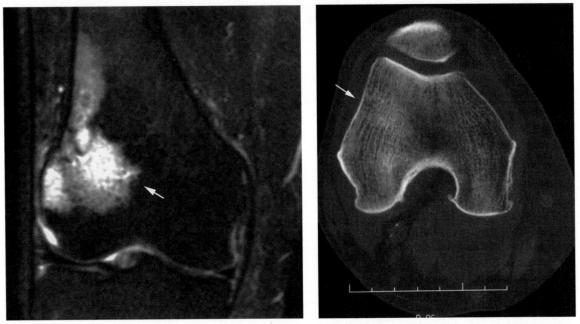

Figure 8.23 Lymphoma of the femur. *A.* Coronal T2-weighted fat-suppressed MRI shows irregular region of high signal (*arrow*). *B.* Axial CT scan shows vague region of sclerosis in the lateral femoral condyle (*arrow*).

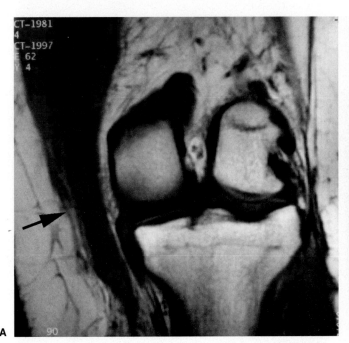 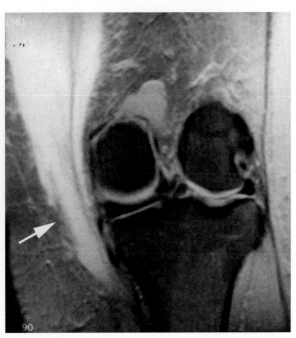

A **B**

Figure 8.24 Intramuscular lymphoma. *A.* Coronal T1-weighted MRI shows enlargement of the gracilis muscle (*arrow*). *B.* Coronal T2-weighted fat-suppressed MRI shows high signal throughout the gracilis muscle (*arrow*).

disease and to the extent of dissemination at presentation. With optimal treatment, the 5-year survival rate is greater than 75%.

SMALL CELL SARCOMAS

The group of small cell sarcomas includes Ewing sarcoma, primitive neuroectodermal tumor (PNET) of bone, and small cell osteosarcoma.

EWING SARCOMA

Ewing sarcoma is a tumor that consists of small, round, undifferentiated cells, probably of neuroectodermal histogenesis. Although 75% of Ewing sarcomas occur in patients younger than 20 years of age, these lesions may develop at any age. They are the most common primary bone tumor in the first decade of life, and the second most common (behind osteosarcoma) in the second decade. Patients present with local pain and swelling, fever, anemia, and elevated erythrocyte sedimentation rate; the clinical impression is often that of osteomyelitis. Up to 30% of patients have metastases at presentation. Ewing sarcoma may develop in practically any bone, although the majority of cases involve the sacrum, innominate bone, and long bones of the lower extremities. Only 3% of tumors affect the hands and feet. Most Ewing sarcomas are found in the metadiaphysis of long bones, mostly the femur, but they also occur in the diaphysis and metaphysis. Approximately one-fourth occur in flat bones (pelvis and scapula). The tumor begins in the medullary space and spreads through the bone, often causing only minimal osseous destruction. The tumor penetrates the cortex by extending through the haversian systems into the subperiosteal space where the tumor may enlarge, lift the periosteum off the bone, and eventually penetrate it to form an extraosseous mass. As further destruction of the cortex occurs, a permeated pattern of bone destruction may become evident. In the long bones, the typical radiographic appearance is that of permeated intramedullary bone destruction with periosteal reactive bone (Figs. 8.25 through 8.28). Sclerotic bone reaction within the bone is usually not seen, but on bone scan, intense radionuclide activity is present.

Although most common in the long bones of children, Ewing sarcomas may develop in virtually any bone at any age.

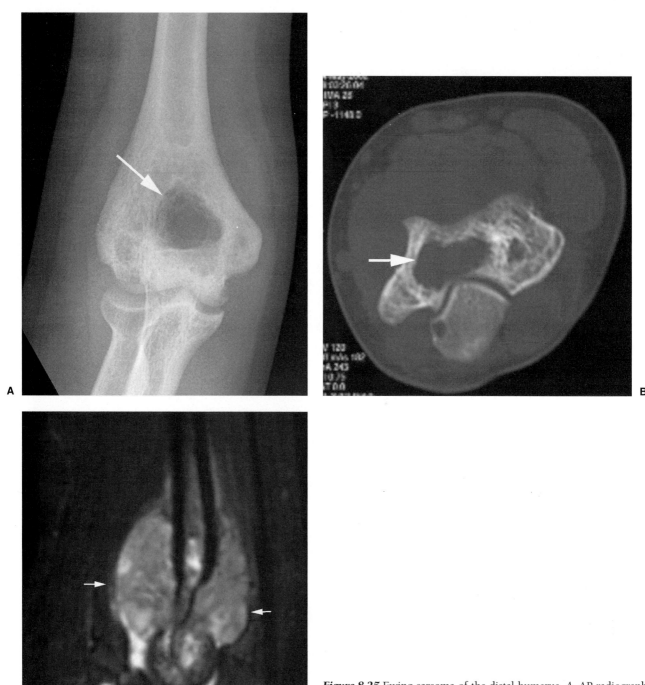

Figure 8.25 Ewing sarcoma of the distal humerus. *A.* AP radiograph shows a lytic lesion in the distal humerus at the olecranon fossa (*arrow*). The margins of the lesion are irregular, and there is no reactive bone formation. *B.* Axial CT scan shows the destructive bone lesion (*arrow*) with anterior and posterior soft tissue extension. *C.* Sagittal T2-weighted MRI shows a mass centered at the distal humerus with large anterior and posterior soft tissue components (*arrows*). The lesion has heterogeneous high signal. An elbow effusion is present.

Pathologic fractures occur in a small number of cases. CT and MRI scanning define the extraosseous and intramedullary components of the tumor and are useful in planning radiation portals and in following response to radiation and chemotherapy. A surrounding zone of edema is commonly present. Ewing sarcoma is highly radiosensitive. Radiation and chemotherapy may be used alone or in combination with surgical excision. However,

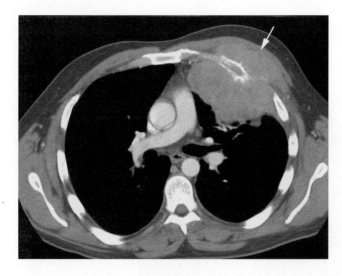

Figure 8.26 Ewing sarcoma of the rib. Enhanced CT scan shows rib destruction and massive soft tissue mass (*arrow*).

the rate of local tumor recurrence ranges from 12% to 25%. Soft tissue extension is associated with increased risk of distant metastases and local recurrence. Five-year survival for nonmetastatic tumor confined to the bone of origin is 87%, but survival drops to 20% with extraosseous extension. Patients who survive for several years may eventually develop secondary, radiation-induced sarcomas.

Hematogenous osteomyelitis spreads through bone in a fashion similar to Ewing sarcoma, leading to a similar radiologic appearance (see Chapter 16). Both may occur in the same age group and have similar clinical presentations.

PRIMITIVE NEUROECTODERMAL TUMOR

PNET is a type of small cell sarcoma closely related to but distinct from Ewing sarcoma and neuroblastoma. They share a number of cytogenetic and molecular biologic features and are identical to the malignant small cell tumor of the thoraco-pulmonary region (Askin tumor).

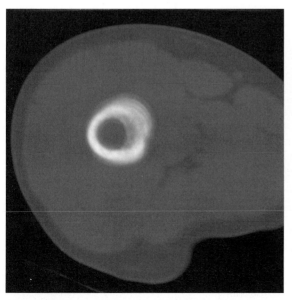
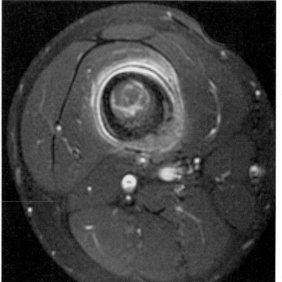

A

B

Figure 8.27 Ewing sarcoma of the femoral shaft. *A.* Axial CT scan shows onion-skin periosteal reaction in the femoral cortex with soft tissue density replacing normal fatty marrow. *B.* Axial T2-weighted fat-suppressed MRI shows onion-skin periosteal reaction and surrounding edema.

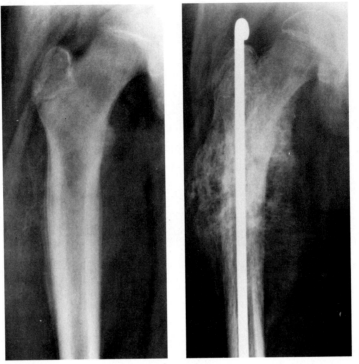

A   B

Figure 8.28 Ewing sarcoma. *A.* AP radiograph at presentation shows permeative destruction of the proximal femur with layered periosteal reaction and soft tissue mass. *B.* AP radiograph 6 months later (after radiotherapy) shows calcifying mass with layered and sunburst periosteal reaction. An intramedullary rod has been placed for fracture prophylaxis.

In the extremities, PNET shares many clinical characteristics with Ewing sarcoma, with similar presentation, peak age (mean, 15 years), and male predominance of 2:1. Metastases to bone, lung, liver, bone marrow, spleen, and lymph nodes are noted at presentation in 50%. It is virtually indistinguishable from Ewing sarcoma on imaging (Fig. 8.29). There is a per-

PNET is virtually indistinguishable from Ewing sarcoma on imaging.

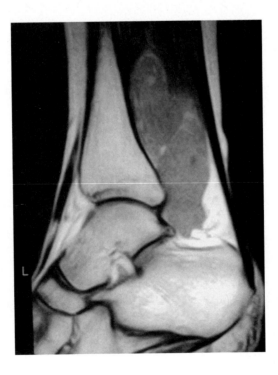

Figure 8.29 Primitive neuroectodermal tumor of ankle. Sagittal T1-weighted MRI shows a lobulated soft tissue mass in the posterior compartment of the ankle.

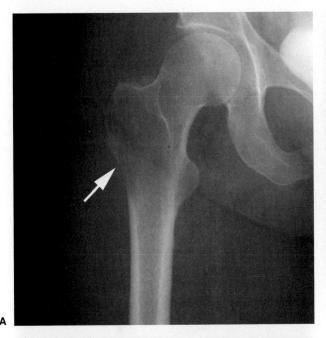

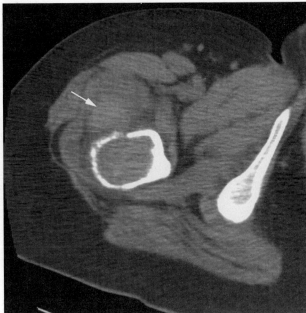

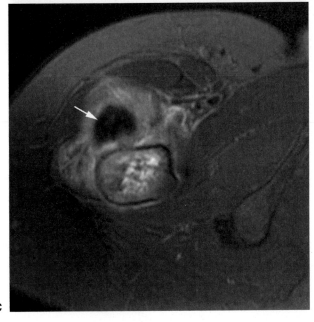

Figure 8.30 Small cell osteosarcoma. *A.* AP hip radiograph shows a lytic lesion in the intertrochanteric region of the femur (*arrow*). *B.* Axial CT scan shows intramedullary lesion with anterior cortical breakthrough and soft tissue mass with hyperdense mineralized region (*arrow*). *C.* Axial T2-weighted fat-suppressed MRI shows the extent of the lesion. The mineralized portion of the soft tissue mass (*arrow*) has low signal.

meated pattern of destruction with early soft tissue extension in a diaphyseal or metadiaphyseal location. There can be extensive periosteal reaction, often with an onion-skin or hair-on-end appearance. CT and MRI can be helpful in clarifying the extent of disease, and the radionuclide bone scan is useful in looking for osseous metastases. PNET has a much poorer prognosis than Ewing sarcoma.

SMALL CELL OSTEOSARCOMA

Small cell osteosarcoma is a variant of osteosarcoma that has a histologic appearance similar to Ewing sarcoma and lymphoma of bone. However, small amounts of mineralized tumor osteoid are present. The radiologic appearance is that of osteosarcoma in the majority of cases, but a significant proportion has an appearance that resembles Ewing sarcoma or lymphoma (Fig. 8.30). Similar to Ewing sarcoma, most patients are young. Small cell osteosarcomas are high-grade lesions that are treated similarly to conventional high-grade intramedullary osteosarcomas.

MALIGNANT FIBROUS HISTIOCYTOMA OF BONE

Although MFH of the soft tissues is common, MFH of bone is rare.

Malignant fibrous histiocytoma (MFH) is a malignant tumor of mesenchymal origin. Although MFH is the most common soft tissue sarcoma of adults, MFH of bone is rare. MFH of bone is most commonly found in the fifth to seventh decades but may occur at any age. Symptoms are nonspecific, often a palpable mass with pain and tenderness. More acute pain can occur secondary to pathologic fractures, which are common. MFH of bone can occur de novo, but 10% to 20% occur in association with other osseous abnormalities such as Paget disease and bone infarct (Fig. 8.31) or after radiation therapy. The most common sites are similar to those in

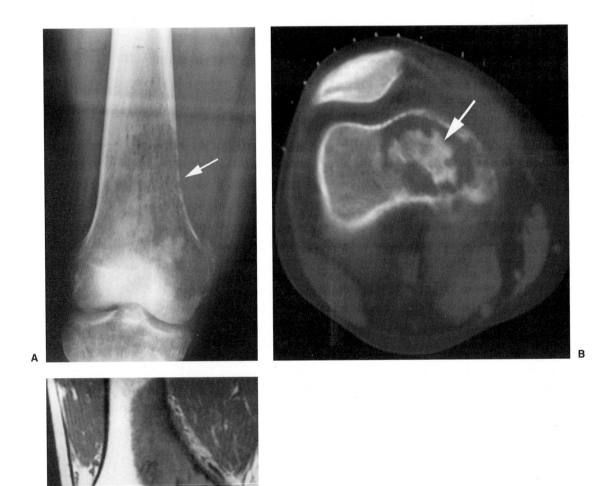

Figure 8.31 Malignant fibrous histiocytoma of bone arising in marrow infarct. *A.* AP radiograph of the distal femur shows permeated bone destruction (*arrow*). *B.* Axial CT scan shows bone destruction surrounding an irregularly shaped sequestrum (*arrow*) of bone. *C.* Coronal T1-weighted MRI shows the lesion (*long arrow*) in the distal femur and a marrow infarct (*short arrow*) in the proximal tibia.

osteosarcoma: the ends of long bones (75%), with a preponderance in the lower extremity. The femur (45%), tibia (20%), and humerus (9%) are the bones most often involved. The metaphyseal region is the most common location within bone, and extension into the epiphysis or diaphysis is frequent. The lesions have an aggressive appearance with permeated or moth-eaten destruction involving a poorly defined unifocal lesion. Cortical destruction and soft tissue mass are almost invariably present, and cortical expansion is unusual except in the flat and irregularly shaped bones (ribs, scapula, sternum). Periostitis is unusual unless a healing pathologic fracture is present. Mottled internal calcifications or sclerotic margins are rarely present. On CT, the lesions are predominantly muscle density (30 to 60 HU), with hypodense regions representing necrosis. MRI may be helpful to assess intraosseous versus extraosseous extension. Increased uptake is seen on bone scan. The treatment is surgical, with no clearly defined role for chemotherapy or radiotherapy. However, the prognosis is poor because of high rates of local recurrence and early metastases to regional lymph nodes and other distant sites. The reported 5-year survival ranges from 0% to 70%, depending on the stage of the lesion.

CHORDOMA

Chordomas are slow-growing malignant neoplasms that arise from notochordal remnants. They are typically seen in middle-aged men, most frequently at the ends of the spine (50% in the sacrum or coccyx, 35% in the clivus, and 15% elsewhere in the spine). Patients present with pain of insidious onset and symptoms caused by mass effect, often of long duration. Grossly, these tumors are multilobular, soft, myxoid, gelatinous masses that infiltrate locally and may eventually metastasize. In the sacrococcygeal region, the radiologic appearance is geographic bone destruction and replacement of bone by nonmineralized tumor. The margins range from sclerotic to ill defined. The cortex is often penetrated with the formation of a large, lobular, extraosseous mass anterior to the spine (Fig. 8.32). The tumors are typically large at presentation. Because of the myxoid matrix, the attenuation on CT is typically lower than cellular soft tissue, and MRI may show high signal on both T1- and T2-weighted images. The treatment is surgical, but complete excision is rarely possible because of their central location. A high rate of local recurrence and progressive difficulties in treating the recurrences result in a poor long-term prognosis. A secondary

Chordomas are slow-growing malignancies that have a high rate of local recurrence.

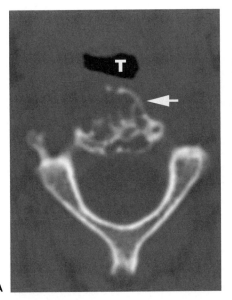 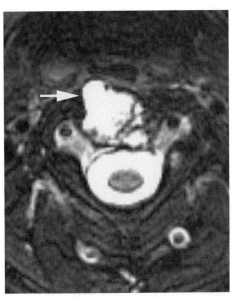

A   B

Figure 8.32 Chordoma. *A.* CT shows bone destruction at the body of C2 (*arrow*) with a soft tissue mass that impinges on the trachea (T). *B.* Axial T2-weighted MRI shows high signal within the lesion (*arrow*). (*continued*)

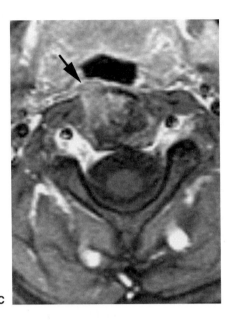

Figure 8.32 *(continued) C.* Axial T1-weighted MRI with fat suppression after gadolinium injection shows heterogeneous enhancement *(arrow).* (Courtesy of Kevin McEnery, MD.)

component of high-grade sarcoma resembling MFH (dedifferentiated chordoma) may appear after multiple recurrences.

ADAMANTINOMA

Adamantinoma is a primary low-grade malignant tumor of bone. It is of epithelial origin, with marked predilection for the tibia. Adamantinoma is often associated with osteofibrous dysplasia, and some authorities believe that they are subsets of the same disease. [Adamantinoma of bone is distinct from gnathic adamantinoma (ameloblastoma), although both share an epithelial origin and a microscopic resemblance.] Although 50% present at ages 10 to 30 years, adamantinoma may be found at any age. Symptoms of pain are often present

Adamantinoma involves the tibia in 90% of cases.

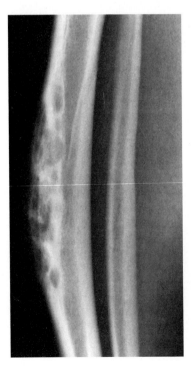

Figure 8.33 Adamantinoma of the tibia. Lateral radiograph shows lobulated, expansile lucent lesion with anterior tibial bowing deformity.

for more than a year, and 90% involve the tibia. A few patients have an ipsilateral fibular tumor. The radiographic appearance is that of an eccentrically located lucent lesion with lobulated expansion of the cortex and sharply defined margins (Fig. 8.33). The most common location is the tibial diaphysis with involvement of the anterior cortex. An anterior tibial bowing deformity is common. Approximately 90% involve the cortex and medullary space, 10% are confined to the cortex, and 15% penetrate the cortex and involve the soft tissues. The treatment is surgical, with a high rate of recurrence after curettage and a lower rate after wide excision. Metastases to lung, nodes, or bone may present many years later.

SOFT TISSUE SARCOMAS

The reported annual incidence of soft tissue sarcomas in the United States is 6,400. Approximately two-thirds of these are found in the extremities and limb girdles (Table 8.3), making them more common than primary bone sarcomas in the same locations. Most are of mesenchymal origin; a minority is of neuroectodermal origin. In adults, the most common lesions are MFH, liposarcoma, synovial sarcoma, leiomyosarcoma, and malignant schwannoma (Table 8.4). Fibrosarcoma is the most common lesion in patients younger than 6 years of age, and MFH (including variants) and synovial sarcoma are most common from ages 6 to 15 years. The majority of soft tissue sarcomas present in adults. Patients complain of a palpable mass of long duration and pain or tenderness of insidious onset. Patients may delay seeking medical attention, and this long chronicity may falsely suggest

> The typical presentation of a soft tissue sarcoma is a large, palpable mass that has been present for months or years.

Table 8.3: Anatomic Distribution of Soft Tissue Sarcomas in the Extremities and Limb Girdles[a]

Location	Frequency (%)
Lower extremity	45
Upper extremity	16
Hip and buttocks	14
Proximal limb girdle	9
Foot and ankle	9
Hand and wrist	7

[a]Based on 6,796 soft tissue sarcomas of the extremities and limb girdles, including all ages and all histologic types. Adapted from Kransdorf MJ. Malignant soft-tissue tumors in a large referral population: distribution of diagnoses by age, sex, and location. *AJR Am J Roentgenol* 1995;164:129–134.

Table 8.4: Most Common Soft Tissue Sarcomas in the Extremities and Limb Girdles at Various Ages[a]

0–5 yr	6–15 yr	≥16 yr
Fibrosarcoma	MFH (including angiomatoid MFH)	MFH
Rhabdomyosarcoma	Synovial sarcoma	Liposarcoma
		Synovial sarcoma
		Malignant schwannoma
		Leiomyosarcoma

MFH, malignant fibrous histiocytoma.
[a]For each age range, the tumors are listed in order of frequency and account for more than 50% of the lesions.
Adapted from Kransdorf MJ. Malignant soft-tissue tumors in a large referral population: distribution of diagnoses by age, sex, and location. *AJR Am J Roentgenol* 1995;164:129–134.

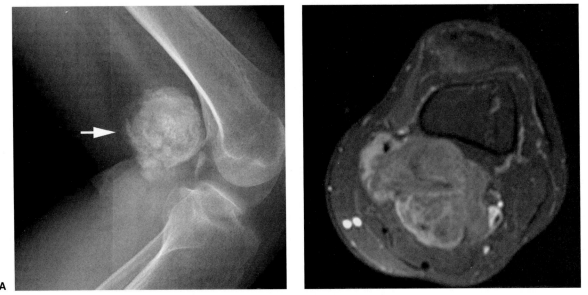

Figure 8.34 Synovial sarcoma. *A.* Lateral radiograph of the knee shows a heavily calcified mass posterior to the knee (*arrow*). *B.* Axial T1-weighted MRI with fat suppression after gadolinium injection shows heterogeneous enhancement. The low signal regions correspond to calcification.

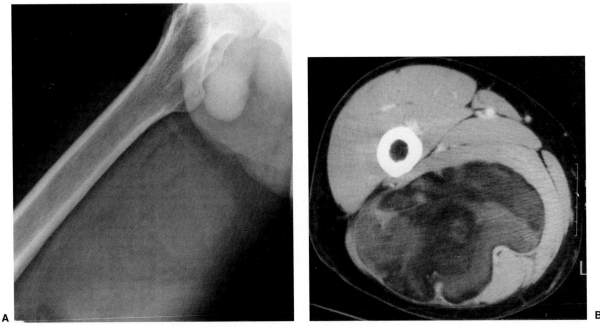

Figure 8.35 Liposarcoma. *A.* Lateral radiograph of the thigh shows a large, lucent lesion in the posterior soft tissues. *B.* Axial CT scan shows a heterogeneous fat-containing soft tissue mass in the posterior compartment of the thigh. (*continued*)

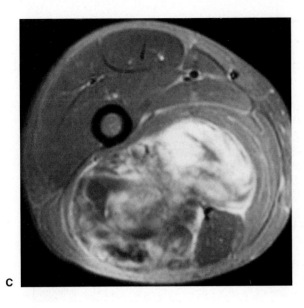

C

Figure 8.35 (*continued*) *C.* Axial T2-weighted MRI with fat suppression shows high signal in some portions of the lesion with low signal resulting from fat suppression in other portions of the lesion.

an indolent process. The majority of lesions present in stage II-B or III (see Chapter 7). Soft tissue sarcomas metastasize to lung, liver, or bone.

Soft tissue sarcomas have nonspecific appearances on imaging, and there are no reliable criteria for distinguishing among them. Once benign soft tissue masses with specific features such as lipoma, elastofibroma, ganglion, myositis ossificans, aneurysm, bursitis, and hematoma have been eliminated as possibilities, factors that suggest sarcoma include older age, location in the thigh, large size, round or ovoid shape, and involvement of adjacent bone. Malignant soft tissue masses usually have areas of inhomogeneity and lower density on CT that correspond to regions of necrosis and hemorrhage. Sarcomas that calcify or ossify include synovial sarcoma (Fig. 8.34), extraskeletal osteosarcoma, extraskeletal chondrosarcoma, rhabdomyosarcoma, MFH, and liposarcoma. The presence of fat within a lesion suggests a well-differentiated liposarcoma (Fig. 8.35), but higher-grade liposarcomas generally do not contain fat. Small amounts of subcutaneous or intermuscular fat may be engulfed by an aggressive sarcoma as it enlarges, so that the presence of fat

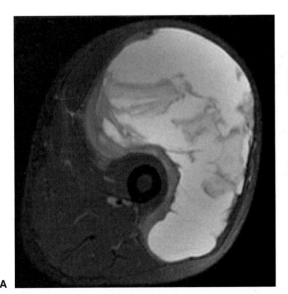

A

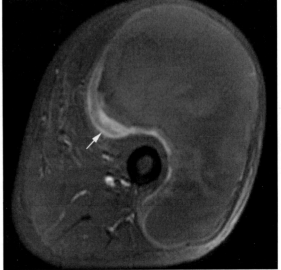

B

Figure 8.36 Preoperative staging for soft tissue sarcoma in the anterior compartment of the thigh. *A.* Axial T2-weighted MRI shows a lesion occupying the entire anterior compartment. Septation and stranding are present within the lesion. *B.* Axial T1-weighted MRI with fat suppression after gadolinium injection shows rim enhancement (*arrow*), indicative of extensive necrosis of the nonenhancing regions.

is not necessarily indicative of liposarcoma. On MRI, soft tissue sarcomas usually have intermediate signal on T1-weighted images and high signal on T2-weighted images. Enhancement with intravenous contrast can be expected on both CT and MRI. The goal of imaging, once the presence of the lesion is confirmed, should be to define the lesion's size and location and the extent and anatomic relation of the lesion to muscle compartments, fascial planes, neurovascular bundles, and bone. Staging follows the system used for bone sarcomas. The treatment of soft tissue sarcomas is surgical, sometimes with neoadjuvant or adjuvant radiation therapy, chemotherapy, or both. Imaging of soft tissue sarcomas for surgical planning after chemotherapy and radiation therapy may reveal extensive areas of liquefaction, hemorrhage, and necrosis (Fig. 8.36). Five-year survival rates of 25% to 60% have been reported.

SOURCES AND READINGS

Askin FB, Perlman EJ. Neuroblastoma and peripheral neuroectodermal tumors. *Am J Clin Pathol* 1998;109[Suppl]:S23–S30.

Bataille R, Chappard D, Klein B. Mechanisms of bone lesions in multiple myeloma. *Hematol Oncol Clin North Am* 1992;6:285–295.

Callander NS, Roodman GD. Myeloma bone disease. *Semin Hematol* 2001;38:276–285.

Durr HR, Muller PE, Hiller E, et al. Malignant lymphoma of bone. *Arch Orthop Trauma Surg* 2002;122:10–16.

Enneking WF. *Musculoskeletal tumor surgery.* Edinburgh: Churchill Livingstone, 1983.

Fechner RE, Mills SE. *Tumors of the bones and joints.* Washington, DC: Armed Forces Institute of Pathology, 1993.

Ferguson WS, Goorin AM. Current treatment of osteosarcoma. *Cancer Invest* 2001;19:292–315.

Fuchs B, Pritchard DJ. Etiology of osteosarcoma. *Clin Orthop* 2002;397:40–52.

George ED, Sadovsky R. Multiple myeloma: recognition and management. *Am Fam Physician* 1999;59:1885–1894.

Goorin AM, Abelson HT, Frei E III. Osteosarcoma: fifteen years later. *N Engl J Med* 1985;313:1637–1643.

Guise TA. Molecular mechanisms of osteolytic bone metastases. *Cancer* 2000;88[Suppl]:2892–2898.

Hallek M, Bergsagel PL, Anderson KC. Multiple myeloma: increasing evidence for a multistep transformation process. *Blood* 1998;91:3–21.

Hemminki K, Li X. A population-based study of familial soft tissue tumors. *J Clin Epidemiol* 2001;54:411–416.

Hudson TM. *Radiologic-pathologic correlation of musculoskeletal lesions.* Baltimore: Williams & Wilkins, 1987.

Hussein MA, Juturi JV, Lieberman I. Multiple myeloma: present and future. *Curr Opin Oncol* 2002;14:31–35.

Huvos AG. *Bone tumors: diagnosis, treatment, and prognosis,* 2nd ed. Philadelphia: WB Saunders, 1991.

Jacobs JJ, Roebuck KA, Archibeck M, et al. Osteolysis: basic science. *Clin Orthop* 2001;393:71–77.

Jemal A, Thomas A, Murray T, et al. Cancer statistics, 2002. *CA Cancer J Clin* 2002;52:23–47.

Jurgens H, Bier V, Harms D, et al. Malignant peripheral neuroectodermal tumors: a retrospective analysis of 42 patients. *Cancer* 1988;61:349–357.

Kransdorf MJ. Malignant soft-tissue tumors in a large referral population: distribution of diagnoses by age, sex, and location. *AJR Am J Roentgenol* 1995;164:129–134.

Kransdorf MJ, Murphey MD. *Imaging of soft tissue tumors.* Philadelphia: WB Saunders, 1997.

Kransdorf MJ, Murphey MD. Radiologic evaluation of soft-tissue masses: a current perspective. *AJR Am J Roentgenol* 2000;175:575–587.

Kumar RV, Mukherjee G, Bhargava MK. Malignant fibrous histiocytoma of bone. *J Surg Oncol* 1990;44:166–170.

Lodwick GS. *Atlas of tumor radiology. The bones and joints.* Chicago: Year Book, 1971.

Meyers PA, Gorlick R. Osteosarcoma. *Pediatr Clin North Am* 1997;44:973–989.

Mulligan ME, Kransdorf MJ. Sequestra in primary lymphoma of bone: prevalence and radiographic features. *AJR Am J Roentgenol* 1993;160:1245–1248.

Mulligan ME, McRae GA, Murphey MD. Imaging features of primary lymphoma of bone. *AJR Am J Roentgenol* 1999;173:1691–1697.

Mundy G. Preclinical models of bone metastases. *Semin Oncol* 2001;28:2–8.

Mundy GR. Mechanisms of osteolytic bone destruction. *Bone* 1991;12[Suppl 1]:1–6.

Munk PL, Sallomi DF, Janzen DL, et al. Malignant fibrous histiocytoma of soft tissue imaging with emphasis on MRI. *J Comput Assist Tomogr* 1998;22:819–826.

Murphey MD, Flemming DJ, Boyea SR, et al. Enchondroma versus chondrosarcoma in the appendicular skeleton: differentiating features. *Radiographics* 1998;18:1213–1237.

Murphey MD, Kransdorf MJ, Smith SE. Imaging of soft tissue neoplasms in the adult: malignant tumors. *Semin Musculoskelet Radiol* 1999;3:39–58.

Murphey MD, Robbin MR, McRae GA, et al. The many faces of osteosarcoma. *Radiographics* 1997;17:1205–1231.

Niesvizky R, Siegel D, Michaeli J. Biology and treatment of multiple myeloma. *Blood Rev* 1993;7:24–33.

Papagelopoulos PJ, Galanis EC, Sim FH, et al. Clinicopathologic features, diagnosis, and treatment of malignant fibrous histiocytoma of bone. *Orthopedics* 2000;23:59–65.

Papagelopoulos PJ, Galanis EC, Vlastou C, et al. Current concepts in the evaluation and treatment of osteosarcoma. *Orthopedics* 2000;23:858–867.

Pitcher JD Jr, Bocklage T, Crooks L, et al. *The pathology, orthopaedics, and radiology of musculoskeletal tumors PORT notes.* Albuquerque, NM: Orthopaedic Oncologic Publishing Services, 2002.

Resnick D. *Diagnosis of bone and joint disorders*, 4th ed. Philadelphia: WB Saunders, 2002.

Ros P, Viamonte M Jr, Rywlin AM. Malignant fibrous histiocytoma: mesenchymal tumor of ubiquitous origin. *AJR Am J Roentgenol* 1984;142:753–759.

Sangueza OP, Requena L. Neoplasms with neural differentiation: a review part II: malignant neoplasms. *Am J Dermatopathol* 1998;20:89–102.

Unni KK. *Dahlin's bone tumors. General aspects and data on 11,087 cases*, 5th ed. Philadelphia: Lippincott–Raven, 1996.

Zahir KS, Quin JA, Brown W, et al. Trends in the incidence of upper extremity soft tissue malignancies: a 40-year review of the Connecticut State Tumor Registry. *Conn Med* 1998;62:9–14.

Zaidi AA, Vesole DH. Multiple myeloma: an old disease with new hope for the future. *CA Cancer J Clin* 2001;51:273–285.

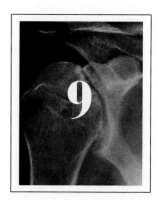

BENIGN LESIONS

This chapter describes benign neoplasms and benign tumor-like lesions that are not neo-plastic in origin. A key decision that becomes easier with experience is whether a radiologic finding represents an actual lesion or merely a normal structure, an anatomic or develop-mental variant, or the result of previous trauma, surgery, or other disease. Atlases of normal variants are often helpful. The principal lesions one should consider in formulating a dif-ferential diagnosis for a benign lesion are listed in Table 9.1.

BENIGN BONE-FORMING LESIONS

OSTEOID OSTEOMA

Osteoid osteoma is a fairly common benign bone-forming neoplasm. The lesion, called a *nidus*, is small, generally ranging in size from 3 to 15 mm. When larger, the lesion is often classified as an osteoblastoma (discussed in the section Osteoblastoma). Approximately 80% of patients are between the ages of 5 and 20 years; few are older than 30 years of age. The location may be cortical, central, or, less frequently, subperiosteal. The femur is the most common site (39% of cases), followed by the tibia (23%) and upper extremity (21%). Patients present with dull, aching pain that has lasted for months to years. When located in the spine, osteoid osteomas may cause painful scoliosis of rapid onset; near a joint, they may cause reac-tive synovitis. The nidus consists of osteoid and fibrovascular connective tissue. The osteoid may be mineralized to a variable extent, usually in the center (Fig. 9.1). The nidus is radiolu-cent but may be obscured by cortical thickening and dense sclerosis from reactive bone. Scle-rosis is usually minimal around lesions located in cancellous bone, near a joint, or in a subperiosteal position (Fig. 9.2). Osteoid osteomas have intensely increased activity on bone scan; the activity may be more intense in the nidus ("double-density" sign). The nidus may enhance on CT and MRI, reflecting the fibrovascular tissue within it. Because of the small size of the nidus and its possible obscuration by reactive sclerosis, CT is commonly used to iden-tify and localize the nidus. Osteoid osteomas have been treated by surgical excision, but their small size makes them amenable to percutaneous radiofrequency ablation or excision under CT guidance. Failure to remove or destroy the entire nidus may lead to recurrence.

Osteoid osteomas located in cancel-lous bone, near a joint, or in the subperiosteum often have minimal reactive sclerosis.

Table 9.1: Benign Bone Lesions

	Solitary[a]	*Solitary or Multifocal*
Common	Osteoid osteoma	Bone island
	Simple bone cyst	Fibrous cortical defect
	Bone (Brodie) abscess	Osteochondroma
		Enchondroma
		Fibrous dysplasia
		Nonossifying fibroma
		Eosinophilic granuloma
Uncommon	Giant cell tumor	
	Osteoblastoma	
	Chondroblastoma	
	Periosteal chondroma	
	Aneurysmal bone cyst	
Rare	Chondromyxoid fibroma	

[a]There may be case reports of multiple lesions.

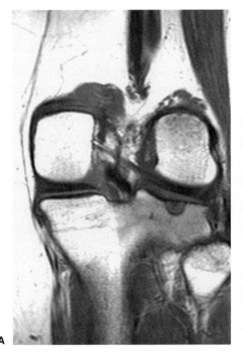
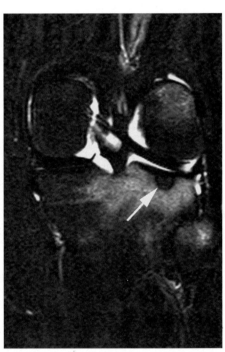

Figure 9.1 Osteoid osteoma in the lateral tibial plateau. *A.* Coronal T1-weighted MRI shows lesion in the subchondral bone of the lateral tibial plateau. *B.* Coronal T2-weighted fat-suppressed MRI shows nidus (*arrow*) with surrounding edema. (*continued*)

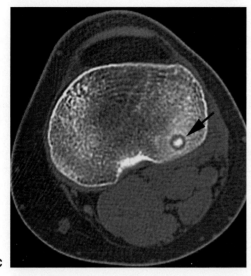

C

Figure 9.1 (*continued*) *C.* Axial CT scan shows central ossification within the nidus (*arrow*).

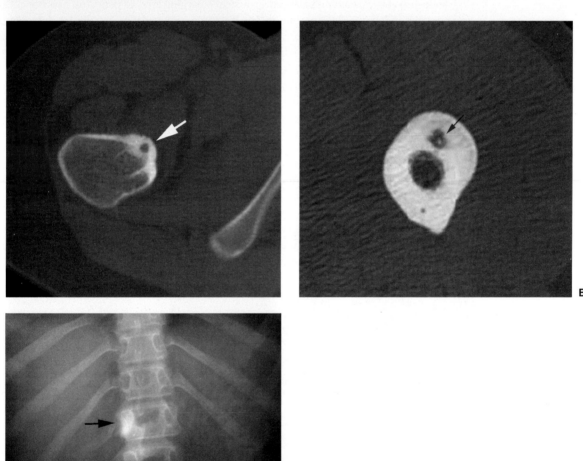

A

B

C

Figure 9.2 Radiologic presentations of osteoid osteoma (different patients). *A.* Axial CT scan shows a round nidus (*arrow*) in the lesser trochanter with moderate reactive bone formation. *B.* Axial CT scan shows a round nidus with central calcification (*arrow*) in the cortex of the femoral shaft, with exuberant reactive sclerosis. *C.* AP radiograph shows reactive scoliosis with an osteoid osteoma in the T12 vertebra (*arrow*).

OSTEOBLASTOMA

Osteoblastomas are uncommon lesions that are considered by some to be giant osteoid osteomas because of their histologic resemblance. They affect young persons; 80% occur in patients younger than 30 years of age. Approximately half are found in the spine and most of the remainder in the femur and tibia. Of those in the spine, most are in the posterior elements; a few also involve the vertebral body, and very few involve the vertebral body alone. Within tubular bones, osteoblastomas may be intracortical, subperiosteal, or central in location. They are larger than osteoid osteomas, generally 1 to 10 cm in diameter. There is usually much less reactive bone surrounding an osteoblastoma than an osteoid osteoma. Patients with osteoblastomas typically present with pain of several months' duration. If the lesion is superficial, localized swelling and tenderness are present. In the spine, lesions may produce painful scoliosis; they may also interfere mechanically with the cord or with nerve roots. The radiographic appearance is a partially lucent expansile lesion with well-defined margins and a variable amount of matrix mineralization (Figs. 9.3 and 9.4). The lucent area of geographic bone destruction corresponds to replacement of bone by nonmineralized tumor tissue. The tumor osteoid may have densely solid or ground-glass mineralization. Large lesions may have an expanded cortical shell from slow endosteal cortical erosion balanced against an enlarging layer of periosteal new bone. Cortical penetration into the soft tissues is absent, but tomography may be required to demonstrate the cortical shell. The tumor tissue may have high attenuation on CT from the diffuse mineralization. Osteoblastomas are hot on bone scan. Osteoblastomas usually grow slowly and respond well to excision; very few have been reported to become locally aggressive.

> Osteoblastomas are found in the spine in approximately 50% of cases.

BONE ISLAND

A bone island (enostosis) is a circular or oblong nodule of cortical-type bone lying within cancellous bone. Bone islands are typically 1 cm in size but range up to 4 cm. They consist of histologically normal compact bone with haversian systems. They may be found anywhere in the skeleton. Radiographically, they are homogeneous and as dense as cortical bone. They are well defined but have peripheral spiculations that merge with the surrounding trabeculae (Fig. 9.5). Occasionally, they may change in size or remodel. On radionuclide bone scan, isotope uptake is absent or minimal. Bone islands are common and may be mistaken for other lesions such as osteoblastic metastases; they have no clinical significance. Small bone islands are common incidental findings on CT and MRI.

> Bone islands may change size or shape.

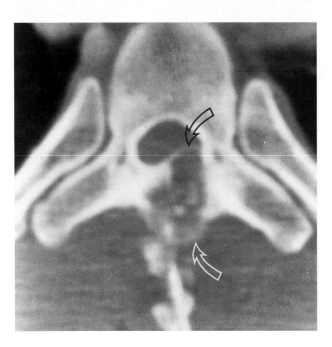

Figure 9.3 Osteoblastoma in the spine. CT shows an expansile lesion in the neural arch of a lower thoracic vertebra (*curved arrows*).

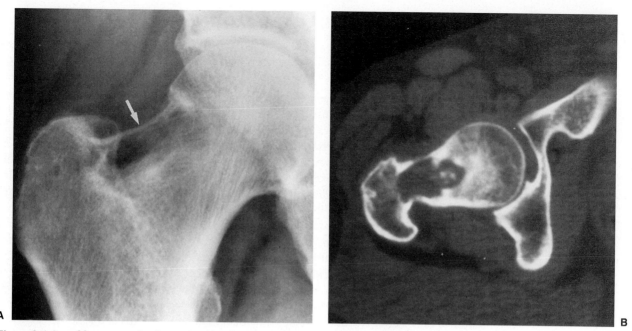

Figure 9.4 Osteoblastoma in the femoral neck. *A.* Radiograph shows lucent lesion (*arrow*) in femoral neck with sclerotic margin. *B.* CT shows partial mineralization.

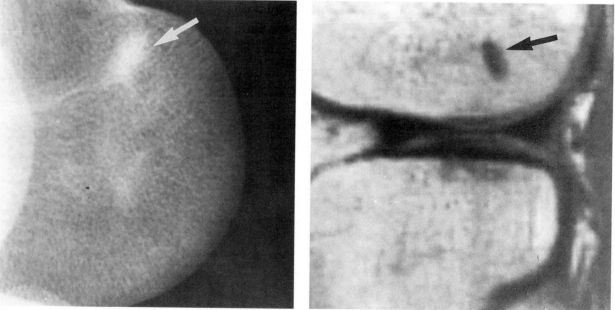

Figure 9.5 Bone islands. *A.* Bone island in the cancellous bone of the femoral metaphysis (*arrow*). The margins appear spiculated where they blend into the normal cancellous bone. The lesion is as dense as the cortex. *B.* Sagittal T1-weighted MRI shows a bone island in the lateral femoral condyle (*arrow*).

BENIGN CARTILAGE LESIONS

ENCHONDROMA

Solitary enchondromas are benign neoplasms located within the medullary cavity that are composed of mature hyaline cartilage. They probably arise from cartilaginous rests displaced from the growth plate. The sex incidence is equal, and most patients are between 10 and 50 years of age. Typically, the lesions are asymptomatic and discovered incidentally, but many patients present with pathologic fractures. The most common locations for solitary enchondromas are the hands (approximately 50% of cases), the proximal and distal femur, and the proximal humerus. In the hands, the middle and distal portions of the metacarpals and the proximal portions of the phalanges are typically involved. Radiographically, these lesions are lucent from replacement of bone by nonmineralized cartilage, but the typical mineralization patterns of cartilaginous matrix may be present: dense punctate or flocculent calcifications or ring- or arc-shaped densities from enchondral ossification of lobular cartilage (Fig. 9.6). Slow endosteal enlargement causes an expanded, thinned cortex, but cortical penetration is absent. On MRI, enchondromas have low signal on T1-weighted and proton density images but high signal on T2-weighted images with foci of low signal intensity corresponding to areas of calcification. A characteristic lobular configuration is virtually diagnostic (Fig. 9.7). On radionuclide bone scan, increased isotope uptake is seen, reflecting enchondral ossification, hyperemia, and reactive bone formation.

Occasionally, it may be difficult to distinguish an enchondroma from a low-grade chondrosarcoma radiographically. Imaging findings that suggest a chondrosarcoma include deep endosteal scalloping (greater than two-thirds of cortical thickness), cortical destruction and soft-tissue mass (at CT or MRI), periosteal reaction (at radiography), marked uptake of radionuclide (greater than the anterior iliac crest) at bone scintigraphy, and destruction of chondroid matrix over time. Development of chondrosarcoma from solitary enchondroma has not been proved conclusively.

Most solitary enchondromas are asymptomatic and discovered incidentally.

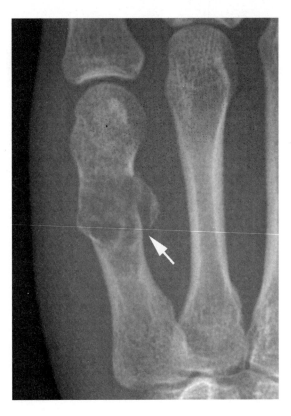

Figure 9.6 Enchondroma with lucent matrix occupying the midshaft of the fifth metacarpal. The overlying cortex is thinned. A pathologic fracture is present (*arrow*).

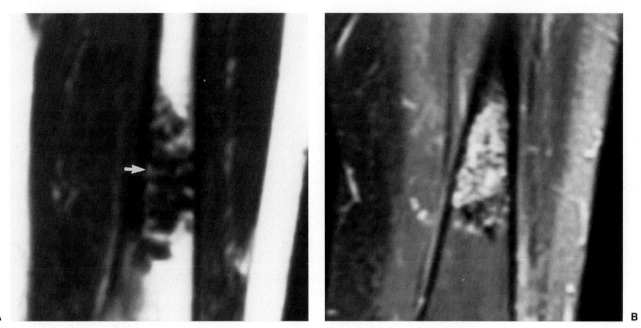

A   B

Figure 9.7 Enchondroma in the femur. *A.* Coronal T1-weighted MRI shows low signal and lobular configuration (*arrow*). *B.* Coronal T2-weighted MRI shows high signal in the lesion.

Multiple enchondromatosis (Ollier disease) is a nonfamilial, nonheritable diffuse growth abnormalityin which the tubular bones may be bowed and shortened to a variable extent and filled with multiple enchondromas (Fig. 9.8). The severity of involvement may range from a few lesions with mild deformities to countless lesions with severe deformities. The lesions often become stable at puberty, but their growth may continue throughout life. Individual lesions are radiologically and histologically identical to solitary enchondromas,

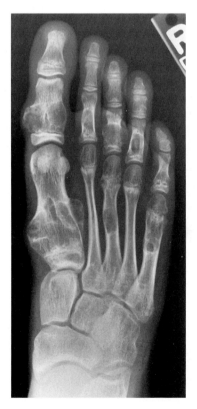

Figure 9.8 Multiple enchondromatosis (Ollier disease) deforming the foot. Some lesions have calcified matrix.

Patients with multiple enchondromatosis are at risk for developing chondrosarcoma.

but patients with multiple enchondromatosis have a 30% to 50% risk of developing chondrosarcoma. A lesion that becomes painful in the absence of pathologic fracture should trigger consideration of malignancy. Multiple enchondromatosis with multiple soft tissue hemangiomas is called *Maffucci syndrome*. The hemangiomatosis may be localized or extensive and may occur anywhere in the skin or subcutaneous tissues.

OSTEOCHONDROMA

Osteochondromas (also called *benign exostoses*) are outgrowths of histologically normal bone that arise in the vicinity of a growth plate. They are exceedingly common and present during late childhood and adolescence. Although any bone with enchondral ossification may be involved, the femur, the proximal tibia, and the proximal humerus account for two-thirds of cases. The typical site is metaphyseal, but osteochondromas may arise anywhere near a growth plate, including accessory ossification centers. Osteochondromas are not thought to be neoplastic but result from the growth of aberrant foci of cartilage on the bony surface. As the cartilage grows, it forms a cap over a bony mass that develops by progressive enchondral ossification. The bony portion contains mature, normal cortical and medullary bone with a marrow space contiguous with the parent bone. Deep lobules of cartilage may be present, often heavily ossified. The lesion may be pedunculated on a stalk, sometimes resembling a cauliflower (Figs. 9.9 and 9.10). Osteochondromas may also be sessile and resemble an expansile lesion. The cartilage cap largely disappears by adulthood. The typical clinical presentation is a firm mass of long duration that may mechanically interfere with function. A bursa may form over the surface and produce pain; in the presence of hemorrhage into a bursa, an enlarging mass develops.

Osteochondromas are not thought to be neoplastic.

OSTEOCHONDROMATOSIS

Osteochondromatosis is a skeletal dysplasia.

Osteochondromatosis (multiple heritable exostoses, multiple osteochondromas, diaphyseal aclasis) is one of the most common skeletal dysplasias. The condition is familial, with more severe manifestations in men. The skeleton is involved symmetrically, and the limbs are affected more than the spine. The number of exostoses varies. Deformities of the tubular bones are present (Fig. 9.11) and cause disproportionately short limbs, but the degree of shortness appears to be unrelated to the number of exostoses. Growth of the lesions slows as the skeleton matures, and new lesions do not appear in adulthood. Multiple exostoses are radiologically and

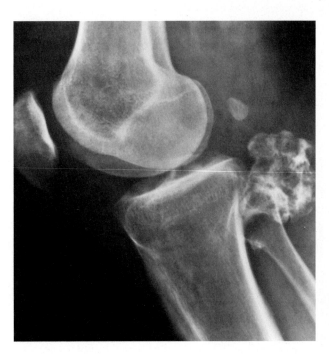

Figure 9.9 Pedunculated osteochondroma arising from posterior tibial cortex that resembles a cauliflower.

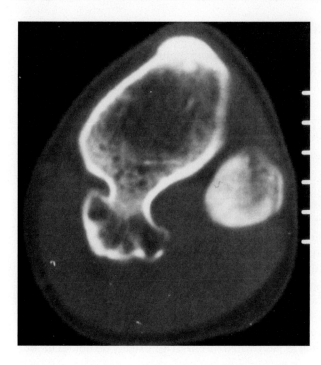

Figure 9.10 Axial CT scan of osteochondroma showing its marrow space to be contiguous with that of the underlying bone.

histologically indistinguishable from solitary exostoses. Secondary development of chondrosarcoma in a solitary exostosis or in one of the multiple exostoses is a small but definite risk, probably on the order of 1% to 2%; the onset of pain or growth in an adult suggests the possibility. The radiologic distinction between a benign exostosis and an exostotic chondrosarcoma is difficult unless growth and change in appearance can be demonstrated on serial films.

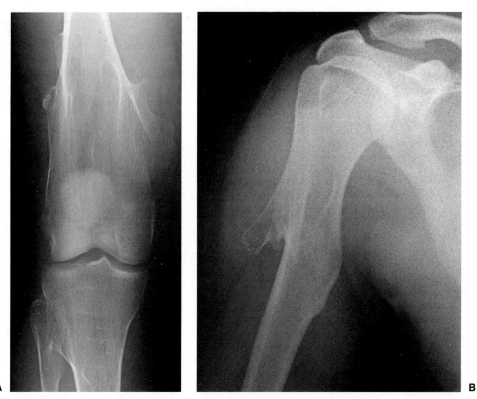

A B

Figure 9.11 Multiple hereditary osteochondromatosis. *A,B.* Radiographs of the knee and shoulder show multiple bony exostoses and deformity of the tubular bones.

Periosteal Chondroma

Periosteal chondroma is a benign neoplasm composed of mature cartilage that is located beneath the periosteum. The cortical surface is eroded, but the medullary cavity is not involved. Most are located in the metaphysis or diaphysis of a long bone; the humerus is the most common site. The lesions are lucent and characteristically surrounded by smoothly contoured, solid, periosteal reactive bone (Fig. 9.12). Cartilage matrix calcification may be present. Symptoms are nonspecific; local excision is curative.

Chondroblastoma

When chondroblastomas occur outside the usual age group, they arise in unusual locations.

Chondroblastoma (Codman tumor) is an uncommon benign neoplasm that consists of chondroid tissue mixed with more cellular tissue. Location in the epiphysis is characteristic (approximately 98%), often with extension into the metaphysis (Fig. 9.13). Two-thirds arise in the lower extremities, and half arise around the knee. Most patients are young; 80% are between 5 and 25 years of age. When chondroblastomas occur outside the usual age group, they arise in unusual locations. The presentation is nonspecific, typically pain. The radiographic appearance is an ovoid or rounded lucent epiphyseal lesion that is eccentrically located. The margins are geographic, usually with a thin, reactive bony rim. Scattered mottled or stippled calcifications, like those of other cartilage tumors, may be present. Chondroblastomas treated by curettage usually do not recur, but some are aggressive locally.

Chondromyxoid Fibroma

Chondromyxoid fibromas are rare, cartilage-forming neoplasms with variable amounts of myxoid and fibrous tissue. Young adults are affected most often, but there is a broad age range. The presentation is usually pain. Most chondromyxoid fibromas are found in the lower extremities. The typical radiographic appearance is an eccentric metaphyseal lucent lesion, ovoid or round and lobulated, with a sclerotic rim (Fig. 9.14). Intralesional matrix mineralization is rare. Sometimes, the rim has thickly trabeculated walls, corresponding to a grossly lobular tumor. Cortical expansion may result in a thin, perhaps imperceptible, cortical shell. The treatment is curettage.

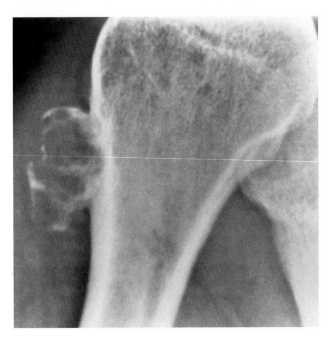

Figure 9.12 Periosteal chondroma of proximal humerus.

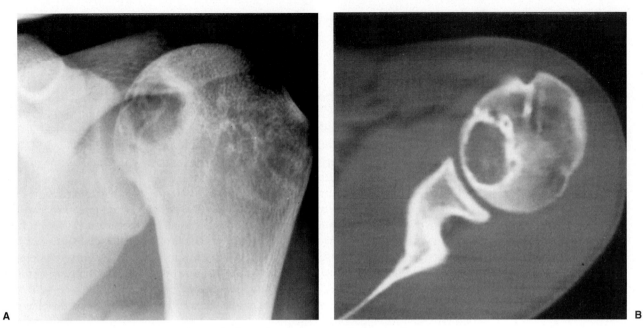

A   B

Figure 9.13 Chondroblastoma. *A.* Radiograph shows lucent lesion with dense sclerotic margin in humeral epiphysis. *B.* Axial CT scan shows faint matrix mineralization.

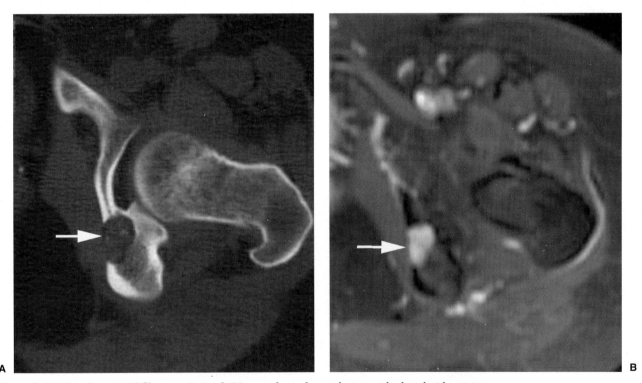

A   B

Figure 9.14 Chondromyxoid fibroma. *A.* Axial CT scan shows lucent lesion with chondroid matrix mineralization in the ischium (*arrow*). *B.* Axial T2-weighted fat-suppressed MRI showing high signal within the lesion (*arrow*).

BENIGN FIBROUS LESIONS

FIBROUS CORTICAL DEFECTS AND NONOSSIFYING FIBROMAS

Fibrous cortical defects and nonossifying fibromas regress spontaneously.

Fibrous cortical defects and nonossifying fibromas (fibroxanthomas) are histologically identical nonneoplastic lesions thought to be the result of faulty ossification at the growth plate. A causal relationship with stress or trauma has been suggested but not proved. These are self-limited, with no potential for growth or spread. Both regress spontaneously, filling in with bone from the periphery and disappearing. The lesions are present at some time in perhaps one-third of all children.

Fibrous cortical defects (metaphyseal fibrous defects) are seen most typically in children aged 4 to 8 years. They are located on the cortical surface of the metaphysis at the attachment of a tendon or ligament, mostly around the knee, and produce a 1- to 4-cm scalloped defect in the underlying bone. They are round or oval, lucent, and sharply marginated by a sclerotic rim (Fig. 9.15). Some have a bubbly appearance. Pathologic fractures may occur, but fibrous cortical defects are usually clinically silent and disappear within 2 years of discovery.

Nonossifying fibromas can be thought of as fibrous cortical defects with somewhat different radiographic appearance; the distinction is not important for the patient. They are less common than fibrous cortical defects and are discovered in older children or adolescents. They are located eccentrically within the medullary cavity but still within an expanded cortex and are lucent with a sclerotic margin. Some lesions have a trabeculated, scalloped, multilocular, or bubbly appearance (Figs. 9.16 and 9.17). The size range is 1 to 7 cm, and larger lesions may fracture or cause pain.

FIBROUS DYSPLASIA

Fibrous dysplasia is a benign fibro-osseous lesion that is neither familial nor hereditary. Fibrous dysplasia appears to be a developmental abnormality involving the proliferation and maturation of fibroblasts in which benign fibrous tissue with abnormally arranged, dysplastic trabeculae of immature woven bone replaces normal bone. The dysplastic trabeculae are no thicker than 0.1 mm, so they are not individually visible on clinical radio-

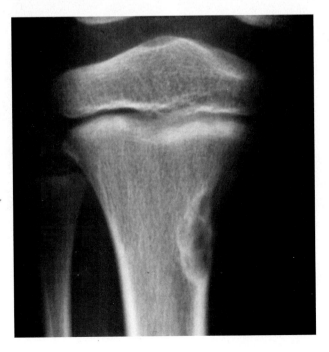

Figure 9.15 Fibrous cortical defect shown on AP radiograph.

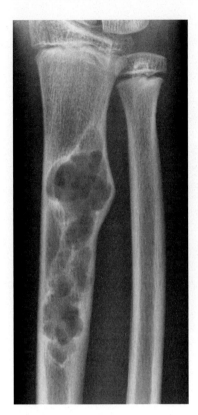

Figure 9.16 Nonossifying fibroma in the distal radial shaft. The lesion has a bubbly appearance with sclerotic margin, expanded cortical shell, and no matrix calcification.

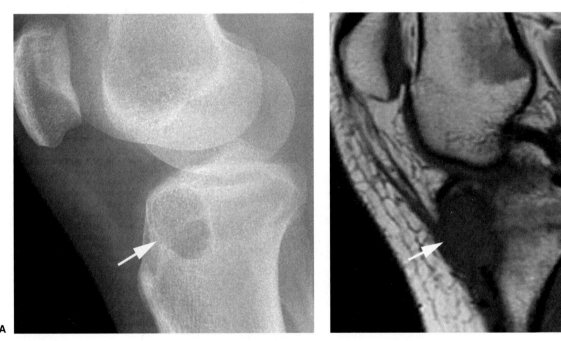

A

B

Figure 9.17 Nonossifying fibroma (*arrows*) in the proximal tibia. *A.* Lateral radiograph. *B.* Sagittal T1-weighted MRI.

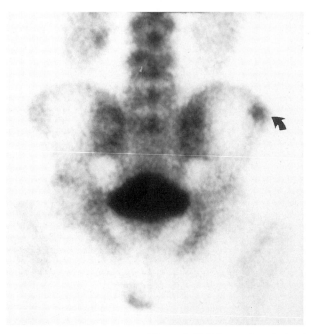

A

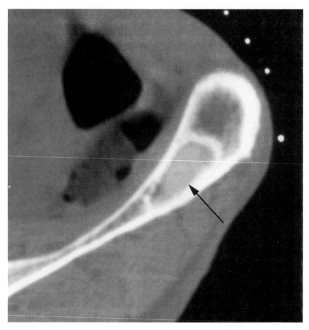

B

Figure 9.18 Fibrous dysplasia. *A.* Hot bone scan in patient with breast carcinoma (*arrow*). *B.* CT shows thick sclerotic rim and ground-glass matrix mineralization (*arrow*).

Fibrous dysplasia may have a ground-glass or radiolucent appearance and may mimic other bone lesions.

graphs. If present in sufficient number, however, they give the lesions a ground-glass density; if not, the lesions are radiolucent. The lesions are medullary but may replace both cancellous and cortical bone. The abnormal area may be sharply circumscribed and marginated by a thick layer of reactive bone, or it may blend gradually with the adjacent normal bone. The cortex may be either thickened or thinned, but the outer size and shape of the affected bone often is unchanged (Fig. 9.18). Bowing deformities result from biomechanically insufficient bone and from malunion of pathologic fractures. Fibrous dysplasia has a variable radiographic appearance and often mimics the appearance of other bone lesions.

Fibrous dysplasia occurs in monostotic and polyostotic forms. Approximately 80% of cases of fibrous dysplasia are monostotic. The peak age of diagnosis is 5 to 20 years. The typical sites of involvement are the proximal femur, tibia, ribs, and facial bones. Monostotic fibrous dysplasia seldom occurs in the spine or pelvis. Lesions in the long bones are often discovered because of fracture or deformity. Therapy is restricted to orthopedic management of complications. The monostotic form is not associated with other abnormalities or disease.

Although fibrous dysplasia does not spread or proliferate, individual lesions in children may enlarge in proportion with skeletal growth.

In polyostotic fibrous dysplasia, the distribution of lesions may be monomelic, unilateral, or widespread (Fig. 9.19). The extent of bone involvement can be documented at presentation by skeletal survey; fibrous dysplasia does not spread or proliferate, although the lesions may enlarge as the skeleton grows. Most bony lesions occur in the lower extremities, including the pelvis, legs, and feet. Rib or skull lesions are also often seen. Common deformities include leg-length discrepancy (lesions are in the longer leg); bowing deformities of long bones and ribs, including varus angulation of the proximal femur (shepherd's crook deformity); and, in the skull, frontal bossing, facial asymmetry, and inferolateral orbital displacement. Most patients have only bone lesions or bone and skin lesions; up to 30% of women with polyostotic fibrous dysplasia may have café-au-lait spots and precocious puberty (McCune-Albright syndrome). The clinical course ranges from asymptomatic (even in the presence of severe skeletal deformities) to multiple pathologic fractures, rapidly progressive deformities, severe pain, debilitation, and even death (Fig. 9.20). Malignant transformation has been documented but is rare. Polyostotic fibrous dysplasia with associated intramuscular myxomas (usually adjacent to the affected bone) is known as *Mazabraud syndrome*.

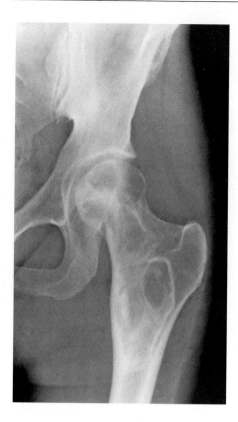

Figure 9.19 Polyostotic fibrous dysplasia involving the proximal femur and iliac wing.

DESMOPLASTIC FIBROMA

Desmoplastic fibromas are rare intraosseous fibrous lesions that are histologically identical to soft tissue fibromatosis. They are usually seen in adolescents and young adults. Their location is typically central in the metaphysis of a long bone. They are geographic, lytic lesions with a narrow zone of transition but often without a sclerotic rim. There is no matrix mineralization, but there can be a sequestrum. Endosteal erosion and modest cortical expansion are present, but cortical breakthrough usually is not. The endosteal margins

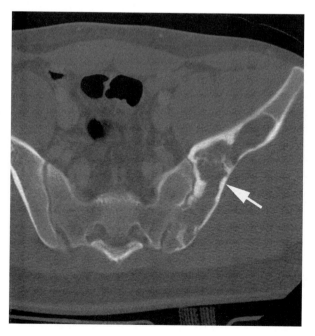

Figure 9.20 Fibrous dysplasia of the pelvis (*arrow*) found incidental to trauma.

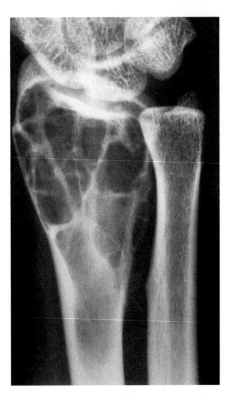

Figure 9.21 Desmoplastic fibroma of the distal radius.

characteristically have thick ridges of bone that may suggest the diagnosis in these otherwise nonspecific-appearing lesions (Fig. 9.21). They may be infiltrative and locally aggressive, but they have no metastatic potential.

AGGRESSIVE FIBROMATOSIS

Aggressive fibromatosis may be locally invasive but not metastatic.

Aggressive fibromatosis is a true neoplasm of soft tissues that arises from fascial and musculoaponeurotic coverings, sometimes at the site of a traumatic or postsurgical scar. Nonencapsulated, poorly circumscribed, and infiltrative, aggressive fibromatosis grows insidiously and invades locally but does not metastasize. The lesion may grow large and become adherent to neighboring structures such as neurovascular bundles. Aggressive fibromatosis grossly

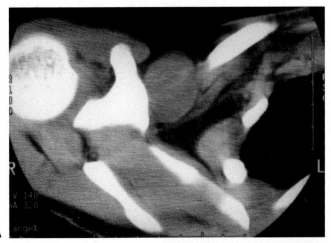
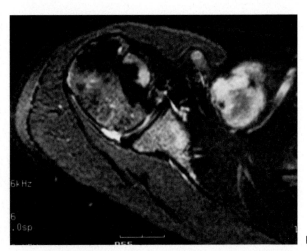

Figure 9.22 Fibromatosis. *A.* Axial CT scan (soft tissue windows) shows a globular mass in the infraclavicular region. *B.* Axial T2-weighted fat-suppressed MRI shows high signal with the lesion. The lesion showed enhancement after gadolinium injection.

resembles scar tissue. It is composed of well-differentiated fibroblasts embedded in abundant collagenous matrix with increased cellularity at the periphery. Radiographs may show soft tissue mass, localized periosteal thickening, and frank bony destruction. Because of variable degrees of cellularity, matrix water content, and infiltration, aggressive fibromatosis may be well or poorly defined and demonstrate variable attenuation and enhancement on CT and variable signal intensity on MRI (Fig. 9.22). The treatment is wide resection. Mortality is low, but local recurrences are frequent (18% to 54%).

BENIGN FATTY LESIONS

INTRAOSSEOUS LIPOMA

Intraosseous lipomas are benign bone lesions. The patients are asymptomatic, and the lesions are usually discovered incidentally. They are seen in young adults, but there is a wide age range (5 to 85 years). They are typically found in the metaphysis or epiphysis of the long bones, skull and jaws, ribs, pelvis, and calcaneus (Fig. 9.23). They are geographic lytic lesions with a sclerotic rim. Central calcific densities are occasionally seen, representing calcification due to fat necrosis. CT and MRI demonstrate attenuation and signal intensity similar to subcutaneous fat with areas of cystic changes. If the structural stability of the bone is compromised by the lesion, treatment is curettage and bone grafting.

LIPOSCLEROSING MYXOFIBROUS TUMOR OF BONE

Liposclerosing myxofibrous tumor of bone is a benign fibro-osseous lesion of bone (Fig. 9.24). These lesions are typically seen in middle-aged adults, but there is a wide age range (15 to 85 years). Pain is the most common presenting symptom, but many lesions are discovered incidentally. The majority of the lesions (85%) are found in the femur, and 91% of the femoral lesions are located in the medullary cavity of the intertrochanteric region. Radiographs show a well-defined, geographic lytic lesion with a sclerotic margin. Most of

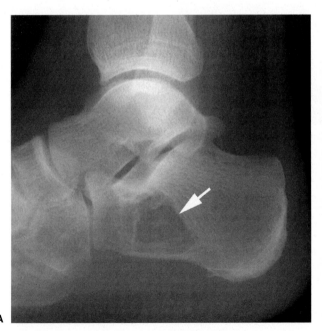 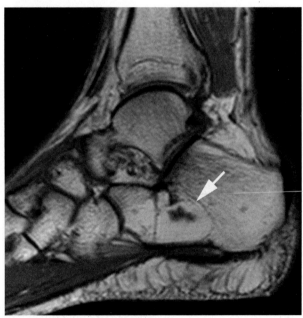

A   B

Figure 9.23 Intraosseous lipoma. *A.* Lateral radiograph shows a geographic lucent lesion in the calcaneus with sclerotic margin and faint calcific densities centrally (*arrow*). *B.* Sagittal T1-weighted MRI shows an intraosseous lipoma with dark, central focus corresponding to calcification (*arrow*).

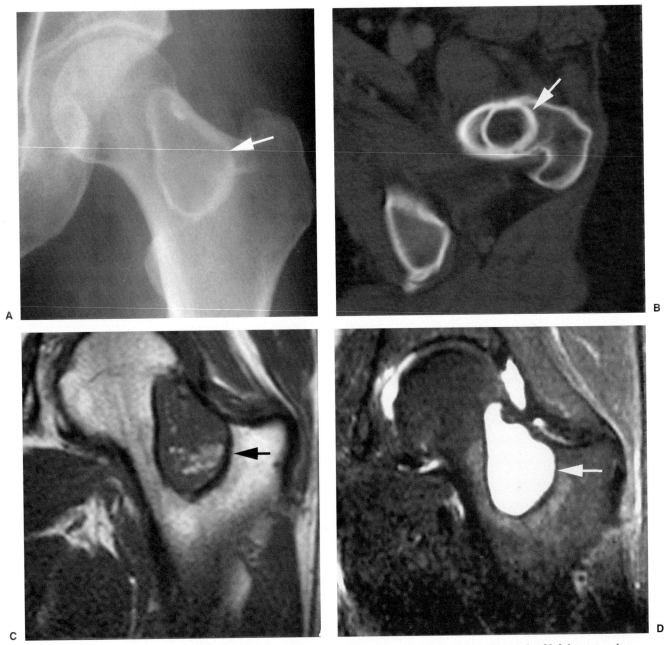

Figure 9.24 Liposclerosing myxofibrous tumor of bone. *A.* AP radiograph of left hip joint shows geographic lytic lesion with sclerotic margin (*arrow*) in femoral neck extending into intertrochanteric region. *B.* Axial CT scan of pelvis shows intramedullary cavity cystic mass with sclerotic margin (*arrow*). *C.* Coronal T1-weighted MRI shows lesion to have both lipomatous and cystic components (*arrow*). *D.* Coronal T2-weighted MRI shows predominant cystic change (*arrow*) of the mass.

Liposclerosing myxofibrous tumor of bone has significant potential for sarcomatous degeneration.

the lesions (72%) have mineralized matrix, which include globular and linear areas of intense opacity as well as regions with small, rounded, and arc-like configurations. The potential for sarcomatous degeneration appears to be significant, perhaps as high as 10% and 16% in two relatively small pathologically proven series.

LIPOMA

Lipomas are common benign tumors consisting of mature fat. They are clinically evident as soft, painless masses that gradually enlarge. Although most are subcutaneous, they may occur in an intramuscular location. A definitive diagnosis is made by CT when the lesion has the attenuation

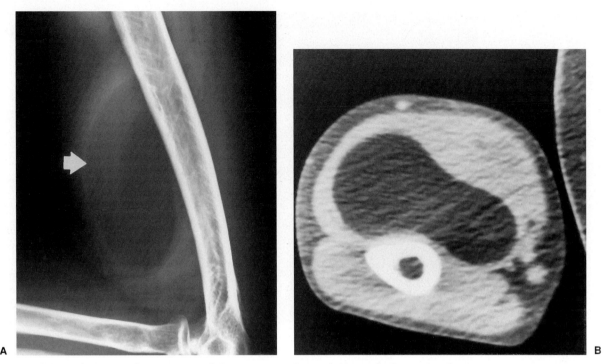

Figure 9.25 Lipoma in the flexor aspect of the arm. *A.* Radiograph shows fat lucency in biceps (*arrow*). *B.* CT shows fat within the lesion.

characteristics of fat (Fig. 9.25). Fat also has distinctive signal characteristics on MRI. Unusual variants of soft tissue lipomas include ossifying lipoma (Fig. 9.26) and parosteal lipoma.

Spindle Cell Lipoma

Spindle cell lipoma is an uncommon lipoma variant that is commonly misdiagnosed as a liposarcoma. The tumor occurs chiefly in men (ratio, 7.3:1.0) between 45 and 70 years of age (mean

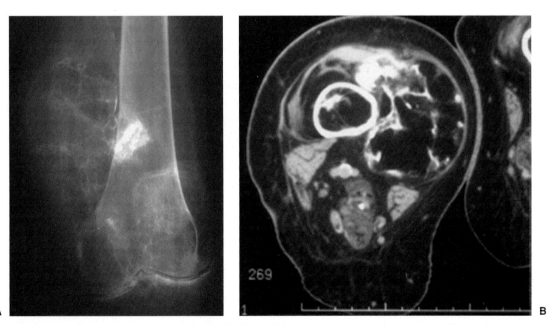

Figure 9.26 Ossifying lipoma. *A.* AP radiograph of distal femur shows an extraosseous ossifying mass. *B.* Axial CT image shows ossification within a fatty mass.

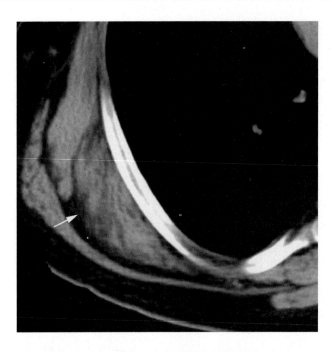

Figure 9.27 Elastofibroma dorsi of the chest wall. Axial CT scan of chest reveals right subscapular soft tissue mass (*arrow*) applied to chest wall with striated appearance caused by alternating bands of soft tissue and fat attenuation.

age, 56 years). Approximately two-thirds of lesions affect the subcutaneous tissue of the shoulder and posterior neck, although they may occur elsewhere in the body. MRI reveals a well-defined, fatty mass with linear and globular nonfatty areas within the mass, which enhance markedly. In the extremity, its large size may erode adjacent bone. Its heterogeneous MRI appearance may mimic that of a liposarcoma. However, because of its uniformly favorable clinical course, local excision is the treatment of choice for spindle cell lipoma.

ELASTOFIBROMA

Elastofibroma is a benign reactive fibrous lesion producing abnormal elastic fibers. This pseudotumor is believed to result from chronic mechanical friction between the tip of the scapula and the chest wall. An incidental prevalence of 2.0% was found in an elderly patient population studied by chest CT, but an autopsy series found a frequency of 11.2% in men and 24.4% in women. The characteristic location is between the chest wall and the inferior tip of the scapula, but 5% of elastofibromas are found elsewhere. Most lesions are asymptomatic, but patients may present with mass or pain. Large lesions may ulcerate or cause brachial plexus impingement. Bilateral lesions are common but are often asymmetric.

On sonography, elastofibroma appears as arrays of interspersed linear or curvilinear hypoechoic strands (elastic fibers) against an echogenic background (entrapped fat). CT shows a mass of soft tissue attenuation with striations of fat attenuation (Fig. 9.27). On MRI, elastofibroma is a poorly circumscribed, semilunar, heterogeneous soft tissue mass with signal intensity similar to that of skeletal muscle interlaced with strands of fat. Elastofibroma may have marked enhancement after administration of gadolinium. Surgery is curative; recurrences (7%) are probably due to incomplete excision.

EOSINOPHILIC GRANULOMA

Eosinophilic granuloma of bone is a granulomatous lesion characterized by a focal proliferation of macrophages (Langerhans' cells) infiltrated with eosinophils and other inflammatory cells. It is a nonmalignant, reactive process of uncertain etiology that is related to other syndromes of proliferative histiocytosis (Langerhans' cell histiocytosis, histiocytosis X), including Hand-Schüller-Christian and Letterer-Siwe diseases. Unlike these other syndromes, the involvement is limited to bone. The lesions are more often solitary than multi-

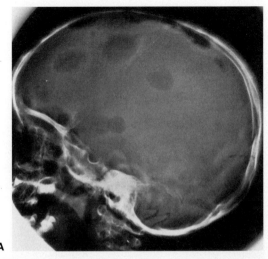
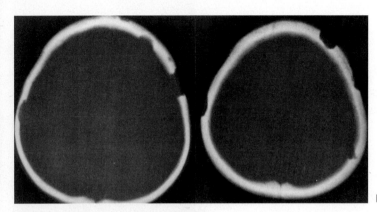

A   B

Figure 9.28 Multiple eosinophilic granulomas. *A.* Lateral skull radiograph shows lesions with beveled edges from variable destruction of inner and outer tables. *B.* Axial CT shows the bone destruction involving inner and outer tables.

ple, and although the peak incidence is at ages 5 to 15 years, lesions may be found at any age. Sites of involvement include the skull and other flat bones; the spine, especially vertebral bodies; and the peripheral skeleton. Involvement of the vertebral bodies characteristically results in flattening of the vertebral body, or vertebra plana. However, vertebra plana is not pathognomonic for eosinophilic granuloma. In long bones, the lesions are usually diaphyseal or metaphyseal, rarely epiphyseal, and may be up to several centimeters in size. Destruction and replacement of bone by eosinophilic granuloma produces a lytic, aggressive-appearing geographic lesion early in the clinical course (Figs. 9.28 through 9.30), sometimes with lamellated periosteal reaction. Late in the clinical course, lesions become well defined as they heal by becoming sclerotic and eventually remodeling. On radionuclide bone scan, the degree of isotope uptake may be high, normal, or low, depending on the bone reaction and the size of the lesion. The clinical presentation is usually localized pain or a limp, but lesions in the spine may cause neurologic syndromes, and lesions in the skull may cause chronic otic drainage. The clinical courses of both solitary and multiple eosinophilic granuloma of bone are benign; lesions may regress spontaneously. Therapy is

Vertebra plana is not pathognomonic for eosinophilic granuloma.

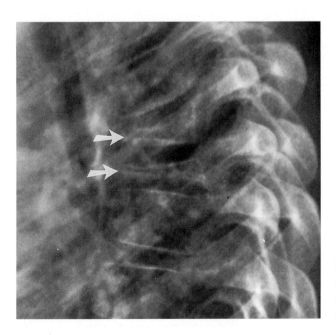

Figure 9.29 Eosinophilic granuloma with pathologic vertebral collapse (vertebra plana). Lateral radiograph shows collapse of T6 and T7 with kyphosis (*arrows*).

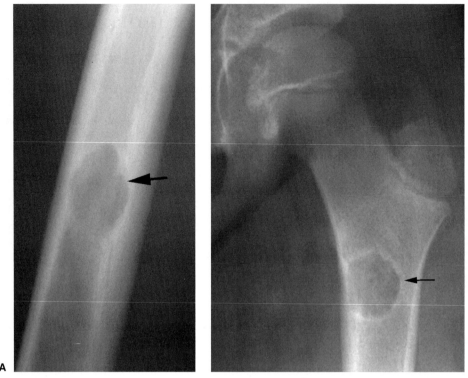

Figure 9.30 Eosinophilic granulomas in the femur (different patients). *A.* Radiograph shows sharply defined lucent lesion without a sclerotic margin (*arrow*). *B.* Radiograph shows lesion with thin sclerotic margin (*arrow*).

curettage, steroid injection, low-dose radiotherapy, and, rarely, chemotherapy. There is no metastatic potential.

GIANT CELL TUMOR

Giant cell tumor of bone (osteoclastoma) is an uncommon lesion thought to arise from osteoclasts. The presence of giant cells is only one histologic component of the tumor, and other types of tumors may have giant cells. Giant cell tumors may occur at any age, but the typical patient is a young adult. Tumors are located almost invariably in the epiphysis, with extension to the subchondral cortex and into the metaphysis. Fewer than 2% occur adjacent to open growth plates. Giant cell tumors probably arise in the cut-back zone of the metaphysis where osteoclasts are plentiful and active. Approximately 50% of tumors are found around the knee, but other long bones and the sacrum are also commonly involved. The typical radiographic appearance is a geographic, lytic tumor near the end of a long bone, extending to or very close to the subarticular cortex (Fig. 9.31). Lytic regions correspond to nonmineralized tumor tissue, destroying and replacing cancellous bone. A lobular pattern of growth may leave ridges or trabeculations in surrounding bone. Giant cell tumors are often expansile and may have cystic blood-filled regions similar to aneurysmal bone cysts (Fig. 9.32). The zone of transition from tumor to normal bone is usually sharp and abrupt, but without a sclerotic margin (growth rate I-B). Some lesions erode from the epiphysis into the joint cavity and provoke synovitis. Approximately 10% of patients present with pathologic fracture. CT or MRI may be required to show the extent of tumor and the relationship to the adjacent joint. Giant cell tumors appear as areas of intense isotope uptake on bone scan and sometimes have a doughnut appearance with greater activity at the margins. The typical treatment of giant cell tumor is curettage; adjuvant treatment of the surgical bed with a high-speed burr, phenol, or cryotherapy; and packing with methylmethacrylate (bone cement). The reported overall rate of recurrence is approximately

Giant cell tumors are often expansile and may have cystic blood-filled regions similar to aneurysmal bone cysts.

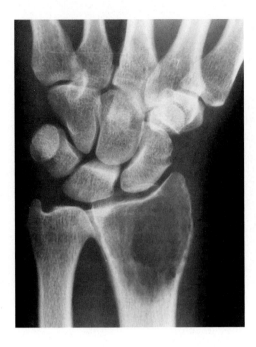

Figure 9.31 Giant cell tumor of the distal radius.

25%. There are case reports of pulmonary metastases from giant cell tumors. Older literature suggests the existence of malignant giant cell tumors, but these likely represent primary malignant lesions such as osteosarcoma or malignant fibrous histiocytoma that have prominent giant cells at histology.

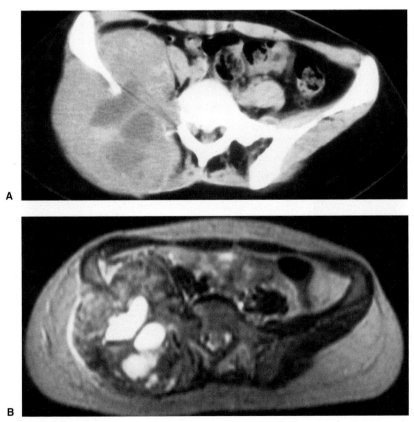

Figure 9.32 Giant cell tumor in the pelvis. *A.* CT shows large destructive lesion with regions of low density. *B.* Axial T2-weighted MRI shows fluid-filled spaces with high signal within the tumor.

CYSTIC LESIONS OF BONE

ANEURYSMAL BONE CYST

Aneurysmal bone cysts are expansile, cystic lesions of bone. They probably result from a vascular disturbance caused by trauma or underlying tumor, and in one-third or more of cases, an adjacent primary benign or malignant bone lesion can be recognized by the pathologist. The most common underlying lesion is giant cell tumor, and many believe that some underlying lesions may be obliterated as the aneurysmal bone cyst forms and expands rapidly. Most occur at ages 10 to 20 years, and patients typically present with pain or swelling of less than 6 months' duration. More than 50% are found in long bones, usually metaphyseal; 12% to 30% are found in the spine, often the posterior elements; and the remainder are found in the pelvis or other flat bones. Aneurysmal bone cysts are eccentric, lucent lesions that expand the host bone and give it a blown-out or ballooned appearance (hence the term *aneurysmal*) (Fig. 9.33). Sometimes, the expanded cortical shell is interrupted when periosteal bone growth is outpaced by expansion of the lesion, but the periosteum remains intact, although radiographically invisible. The walls may have trabeculations, but true septations are rare. The lesion consists of sponge-like fibrovascular tissue with cystic spaces or cavities filled with blood or serosanguineous fluid. The growth plate may be invaded. Vertebral lesions commonly involve contiguous levels or adjacent ribs. Fluid-fluid levels may be demonstrated by CT or MRI; CT attenuation values of 20 to 78 Hounsfield units (HU) reflect the fluid, blood, and solid tissue components of the lesion (Fig. 9.34). Bone scans show increased uptake around the periphery of the lesion but none within the lesion itself. Aneurysmal bone cysts are treated in a manner similar to giant cell tumors, unless an underlying lesion is found that requires more aggressive treatment. The clinical course may vary from indolent and self-healing to rapid, relentless growth. Aneurysmal bone cysts have no metastatic potential.

Aneurysmal bone cysts may have trabeculated walls.

SIMPLE BONE CYST

Simple (unicameral) bone cysts are fairly common nonneoplastic fluid-filled lesions in the medullary cavity that may be related to venous outflow obstruction. Nearly all are found

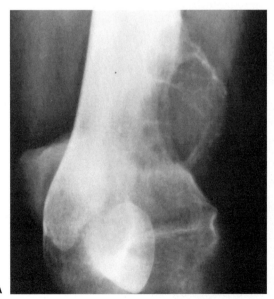 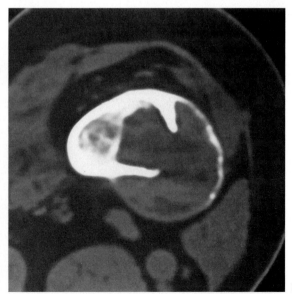

Figure 9.33 Aneurysmal bone cyst in the femur. *A.* Radiograph shows an expansile cortical lesion. *B.* CT shows a thin, expanded cortical rim around the lesion.

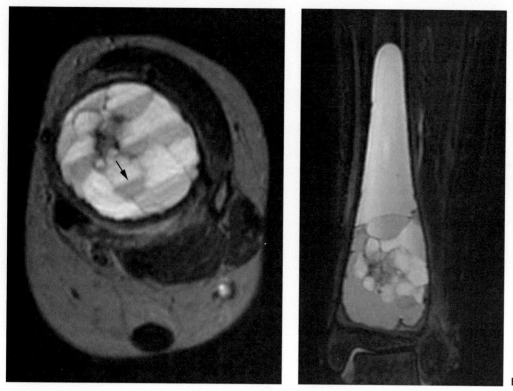

Figure 9.34 Aneurysmal bone cyst of distal tibia. *A*. Axial T2-weighted MRI shows fluid-fluid levels (*arrow*). *B*. Coronal T2-weighted fat-suppressed MRI shows the septations.

in patients between 2 and 20 years of age, and they disappear with maturity. Men are affected more often than women by a 3:1 ratio. The most common sites are the proximal humerus and the proximal femur. The location transversely is intramedullary, usually occupying the entire cross section of the bone; the location longitudinally is metaphyseal, sometimes extending to the diaphysis. In young adults, cysts may be found in the flat bones. Simple cysts have a thin lining with serous or serosanguineous fluid inside and sparse solid tissue. The internal pressure is greater than that in normal marrow. Most are unicameral (having a single compartment), but some have fibrous septa that make them multilocular. Bony ridges in the cyst wall may give the false impression of multiple cysts. The cortex is thinned and expanded, but cortical penetration or soft tissue involvement never occurs (Fig. 9.35). The lesion is considered active if it abuts the growth plate. After the lesion has become inactive, it becomes separated from the physis as normal bone formation resumes. The lesions are radiolucent and may reach large size. A CT scan shows a homogeneous avascular lesion with attenuation values typical of cysts (15 to 20 HU). MRI shows fluid (Fig. 9.36). Pathologic fracture may lead to the discovery of an unsuspected cyst (Fig. 9.37). These fractures heal with a solid layer of periosteal bone that eventually thickens the cortex. Occasionally, a bone fragment may actually fall into the cyst; such a fallen fragment is indicative of a fluid-filled lesion. Treatment of simple bone cysts may be necessary to avoid pathologic fracture and deformity. The therapy is intralesional steroid injection, curetting, and packing with bone chips. Approximately 20% recur after curetting; recurrent lesions may have been unrecognized multilocular lesions.

Simple bone cysts may present with pathologic fracture.

INTRAOSSEOUS GANGLION

An intraosseous ganglion (juxta-articular bone cyst) is a nonneoplastic, mucin-filled cyst lined by fibrous tissue. Of uncertain pathogenesis, it is usually found in patients between 30 and 60 years of age. It is always located in the epiphysis and tends to be

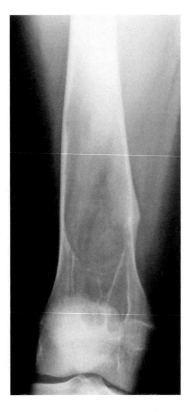

Figure 9.35 Simple bone cyst in distal femur.

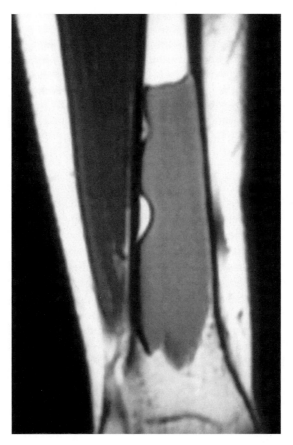

Figure 9.36 Coronal T1-weighted MRI of simple bone cyst in the distal tibial shaft.

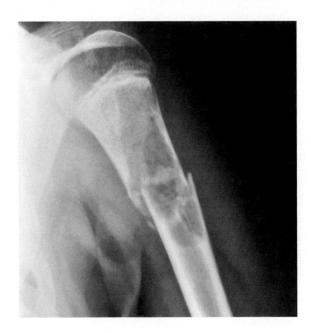

Figure 9.37 Simple bone cyst presenting with pathologic fracture.

eccentric, lucent, and sharply defined, with a thin sclerotic margin. Unlike a subchondral cyst, an intraosseous ganglion does not communicate with the adjacent joint space. Curettage, with bone graft packing, if necessary, is curative.

EPIDERMOID INCLUSION CYST

An epidermoid inclusion cyst may develop after penetrating trauma displaces epidermoid elements into the substance of the bone. These cysts are usually seen at the terminal phalanx of the hand after remote trauma to the finger. They are radiolucent, sclerotically marginated, and nearly perfectly round.

CYSTIC MASSES OF SOFT TISSUES

GANGLION

Ganglia are cystic tumor-like lesions that are usually attached to a tendon sheath, commonly found in the hands, wrists, and feet. They may be found near a joint, such as a meniscal cyst or cruciate ligament ganglion of the knee and paralabral cyst of the shoulder or hip. Ganglia can be either unilocular or multilocular cystic masses. MRI reveals a cystic mass with peripheral enhancement after the administration of gadolinium. There is a high association of meniscal and paralabral cysts with meniscal and labral tears. Once they become large, they may erode the adjacent bone, stimulate periosteal new bone formation, or cause compressive neuropathy.

SYNOVIAL CYSTS

Synovial cysts are fluid-filled juxta-articular masses. Unlike ganglia, synovial cysts are lined by a synovial membrane that may or may not communicate with the adjacent joint. The most common symptomatic synovial cyst is the Baker cyst, found in the popliteal fossa (see Chapter 13).

BURSITIS

Bursae are enclosed, flattened sacs consisting of synovial lining and a thin film of synovial fluid. They facilitate motion between apposing tissues. Bursitis is inflammation of the bursae due to trauma, repetitive stress, infection, or arthritis. In addition to normal anatomic sites, adventitial bursae may develop at sites where there is movement between apposing tissues. For example, bursae may develop over osteochondromas or other bony prominences. Similar to bursae elsewhere, adventitial bursae may become inflamed and cause symptoms.

Myxoma

Myxomas are connective tissue tumors characterized by an abundant myxoid matrix and a paucity of stromal cells. Myxomas may appear at any age. They may be found in the subcutaneous tissue, within a muscle, or near a joint. Intramuscular myxomas predominate in women in the fifth through seventh decades of life and in the thigh. Intramuscular myxomas are well-circumscribed cystic masses of homogeneous low signal intensity on T1-weighted imaging, high signal intensity on T2-weighted imaging, and peripheral and septal enhancement after gadolinium administration. Often, myxomas have a perilesional fat rind (65% to 71%), corresponding histologically to atrophy of surrounding muscle.

Miscellaneous Benign Lesions

Vascular Lesions

Osseous Hemangioma

Benign vascular lesions of bone are common and usually discovered incidentally in adults. Hemangioma is a benign proliferation of blood vessels, and lymphangioma is a benign proliferation of lymphatic channels; histologically, they are indistinguishable from their soft tissue counterparts. The typical appearance of bone involvement by these lesions on radiographs is a focal, well-defined, lucent lesion surrounded by irregular, coarse, thickened trabeculae (Fig. 9.38). The abnormal vascular spaces infiltrate and replace the bone and are surrounded by irregular, reactively thickened trabeculae. Any part of the skeleton may be affected, but most of these lesions are found in the vertebral bodies, where the thickened

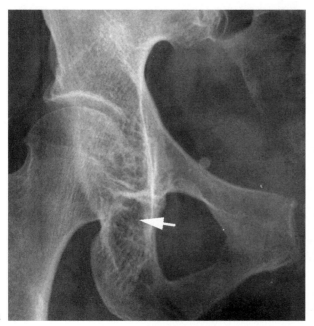
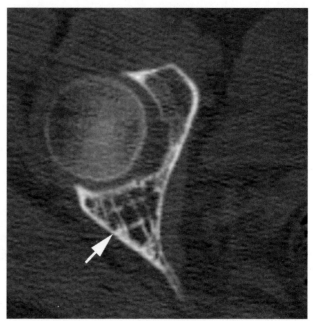

A   B

Figure 9.38 Hemangioma involving the bony pelvis. *A.* AP radiograph shows a prominent trabecular bone pattern (*arrow*) in the right ischium. *B.* Axial CT scan shows the prominent trabeculae within a lucent, fat-filled lesion (*arrow*).

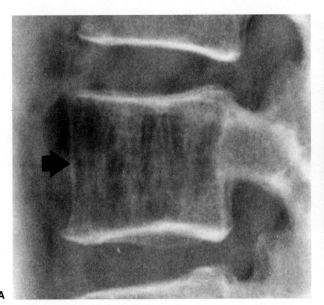
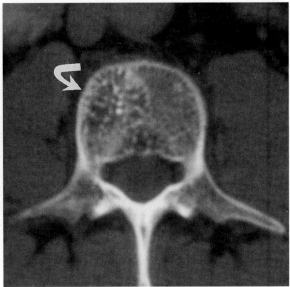

A

B

Figure 9.39 Vertebral body hemangioma. *A.* "Corduroy" appearance (*arrow*). *B.* CT shows fat and thickened trabeculae (*arrow*).

trabeculae are vertically oriented and give the lesion a "corduroy" appearance (Fig. 9.39). On CT, they appear as a localized region of thick, vertical trabeculae interspersed with fat. This appearance is diagnostic. MRI shows the presence of fat and vascular spaces. Diffuse skeletal angiomatosis, with or without soft tissue angiomatosis, is rare. There is no potential for malignant degeneration.

> On CT, hemangiomas appear as localized regions of thick vertical trabeculae interspersed with fat.

Soft Tissue Hemangioma

Hemangioma is one of the most common soft tissue tumors, accounting for 7% of all benign tumors. Hemangioma is a benign vascular lesion that may contain nonvascular elements such as fat, fibrous and myxoid tissue, smooth muscle, thrombus, and even bone. Hemangiomas are classified histologically by the predominant type of vascular channel (capillary, cavernous, arteriovenous, or venous). Hemangiomas may be found in the subcutaneous tissue, within a muscle, or in a joint. At radiography, hemangiomas appear as a nonspecific soft tissue mass. Phleboliths are seen in 30% of the hemangiomas, most frequently in cavernous hemangiomas. CT reveals a soft tissue mass with associated fat overgrowth and serpentine vascular components, which may enhance after administration of contrast. Sonography shows a complex mass with high vessel density (more than five per cm²) and a peak arterial Doppler shift exceeding 2 kHz (sensitivity, 84%; specificity, 98%). MRI is considered the best modality for evaluating hemangiomas. Characteristic MRI features include lobulation, septation, central low-signal-intensity dots, and marked enhancement after gadolinium administration (Fig. 9.40). The septate-lobulated appearance on T2-weighted images correlates with fibrous and fatty septa (low signal) between endothelial-lined vascular channels (high signal). The central low-intensity dot sign on T2-weighted imaging may represent fibrofatty septa seen in cross section, hyalinized or thrombosed vascular channels, smooth muscle components, fast flow within blood vessels, calcification, or ossification. Many forms of therapy have been used to control or cure hemangiomas: steroids, radiation therapy, sclerosing agents, interferon alpha-2a, pentoxifylline, and surgical excision. Hemangiomas may have association with several syndromes or bone lesions.

> MRI is considered the best modality for evaluating soft tissue hemangiomas.

NEUROGENIC LESIONS

Peripheral Nerve Sheath Tumors

Benign peripheral nerve sheath tumors (schwannoma and neurofibroma) can arise from any central or peripheral nerve. They are found in young adults between the third to fifth

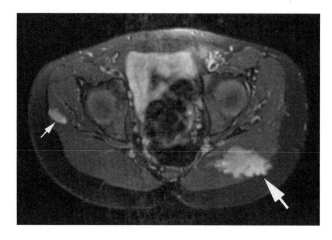

Figure 9.40 Intramuscular hemangioma. Axial T2-weighted MRI of the pelvis shows a large hemangioma (*large arrow*) in the left gluteus maximus and a smaller hemangioma (*small arrow*) in the right tensor fascia lata.

decades of life. Most are found incidentally, but others, when large, may cause pain, soft tissue mass, and neurologic findings. They present as a fusiform soft tissue mass related to the neurovascular bundle. The affected nerve is seen entering and exiting the mass. In neurofibroma, the nerve is central or obliterated by the mass. In schwannoma, the nerve is eccentric to the mass (Fig. 9.41). On T1-weighted images, the "split fat" sign describes a rim of fat around the tumor. On T2-weighted images, the "fascicular" or "target" sign describes a ring-like structure with central low signal intensity and peripheral high signal intensity. Treatment is surgical excision.

Morton Neuroma

Morton neuroma is a benign tumor-like lesion that is perineural fibrosis of the plantar digital nerve. It has a marked predilection for middle-aged women (as high as 18:1). It has been hypothesized that the wearing of high-heeled shoes compresses the nerve against the

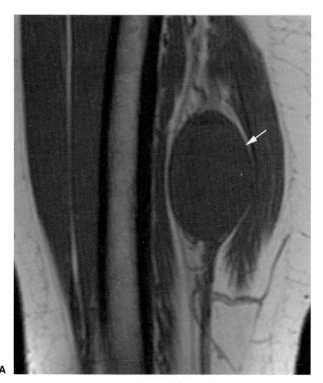

A

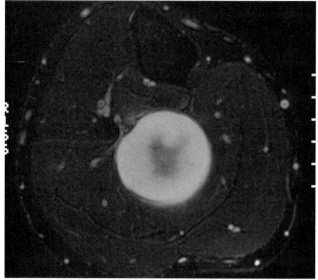

B

Figure 9.41 A. Sagittal T1-weighted MRI shows sciatic nerve schwannoma (*arrow*). B. Axial T2-weighted MRI shows tibial nerve schwannoma with high signal surrounding a lower-signal center, the target sign.

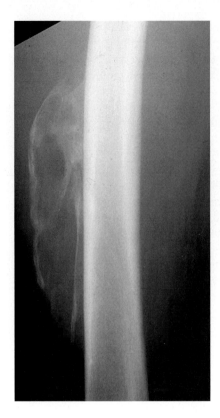

Figure 9.42 Thigh radiograph 6 months after blunt trauma shows myositis ossificans.

intermetatarsal ligaments. Patients complain of pain radiating into the toes or leg that is elicited by exercise and relieved with rest. Sonography reveals a hypoechoic mass that shows increased vascularity on power Doppler mode. MRI shows a focal low-intensity mass surrounded by fat on T1-weighted images, high signal on T2-weighted images, and intense enhancement after gadolinium administration. A fluid-filled intermetatarsal bursa is often seen proximal to the neuroma. Various treatment options exist, including modification of the patient's footwear, neurolysis, steroid injection, ultrasound therapy, surgical release of the transverse metatarsal ligament for decompression, and surgical excision of the neuroma.

POSTTRAUMATIC LESIONS

Myositis Ossificans

Myositis ossificans commonly refers to posttraumatic heterotopic ossification in the muscles and other soft tissues after blunt trauma and hemorrhage. Most common in the quadriceps muscles or around the elbow, it progresses over a few weeks from hematoma to ill-defined calcification to well-organized cortical and trabecular bone. The process is similar to the formation and maturation of fracture callus (Fig. 9.42) and may be initially confused with sarcoma. However, myositis ossificans evolves over a period of weeks into an organized, peripherally calcified mass as it begins to ossify. The ectopic bone may ultimately blend with underlying bone, sometimes causing mechanical problems. Myositis ossificans may complicate acute or chronic bony or soft tissue trauma and may occur in association with neurologic diseases of a wide variety, including paralysis and coma. A localized form that occurs without a history of significant trauma is called *myositis ossificans circumscripta*. Treatment is rarely indicated.

Bizarre Parosteal Osteochondromatous Proliferation

Bizarre parosteal osteochondromatous proliferation (BPOP), or Nora lesion, is a form of heterotopic ossification observed most commonly in the bones of the hands and feet. It may also occur in the long tubular bones and rarely in the skull. It presents as a painless, palpable mass. A history of trauma is inconstant. Radiographically, it mimics a pedunculated or sessile osteochondroma. The main distinction is the absence of medullary continuity between the lesion and the adjacent bone. Yuen et al. proposed a hypothesis uniting the concepts of florid reactive periostitis and BPOP. The initial stimulus is often due to trauma. Hematoma in the soft tissue develops into myositis ossificans. Subperiosteal hemorrhage or proliferation matures into a localized fusiform periostitis. If the periosteum is breached, the reactive process can extend into the soft tissue, forming a BPOP.

Foreign Body Granuloma

Foreign body granuloma is a common cause of a soft tissue mass in an extremity, particularly in the plantar aspect of the foot. A granulomatous reaction may be provoked by organic material such as wood or plant thorns as well as glass, plastic, or metal. The patient often does not recall the episode of penetrating trauma. CT is better than MRI for identification of a foreign body. On MRI, a metallic foreign body is suggested when there is a blooming artifact on gradient echo sequences. In bone, foreign body granuloma causes osteolysis and is usually associated with total joint replacements (see Chapter 17).

> Foreign body granuloma is a common cause of a soft tissue mass in an extremity.

SOURCES AND READINGS

Arceci RJ. The histiocytoses: the fall of the Tower of Babel. *Eur J Cancer* 1999;35:747–767.

Bancroft LW, Kransdorf MJ, Menke DM, et al. Intramuscular myxoma: characteristic MR imaging features. *AJR Am J Roentgenol* 2002;178:1255–1259.

Blackley HR, Wunder JS, Davis AM, et al. Treatment of giant-cell tumors of long bones with curettage and bone-grafting. *J Bone Joint Surg Am* 1999;81A:811–820.

Boutou-Bredaki S, Agapios P, Papachristou G. Prognosis of giant cell tumor of bone. Histopathological analysis of 15 cases and review of the literature. *Adv Clin Path* 2001;5:71–78.

Bui-Mansfield LT, Chew FS, Stanton CA. Elastofibroma dorsi of the chest wall. *AJR Am J Roentgenol* 2000;175:244.

Bui-Mansfield LT, Kaplan KJ. Spindle cell lipoma of the upper back. *AJR Am J Roentgenol* 2002; 179:1158.

Bui-Mansfield LT, Myers CP, Chew FS. Parosteal lipoma of the fibula. *AJR Am J Roentgenol* 2000; 174:1698.

Campbell SE, Sanders TG, Morrison WB. MR imaging of meniscal cysts: incidence, location, and clinical significance. *AJR Am J Roentgenol* 2001;177:409–413.

Cheng JC, Johnston JO. Giant cell tumor of bone. Prognosis and treatment of pulmonary metastases. *Clin Orthop* 1997;338:205–214.

de Kleuver M, van der Heul RO, Veraart BE. Aneurysmal bone cyst of the spine: 31 cases and the importance of the surgical approach. *J Pediatr Orthop* 1998;7:286–292.

Ehara S, Shiraishi H, Abe M, et al. Reactive heterotopic ossification. Its patterns on MRI. *Clin Imag* 1998;22:292–296.

Enneking WF. *Musculoskeletal tumor surgery.* Edinburgh: Churchill–Livingstone, 1983.

Fechner RE, Mills SE. *Tumors of the bones and joints.* Washington, DC: Armed Forces Institute of Pathology, 1993.

Gogusev J, Nezelof C. Malignant histiocytosis—histologic, cytochemical, chromosomal, and molecular data with a nosologic discussion. *Hematol Oncol Clin North Am* 1998;12:445–463.

Hudson TM. *Radiologic-pathologic correlation of musculoskeletal lesions.* Baltimore: Williams & Wilkins, 1987.

Huvos AG. *Bone tumors: diagnosis, treatment, and prognosis,* 2nd ed. Philadelphia: WB Saunders, 1991.

Keats TE, Anderson MW. *Atlas of normal roentgen variants that may simulate disease,* 7th ed. St. Louis: Mosby–Year Book, 2001.

Keats TE. *Atlas of normal variants that may simulate disease,* 5th ed. St. Louis: Mosby–Year Book, 1996.

Kransdorf MJ, Murphey MD. *Imaging of soft tissue tumors.* Philadelphia: WB Saunders, 1997.

Kransdorf MJ, Sweet DE. Aneurysmal bone cyst: concept, controversy, clinical presentation, and imaging. *AJR Am J Roentgenol* 1995;64:573–580.

Ladisch S. Langerhans cell histiocytosis. *Curr Opin Hematol* 1998;5:54–58.

Leithner A, Windhager R, Lang S, et al. Aneurysmal bone cyst. A population based epidemiologic study and literature review. *Clin Orthop* 1999;363:176–179.

Lodwick GS. *Atlas of tumor radiology. The bones and joints.* Chicago: Year Book, 1971.

Magee T, Hinson G. Association of paralabral cysts with acetabular disorders. *AJR Am J Roentgenol* 2000;174:1381–1384.

Meyer JS, De Camargo B. The role of radiology in the diagnosis and follow-up of Langerhans cell histiocytosis. *Hematol Oncol Clin North Am* 1998;2:307–326.

Murphey MD, Choi JJ, Kransdorf MJ, et al. Imaging of osteochondroma: variants and complications with radiologic-pathologic correlation. *Radiographics* 2000;20:1407–1434.

Murphey MD, Nomikos GC, Flemming DJ, et al. Imaging of giant cell tumor and giant cell reparative granuloma of the bone: radiologic-pathologic correlation. *Radiographics* 2001;21:1283–1309.

Nezelof C, Basset F. Langerhans cell histiocytosis research. Past, present, and future. *Hematol Oncol Clin North Am* 1998;12:385–406.

Pitcher JD Jr, Bocklage T, Crooks L, et al. *The pathology, orthopaedics, and radiology of musculoskeletal tumors PORT notes.* Albuquerque: Orthopaedic Oncologic Publishing Services, 2002.

Propeck T, Bullard MA, Lin J, et al. Radiologic-pathologic correlation of intraosseous lipomas. *AJR Am J Roentgenol* 2000;175:673–678.

Resnick D. *Diagnosis of bone and joint disorders,* 4th ed. Philadelphia: WB Saunders, 2002.

Schick S, Zembsch A, Gahleitner A, et al. Atypical appearance of elastofibroma on MRI: case reports and review of the literature. *J Comput Assist Tomogr* 2000;24:288–292.

Schmidt H, Freyschmidt J. *Köhler/Zimmer borderlands of normal and early pathologic findings in skeletal radiography,* 4th ed. New York: Thieme, 1993.

Stull MA, Kransdorf MJ, Devaney KO. Langerhans' cell histiocytosis of bone. *Radiographics* 1992;12:801–823.

Sundaram M, Wang LH, Rotman M, et al. Florid reactive periostitis and bizarre parosteal osteochondromatous proliferation: pre-biopsy imaging evaluation, treatment and outcome. *Skeletal Radiol* 2001;30:192–198.

Tung GA, Entzian D, Stern JB, et al. MR imaging and MR arthrography of paraglenoid labral cysts. *AJR Am J Roentgenol* 2000;174:1707–1715.

Turcotte RE, Wunder JS, Isler MH, et al. Giant cell tumor of long bone: a Canadian Sarcoma Group study. *Clin Orthop* 2002;397:248–258.

Unni KK. *Dahlin's bone tumors. General aspects and data on 11,087 cases,* 5th ed. Philadelphia: Lippincott–Raven, 1996.

Yuen M, Friedman L, Orr W, et al. Proliferative periosteal processes of phalanges: a unitary hypothesis. *Skeletal Radiol* 1992;21:301.

METASTATIC TUMORS

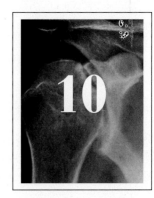

This chapter describes the radiology of tumors that are metastatic to bone or soft tissue.

INCIDENCE

More than 95% of adult patients with malignant disease involving bone have metastases rather than myeloma or primary bone sarcomas. The prevalence of bone involvement in autopsy series of cancer patients ranges from 3% to 85%, depending on the site of origin and the thoroughness of the postmortem search (Table 10.1). With improving cancer treatments and longer patient survival, more and more cancer patients will have skeletal involvement by the end of their clinical course. Most skeletal metastases occur in middle-aged and elderly patients with primary cancers of the prostate, breast, lung, or kidney. In men, prostate malignancies account for 60% of patients with skeletal metastases; in women, breast malignancies account for 70% (Table 10.2). In children with osseous metastases, neuroblastoma is the most common primary lesion (Table 10.3). The relative incidence of primary tumors that are likely to metastasize to bone may be affected in the future by the rising incidence of lung cancer among women (due to smoking), the decrease in the proportion of advanced breast cancers (due to screening mammography), and the increasing incidence of breast and prostate cancers overall (due to an aging population). Most skeletal metastases are subclinical and asymptomatic. When symptomatic, they present as bone pain or pathologic fractures. Bone pain ranges in severity from minimal to extreme and intolerable, but skeletal metastases are themselves rarely a cause of death.

In the radiologic evaluation of metastatic bone tumors, less emphasis is placed on complete anatomic delineation of individual lesions and more on discovering sites of disease and planning and following the course of palliative therapy. Sometimes, a skeletal metastasis is the initial presentation of malignant disease in a patient whose primary site is asymptomatic or minimally symptomatic. Occult primary tumors that present with bone metastases are usually kidney, lung, and gastrointestinal tract lesions. Only in select cases does locating the primary tumor benefit the patient, because in most instances, the prognosis has already become unalterable by metastatic dissemination. In most cases, the primary tumor is never located, even at autopsy. Biopsy of the skeletal metastasis in these circumstances often shows adenocarcinoma without organ-specific features.

More than 95% of malignant bone lesions are metastases.

Table 10.1: Prevalence of Skeletal Metastases at Autopsy for Various Primary Sites in Adults

Primary Site	Prevalence (%)
Breast	65
Prostate	64
Lung	40
Renal	36
Uterus	50
Thyroid	43
Gastrointestinal tract	8

Adapted from Galasko CSB. *Skeletal metastases.* London: Butterworths, 1986:15.

Table 10.2: Frequency of Primary Sites among Adults with Skeletal Metastases

Primary Site	Frequency (%)
Women	
Breast	70
Lung	6
Kidney	4
Uterus	4
Thyroid	3
Others/unknown	13
Total	100
Men	
Prostate	60
Lung	14
Kidney	6
Gastrointestinal tract	3
Others/unknown	17
Total	100

Table 10.3: Primary Tumors in Children That May Metastasize to Bone

Neuroblastoma
Leukemia
Lymphoma
Ewing sarcoma
Osteosarcoma
Malignant soft tissue sarcoma
Retinoblastoma
Embryonal rhabdomyosarcoma
Medulloblastoma
Wilms' tumor

TUMOR SPREAD

Tumor cells gain access to the skeleton by (a) hematogenous spread through the arterial circulation, (b) retrograde venous flow, and (c) direct extension. The portions of the skeleton that contain red marrow have a rich vascular supply, and tumor emboli frequently lodge within the sinusoidal channels found there. Tumor spread through retrograde venous flow occurs in the valveless vertebral plexus of Batson. This venous plexus interconnects the spine, the ribs, and the pelvis, providing access to the axial skeleton. Blood flow through the plexus may be transiently reversed by increased intra-abdominal pressure caused by activities such as coughing. Direct extension is much less frequent than hematogenous spread; when it occurs, it is usually extension of an intrathoracic tumor to the chest wall, an intrapelvic tumor to the pelvic wall, or a retroperitoneal process to the lumbar spine. For practical purposes, lymphatic spread of tumor to bone does not occur.

Metastases in the cancellous bone of the axial skeleton and in the cancellous metaphyseal bone of the proximal femur and proximal humerus account for nearly 90% of lesions, a distribution that is related to hematogenous spread. Metastases to the spinal column usually involve the vertebral body rather than the posterior elements. They are more common in the lumbar region than the thoracic region and least common in the cervical region. Metastases are distinctly uncommon distal to the knees or elbows. Approximately 90% of patients with bone metastases have multifocal involvement.

Skeletal metastases are common around joints, especially the hips, shoulders, knees, and intervertebral discs. Periarticular metastases with subchondral, intra-articular, or synovial extension may have a clinical presentation that simulates inflammatory arthritis. Lesions in the hands or feet are relatively rare and usually come from primary lung cancers. The intervertebral disc is a relative barrier to the spread of tumor, so that the usual pattern of vertebral metastatic involvement is vertebral destruction with preservation of the disc, even when multiple contiguous vertebral levels have tumor. It is very unusual for the disc to be involved by tumor. Coexistent degenerative disc disease is frequent and may be caused or exacerbated secondarily by the presence of tumor. In the subchondral region of the vertebral body, a metastasis may interfere with the nutrition of the disc or weaken the end plate so that disc material herniates through. The former process produces degenerative disc disease, and the latter produces a Schmorl node.

> Approximately 90% of patients with bone metastases have multifocal involvement.

> The intervertebral disc is a relative barrier to the spread of tumor.

RADIOLOGIC APPEARANCE

The appearance of a bone metastasis on radiographs reflects the balance of bone destruction and bone formation (Table 10.4). Metastatic tumors secrete osteoclast-stimulating factors; the osteoclasts excavate a defect in the bone where the metastasis establishes itself. The osteoclasts are not part of the tumor mass but can be found at the periphery, some-

Table 10.4: Typical Radiologic Appearances of Metastases from Specific Primary Tumors

Primary Tumor Site	Appearance on Plain Radiographs	Appearance on Bone Scan
Breast	Lytic, mixed, or blastic	Increased isotope uptake
Prostate	Blastic, occasionally mixed, or lytic	Increased isotope uptake
Lung	Lytic, mixed, occasionally blastic	Increased isotope uptake
Kidney	Lytic, expansile, or blow-out	Often decreased isotope uptake
Thyroid	Lytic, expansile, or blow-out	Often decreased or normal isotope uptake

times separated by fibrous tissue. Growth of the tumor is preceded by osteoclastic bone resorption. When bony trabeculae have been completely engulfed, tumor can destroy bone directly by elaborating enzymes. Osteoclast proliferation and osteoclastic bone resorption occur in all bone metastases, regardless of whether they also form bone. Bone formation may occur as stromal bone formation or as reactive bone formation. In those tumors associated with an acellular fibrous stroma, osteoprogenitor cells form bone under the influence of osteoinductive humoral factors secreted by the tumor. Metastases from prostatic carcinoma produce a fibrous stroma and form bone in this way; metastases from breast and lung carcinomas do not. In reactive bone formation, immature woven bone forms at the same time that bone destruction occurs. Proposed mechanisms for reactive bone include a mechanical response to weakening of the bone by the growing metastasis, an attempt by the bone to contain the lesion, or perhaps an uncoupling of the humoral factors that normally control bone formation and resorption.

| The pattern of destruction may be geographic, permeated, or moth-eaten. | Lytic lesions correspond to destruction and replacement of bone by nonmineralized tumor, without appreciable bone formation. The pattern of destruction may be geographic, permeated, or moth-eaten, and although there is a rough correspondence to increasing biologic aggressiveness, all patterns may be present in the same patient when extensive disease is present (Figs. 10.1 through 10.3). Because 30% to 50% of the bone mineralization must be lost before a lesion becomes visible on plain film, widespread lytic metastases may be inapparent on radiographs. Blastic lesions correspond to bone formation in or around tumor implants through reactive bone proliferation or ossification in fibrous stroma. Reactive apposition of new bone on cancellous bone surfaces results in a dense, blastic appearance. Proliferation of new endosteal bone is seen as endosteal thickening or irregular densities projected over the marrow cavity. Deposition of periosteal new bone causes cortical thickening or layers of periosteal new bone. Metastatic lesions usually do not stimulate periosteal new bone, and when they do, the periosteal bone tends to be scanty. The |

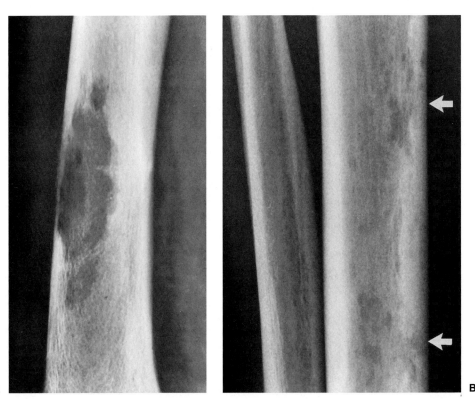

A   B

Figure 10.1 Lytic metastases from lung carcinoma. A. Geographic destruction in femoral shaft. The edges of the lesion are poorly defined. B. Moth-eaten destruction in the tibial shaft (*arrows*). (*continued*)

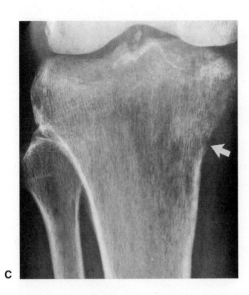

C

Figure 10.1 (*continued*) *C.* Permeated bone destruction in the proximal tibia (*arrow*). The region of destruction merges imperceptibly with normal bone.

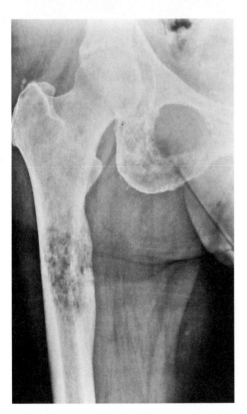

Figure 10.2 Lytic metastases from breast carcinoma. Permeated destruction is evident in the proximal femoral shaft and ischium.

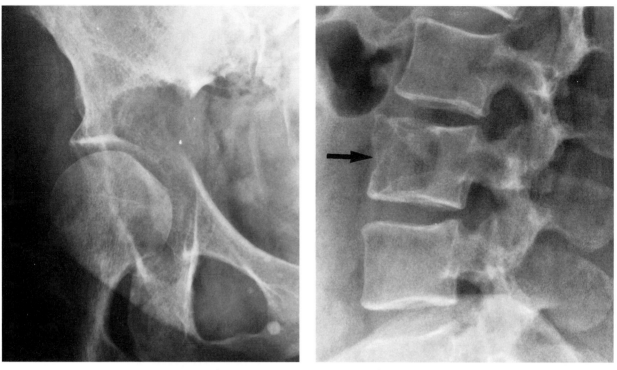

Figure 10.3 Lytic metastases from breast carcinoma. *A.* Huge destructive lesion in the ilium. *B.* Lytic lesion in the anterior two-thirds of the L3 vertebral body (*arrow*).

pattern of reactive bone proliferation generally reflects the tumor's growth rate, with highly anaplastic, fast-growing tumors and marrow element malignancies (myeloma and leukemia) provoking no radiographically appreciable reactive bone. Blastic metastases tend to have a dense homogeneous appearance with margins that fade imperceptibly into normal bone (Figs. 10.4 and 10.5). Mixed lesions contain both lytic and blastic areas, reflecting

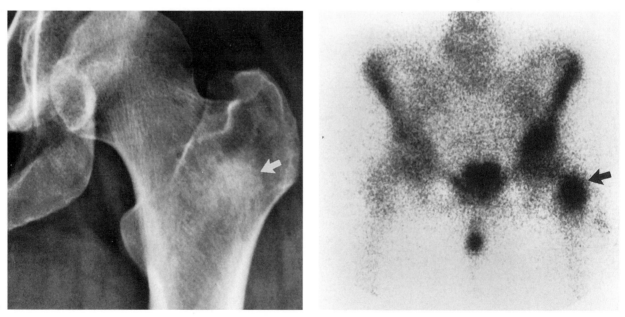

Figure 10.4 Blastic metastases from breast carcinoma in the intertrochanteric region of the femur. *A.* A homogeneously dense blastic lesion with poorly defined margins (*arrow*). *B.* Bone scan shows increased radionuclide accumulation in the lesion and in the ipsilateral acetabulum (*arrow*).

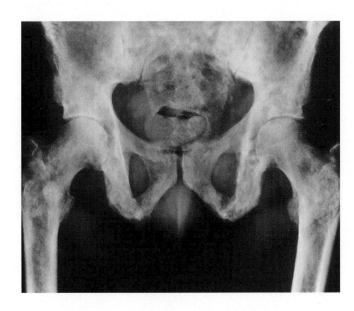

Figure 10.5 Diffuse blastic metastases from prostate carcinoma throughout the pelvis and proximal femurs.

bone destruction and bone formation in different portions of the same lesion (Fig. 10.6). In fact, both processes occur simultaneously in virtually all metastases.

The bone scan is more sensitive than radiographs for detecting metastases but has lower specificity. Radionuclide bone scanning agents such as technetium-99m methylene diphosphonate accumulate in new reactive or stromal bone (Fig. 10.4B). The metastasis itself may not accumulate the tracer unless the primary lesion forms bone or cartilage. Most lytic lesions, as well as all blastic and mixed lesions, have enough new bone formation to appear as areas of intense uptake on scan. If the activity in the reactive and stromal bone is equal to that of normal bone, or if the metastasis is in the marrow space but does not affect the bone, the scan is falsely negative. If bone is destroyed and replaced by tumor without provoking detectable reactive bone, an area of decreased uptake may result. Anaplastic, purely lytic lesions tend to have decreased uptake. A "superscan," that is, diffuse increased radionuclide accumulation throughout the entire skeleton, can indicate diffuse osseous metastatic disease.

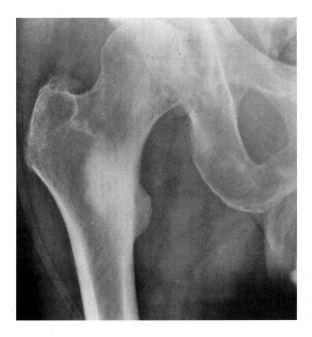

Figure 10.6 Metastases from breast carcinoma. Mixed lytic and blastic lesions in the pelvis and blastic lesions in the proximal femur.

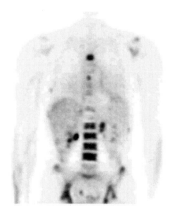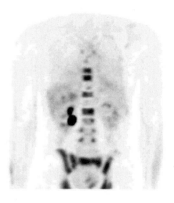

Figure 10.7 Metastases from adenocarcinoma detected by PET. Coronal tomographic images show multiple hypermetabolic lesions in the spine, pelvis, liver, and abdominal lymph nodes.

Positron emission tomography (PET) using 18-fluorodeoxyglucose (18-FDG), a radioactive-labeled glucose analog that permits imaging based on metabolic rate, has demonstrated considerable utility in oncologic imaging. With regard to screening for skeletal metastases, compared with the radionuclide bone scan, PET with 18-FDG appears to have higher sensitivity and higher specificity for detection of osteolytic metastases. Osteoblastic metastases and osteosarcoma metastases appear to have lower metabolic rates than osteolytic metastases, and the radionuclide bone scan appears better than PET in these circumstances (Fig. 10.7).

CT may show the extent of bone involvement more clearly than radiographs (Fig. 10.8). Delineation of the extent of cortical involvement is important when prophylactic internal fixation is contemplated. In addition, CT may show tumor in the marrow spaces in the absence of bone destruction. Increased attenuation in the medullary cavity reflects replacement of fatty marrow by tumor, edema, or reactive mesenchymal tissue (Fig. 10.9). CT is helpful for problem solving when routine imaging is discordant with the clinical situation (Fig. 10.10).

On MRI, metastatic lesions are seen as focal areas of abnormal signal replacing the normal marrow signal (Fig. 10.11). They are easily distinguished from normal tissue unless the metastases are so extensive that normal marrow signal is absent. On T1-weighted images, metastatic foci have low signal intensity; on T2-weighted images, they have high signal intensity (Figs. 10.12 and 10.13); following intravenous gadolin-

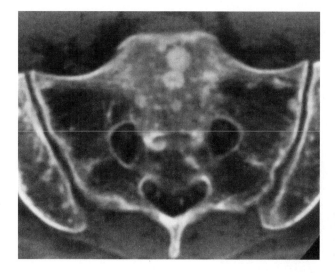

Figure 10.8 Multiple blastic metastases from thyroid carcinoma. Radiographs and bone scan were normal.

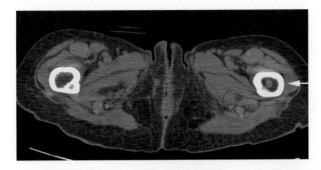

Figure 10.9 Marrow space metastasis in the left femur (*arrow*) from lung cancer demonstrated by CT. The bone scan was negative in the region of this lesion.

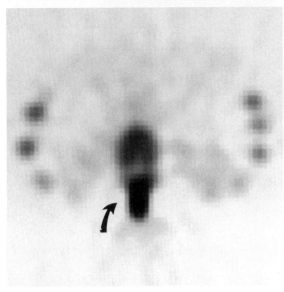

A

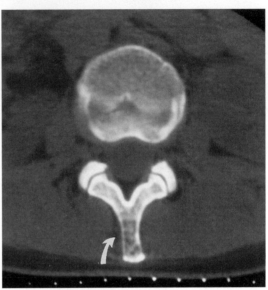

B

Figure 10.10 Solitary lesion found on bone scan in a woman with breast carcinoma with no other evidence of disease. *A.* Axial SPECT image shows increased activity in a thoracic spinous process (*arrow*). *B.* CT scan at time of percutaneous needle biopsy shows destructive lesion confined to spinous process (*arrow*).

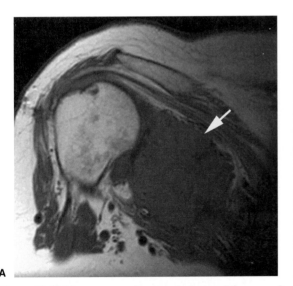

A

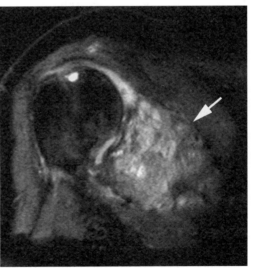

B

Figure 10.11 Metastases to the scapula (*arrows*) from renal cell carcinoma. *A,B.* Oblique coronal T1-weighted and T2-weighted fat-suppressed MRIs of the scapula show bone destruction and replacement with a heterogeneous mass.

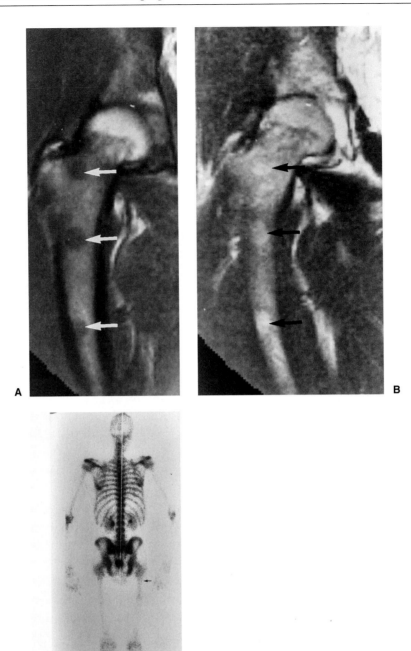

A

B

C

Figure 10.12 Metastases not evident on plain films. *A.* Coronal T1-weighted MRI shows three discrete rounded low-signal lesions in the proximal femoral shaft (*arrows*). *B.* Coronal T2-weighted MRI shows that all lesions have high signal (*arrows*), typical of tumor. *C.* Posterior bone scan demonstrates vague increase in tracer uptake in right proximal femur (*arrow*).

MRI is more sensitive for detecting marrow lesions than the radionuclide bone scan.

ium, they enhance. MRI is more sensitive than bone scan and has superior anatomic detail. Whole-body MRI has been used for detection of bone metastases in children and young adults, using spin-echo T1-weighted and STIR sequences. MRI is the best examination for investigating acute spinal cord symptoms in patients with known metastatic disease and for screening the spine when the bone scan is negative and profound osteopenia is present (Fig. 10.14). MRI may also be particularly helpful in making decisions

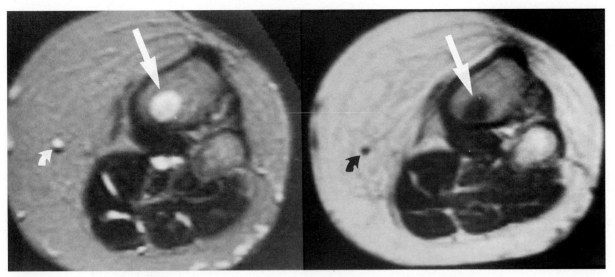

Figure 10.13 Metastasis from rhabdomyosarcoma. Axial MRI shows a round lesion in the tibial marrow space that has high signal on T2-weighted images and low signal on T1-weighted images (*long arrows*). Blood vessels (*short arrows*) have similar signal characteristics on this image but have predictable anatomic locations.

about staging and treatment when a solitary lesion is found on a screening bone scan and radiographs are normal.

Metastases may appear in any transverse or longitudinal location within an involved bone, including marrow space, cortex, or surface, and epiphysis, metaphysis, or diaphysis.

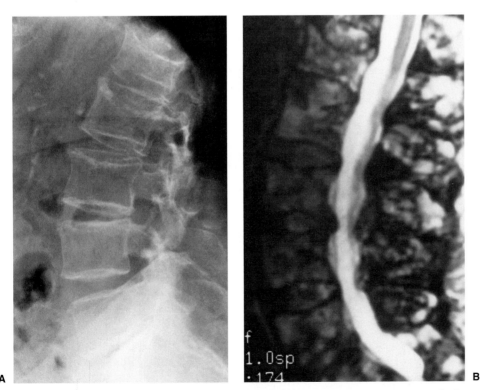

Figure 10.14 Widespread spine metastases from breast carcinoma. *A*. Lateral radiograph shows osteopenia and compression fractures in the upper lumbar spine. *B*. Sagittal T2-weighted MRI shows widespread replacement of the normal marrow signal by multiple high signal lesions.

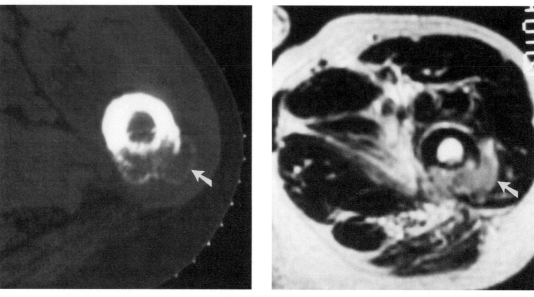

Figure 10.15 Cortical metastasis not involving the marrow space. *A.* CT shows destructive lesion in posterior cortex of femur with irregular periosteal reaction (*arrow*). *B.* Axial T2-weighted MRI shows the lesion (*arrow*) with surrounding edema.

Intracortical or subperiosteal locations are common for metastases (Fig. 10.15) but rare for primary bone tumors.

In young children, skeletal metastases tend to be widespread and generally symmetric in their involvement of the skeleton (Fig. 10.16). Osteolysis and permeated destruction are prominent, and collapse of vertebral bodies is frequent.

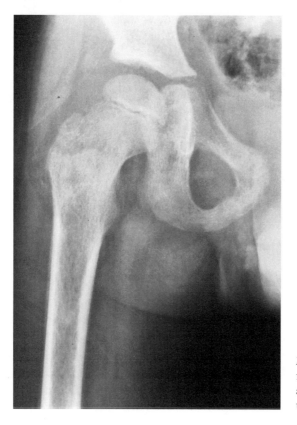

Figure 10.16 Child with metastases from neuroblastoma. The bones are diffusely abnormal with loss of the normal trabecular pattern and cortical edges.

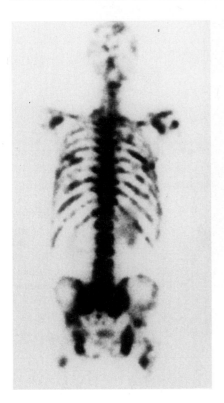

Figure 10.17 Bone scan shows multiple metastases from prostate carcinoma.

SCREENING FOR METASTASES

Screening for skeletal metastases in patients with known primary malignancies is usually accomplished with bone scanning; 30% of metastatic lesions detected by bone scan are missed by radiographs, and 2% of metastatic lesions detected by radiographs are missed by scans. Because most patients have multiple lesions, it is rare for a patient with osseous metastases to have an entirely normal bone scan (Fig. 10.17). The bone scan can be falsely negative or nondiagnostic in debilitated patients with a poor host response or in patients who have had radiotherapy.

When bone metastases are known to be present, response to therapy can be documented by serial bone scans. With successful treatment, lesions with increased isotope uptake tend to become normal, and the number of lesions decreases. Sometimes, in the presence of clinical improvement, an increase in lesion intensity is seen after therapy. This "flare phenomenon" presumably corresponds to healing of metastatic lesions with increasing formation of reactive bone. Follow-up scans in 2 to 3 months clarify the situation by showing the expected decrease in activity. Growth of lesions and the onset of new lesions indicate worsening disease. When additional lesions are suspected in specific areas of new, worsening, or recurrent pain, plain radiographs are usually obtained first. If these are negative, a bone scan is indicated, and if that, too, is negative, CT or MRI may be necessary.

HEMATOLOGIC MALIGNANCIES INVOLVING BONE SECONDARILY

Marrow element malignancies tend to infiltrate and involve the skeleton diffusely and do not have the discrete multifocal tumor deposits more typical of metastases from primary tumors of parenchymal organs. Primary marrow element tumors (multiple myeloma, Ewing sarcoma, primitive neuroectodermal tumor, and primary lymphoma of bone) are discussed in Chapter 8.

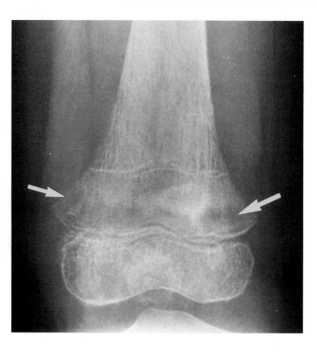

Figure 10.18 Child with leukemia. Transverse metaphyseal lucencies are present (*arrows*), corresponding to marrow space packing with leukemic infiltrates.

LEUKEMIA

Leukemia is a neoplasm of leukocytes that may involve bone secondarily. Leukemia is the most common malignancy in children. Leukemic infiltration of many organs and tissues, including the marrow spaces, is present and may have a diffuse or nodular character. Packing of the marrow spaces with leukemic cells causes pressure atrophy of cancellous trabeculae and is seen radiographically as diffuse osteopenia. In children, lucent metaphyseal bands may occur, reflecting zones of trabeculae that are thinner and sparser than normal in areas of rapid bone growth (Fig. 10.18). Although often seen in children with leukemia,

Packing of the marrow spaces with leukemic cells causes pressure atrophy of cancellous trabeculae and is seen radiographically as osteopenia.

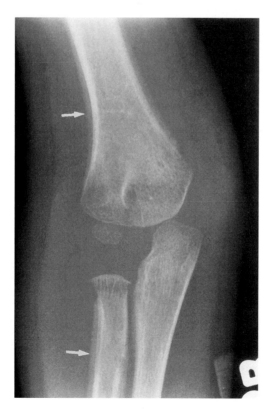

Figure 10.19 Child with leukemia. Diffuse periosteal reaction (*arrows*) and metaphyseal lucencies are present.

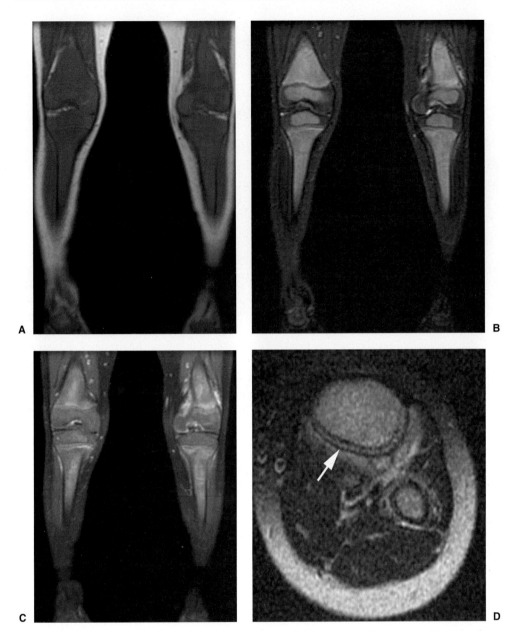

Figure 10.20 Acute lymphoblastic leukemia in a young child. *A.* Coronal T1-weighted MRI (without fat suppression) shows replacement of the marrow. *B.* Coronal T2-weighted fat-suppressed MRI shows high signal throughout the marrow spaces. *C.* Coronal T1-weighted fat-suppressed MRI following gadolinium injection shows diffuse enhancement. *D.* Axial T2-weighted MRI through the leg shows periosteal reaction (*arrow*) and surrounding edema.

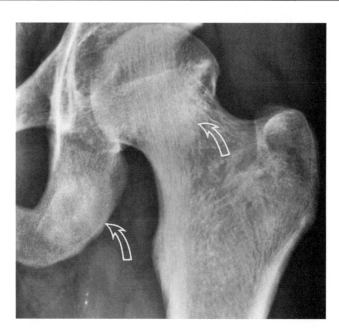

Figure 10.21 Eighteen-year-old man with Hodgkin disease. Blastic lesions in femoral neck and ischium (*arrows*).

these lucent metaphyseal bands are nonspecific and simply reflect the presence of systemic disease or even normal variation. Nodular collections of leukemic cells cause focal areas of medullary, cortical, or subperiosteal bone destruction.

Leukemic infiltration can extend through the cortex by way of the haversian systems, enlarging them by eroding the bone. This causes the cortex to appear fuzzy and osteopenic, often with lucent streaks. Infiltration of subperiosteal spaces lifts the periosteum and stimulates bone formation (Fig. 10.19). Periosteal bone formation that occurs as the periosteum is being lifted results in perpendicular sunburst bone spicules as the periosteum leaves a trail of reactive bone behind. Even if radiographs of bone are normal, widespread marrow space involvement is the rule and can be confirmed by MRI bone marrow aspiration. On MRI, leukemia is evident as marrow replacement and periosteal reaction (Fig. 10.20).

HODGKIN DISEASE

Hodgkin disease is a malignant tumor of lymph nodes. Secondary bone involvement is detected clinically in 5% to 21% of patients, but a much higher incidence can be demonstrated by marrow biopsy or at autopsy. Bone involvement usually occurs by direct extension from tumor-filled nodes so that the lumbar spine is affected most commonly. Pressure erosion of the cortical surface by enlarged periaortic nodes, without actual invasion, causes scalloping of the anterior aspects of the vertebral bodies. Hematogenous spread may occur as well. Extensive osteoblastic reaction is usual, but lytic and mixed lesions may occur. Ill-defined permeating lesions reflect spread of tumor through the medullary spaces and haversian systems (Fig. 10.21). Partial collapse of involved vertebral bodies is possible, representing pathologic compression fractures. A densely sclerotic vertebral body, a so-called ivory vertebra, is a classic radiographic sign with the differential diagnosis of lymphoma, blastic metastasis, Paget disease, and, rarely, myelosclerosis, fluorosis, or osteopetrosis.

NON-HODGKIN LYMPHOMA

Bone involvement is seen in 5% to 15% of patients with non-Hodgkin (extranodal) lymphoma. The prevalence of bone marrow involvement in autopsy series is much higher. The radiographic appearance of secondary involvement of bone by lymphoma is identical to that of primary involvement (see Chapter 8).

PATHOLOGIC FRACTURE

Pathologic fractures through bones involved by metastases are common. The most common sites of pathologic fracture are the vertebral bodies, ribs, pelvis, proximal femur, and proximal humerus (Figs. 10.22 and 10.23). Metastases of lytic, blastic, and mixed radiographic appearance all cause weakening of the bone.

> Metastases of lytic, blastic, and mixed radiographic appearance all cause weakening of the bone.

In the spine, compression fractures with vertebral collapse occur, presumably as a result of gradual destruction of the trabeculae that bear the compressive loads. Involvement of the posterior elements may render some vertebral fractures unstable. An epidural mass may be present and may block the spinal canal. MRI or myelography with CT can demonstrate the epidural mass, indicate the status of the spinal cord, and delineate the extent of vertebral disease.

In the long bones, destructive lesions with full-thickness cortical penetration lead to pathologic fractures. Gaps in the cortex weaken the bone by causing uneven and aberrant distribution of the stresses of loading, impeding the normal biomechanical dispersion of force. Weakening is gradual as cortical bone is infiltrated, eroded, and destroyed. Blastic lesions also destroy cortex, and the reactive bone and stromal bone that give blastic lesions their radiodensity are structurally unsound. The bone may fracture under the stresses of normal activity. Cortical weakening makes bone most vulnerable to tensile forces; therefore, in the long bones, pathologic fractures are usually transverse. The onset of pain at a site of metastatic involvement may indicate the presence of microfractures in a weakened cortex.

The goal of treatment of osseous metastases is to palliate pain and prevent pathologic fracture; curative resection is generally not realistic. Prophylactic internal fixation of metastatically involved bone is often considered. The clinical decision revolves around the patient's concerns and level of activity, the localization and multiplicity of bone involvement, and the extent of destruction. Fixation is generally indicated for lytic lesions if they are greater than 2.5 cm in size or involve more than half the circumference of the bone. Pathologic fractures are usually treated surgically. Prosthetic replacements allow the removal of the tumor-destroyed bone. Methylmethacrylate is often used

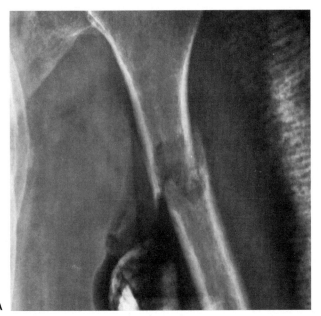
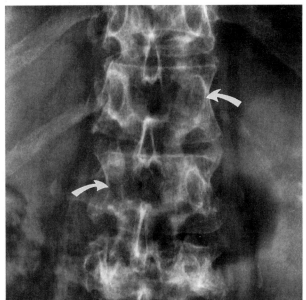

A   B

Figure 10.22 Metastatic breast carcinoma. *A.* Pathologic fracture transversely through lytic lesion in proximal humeral shaft. *B.* Left T12 pedicle has lost medial cortical margin, and right L1 pedicle is missing, both involved by metastases (*arrows*). L2 vertebral body is also involved and has collapsed (pathologic compression fracture).

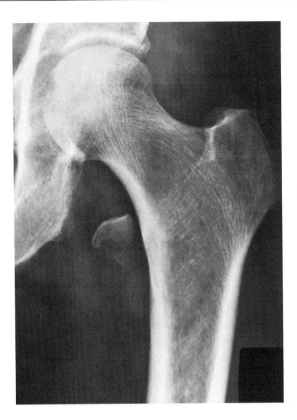

Figure 10.23 Breast carcinoma with pathologic avulsion fracture of lesser trochanter. Avulsion fractures of the lesser trochanter in adults are usually pathologic.

to buttress destroyed portions of bone and fill in bony defects. Radiotherapy can interfere with secondary healing by destroying chondrogenesis. The primary osteogenesis that occurs with internal fixation is more resistant to radiation, so that radiotherapy generally does not interfere with healing of internally fixed fractures. If the patient's life span is long enough, pathologic fractures will heal, but the healing process may be prolonged. Median survival after discovery of a pathologic fracture through an osseous metastasis, combined for all primary sites, is approximately 18 months.

SOFT TISSUE AND MUSCLE METASTASES

Although the skeletal muscle mass of the human body accounts for a large percentage of the total body weight, nearly 50%, in clinical experience, skeletal muscle is a rare site for metastases. Muscle is highly resistant to both primary and metastatic cancer. The cited factors for this high resistance include contractile activity, local changes in pH, oxygenation, accumulation of lactic acid and other metabolites, blood flow per unit weight (mL/minute/g), intramuscular blood pressure, and local temperature. Weiss experimentally showed that cancer cell survival is greatest in denervated muscle that is unable to contract as opposed to electrically stimulated muscle. His experimental work supports the hypothesis that the rapid death of most cancer cells after delivery to some target organs is a consequence of their mechanical interactions within the microvasculature. Muscle metastases have been reported in sites of previously documented skeletal muscle trauma.

Autopsies in two series of patients showed that the prevalence of metastases to muscle was 16.0% and 17.5%. Neoplasms with the highest incidence of metastases to muscle were carcinoma, leukemia, and lymphoma. The diaphragm, rectus muscle of the abdomen, deltoid muscle, psoas muscle, and intercostal muscles were most commonly involved. The patients with muscle metastases were 26 to 84 years old (mean age, 62 years old). Most patients present with pain in the involved muscles or a clinically palpable mass and have

Muscle is highly resistant to both primary and metastatic cancer.

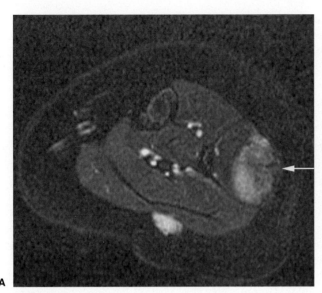 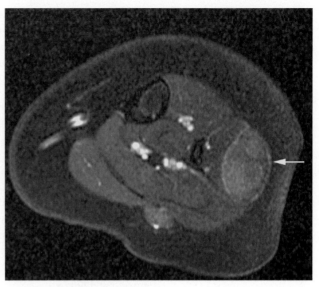

A   B

Figure 10.24 Metastases to muscle from lung cancer. *A.* Axial T2-weighted fat-suppressed MRI shows high signal (*arrow*) in the lateral compartment muscles of the leg. *B.* Axial T1-weighted fat-suppressed MRI after gadolinium injection shows moderate enhancement (*arrow*) in the lesion.

advanced-stage neoplasms. On unenhanced CT scans, muscle metastasis is revealed as an enlargement of a muscle.

Occasionally, the findings may be subtle because the tumor is isodense to the surrounding muscle, and contralateral asymmetry is necessary to make the diagnosis. On contrast-enhanced CT, skeletal muscle metastases appear as rim-enhancing intramuscular lesions with central hypoattenuation (Fig. 10.24). On MRI, muscle metastases have high signal intensity on T2-weighted sequence, lobulated morphology, large areas of central necrosis, and extensive peritumoral edema (Fig. 10.25). MRI findings of carcinoma metastatic to muscle are not pathognomonic, and the differential diagnosis must include soft tissue sarcoma, hematoma, and abscess.

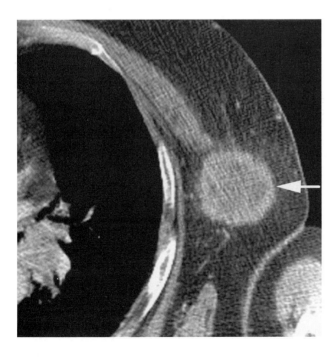

Figure 10.25 Soft tissue metastasis from lung cancer. Contrast-enhanced CT scan shows a rim-enhanced soft tissue metastasis (*arrow*).

Metastases to skin, subcutaneous tissues, and lymph nodes may present as soft tissue masses. On CT, such lesions tend to be isodense to muscle and may enhance. On MRI, soft tissue metastases typically have low signal on T1-weighted images, high signal on T2-weighted images, and enhancement after gadolinium injection.

PERCUTANEOUS NEEDLE BIOPSY

In the evaluation of a patient with one or more focal lesions in the setting of a known primary tumor or no known primary tumor, percutaneous needle biopsy is often the invasive procedure of choice. Typically performed under CT guidance, the diagnostic yield is high, and the morbidity is low. Virtually any anatomic site may be accessible to needle biopsy, and some sites that would be problematic for the surgeon are straightforward for the interventional bone radiologist. A variety of specialized needles is available for obtaining core specimens of bone or soft tissue lesions. An extraosseous component of a malignant bone tumor is as representative of the tumor as is the bone tumor itself. A frozen section of a core biopsy or cytologic preparation of a fine-needle aspiration may provide an immediate pathologic diagnosis. Specific benign diagnoses that may account for clinical symptoms or radiologic abnormalities may be made from needle biopsy specimens by the experienced pathologist. Aspiration of bone marrow from the iliac crest in many patients may find tumor cells, but these correspond to circulating tumor cells that have been shed into the bloodstream. They do not necessarily become established skeletal metastases. Aspiration specimens should also be sent for culture and sensitivity.

The diagnostic yield of CT-guided percutaneous needle biopsy is high, and the morbidity is low.

TREATMENT

The basic treatment modalities for osseous metastases, with or without pathologic fractures, are radiation therapy, chemotherapy, and surgical stabilization. Palliative radiation of symptomatic lesions without pathologic fracture provides pain relief in approximately 80% of patients. If a pathologic fracture is present, pain relief may be experienced by approximately 60% of patients; without internal fixation, the pathologic fractures may progress to nonunion.

RADIOTHERAPY CHANGES IN BONE

Therapeutic irradiation is a common means of treating osseous metastases. Sites of bone pain confirmed as abnormal by roentgenography or bone scan in patients with known metastases are often treated palliatively by radiation. Irradiated osseous lesions heal by sclerosis and filling-in of lytic areas. Radiation effects are independent of the radiation source. In the immature skeleton, radiation in total doses of 2,000 cGy or greater impairs bone growth. The epiphysis is especially sensitive; radiation causes direct cellular injury to chondrocytes and possibly vascular damage to fine physeal blood vessels. The greater the growth potential at the time of irradiation, the more profound is its effect. If an entire growing bone is irradiated, loss of bone growth in the whole bone results in a small bone. Focal doses affect the irradiated portion; for example, angular deformities could result from an asymmetrically irradiated growth plate. Radiotherapy also increases the risk for epiphyseal plate trauma, including the occurrence of slipped capital femoral epiphysis and avascular necrosis. Scoliosis may follow irradiation of the spine (Fig. 10.26).

In the mature skeleton, the primary change is radiation necrosis (Fig. 10.27). This osteonecrosis is dose related. Radiographs and CT show irregular sclerosis in the irradiated bone. Insufficiency fracture is a relatively common complication of radiation necrosis (Fig. 10.28).

Radiation-induced tumors in patients who received radiotherapy before 2 years of age are usually benign.

In patients who received radiotherapy before 2 years of age, induced tumors (Table 10.5) are usually benign. The most common are exostoses (osteochondromas); these are

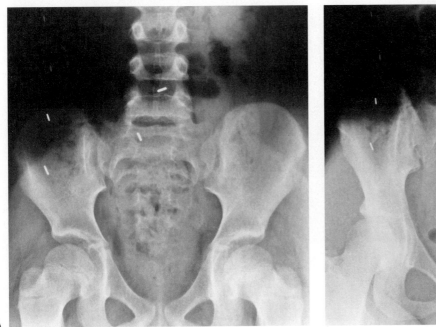
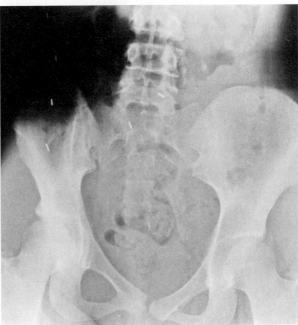

A

B

Figure 10.26 Radiation hypoplasia. *A.* After radiation to right lower abdomen for Wilms' tumor. *B.* Ten years later, hypoplasia of the right iliac wing and the right half of the lumbar spine is evident.

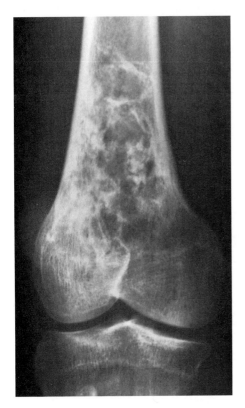

Figure 10.27 Radiation changes in the distal femur in a 30-year-old woman who was treated 6 years previously for lymphoma. There are sclerotic and cystic-appearing changes in distal femoral metaphysis.

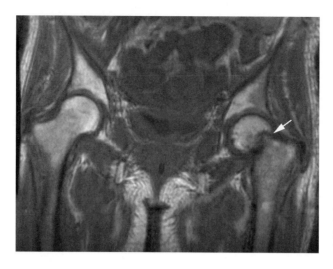

Figure 10.28 Insufficiency fracture (*arrow*) of the femoral neck in an irradiated hip on coronal T1-weighted MRI.

Table 10.5: Radiation-Induced Tumors

Benign
  Osteochondroma
  Osteoblastoma
Malignant
  Squamous cell carcinoma of skin
  Osteosarcoma
  Fibrosarcoma
  Malignant fibrous histiocytoma
  Chondrosarcoma

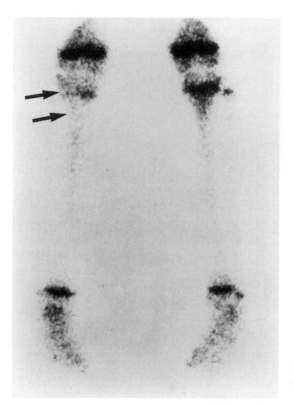

Figure 10.29 Decreased radionuclide activity in the area of a radiation portal (*arrows*).

histologically and biologically indistinguishable from those that occur naturally. Fibrosarcoma or malignant fibrous histiocytoma, chondrosarcoma, and other unusual sarcomas are much less likely to occur. Malignant tumors may occur in older patients who have received radiotherapy. The following criteria must be satisfied to make the diagnosis of a radiation-induced sarcoma: (a) the sarcoma arises within the irradiated field, (b) the latent period is at least 4 years, and (c) the sarcoma is histologically different from a previous tumor or the radiation was delivered in the absence of a malignant diagnosis. The latent period averages 11 years. The presence of pain, soft tissue mass, and progression on serial films should raise suspicion and lead to biopsy.

On bone scan, irradiated bone may initially show increased radionuclide accumulation from hyperemia and new bone formation. After several weeks or months, the bone scan shows decreased radionuclide accumulation because of decreased bone formation and decreased vascularity (Fig. 10.29). On MRI, irradiated bone has the signal characteristics of fatty marrow. The anatomic location and extent of these changes conform to the size and shape of the radiation portal.

SOURCES AND READINGS

Berger FH, Verstraete KL, Gooding CA, et al. MR imaging of musculoskeletal neoplasm. *Magn Reson Imaging Clin North Am* 2000;8:929–951.

Bui-Mansfield LT, Chew FS, Lenchik L, et al. Nontraumatic avulsions of the pelvis. *AJR Am J Roentgenol* 2001;178:423–427.

Cook GJ, Houston S, Rubens R, et al. Detection of bone metastases in breast cancer by 18FDG PET: differing metabolic activity in osteoblastic and osteolytic lesions. *J Clin Oncol* 1998;16:3375–3379.

Daldrup-Link HE, Franzius C, Link TM, et al. Whole-body MR imaging for detection of bone metastases in children and young adults: comparison with skeletal scintigraphy and FDG PET. *AJR Am J Roentgenol* 2001;177:229–236.

Damron TA, Heiner J. Management of metastatic disease to soft tissue. *Orthop Clin North Am* 2000;31:661–673.

Galasko CSB. *Skeletal metastases*. London: Butterworths, 1986.

Glockner JF, White LM, Sundaram M, et al. Unsuspected metastases presenting as solitary soft tissue lesions: a fourteen-year review. *Skeletal Radiol* 2000;29:270–274.

Herring CL, Harrelson JM, Scully SP. Metastatic carcinoma to skeletal muscle—a report of 15 patients. *Clin Orthop* 1998;355:272–281.

Hudson TM. *Radiologic-pathologic correlation of musculoskeletal lesions*. Baltimore: Williams & Wilkins, 1987:421–440.

Kagan AR, Bassett LW, Steckel RJ, et al. Radiologic contributions to cancer management. Bone metastases. *AJR Am J Roentgenol* 1986;147:305–312.

Magee T, Rosenthal H. Skeletal muscle metastases at sites of documented trauma. *AJR Am J Roentgenol* 2002;178:985–988.

Mollabashy A, Scarborough M. The mechanism of metastasis. *Orthop Clin North Am* 2000;31:529–535.

Orr FW, Lee J, Duivenvoorden WC, et al. Pathophysiologic interactions in skeletal metastasis. *Cancer* 2000;88[Suppl]:2912–2918.

Panicek DM, Schwartz LH. MR imaging after surgery for musculoskeletal neoplasm. *Semin Musculoskelet Radiol* 2002;6:57–66.

Podoloff DA. Malignant bone disease. In: Henkin RE, Boles MA, Dillehay GL, et al., eds. *Nuclear medicine*. St. Louis: Mosby–Year Book, 1996:1208–1222.

Pretorius ES, Fishman EK. Helical CT of skeletal muscle metastases from primary carcinomas. *AJR Am J Roentgenol* 2000;174:401–404.

Resnick D. *Diagnosis of bone and joint disorders*, 4th ed. Philadelphia: WB Saunders, 2002.

Rubens RD, Fogelman I, eds. *Bone metastases: diagnosis and treatment*. London: Springer-Verlag New York, 1991.

Seely S. Possible reasons for the high resistance of muscle to cancer. *Med Hypotheses* 1980;6:133–137.

Sim FH, ed. *Diagnosis and management of metastatic bone disease. A multidisciplinary approach*. New York: Raven Press, 1988.

Thrall JH, Ellis BI. Skeletal metastasis. *Radiol Clin North Am* 1987;25:1155–1170.

Weatherall P. Imaging of muscle tumors. *Semin Musculoskelet Radiol* 2000;4:435–458.

Weiss L. Biomechanical destruction of cancer cells in skeletal muscle: a rate-regulator for hematogenous metastasis. *Clin Exp Metastasis* 1989;7:483–491.

Williams JB, Youngberg RA, Bui-Mansfield LT, et al. MR imaging of skeletal muscle metastases. *AJR Am J Roentgenol* 1997;168:555–557.

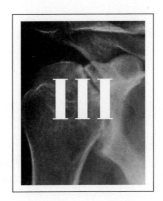

JOINT DISEASE

APPROACH TO JOINT DISEASE

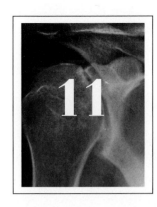

- General Principles
- Synovial Joints
- Intervertebral Disc Joints
- Entheses
- Distribution of Disease
- Laboratory Findings
- Sources and Readings

This chapter describes a pragmatic approach to the radiology of joint disease, based on anatomy, pathophysiology, and radiographic analysis. This approach draws heavily on the work of Forrester, Brower, and Resnick (Tables 11.1 and 11.2). Detailed discussions of specific clinical forms of arthritis are presented in Chapters 12 and 13.

GENERAL PRINCIPLES

Radiographs mirror the pathologic processes that affect the joints and the functional adaptations that may follow. In general, the radiologic diagnosis of arthritis can be highly specific and reliable when classic changes are present in the expected distributions but much less specific in the early stages before the disease process has fully evolved. Regardless of approach, however, several frustrations are unavoidable: A specific radiologic diagnosis is not always possible; many types of joint disease overlap in their radiologic and clinical features; two or more diseases may coexist in the same patient; and, finally, clinical disease may precede radiologic abnormalities and vice versa, sometimes by years.

Diseases that affect joints do so by three broad pathophysiologic mechanisms, each with a distinctive radiographic appearance: degeneration, inflammation, and metabolic deposition. For practical purposes, one mechanism is usually predominant. Degeneration of a joint refers to mechanical damage and reparative adaptations; in essence, the joint is worn away. Inflammation of a joint may be acute, chronic, or both; the joint is dissolved by the inflammatory process. Metabolic deposition refers to infiltration of a joint by aberrant metabolic products. Each of these mechanisms affects joints in radiographically distinctive ways (Table 11.3).

Imaging mirrors the pathophysiology of arthritis.

SYNOVIAL JOINTS

Most articulations of the appendicular skeleton are synovial joints. In the axial skeleton, the facet joints of the spine, the atlantoaxial (C1-C2) joint, the uncovertebral joints of the cervical spine, and the lower two-thirds of the sacroiliac joints are synovial.

Table 11.1: Forrester's ABCS Approach to Radiographic Changes in the Hand

Alignment
Bone
Cartilage
Soft tissues

Adapted from Forrester DM, Brown JC. *The radiology of joint disease*, 3rd ed. Philadelphia: WB Saunders, 1987.

Table 11.2: Brower's Black-and-White Approach to Radiographic Changes in the Hand

Soft tissue swelling
   Symmetric around involved joint
   Asymmetric around involved joint
   Diffuse, involving entire digit
   Lumpy-bumpy
Subluxation
Mineralization
   Normal
   Juxta-articular osteoporosis
   Diffuse osteoporosis
Calcification
   Within soft tissue mass
   Tendinous and soft tissue (no mass)
   Chondrocalcinosis
Joint space
   Normal
   Uniform narrowing
   Asymmetric narrowing
Erosions
   Aggressive (without reactive bone)
   Nonaggressive (with reactive bone)
   Location
Bone production
   Periosteal new bone
   Bone ankylosis
   Overhanging cortical edge
   Subchondral sclerosis
   Osteophytes

Adapted from Brower AC. *Arthritis in black and white*, 2nd ed. Philadelphia: WB Saunders, 1997.

Table 11.3: Characteristic Radiographic Signs of Arthritis

Pathophysiology	*Characteristic Radiographic Signs*
Inflammation	Acute erosions
	Osteoporosis
	Soft tissue swelling
	Uniform loss of articular space
Degeneration	Osteophytes
	Subchondral sclerosis
	Uneven loss of articular space
	Chondrocalcinosis
Metabolic deposition	Lumpy-bumpy soft tissue swelling
	Chronic bony erosions with overhanging edges

SOFT TISSUES

Synovial joints have a joint cavity and are enclosed by a joint capsule consisting of an inner synovial layer (the synovium), a middle subsynovium, and an outer fibrous layer (Fig. 11.1). The synovium is a cellular secretory mucosa that produces synovial fluid. Synovial fluid is viscous because of a high concentration of hyaluronic acid. Joint capsules have an active blood supply with a large capillary surface area. The synovium has a mesenchymal rather than epithelial origin; therefore, no basement membrane or other structural barrier is present between the synovial fluid and the capillary bed. The change from synovium to fibrous capsule is gradual; there are no distinct boundaries between the layers. Joint capsules are densely innervated. Tendon sheaths invest tendons and reduce friction during motion. Bursae are located where complete freedom of motion between structures is necessary, for example, where a tendon passes directly over the periosteum. Because tendon sheaths and bursae are synovial structures, diseases that affect synovial joints may also involve them.

Soft tissue swelling at a joint may reflect capsular distention from effusion, synovial hypertrophy, soft tissue edema, or a mass. Symmetric, fusiform swelling suggests an inflammatory process with effusion, synovial edema, synovial hypertrophy, or some combination thereof (Fig. 11.2). Inflammatory distention of a tendon sheath may also produce soft tissue swelling, but the swelling extends beyond the joint. In a digit, this kind of swelling produces an appearance that has been likened to a sausage ("sausage digit"). Generalized soft tissue swelling may be caused by subcutaneous edema or hyperemia and suggests inflammation (Fig. 11.3). A lumpy-bumpy swelling that is not symmetric or centered near a joint suggests masses and may be caused by metabolic deposition disease with mass-like deposits of metabolic products in the periarticular soft tissues (Fig. 11.4). Soft tissue prominences at joints that are found on physical examination may actually result from bony or cartilaginous enlargements; the overlying soft tissues may be normal. Heberden and Bouchard nodes are swellings of this kind at the distal interphalangeal (DIP) and proximal interphalangeal (PIP) joints of the hand, respectively, and are characteristic of a degenerative process. Calcification in the soft tissues may affect cartilage, skin, muscles, tendons, or other connective tissues and is associated with connective tissue diseases. Soft tissue atrophy or loss is present in various conditions.

> Joint capsules are densely innervated.

> Heberden nodes result from osteophytes at the DIP joints.

> Bouchard nodes result from osteophytes at the PIP joints.

CARTILAGE

The ends of the articulating bones, that is, the joint surfaces, are covered with hyaline articular cartilage. Hyaline cartilage is composed of a collagen fibril framework and a ground substance. One set of densely packed collagen fibrils is oriented parallel to the articular sur-

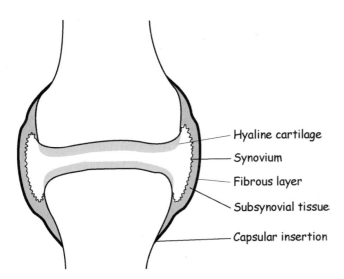

Figure 11.1 Anatomy of a synovial joint.

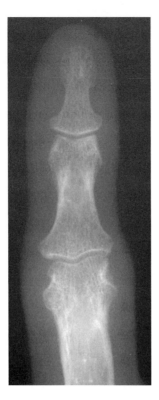

Figure 11.2 Fusiform soft tissue swelling at the proximal interphalangeal joint (rheumatoid arthritis).

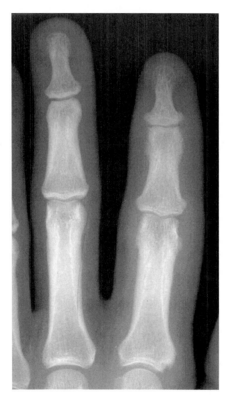

Figure 11.3 "Sausage digit" soft tissue swelling (psoriatic arthritis).

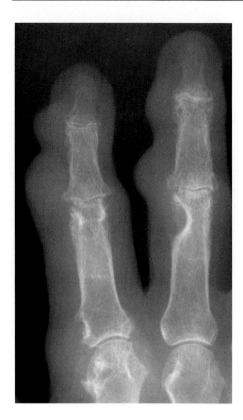

Figure 11.4 Lumpy-bumpy soft tissue swelling (tophaceous gout).

face, forming an armor-plate layer with tiny surface pores that allow the passage of water and small electrolytes. A second, less densely packed set of collagen fibrils is oriented in arcades, linking the armor-plate layer to the subchondral bone (Fig. 11.5). The ground substance is a gel that consists of water and large proteoglycan aggregate macromolecules that are loosely fixed to the collagen framework. The proteoglycan macromolecules are too large to pass through the pores of the armor-plate layer. The physical and chemical properties of these macromolecules allow them to attract and bind water, providing sufficient swelling pressure beneath the armor-plate layer to "inflate" the articular cartilage, even during weight bearing. During motion, a thin layer of water is expressed through the small surface pores, providing a frictionless surface for a lifetime of mobility. Articular cartilage has a load-dampening ability that spreads transmitted loads over a greater area of the subchondral bone. Under rapid, transient loading, articular cartilage has elastic properties. Under a steady load, it creeps and deforms like a sponge. The portion of cartilage that is adjacent to the subchondral bone is calcified. Interdigitations between the calcified cartilage and the subchondral bone provide a strong mechanical coupling. Chondrocytes are the cells whose metabolic activity maintains the specialized structures of articular cartilage. Less than 1% of articular cartilage volume is composed of cells. Because cartilage is avascular and alymphatic, chondrocytes derive their nutrients by diffusion from the synovial

> Normal articular cartilage is inflated by hydrostatic pressure.

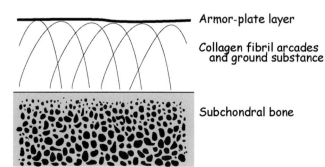

Armor-plate layer

Collagen fibril arcades and ground substance

Subchondral bone

Figure 11.5 Structure of articular cartilage.

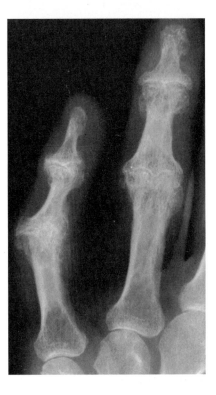

Figure 11.6 Asymmetric joint space narrowing, osteophytes, and subchondral sclerosis (osteoarthritis).

fluid. Articular cartilage has only a limited ability to repair itself. Deep injuries may repair with cartilage that is densely fibrous.

Cartilage abnormalities are inferred from the radiolucent gap between articulating bones, the articular space, or joint space. The articular cartilage fills this space. A potential space exists where the articulating surfaces meet. Loss of articular cartilage causes the joint space to narrow. Cartilage loss within a joint can be diffuse and concentric—indicating an inflammatory process (with enzymatic dissolution of cartilage)—or focal and uneven, indicating a mechanical one (Figs. 11.6 and 11.7). If there is complete cartilage loss, the ends

Loss of articular cartilage causes the joint spaces to narrow.

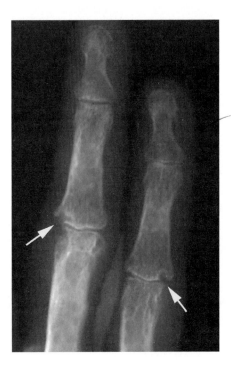

Figure 11.7 Acute marginal erosions (*arrows*), diffuse joint space narrowing, and osteoporosis (rheumatoid arthritis).

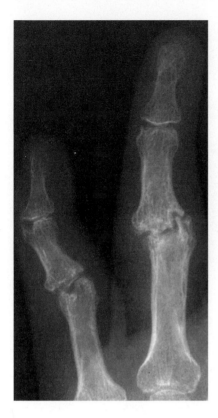

Figure 11.8 Severe proximal interphalangeal joint sub-chondral bone erosions (psoriatic arthritis).

of the bones may become eroded, making the joint space appear wider. The ends of the bone may form a pseudoarthrosis (Fig. 11.8), or fibrous or bony ankylosis (fusion) of the joint may occur (Fig. 11.9). Widening of the articular space may indicate abnormal carti-lage proliferation or intra-articular fluid. Weight-bearing views may be necessary to assess

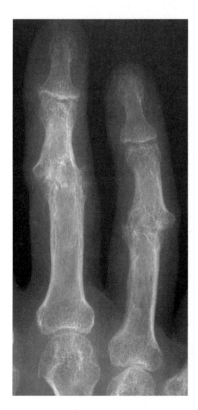

Figure 11.9 Bony ankylosis (psoriatic arthritis).

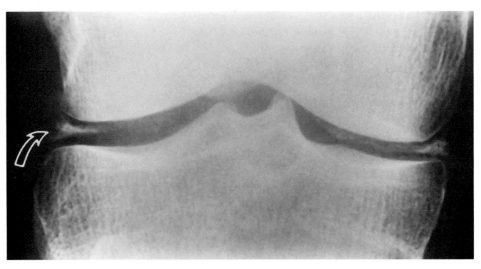

Figure 11.10 Chondrocalcinosis of the menisci (*arrow*).

accurately the degree of cartilage loss at the knee. Asymmetric cartilage loss may result in changes in radiographic joint space narrowing with changes in position.

Calcification of cartilage is called *chondrocalcinosis*. Chondrocalcinosis may involve fibrocartilage structures such as the menisci of the knee (Fig. 11.10) or the triangular fibrocartilage complex of the wrist. Articular cartilage also may calcify (Fig. 11.11).

BONE

Bone changes in arthritis include bone loss and bone proliferation. Osteoporosis is loss of bone through osteoclast action and may be generalized or regional, acute or chronic. Osteoporosis reflects hyperemia from synovial inflammation or from disuse of a body part. Acute osteoporosis is recognized by resorption of bone from subchondral trabeculae, a location where blood flow and metabolic activity are the greatest. The process of osteoporosis affects the trabecular bone and the cortex. However, because the surface area subject to osteoclastic resorption is greater in trabecular bone, the acute process is more evident there. If the process continues, tunneling may become evident in the cortex and can be rec-

Acute osteoporosis is recognized by resorption of subchondral bone.

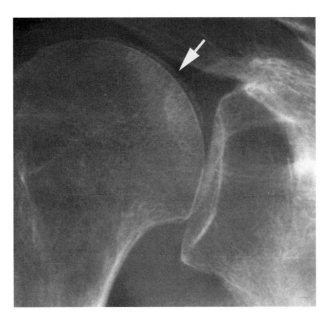

Figure 11.11 Chondrocalcinosis of the articular cartilage (*arrow*).

ognized as being porotic and thin. In noninflammatory articular disease, the normal mineralization of bone is maintained. Arthritic conditions are commonly treated with corticosteroids, which may cause osteoporosis.

Bone erosions represent focal losses of bone from the cortical surface. Erosions with loss of the cortex indicate an acute, aggressive process. In rheumatoid arthritis, for example, cortical bone is eroded by the action of enzymes produced by inflamed synovial tissues (pannus). These enzymes literally dissolve the bone and produce acute erosions without cortex. Erosions with cortex indicate a nonaggressive, chronic process in which bone remodels along the border of the erosion. The chronic erosions seen in metabolic deposition disease are caused by abnormal masses of metabolic products causing adjacent bone to remodel because of mechanical pressure. The bone may attempt to encircle the deposit; such an incomplete attempt leaves an overhanging edge (Fig. 11.12). Other mass-like processes in the joint may also cause chronic erosions of the bone. The characteristic initial site of erosions in arthritis is at the margin of the articular cartilage where a gap between the cartilage and the attachment of the synovium leaves a "bare area" of bone contained within the joint capsule. Once cartilage has been destroyed, erosions may extend over the entire articular surface.

Subchondral cysts, also called *geodes*, occur when cracks or fissures in the articular surface allow the intrusion of synovial fluid into the subchondral cancellous bone or when necrosis of subchondral bone is followed by collapse (Fig. 11.13). Subchondral cysts may also result from erosion of the articular surface by inflamed synovial tissues. Subchondral cysts are seen in virtually all types of arthritis and have no particular differential diagnostic significance. Proliferative new bone may represent attempts at cyst healing.

Proliferative bone formation at arthritic synovial joints occurs in four ways. Periostitis is periosteal apposition of new bone to the cortical surface (Fig. 11.14). Sclerosis, also called *eburnation*, is new bone apposed to the trabeculae of existing bone, usually in a subchondral location (immediately beneath the articular cartilage) but sometimes on the surface after the cartilage is gone. Osteophytes occur in the presence of cartilage loss and

Erosions with loss of the cortex indicate an acute, aggressive process.

Subchondral cysts are seen in virtually all types of arthritis.

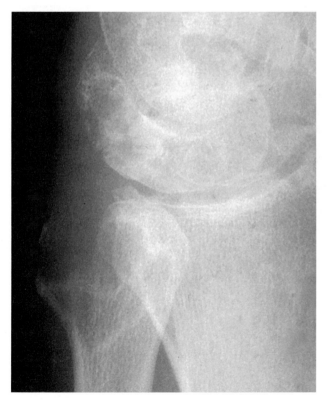

Figure 11.12 Chronic erosion and overhanging edges (tophaceous gout).

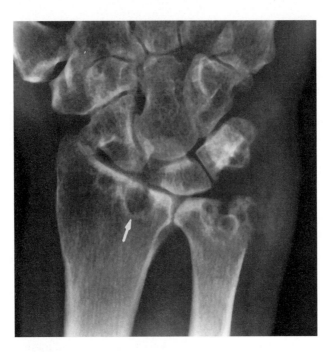

Figure 11.13 Subchondral cyst formation (rheumatoid arthritis) (*arrow*).

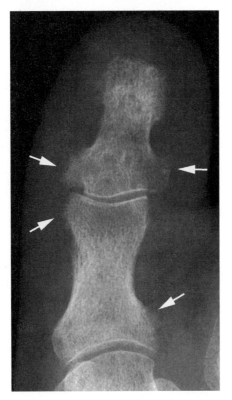

Figure 11.14 Periostitis (psoriatic arthritis) (*arrows*).

represent new excrescences of cartilage and bone that enlarge the articular surface at its margins. Bony proliferation may also occur at the attachment of joint capsules (discussed in the section Entheses).

ALIGNMENT

Alignment becomes abnormal when joint capsules or ligaments are torn or lax, the normally balanced tension across joints becomes unbalanced, or articular surfaces lose their normal size or shape. The result is deformity, subluxation, dislocation, and loss of function. Continued use of a damaged, malaligned joint leads to functional adaptation and secondary anatomic changes; ultimately, it may become difficult to distinguish these functional adaptations from the primary arthritic process. Loss of function and pain are the major causes of morbidity in arthritis.

> Continued use of a damaged, malaligned joint leads to secondary osteoarthritis.

Alignment deformities in the hand may lead to functional disability of great clinical significance. Deformities of the hand result from loss of the balanced muscular tension and ligamentous restriction that maintain its normal alignment. Common deformities of the digit include the swan neck deformity (PIP hyperextension with DIP flexion) (Fig. 11.15), the boutonniere deformity (PIP flexion with DIP hyperextension) (Fig. 11.16), the mallet finger (isolated DIP flexion), and the hitchhiker thumb or Z-shaped collapse of the thumb [metacarpophalangeal (MCP) joint flexion, interphalangeal (IP) joint hyperextension]. Subluxations and dislocations of individual joints may be seen, or the entire hand may collapse into a zigzag deformity (radial deviation of wrist with ulnar deviation of the MCP joints). These deformities reflect loss of normal functional anatomy from any underlying cause, one of which may be arthritis.

Abnormalities of alignment resulting from articular disease are common at the wrist, knee, and foot. Alignment deformities of the wrist may follow or precede actual articular changes on radiographs; these misalignments may have great clinical significance because normal wrist function is a prerequisite for normal hand function. The ligamentous instability patterns that may follow traumatic disruption of the carpal ligaments (see Chapter 2)

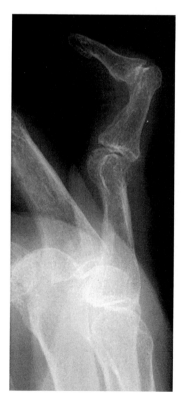

Figure 11.15 Swan neck deformity (rheumatoid arthritis).

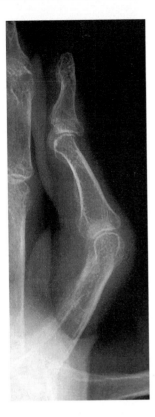

Figure 11.16 Boutonniere deformity (rheumatoid arthritis).

may also result from arthritic involvement of the carpal ligaments. Selective involvement of the medial or lateral tibiofemoral compartment of the knee with asymmetric thinning of cartilage may lead to varus or valgus deformity. In the foot, various digital deformities similar to those occurring in the hand may be found.

INTERVERTEBRAL DISC JOINTS

Intervertebral disc joints are present along the anterior portion of the spine. An intervertebral disc joint comprises cartilaginous end plates covering the articulating surfaces of adjacent vertebral bodies, a central nucleus pulposus, and a circumferential annulus fibrosus (Fig. 11.17). In the child, the nucleus pulposus has a gelatinous character; in the adult, the nucleus pulposus has converted to fibrocartilage. The annulus fibrosus contains an outer zone of collagenous fibers and an inner zone of fibrocartilage. The annulus fibrosus is

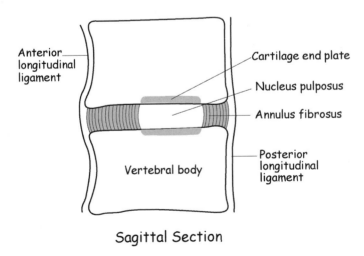

Figure 11.17 Anatomy of an intervertebral disc joint.

Table 11.4: Vertebral Phytes: Associations with Specific Diseases

Type of Phyte	Associated Condition
Syndesmophytes	Ankylosing spondylitis
Diffuse, flowing paravertebral ossification	Diffuse idiopathic skeletal hyperostosis
Osteophytes	Degenerative disc disease, spondylosis deformans
Focal paravertebral ossification	Psoriatic arthritis (common), Reiter syndrome (uncommon)

anchored to the cartilaginous end plates, the vertebral rim, and the periosteum of the vertebral body. The anterior longitudinal ligament is applied to the anterior aspect of the vertebral column with firm attachments to the periosteum near the corners of the vertebral bodies. A posterior longitudinal ligament is applied to the posterior aspect of the vertebral bodies. This same structure and physiology are found at the symphysis pubis.

In the anterior column of the spine, one may evaluate alignment, intervertebral spaces, and bone changes. Soft tissue changes in the axial skeleton are difficult to recognize. Abnormalities of alignment include intervertebral subluxation, exaggerated kyphosis or lordosis, kyphosis or lordosis at inappropriate levels, and scoliosis. Films of the patient in flexion, extension, or lateral bending may be required to demonstrate abnormal mobility or loss of mobility.

The intervertebral disc spaces should be proportionate to the width of the vertebral body. They are relatively small in the cervical region but gradually become thicker in the thoracic and lumbar regions. Narrowing is characteristic of degenerative disc disease, and calcification or gas in the disc space is pathognomonic.

> Gas in the disc space is pathognomonic of degenerative disc disease.

The morphology of bony outgrowths along the spine, called *vertebral phytes*, may be of great diagnostic value (Table 11.4). Ossification in the periphery of the annulus fibrosus may lead to a shell of bone that bridges the intervertebral space (Fig. 11.18). These are

> Ankylosing spondylitis, DISH, degenerative disc disease, and psoriatic arthritis may be distinguished from each other by the morphology of their vertebral phytes.

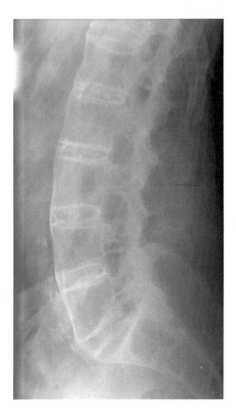

Figure 11.18 Syndesmophytes formed by ossification of the outer layers of the annulus fibrosus (ankylosing spondylitis).

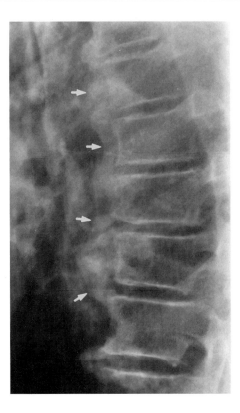

Figure 11.19 Diffuse, flowing ossification of the paravertebral soft tissues over multiple contiguous levels (diffuse idiopathic skeletal hyperostosis) (*arrows*).

called *bridging syndesmophytes* and are characteristic of ankylosing spondylitis. Ossification of the anterior longitudinal ligament along multiple contiguous levels is characteristic of diffuse idiopathic skeletal hyperostosis (DISH). This ossification is often exuberant and adjacent to, but separate from, the vertebral body (Fig. 11.19). Osteophytes are horizontal extensions of the vertebral end plates that have a triangular configuration. If sufficiently large osteophytes are present at adjacent end plates, they may form an extra-articular bridge across the intervertebral space (Fig. 11.20). Small osteophytes are associated with degenerative conditions. Large,

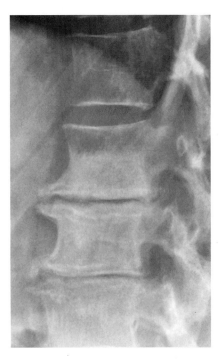

Figure 11.20 Triangular osteophytes (spondylosis deformans and degenerative disc disease). The disc space is narrowed, and the subchondral bone is sclerotic.

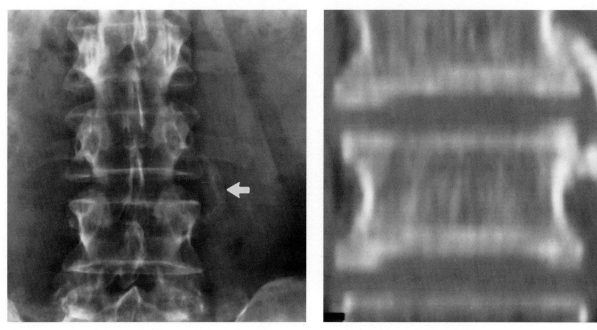

Figure 11.21 Ossification in the paraspinal soft tissues leading to a bridging phyte (*arrow*) (Reiter syndrome). *A.* AP radiograph. *B.* Coronal CT reconstruction.

focal, paravertebral soft tissue ossifications are seen in psoriatic arthritis and Reiter syndrome. These bony excrescences often become coalescent and contiguous with the vertebral bodies, resulting in extra-articular bridges along the lateral aspect of the spinal column (Fig. 11.21). Typically, they occur along the lateral aspects of the vertebral bodies and do not involve multiple, contiguous levels on the same side.

ENTHESES

An enthesis is the site of bony insertion of a tendon, ligament, or articular capsule. Tendons, ligaments, and articular capsules are strong bands or sheets of collagen fibers in a parallel arrangement. Near the attachment to bone, chondrocytes are interspersed between the collagen fibers. The collagen fibers in the bands or sheets become more compact, then cartilaginous, and finally calcified as they enter the bone (Fig. 11.22). The interdigitation

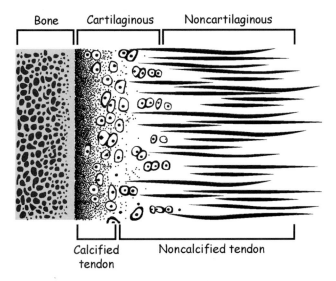

Figure 11.22 Anatomy of an enthesis.

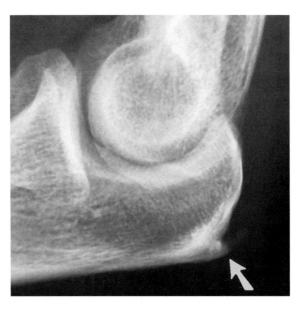

Figure 11.23 Enthesophyte at triceps muscle insertion (*arrow*).

Enthesopathy is disease at the site of the bony attachment of a tendon, ligament, or joint capsule.

of calcified cartilage and bone provides a strong attachment. Entheses have an active blood supply and a prominent innervation. Enthesopathy is disease at an enthesis. Enthesophytes and calcification and ossification of an enthesis are the principal radiographic signs of enthesopathy (Fig. 11.23). Ossification usually proceeds from the bony attachment into the substance of the inserting structure. MRI may directly demonstrate inflammatory and degenerative changes of tendons and ligaments much earlier than radiographs. Normal tendons and ligaments have low signal on both T1- and T2-weighted MRI. Fluid, edema, and myxoid change within tendons or ligaments are identifiable as regions of high signal.

DISTRIBUTION OF DISEASE

There are two clinical situations: monarticular arthritis (one joint affected) and polyarticular arthritis (many joints affected). The differential diagnosis of monarticular arthritis is rather limited (Table 11.5). Each type of polyarticular arthritis has a predilection for specific sites in the skeleton and can often be recognized simply from the distribution of involvement (Table 11.6). The explanation for the highly specific distributions of disease is unknown. There are some joints in the hand and foot where involvement can be virtually diagnostic of specific types of degenerative or inflammatory polyarticular arthritis (Table 11.7).

Different forms of polyarticular arthritis may often be recognized from the distribution of involvement.

In the hand, degenerative involvement of multiple DIP joints suggests osteoarthritis, whereas inflammatory involvement suggests psoriatic arthritis. Degenerative involvement of multiple MCP joints suggests pyrophosphate arthropathy, whereas inflammatory involvement of the MCP joints suggests rheumatoid arthritis. Degenerative involvement of the first carpometacarpal (CMC) joint suggests osteoarthritis. Inflammatory involvement of multiple intercarpal joints suggests rheumatoid arthritis, psoriatic arthritis, or gouty

Table 11.5: Causes of Monarticular Arthritis

Crystal related
Hemophiliac arthropathy
Rheumatoid (including juvenile chronic arthritis)
Infectious
Synovial lesions (chondromatosis, pigmented villonodular synovitis)
Traumatic

Table 11.6: Distribution of Polyarticular Arthritis

Arthritis	Symmetry	Predominant Sites of Involvement
Rheumatoid arthritis	Symmetric	Hand (PIPs, MCPs), wrist (pancompartmental), elbow, shoulder, hip, knee, foot (multiple intertarsal, MTPs), cervical spine
Ankylosing spondylitis	Symmetric	SI, ascending to lumbar, thoracic, cervical spine, hip, foot (MTPs)
Reiter syndrome	Asymmetric	SI, foot (MTPs, IPs, calcaneus), lumbar spine
Psoriatic arthritis	Asymmetric	Hand (often entire rays), wrist, foot (MTPs, IPs, calcaneus), lumbar spine, SI
Primary osteoarthritis	Asymmetric	Hand (DIPs, PIPs, first CMC), knee (especially medial compartment), hip (superolateral or medial), foot (first MTP, first TMT)
CPPD deposition disease	Asymmetric	Wrist (radiocarpal), shoulder (glenohumeral), knee (especially patellofemoral), elbow, ankle, foot (talonavicular)
Gout	Asymmetric	Hand (random joints), elbow, knee, foot (first MTP and random joints)

CMC, carpometacarpal joint; CPPD, calcium pyrophosphate dihydrate; DIP, distal interphalangeal joint; IP, interphalangeal joint; MCP, metacarpophalangeal joint; MTP, metatarsophalangeal joint; PIP, proximal interphalangeal joint; SI, sacroiliac joint; TMT, tarsometatarsal joint.

arthritis. Degenerative involvement of the radiocarpal joint suggests pyrophosphate arthropathy. In the foot, degenerative involvement of the first metatarsophalangeal (MTP) joint suggests osteoarthritis. Inflammatory involvement of the combination of multiple MTP and IP joints suggests psoriatic arthritis or Reiter syndrome, whereas inflammatory

Table 11.7: Polyarticular Arthritis: Sites That Suggest Specific Diseases When Involved by Degenerative or Inflammatory Changes

Involved Site(s)	Type of Joint Changes	
	Degenerative	Inflammatory
Hand and wrist		
Multiple DIP joints	Osteoarthritis	Psoriatic arthritis
Multiple MCP joints	CPPD deposition disease	Rheumatoid arthritis
First CMC joint	Osteoarthritis	—
Multiple intercarpal joints	—	Rheumatoid arthritis Psoriatic arthritis Gouty arthritis
Radiocarpal joint	CPPD deposition disease	—
Foot		
First MTP joint	Osteoarthritis	—
Multiple MTP and IP joints	—	Psoriatic arthritis Reiter syndrome
Multiple MTP joints	—	Ankylosing spondylitis Rheumatoid arthritis
First TMT joint	Osteoarthritis	—
Multiple intertarsal joints	—	Rheumatoid arthritis
Talonavicular joint	CPPD deposition disease	—

CMC, carpometacarpal; CPPD, calcium pyrophosphate dihydrate; DIP, distal interphalangeal; IP, interphalangeal; MCP, metacarpophalangeal; MTP, metatarsophalangeal; TMT, tarsometatarsal.

involvement of multiple MTP joints without IP joint involvement suggests ankylosing spondylitis or rheumatoid arthritis. Degenerative involvement of the first tarsometatarsal (TMT) joint suggests osteoarthritis. Inflammatory involvement of multiple intertarsal joints suggests rheumatoid arthritis. Degenerative involvement of the talonavicular joint suggests pyrophosphate arthropathy.

LABORATORY FINDINGS

Abnormal findings on laboratory examinations are integral to the diagnosis of joint diseases. They are most valuable when correlated with radiographs and other clinical information. Material for laboratory analysis is usually obtained from blood or the joint. Synovial fluid can be obtained by needle aspiration. Samples of the synovial membrane, articular cartilage, or periarticular soft tissues are usually obtained by biopsy.

Rheumatoid factor (RF) is a group of nonspecific autoantibodies found not only in the serum of patients with rheumatoid arthritis but also in that of patients with other acute and chronic inflammatory diseases. These include viral infections such as AIDS, mononucleosis, and influenza; chronic bacterial infections such as tuberculosis and subacute bacterial endocarditis; parasitic infections; neoplasms after chemotherapy or radiotherapy; and various hyperglobulinemic states. The sensitivity and specificity of detecting RF vary with the particular method of measurement. The most common method is the latex fixation test, in which the patient's serum is challenged with latex particles coated with heat-treated human immunoglobulin G. A positive result—that is, agglutination of the latex particles because of the presence of RF—makes the patient seropositive or RF positive. A negative result also has clinical importance because it is one factor that distinguishes rheumatoid arthritis from the clinically overlapping group of seronegative spondyloarthropathies. The strength of a positive result has therapeutic and prognostic significance. Nevertheless, only 80% of patients with classic rheumatoid arthritis are RF positive, as are 30% of patients with nonrheumatic diseases, 25% of patients with other rheumatic diseases, and 5% of the normal population.

> The RF is positive not only in 80% of patients with classic rheumatoid arthritis but also in 30% of patients with nonrheumatic disease and 5% of the normal population.

ANA are a heterogeneous population of serum antibodies that react to various human nuclear components, including DNA. They are detected by an immunofluorescence screening test. A positive ANA test is an empiric marker for connective tissue disease. The test is positive in nearly all patients with systemic lupus erythematosus, scleroderma, and mixed connective tissue disease and in approximately 80% of patients with polymyositis/dermatomyositis. The actual pathogenetic significance is unclear. Changes in serum ANA levels may parallel the clinical course and be used to follow the activity of disease.

HLA antigens represent a polymorphic group of inherited antigens found on the surface membranes of cells; HLA antigens have an uncertain biologic role. The genes for HLA antigens are located on the sixth chromosome in the major histocompatibility complex. Although it is well established that certain specific HLA antigens are associated with certain rheumatic diseases, the precise relationship of these genetic markers to disease is unclear. HLA antigens may influence not only the likelihood of disease but also the age of onset, severity, and individual clinical features. There are three major associations of HLA antigens with rheumatic diseases: (a) HLA-B27 with ankylosing spondylitis, Reiter syndrome, psoriatic arthritis, and enteropathic arthritis; (b) HLA-Cw6 with psoriasis and psoriatic arthritis; and (c) HLA-DR4 with rheumatoid arthritis. The strongest association is between HLA-B27 and ankylosing spondylitis. The prevalence of this antigen in patients with ankylosing spondylitis is 90%, compared with 9% in the general white population.

> HLA-B27 is present in 90% of patients with ankylosing spondylitis and 9% of the general white population.

SOURCES AND READINGS

Akeson WH, Chu CR, Bugbee W. Articular cartilage: morphology, physiology, and function. In: Resnick D, ed. *Diagnosis of bone and joint disorders*, 4th ed. Philadelphia: WB Saunders, 2002:793–816.

Brower AC. *Arthritis in black and white*, 2nd ed. Philadelphia: WB Saunders, 1997.

Forrester DM, Brown JC. *The radiology of joint disease*, 3rd ed. Philadelphia: WB Saunders, 1987.

Frediani B, Falsetti P, Storri L, et al. Quadricepital tendon enthesitis in psoriatic arthritis and rheumatoid arthritis: ultrasound examinations and clinical correlations. *J Rheumatol* 2001;28:2566–2568.

Groshar D, Rozenbaum M, Rosner I. Enthesopathies, inflammatory spondyloarthropathies and bone scintigraphy. *J Nucl Med* 1997;38:2003–2005.

Kelley WN, Ruddy S, Harris ED Jr, et al., eds. *Textbook of rheumatology*, 5th ed. Philadelphia: WB Saunders, 1997.

McCarty DJ, Koopman WJ, eds. *Arthritis and allied conditions: a textbook of rheumatology*, 12th ed. Philadelphia: Lea & Febiger, 1993.

McGonagle D, Gibbon W, Emery P. Classification of inflammatory arthritis by enthesitis. *Lancet* 1998;352:1137–1140.

Olivieri I, Barozzi L, Padula A. Enthesiopathy: clinical manifestations, imaging and treatment. *Bailliere Clin Rheum* 1998;12:665–681.

Resnick D. Articular anatomy and histology. In: Resnick D, ed. *Diagnosis of bone and joint disorders,* 4th ed. Philadelphia: WB Saunders, 2002:688–707.

Resnick D. Target area approach to articular disorders. In: Resnick D, ed. *Diagnosis of bone and joint disorders*, 4th ed. Philadelphia: WB Saunders, 2002:1755–1780.

Resnick D, Niwayama G. Entheses and enthesopathy. Anatomical, pathological, and radiological correlation. *Radiology* 1983;146:1–9.

Salvarani C, Cantini F, Olivieri I, et al. Magnetic resonance imaging and polymyalgia rheumatica. *J Rheumatol* 2001;28:918–919.

INFLAMMATORY ARTHRITIS

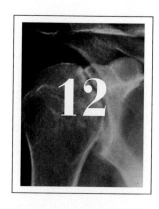

This chapter covers those clinical forms of arthritis and connective tissue disease that present on radiographs with a preponderance of inflammatory changes.

RHEUMATOID ARTHRITIS

Rheumatoid arthritis is a systemic autoimmune disease manifested in the musculoskeletal system by inflammatory polyarthritis of the small synovial joints. The pathogenesis is not understood, and no causative agent has been proved. Genetic factors affect susceptibility to and expression of the disease. Rheumatoid arthritis is usually distinguished from other arthritides by the presence of rheumatoid factor (RF) in the serum (see Chapter 11). Rheumatoid arthritis has a prevalence of 1% in the general population, with women affected more often than men by a 3:1 ratio. High RF titers often correlate with more severe disease. The typical age range of presentation is 25 to 55 years. In 70% of cases, the onset is insidious and occurs over weeks to months; in 20%, the onset occurs over days to weeks; and in 10%, the onset is acute and occurs over hours to days. The acute onset mimics the onset of septic arthritis. The clinical course of rheumatoid arthritis is progressive in 70% of cases, leading to disabling, destructive disease. The clinical progression may be rapid or slow. In 20%, the disease is intermittent with remissions generally lasting longer than exacerbations, and in 10%, remissions last several years. The clinical diagnosis is based on criteria that include morning stiffness, symmetric swelling of the proximal interphalangeal (PIP) joint, metacarpophalangeal (MCP) or wrist joints, rheumatoid nodules, serum RF, and specific radiographic findings.

Rheumatoid arthritis has a prevalence of 1% in the general population, with women affected more often than men by a 3:1 ratio.

PATHOLOGIC-RADIOLOGIC FEATURES

The underlying pathologic change in rheumatoid arthritis is chronic synovial inflammation with hyperemia, edema, and production of excess fluid. Chronicity leads to hypertro-

Table 12.1: Radiologic Features of Rheumatoid Arthritis
Periarticular osteoporosis progressing to generalized osteoporosis
Fusiform periarticular soft tissue swelling
Uniform loss of joint space
Marginal erosions progressing to severe erosions of subchondral bone
Synovial cyst formation
Subluxations
Lack of reactive bone formation (distinguish it from seronegative spondyloarthropathy)
Bilateral symmetric distribution
Distribution: hands (metacarpophalangeal joint, proximal interphalangeal joint), feet, knees, hips, upper cervical spine, shoulder, and elbows, in decreasing order of frequency
Adapted from Brower AC. *Arthritis in black and white*, 2nd ed. Philadelphia: WB Saunders, 1997.

phy and fibrosis. Hypertrophic, chronically inflamed synovium is called *pannus*. Pannus dissolves cartilage and bone by the actions of enzymes along its advancing margin. Commonly seen early radiographic findings include fusiform periarticular soft tissue swelling—corresponding to synovial hypertrophy and joint effusion—and acute erosions at the margins of the joint. Articular cartilage may also be dissolved by enzymes released into the joint space, causing uniform narrowing of the joint space on radiographs. Synovial hyperemia causes juxta-articular osteoporosis. There is a characteristic lack of reactive bone formation (Table 12.1). Common late radiologic findings include chronic generalized osteoporosis, progression of marginal erosions to severe erosions involving subchondral bone, synovial cyst formation, subluxations and abnormalities of alignment, and secondary osteoarthritis. Not all findings are present at any one time in individual patients; observation of combinations of these findings should lead to the correct diagnosis. The distinctive radiographic pattern of chronic osteoporosis, marginal erosions, and little if any reactive bone formation is the hallmark of rheumatoid arthritis. Although the appendicular skeleton tends to be extensively involved, the axial skeleton is usually spared except for the upper cervical spine. Bilaterally symmetric clinical involvement is usual, but the severity of radiologic involvement is not necessarily symmetric, especially when radiographs are obtained early in the clinical course. Secondary degenerative changes may occur if the inflammatory process remits for several years. Both rheumatoid arthritis and primary osteoarthritis are common conditions; patients with both diseases may have confusing radiographic findings.

> Rheumatoid arthritis has the distinctive radiographic pattern of chronic osteoporosis, marginal erosions, and little if any reactive bone formation.

MRI has proved more sensitive than radiography in the detection of the early stage of rheumatoid arthritis. Coronal T1-weighted MRI with fat suppression and gadolinium administration is the most useful sequence. MRI criteria for diagnosing rheumatoid arthritis include periarticular contrast enhancement of the wrist or the MCP or PIP joints in both hands, bone erosions, joint effusion, synovial sheath effusion, and cartilage irregularity and thinning. Gadolinium helps distinguish nonenhancing joint fluid from enhancing synovial proliferation and pannus. MRI is also helpful in the evaluation of the complications of rheumatoid arthritis, the craniocervical junction, and the temporomandibular joint.

HAND AND WRIST

There is considerable variability in the distribution of radiographic abnormalities in rheumatoid arthritis, and the findings on radiographs may not correlate with the clinical features. The earliest radiographic changes are fusiform soft tissue swelling and juxta-articular osteoporosis (Figs. 12.1 and 12.2). In the hand, rheumatoid arthritis classically involves the MCP and PIP joints. The earliest bone erosions are generally at the MCP joints (Fig. 12.3), often the second and third on the radial side. The PIP joint of the middle finger is another site of typical early involvement. Oblique radiographs may show subtle subchondral bone resorption. Fusiform soft tissue swelling, juxta-articular osteoporosis, concentric loss of cartilage space, and acute marginal erosions may be seen (Fig. 12.4). Compressive erosions and

> In the hand, rheumatoid arthritis classically involves the MCP and PIP joints.

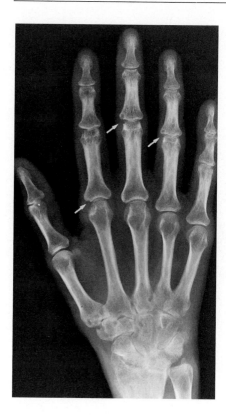

Figure 12.1 Rheumatoid hand. Juxta-articular osteoporosis is present. Small erosions and fusiform soft tissue swelling are present at the proximal interphalangeal joints of the middle and ring fingers and the metacarpophalangeal joint of the index finger (*arrows*). Uniform joint space loss is present throughout the wrist.

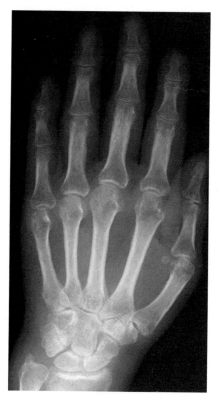

Figure 12.2 Rheumatoid arthritis with early erosive changes at the metacarpophalangeal joints.

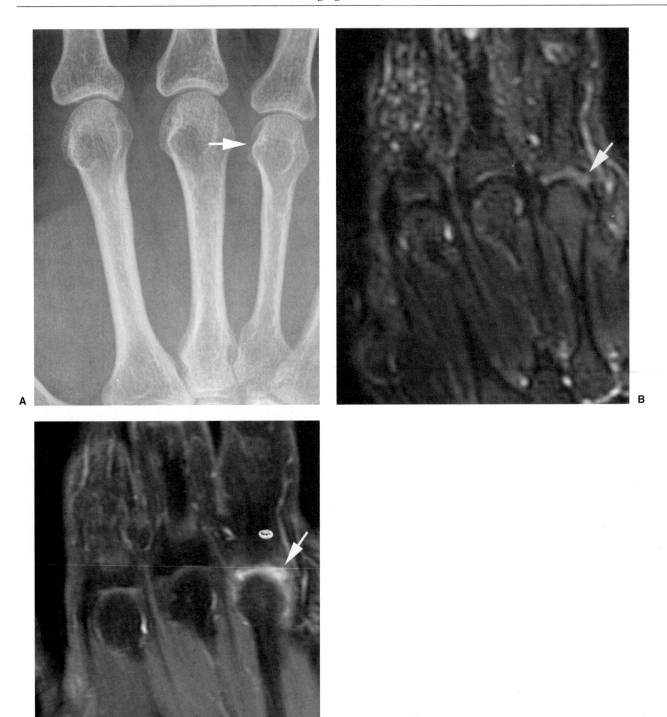

Figure 12.3 Rheumatoid arthritis involving the metacarpopha-langeal joint of the ring finger. *A.* Radiograph shows early subchondral bone erosion (*arrow*). *B.* Coronal T2-weighted fat-suppressed MRI shows effusion (*arrow*). *C.* Coronal T1-weighted fat-suppressed MRI after gadolinium injection shows enhancement (*arrow*).

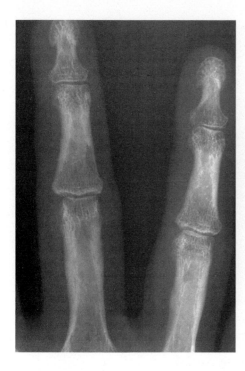

Figure 12.4 Rheumatoid arthritis with juxta-articular osteoporosis.

remodeling of bone may result from the collapse of osteoporotic bone by muscle tension; this is especially common at the MCP joints. Loss of the normal balanced tension at the digits results in various alignment deformities, including the swan neck and boutonniere deformities of the fingers and the Z-shaped deformity of the thumb (Fig. 12.5). Superficial erosions

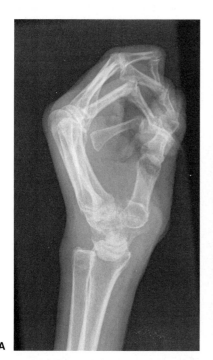

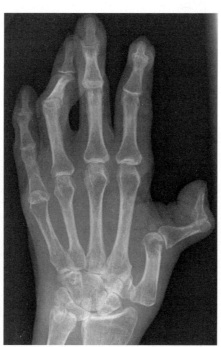

A   B

Figure 12.5 Hand deformities in rheumatoid arthritis. *A,B.* Lateral and PA radiographs of the hand show a swan neck deformity of the index finger, boutonniere deformity of the ring finger, Z-shaped deformity of the thumb, proximal dislocation of the first carpometacarpal joint, volar dislocation of the metacarpophalangeal joint of the little finger, dorsal subluxation of the ulna, and ulnar translocation of the carpus.

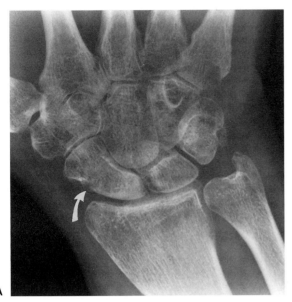 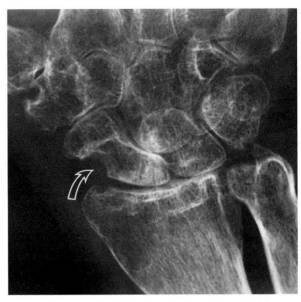

Figure 12.6 Rheumatoid wrist. *A.* Early findings include juxta-articular osteoporosis and subtle erosions, including the scaphoid waist (*arrow*). *B.* The same patient 6 years later has severe erosions and subluxations. Ulnar translocation is present. The bones are diffusely osteoporotic, with no proliferative changes. The scaphoid waist erosion has become large (*arrow*).

In the wrist, rheumatoid arthritis usually involves all three compartments.

of the cortex may occur beneath inflamed tendon sheaths, especially along the outer aspect of the distal ulna, the dorsal aspect of the first metacarpal, and the proximal phalanx of the first digit.

In the wrist, pancompartmental involvement is usual (Fig. 12.6). The earliest bone changes are erosions at the ulnar and radial styloid processes and the waists of the capitate and scaphoid bones. On MRI, erosions are evident as focal defects in the bone that are low to intermediate signal on T1-weighted images and high signal on T2-weighted images (Fig. 12.7). On

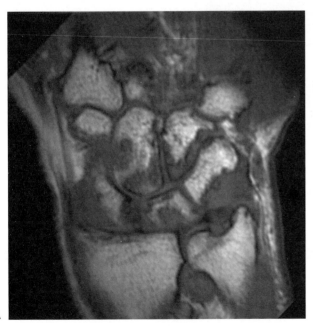 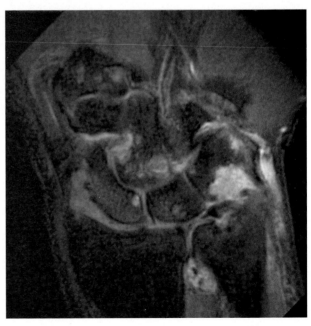

Figure 12.7 Rheumatoid arthritis of the carpal bones. *A.* Coronal T1-weighted MRI shows erosions. *B.* Coronal T1-weighted fat-suppressed MRI after gadolinium injection shows enhancement in the erosions, corresponding to inflammatory pannus.

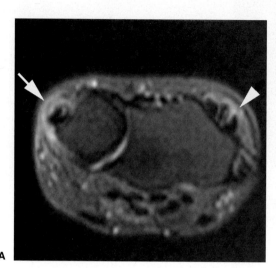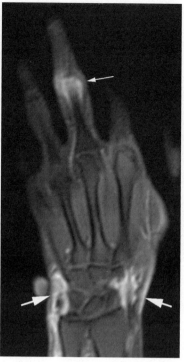

A   B

Figure 12.8 Rheumatoid arthritis with tenosynovitis. *A.* Axial T2-weighted fat-suppressed MRI shows tenosynovitis in the extensor carpi ulnaris tendon (*arrow*) and the extensor carpi radialis brevis and longus tendons (*arrowhead*). *B.* Coronal T1-weighted fat-suppressed MRI after gadolinium injection shows enhancement of tendon sheaths at the wrist (*large arrows*) and of the proximal interphalangeal joint of the middle finger (*small arrow*).

T1-weighted images after gadolinium enhancement, the pannus within the erosions enhances. Malalignment in advanced disease results from loss of balanced muscular tension and ligamentous restriction. Involvement of tendons can be demonstrated by MRI (Fig. 12.8). On T2-weighted images, the synovial sheaths show fluid and high signal. On T1-weighted images after gadolinium injection, the inflamed synovium shows enhancement. The posttraumatic ligamentous instability patterns of the wrist described in Chapter 2 are often seen in advanced rheumatoid arthritis.

OTHER PERIPHERAL JOINTS

In the elbow, synovial hypertrophy and effusion provide a fat pad sign. As in other joints, periarticular osteoporosis, uniform joint space narrowing, and erosions are seen. In the glenohumeral joint, erosions are especially prominent around the proximal humerus, and rotator cuff tear or atrophy causes superior subluxation of the humeral head and adaptive changes in the inferior surface of the acromion from the humeral head (Figs. 12.9 and 12.10). Resorption of the distal clavicle and widening of the acromioclavicular joint are frequently observed in rheumatoid arthritis. In the knee, meniscal invasion by pannus occurs early and may be detectable on MRI. The typical inflammatory changes may be superimposed on secondary degenerative changes, but the proliferative bone response is disproportionately modest in comparison to the loss of joint space (Fig. 12.11). On MRI, effusions, erosions, diffuse cartilage loss, bone marrow edema, and pannus may be demonstrated at the knee (Fig. 12.12). The hip is less frequently involved than the knee. Concentric uniform loss of joint space with axial migration is usual, but superior migration similar to that in osteoarthritis may also occur. Acetabular protrusion (protrusio acetabuli), fibrous ankylosis, subchondral cysts, erosions, and secondary reparative and degenerative changes are common. If steroids are administered, osteonecrosis of the femoral head is a potential com-

Rheumatoid arthritis commonly causes resorption of the distal clavicle.

Acetabular protrusion is a common but nonspecific feature of rheumatoid arthritis involving the hip.

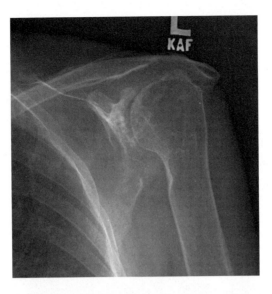

Figure 12.9 Radiograph of shoulder in advanced rheumatoid arthritis shows osteopenia, erosion of the distal clavicle, and remodeling of the undersurface of the acromion and medial humeral shaft.

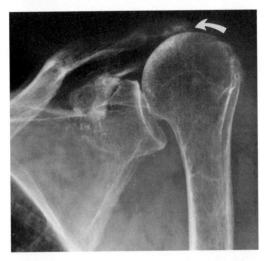

Figure 12.10 Rheumatoid shoulder with osteoporotic bones and superior subluxation of the humeral head, indicative of rotator cuff tear or atrophy (*arrow*).

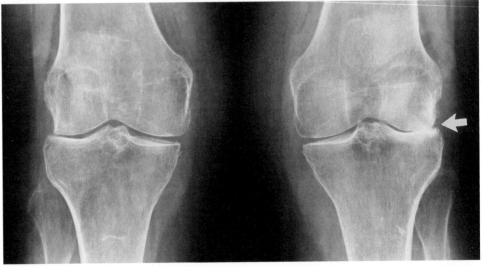

Figure 12.11 Rheumatoid knees. The bones are osteoporotic. Uniform joint space loss is present with minimal proliferative bone changes. Some secondary osteoarthritic changes are present in the lateral compartment of the left knee (*arrow*).

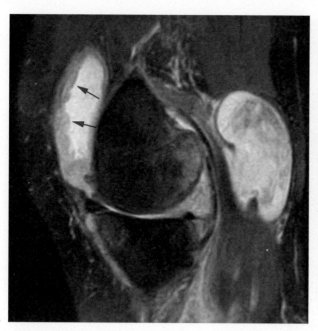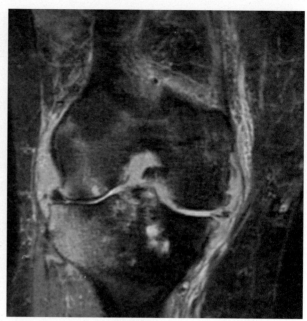

A   B

Figure 12.12 Rheumatoid knee. *A.* Sagittal T2-weighted fat-suppressed MRI shows large effusion and Baker cyst with synovial thickening (*arrows*). Diffuse cartilage loss and subchondral edema are present. *B.* Coronal T1-weighted fat-suppressed MRI after gadolinium injection shows synovial and subchondral enhancement.

plication. In the foot, changes may be seen early at the metatarsophalangeal (MTP) and interphalangeal (IP) joints of the great toe (Fig. 12.13). Although the usual changes of rheumatoid arthritis that are found elsewhere in the skeleton may be present in the foot, erosions tend to be small and infrequent. Soft tissue involvement may lead to hallux valgus

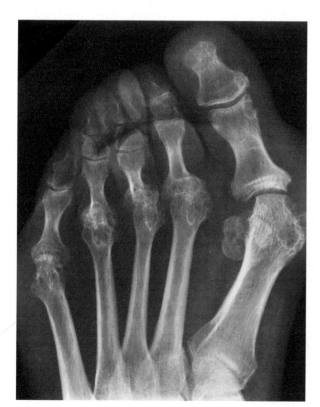

Figure 12.13 Rheumatoid foot. The great toe is deviated laterally, and the remaining metatarsophalangeal (MTP) joints are subluxated. Erosions are present at all of the MTP joints and the interphalangeal joint of the great toe; the other joints appear spared. Some erosions appear sclerotic, suggesting clinical quiescence.

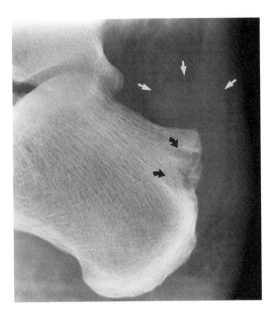

Figure 12.14 Rheumatoid arthritis. Swelling of the retrocalcaneal bursa is present (*white arrows*) with a large erosion in the adjacent bone (*black arrows*).

and planovalgus deformity of the foot. In the heel, retrocalcaneal bursitis, Achilles tendonitis, and plantar fasciitis may cause swelling and calcaneal erosions (Fig. 12.14). Spontaneous Achilles tendon rupture may occur.

SPINE

In the spine, the upper cervical spine is the only common site of involvement. As many as 70% of patients with rheumatoid arthritis are affected symptomatically at some time, and up to 85% of those with classic rheumatoid arthritis have radiographic changes at the upper cervical spine. The atlantoaxial articulation (C1-C2) has a synovial joint anteriorly where the odontoid process articulates with the anterior arch of C1 and is stabilized posteriorly by the transverse ligament. A bursa is interposed between the odontoid process and the transverse ligament. Synovitis at these sites may cause erosions of the odontoid process and rupture of the transverse ligament (Figs. 12.15 and 12.16), resulting in widened predental interval. One

Atlantoaxial instability may result in quadriplegia or death.

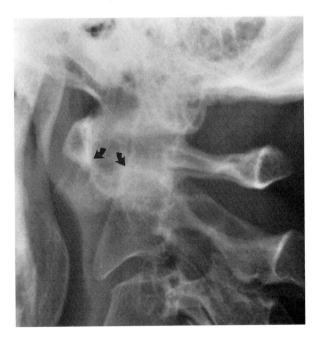

Figure 12.15 Rheumatoid arthritis. Atlantoaxial subluxation is present with a wide gap between the anterior arch of C1 and the odontoid process (*arrows*).

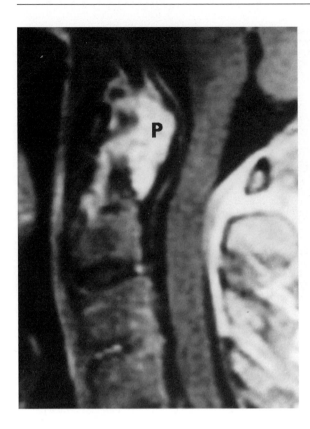

Figure 12.16 Rheumatoid arthritis. Sagittal T1-weighted enhanced MRI scan shows pannus (P) eroding the odontoid process and causing mass effect on spinal cord.

consequence is atlantoaxial instability, with imminent danger of quadriplegia or death. Below the level of C2, the cervical spine may be diffusely involved by joint space narrowing. Inflammatory pannus at the synovial uncovertebral joints (joints of Luschka) may extend into the intervertebral discs. The thoracic spine and lumbar spine are usually spared. Sacroiliac joint involvement is infrequent and, when present, is mild and asymmetric.

EXTRA-ARTICULAR MANIFESTATIONS

Extra-articular manifestations of rheumatoid arthritis include rheumatoid nodules, development of cutaneous fistulas, infections, hematologic abnormalities, vasculitis, renal disease, pulmonary disease, and cardiac complications.

CONNECTIVE TISSUE DISEASE

SYSTEMIC LUPUS ERYTHEMATOSUS

Systemic lupus erythematosus (SLE) is a chronic systemic disease, the pathogenesis of which is related to immune complex deposition. It is more common in women by an 8:1 ratio, and there is a component of genetic susceptibility. The fluorescent ANA test is virtually always positive at the onset of clinical disease. Manifestations in the musculoskeletal system are common and may precede other systemic manifestations by months or years. Nonerosive symmetric polyarthritis with a distribution similar to that of rheumatoid arthritis is present in 75% to 90% of patients with SLE. Early findings on radiographs are fusiform soft tissue swelling and juxta-articular osteoporosis, but there should be no joint space narrowing or erosions. A deforming nonerosive arthropathy is also common in SLE. The hands are typically involved at the MCP and IP joints (Figs. 12.17 and 12.18). Thumb, wrist, and foot involvement are more common than shoulder and knee involvement, and 10% of patients may develop atlantoaxial subluxation. These deformities are initially reducible, and radiographs may be normal.

Manifestations of SLE in the musculoskeletal system are common and may precede other manifestations by months or years.

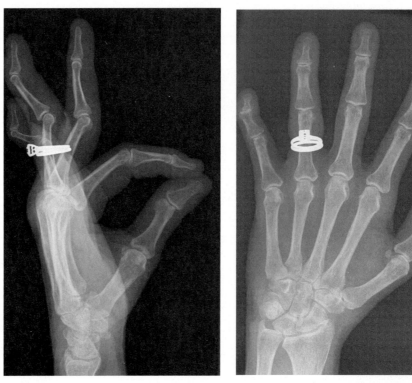

A   **B**

Figure 12.17 Systemic lupus erythematosus with alignment deformities. *A,B.* Lateral and PA radiographs show swan neck deformities of the ring and little fingers, with proximal interphalangeal hyperextension of the middle finger.

Fixed deformities and secondary degenerative changes may develop with time. Osteonecrosis may involve the femoral head, femoral condyle, humeral head, and other sites and commonly has a symmetric distribution. Myositis, tendon weakening and spontaneous rupture, and soft tissue calcification are other musculoskeletal manifestations.

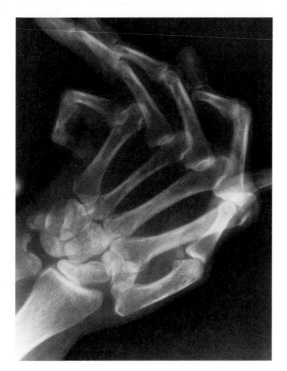

Figure 12.18 Systemic lupus erythematosus with severe subluxations. Erosions are absent.

SCLERODERMA

Scleroderma (progressive systemic sclerosis) is a multisystem fibrosing autoimmune connective tissue disease of variable clinical course. Characteristically, the skin becomes fibrotic, thickened, and taut. Gastrointestinal and renal involvement is prominent. Radiologic manifestations in the musculoskeletal system are present in most patients. These abnormalities are usually seen in the hands and consist of soft tissue atrophy, soft tissue calcification, resorption of the phalangeal tufts, and distal interphalangeal (DIP) joint erosions. Osseous destruction and bony erosions are common in the phalangeal tufts (Fig. 12.19). The soft tissue atrophy results in cone-shaped fingertips. Subcutaneous calcifications are typically present in multiple digits and elsewhere in the extremities; the calcium deposits are dystrophic and consist of calcium hydroxyapatite deposits at sites of local tissue damage. Calcification may also occur in tendons and tendon sheaths, in joint capsules, and even within the joint cavity. Synovial fibrosis without inflammation may cause flexion contractures.

> Most scleroderma patients have musculoskeletal manifestations evident on radiographs.

DERMATOMYOSITIS AND POLYMYOSITIS

Dermatomyositis and polymyositis are diseases of unknown etiology affecting striated muscle by diffuse, nonsuppurative inflammation and degeneration. The pathogenesis involves an autoimmune mechanism. In dermatomyositis, the skin is also involved. Multiple clinical classifications are based on various features, particularly progressive muscle weakness and rash. There is an associated risk of malignancy in patients older than 40 years of age with dermatomyositis, especially men. The diagnosis is made by serum enzyme studies, electromyography, and muscle biopsy. The early imaging findings of dermatomyositis and polymyositis can be made on MRI. T2-weighted MRI shows high signal in the involved muscles (Fig. 12.20). Involvement is generally symmetric bilaterally, and the course of the disease can be followed by MRI. On radiographs, the characteristic abnormality is widespread soft tissue calcification, particularly of intermuscular fascial planes between large proximal limb muscles (Figs. 12.21 and 12.22). There may also be subcutaneous calcifica-

> Patients with dermatomyositis, especially men older than 40 years of age, have an increased risk of developing a malignancy.

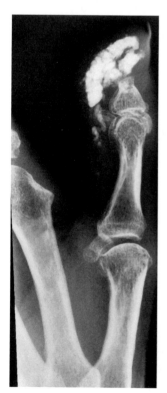

Figure 12.19 Scleroderma with calcium hydroxyapatite deposits in thumb and destruction of the phalangeal tuft.

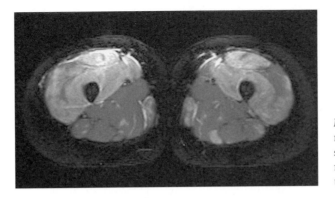

Figure 12.20 Inflammatory myositis. Axial T2-weighted fat-suppressed MRI shows high signal symmetrically distributed in the thigh muscles.

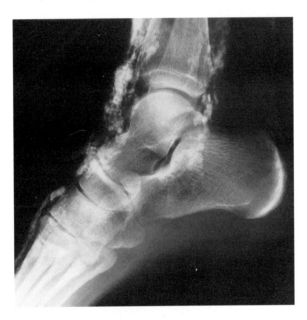

Figure 12.21 Dermatomyositis at the ankle with soft tissue calcification.

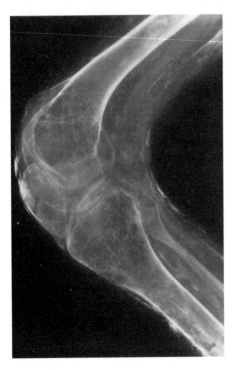

Figure 12.22 Dermatomyositis at the knee with soft tissue calcification, soft tissue atrophy, and osteoporosis.

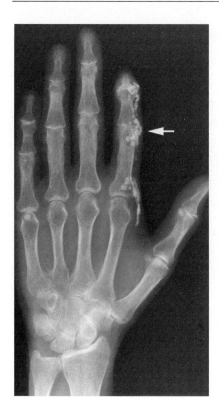

Figure 12.23 Polymyositis with soft tissue calcification (*arrow*) involving the index finger.

tions similar to those in scleroderma (Fig. 12.23). Muscle atrophy, contractures, and chronic osteoporosis are findings late in the clinical course.

OVERLAP SYNDROMES

Patients may have rheumatic diseases with clinical features that overlap those of several of the more well-defined rheumatoid diseases, particularly at the beginning or end of the clinical course. The radiographic features of disease may also overlap so that an individual case may show combinations of features of rheumatoid arthritis, scleroderma, SLE, and dermatomyositis. These overlap syndromes may also be called *mixed connective tissue disease.*

SPONDYLOARTHROPATHY

The spondyloarthropathies are a heterogeneous group of interrelated conditions. Musculoskeletal manifestations common to these diseases include spinal involvement, especially of the sacroiliac joints, enthesopathy, and asymmetric peripheral arthritis of the lower limbs. Additional common features are genetic predisposition; extra-articular manifestations in the skin, gut, urogenital tract, or eyes; negative serum RF; and an association with HLA-B27 (Table 12.2). These conditions have in the past been called *rheumatoid variants* to distinguish them from rheumatoid arthritis and *seronegative spondyloarthropathy* to reflect the negative serum RF.

ANKYLOSING SPONDYLITIS

Ankylosing spondylitis is a chronic inflammatory disease of the spine and sacroiliac (SI) joints. The etiology is unknown, but there is a genetic component; 90% to 95% of white patients with classic ankylosing spondylitis have HLA-B27 (compared with 9% of all white patients). Symptomatic disease affects approximately 1% of the general population; the prevalence of severe disease is approximately 0.1%. The typical onset is insidious lower

Ankylosing spondylitis affects approximately 1% of the general population.

Table 12.2: Common Features of Spondyloarthropathy

Spinal involvement, especially sacroiliac joints
Enthesopathy
Asymmetric peripheral arthritis of the lower limbs
Genetic predisposition
Extra-articular manifestations in the skin, gut, urogenital tract, or eyes
Serum rheumatoid factor negative
HLA-B27 positive

back pain and stiffness in adolescent men. In the severe classic form, there is gross anky-losis and deformity of the spine; in mild forms, there may be only occasional arthralgias. In most cases, ankylosing spondylitis is a benign, self-limited, and undiagnosed disease with absent or minimal radiographic changes. The overall sex distribution is probably equal, but men generally have severe, progressive disease, whereas women have mild, self-limited disease.

Ankylosing spondylitis begins in the lumbosacral region and ascends to the cervical spine. Radiographically, the involved vertebral bodies become squared off by erosions from inflammation in the prevertebral soft tissues (Fig. 12.24). The facet joints become inflamed and then fused, and syndesmophytes—ossifications in and around the periphery of the annulus fibrosus—form at multiple contiguous levels, eventually leading to a spine that looks like bamboo (Figs. 12.25 and 12.26). Back pain diminishes or disappears as the spine fuses, but the fused spine becomes osteoporotic, fragile, and subject to insufficiency frac-tures. In the pelvis, the sacroiliac joints become symmetrically blurred, sclerotic, and fused (Fig. 12.27). Early in this process, the sacroiliac joints have subchondral granulation tis-sue, and the joint cartilage becomes replaced by fibrous tissue. Ankylosis follows the for-mation of new cartilage and bone in the joint space.

In ankylosing spondylitis, back pain diminishes or disappears as the spine fuses.

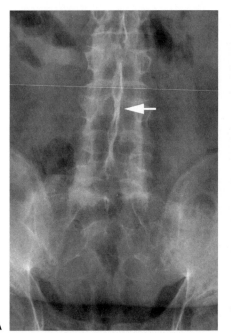 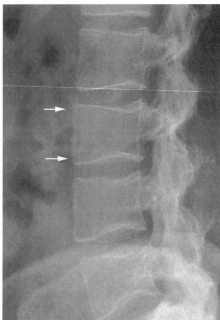

A   B

Figure 12.24 Ankylosing spondylitis. *A.* AP radiograph of the lumbar spine shows that the sacroiliac joints and the posterior elements of the spine (*arrow*) are ankylosed. *B.* Lateral radiograph of the lum-bar spine shows squaring (*arrows*) of the anterior aspects of the lumbar vertebral bodies and ankylo-sis of the posterior elements.

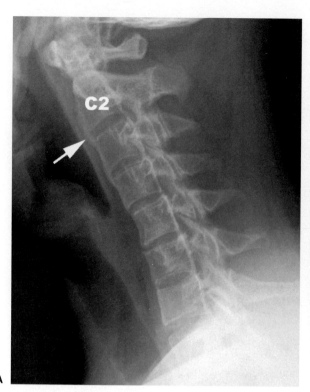
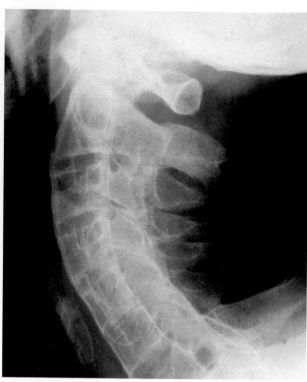

Figure 12.25 Ankylosing spondylitis of the cervical spine (different patients). *A.* Lateral radiograph shows syndesmophytes (*arrow*) bridging the C2 through C4 vertebral bodies. *B.* Lateral radiograph shows syndesmophytes bridging the entire cervical spine and ankylosis of the posterior elements.

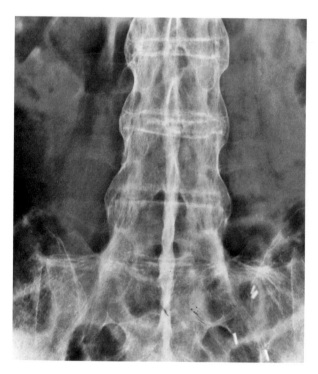

Figure 12.26 Ankylosing spondylitis with syndesmophytes and ossification of the posterior ligamentous structures. The sacroiliac joints have fused.

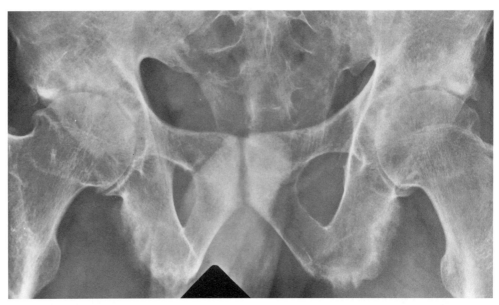

***Figure* 12.27** Ankylosing spondylitis with symmetric, inflammatory arthritis of the hips, ankylosis of the sacroiliac joints, and hyperostosis at the ischial rami.

Approximately 20% of patients with ankylosing spondylitis present initially with peripheral polyarthritis, and, ultimately, approximately 35% will have peripheral disease. This peripheral polyarthritis is similar to rheumatoid arthritis in clinical manifestations, radiographic appearance, and pathophysiology, but the distribution of disease tends to be different. The feet, ankles, knees, hips, and shoulders are typically involved in an asymmetric fashion; the hands are usually spared. Permanent stiffness or bony ankylosis is likely. Peripheral polyarthritis may precede, coincide with, or follow the onset of spinal manifestations.

MRI has proved more sensitive than radiography in the early detection of sacroiliitis. T1-weighted fat suppression with gadolinium administration and fast STIR are superior to T1- and T2-weighted images. MRI findings of sacroiliitis include abnormal cartilage signal intensity, erosions, increased intensity in the joint, and subchondral bone marrow edema. MRI may also be able to distinguish sacroiliitis due to spondyloarthropathy from septic arthritis of the sacroiliac joint.

The fused spine in ankylosing spondylitis is biomechanically fragile and easily fractured.

One major orthopedic complication of ankylosing spondylitis is increased biomechanical fragility of the spine. Syndesmophytes bridging the vertebral bodies and ankylosis of the posterior elements result in a stiff spine that cannot move or dissipate traumatic forces. Bony remodeling of an ankylosed spine does not improve its biomechanical strength as a unit. When patients with ankylosing spondylitis are involved in falls or other accidents, fractures and fracture-dislocations of the spine are common (Figs. 12.28 and 12.29). These fractures may progress to nonunion.

REACTIVE ARTHRITIS AND REITER SYNDROME

Reactive arthritis is an acute inflammatory arthritis that follows an infection elsewhere in the body, but infectious organisms cannot be cultured from the joint fluid or synovium. The pathogenesis of the disease is thought to be immunologic in nature, with a genetic predisposition. Reiter syndrome is a form of reactive arthritis. After gastrointestinal infections by *Shigella, Salmonella, Yersinia,* or *Campylobacter,* or a genitourinary infection with *Chlamydia,* approximately 1% to 4% of patients develop reactive arthritis. Although Reiter syndrome has been classically defined as the triad of peripheral arthritis, conjunctivitis, and urethritis, the current definition generally includes cases of arthritis that occur within 2 months of an episode of venereal infection or epidemic dysentery. The classic triad is present in only one-third

Reactive arthritis includes cases of arthritis that occur within 2 months of an episode of venereal infection or epidemic dysentery.

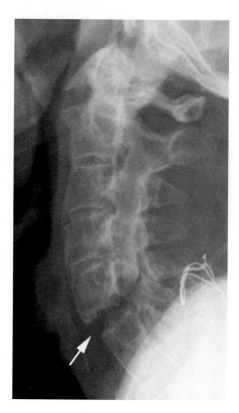

Figure 12.28 Ankylosing spondylitis with traumatic cervical spine fracture at C5-C6 (*arrow*).

of cases that have been called Reiter syndrome. The diagnosis may be difficult to make because there is no definite laboratory test, and the dysenteric or venereal episode may be mild or silent. There is a marked male predominance of at least 5:1. The typical age of onset is 15 to 40 years. HLA-B27 is present in 70% to 80% of cases, and the serum RF is negative. Clinically, Reiter syndrome is an asymmetric lower extremity oligoarthritis manifested by

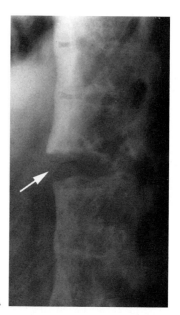

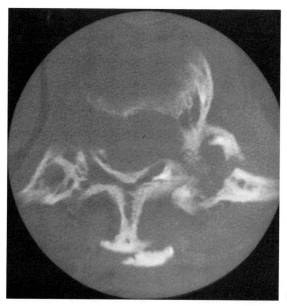

A   B

Figure 12.29 Ankylosing spondylitis with traumatic fracture. *A.* Lateral lumbar spine radiographs show changes of ankylosing spondylitis with fracture at T12-L1 (*arrow*). *B.* Axial CT scan shows the level of fracture and the ankylosed, remodeled spine.

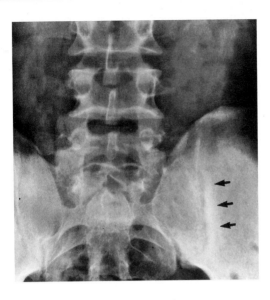

Figure 12.30 Reiter syndrome with sacroiliitis, greater on the left than the right (*arrows*).

sausage digits, heel pain and swelling, low back pain, and sacroiliac joint tenderness. Early clinical signs include effusion, periarticular edema, bursitis, and tendinitis. Fluffy periostitis, enthesopathy, paravertebral comma-shaped ossification, and asymmetric sacroiliitis often develop. Bone density is preserved in chronic disease.

Radiographic abnormalities develop in 60% to 80% of cases, with involvement of synovial joints, symphyses, and entheses. The disease has a predilection for the foot—especially the great toe, ankles, knees, and sacroiliac joints—and manifestations are rarely seen above the level of the umbilicus. Bony erosions combined with bony proliferation characterize an asymmetric arthritis. Erosions first appear at the joint margins and may progress to involve the subchondral bone in the central portion of the articulation. Bony proliferation may take the form of periostitis (linear or fluffy), calcification and ossification at entheses, and intra-articular bone production with bony ankylosis. Additional abnormalities may include fusiform soft tissue swelling, effusions, regional or periarticular osteoporosis, and symmetric and concentric joint space narrowing.

Sacroiliitis is the most common manifestation. The incidence of sacroiliitis increases with chronicity of disease, rising from 5% to 10% of cases at onset to perhaps 75% after several years. Sacroiliitis is evident on radiographs as blurring and eburnation of the adjacent sacral and iliac articular surfaces, initially worse on the iliac side (Fig. 12.30). Bilateral changes are typical, and these may be symmetric or asymmetric.

Spinal involvement in Reiter syndrome is much less frequent than in ankylosing spondylitis or psoriasis. Asymmetric paravertebral ossification about the lower three thoracic and upper three lumbar vertebrae in Reiter syndrome is indistinguishable from the corresponding changes in psoriatic spondylitis. These ossifications are thought to result from inflammatory changes in the paravertebral connective tissue that lead to calcification and ossification. Unlike ankylosing spondylitis, squaring of the vertebral bodies, facet joint erosion, sclerosis, and osseous fusion are unusual in Reiter syndrome.

PSORIATIC ARTHRITIS

Psoriasis is a common skin disease characterized by dry, pink, scaly, nonpruritic lesions with a genetic predisposition. As many as 5% of patients with psoriasis have an associated arthritis. The onset and clinical course of skin lesions and arthritis are generally asynchronous and independent, but 80% to 85% have skin involvement first. There is some evidence that psoriatic arthritis may be a form of reactive arthritis incited by streptococcal and staphylococcal infection of psoriatic plaques and affected nails. HLA-B27 is found in 60% to 80% of patients with psoriatic spondylitis but in only 20% of patients with psoriatic peripheral arthritis. Serum RF is absent. Psoriatic arthritis has five patterns of clinical presentation: (a) asymmetric oligoarthritis,

Psoriatic arthritis may be a form of reactive arthritis incited by streptococcal and staphylococcal infection of psoriatic plaques and affected nails.

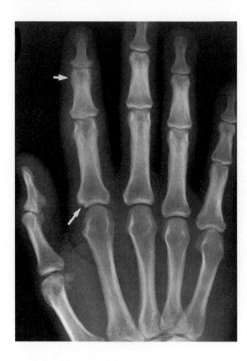

Figure 12.31 Psoriatic arthritis with "sausage digit" swelling, erosions (*long arrow*), and periostitis (*short arrow*) of the index finger.

seen in more than 50% of cases; (b) polyarthritis with predominantly DIP joint involvement, the classic presentation, which is seen in 5% to 19%; (c) symmetric seronegative polyarthritis simulating rheumatoid arthritis, seen in up to 25%; (d) sacroiliitis and spondylitis resembling ankylosing spondylitis, seen in 20% to 40%; and (e) arthritis mutilans with resorption of phalanges, seen in 5%. Individual patients may change from one clinical pattern to another. Two-thirds of patients have an insidious onset, whereas one-third have an acute onset mimicking gout or septic arthritis. The age of onset is 35 to 45 years, and there is no sex predominance.

The predominant radiologic abnormalities are found asymmetrically in the upper extremities and result from a synovitis that is similar in pathophysiology to rheumatoid arthritis. The distribution of articular involvement in the hands tends to be distal, commonly the DIP joints of the fingers, and usually accompanies fingernail involvement. Soft tissue swelling of the digits tends to be of the "sausage" variety, in which the entire digit is swollen, not just the joints (Fig. 12.31). Dramatic joint space loss to the point of erosion and resorption of the articulating ends of bones may occur. Pencil-in-cup erosions (Fig. 12.32) and peri-

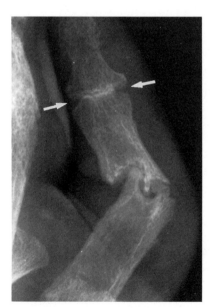

Figure 12.32 Psoriatic arthritis of the finger with interdigitating erosions at the proximal interphalangeal joint (pencil-in-cup appearance). Smaller erosions (*arrows*) are present at the distal interphalangeal joint.

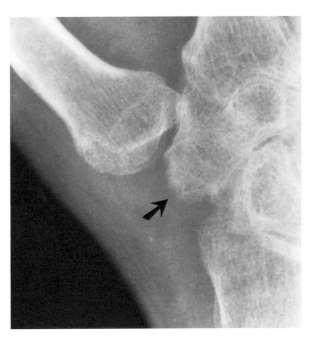

Figure 12.33 Psoriatic arthritis with inflammatory periostitis (*arrow*).

osteal bony excrescences (Fig. 12.33) are other typical findings. The arthritis is highly erosive and in the hands or feet may lead to *arthritis mutilans*, which is severe resorptive arthritis of the phalanges (Figs. 12.34 and 12.35). In the spine, irregular, asymmetric paravertebral excrescences of bone appear; these may be quite bulky and merge with the underlying vertebral bodies and discs. The changes in the spine and SI joints in psoriatic arthritis tend to be more marked than in Reiter syndrome, but they are often indistinguishable. Sacroiliitis may progress to ankylosis.

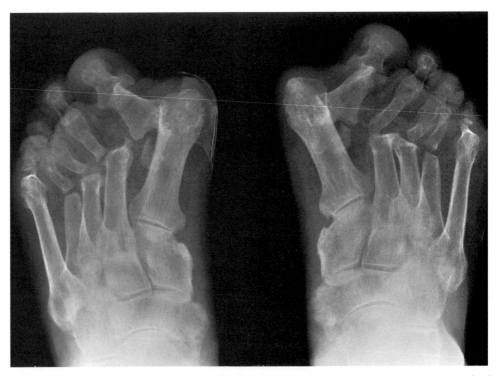

Figure 12.34 Psoriatic arthritis in the feet. All of the metatarsophalangeal joints are severely involved and subluxated.

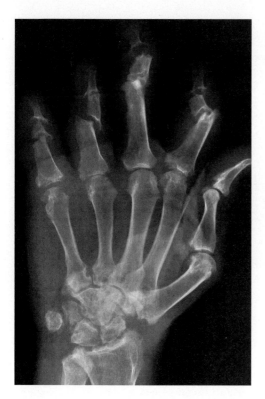

Figure 12.35 Arthritis mutilans presentation of psoriatic arthritis in the hand and wrist. The distal interphalangeal and proximal interphalangeal joints of all of the fingers are severely involved. There is pancompartmental involvement of the wrist, with erosions and mature periosteal bone.

ENTEROPATHIC SPONDYLOARTHROPATHY

Patients with inflammatory bowel disease (Crohn disease, ulcerative colitis) may have spondyloarthropathy associated with their disease. The prevalence of articular disease in patients with ulcerative colitis is approximately 10% to 15%; occasionally, it precedes the gastrointestinal disease. Common articular manifestations include peripheral joint arthralgias, soft tissue swelling, and periarticular osteoporosis; less common manifestations include erosive changes similar to rheumatoid arthritis. The peripheral arthritis may wax and wane in tandem with exacerbations and remissions in the bowel disease. Sacroiliitis and spondylitis resembling or identical to ankylosing spondylitis may also occur in ulcerative colitis. Up to 20% of patients with Crohn disease may have bilateral sacroiliitis, and 25% of these develop ankylosing spondylitis. The sacroiliitis and spondylitis tend to be progressive and not particularly related to the bowel disease (Fig. 12.36). Certain dysen-

Articular disease in patients with ulcerative colitis may precede the gastrointestinal disease.

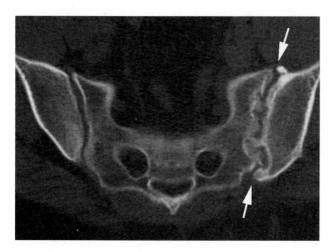

Figure 12.36 Unilateral inflammatory sacroiliitis in a patient with inflammatory bowel disease. Axial CT scan shows erosions of the left sacroiliac joint (*arrows*).

Table 12.3: Distinguishing Features of Spondyloarthropathy

Feature	Ankylosing Spondylitis	Reiter Syndrome	Psoriatic Arthritis
Clinical setting	Low back pain, adolescents	After dysenteric or venereal infection	Psoriasis
Sex predominance	Male (classic disease)	Male	None
Joint distribution	Sacroiliac joint, entire spine	Sacroiliac joint, lumbar spine, feet	Hands, feet, thoracolumbar spine
Severity of involvement	Severe ankylosis	Mild	Severe erosions
Sacroiliac joint involvement	Bilateral, symmetric sacroiliitis invariably leading to ankylosis	Bilateral, asymmetric sacroiliitis	Bilateral, asymmetric sacroiliitis, may progress to ankylosis
Type of phytes	Delicate syndesmophytes	Paravertebral ossification	Paravertebral ossification

teric infections are associated with reactive arthritis and Reiter syndrome, discussed earlier in this chapter.

DIFFERENTIAL DIAGNOSIS

Although the spondyloarthropathies have common features, it is frequently possible to distinguish one from the other in individual patients (Table 12.3). The manifestations of ankylosing spondylitis are usually severe in the spine and sacroiliac joints and less severe in the peripheral joints. The manifestations of psoriatic arthritis are usually severe in the small peripheral joints and less severe in the large peripheral joints, spine, or sacroiliac joints. The manifestations of reactive arthritis and Reiter syndrome are usually mild and rarely involve the upper body. When disease is mild and radiographic findings are minimal, it may be difficult to recognize a specific form of spondyloarthropathy.

JUVENILE IDIOPATHIC ARTHRITIS

In juvenile idiopathic arthritis, the earlier the age of onset, the more severe the radiographic features.

Juvenile idiopathic arthritis (formerly called *juvenile chronic arthritis*) is a designation that includes Still disease (seronegative juvenile-onset rheumatoid arthritis), juvenile onset of seropositive adult-type rheumatoid arthritis, and the seronegative spondyloarthropathies (Table 12.4). The radiologic findings in juvenile idiopathic arthritis reflect the effect of a chronic inflammatory arthritis on a growing skeleton and are generally not specific for a particular clinical entity. The radiographic findings include soft tissue swelling, osteoporosis, periostitis, erosions, ankylosis, and growth disturbances (Fig. 12.37). The earlier the age of onset, the more severe the findings are. Not all findings are likely to be present together, but combinations of these findings should point to the diagnosis. The disease may remit in adulthood, but permanent muscle wasting, growth deformities, loss of function from ankylosis, and secondary osteoarthritis are common sequelae (Fig. 12.38).

Table 12.4: Clinical Types of Juvenile Idiopathic Arthritis

Seronegative chronic arthritis (Still disease, 70%)
Juvenile-onset seropositive rheumatoid arthritis (adult type)
Juvenile-onset ankylosing spondylitis
Psoriatic arthritis
Arthritis of inflammatory bowel disease
Other seronegative spondyloarthropathies
Miscellaneous arthritis

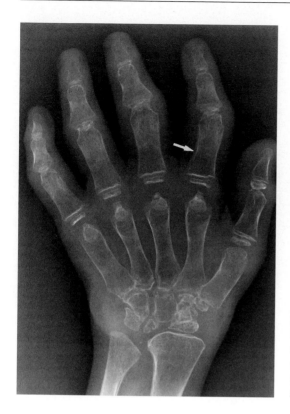

Figure 12.37 Juvenile idiopathic arthritis (Still disease) in the hand. The bones are osteopenic. Soft tissue swelling is evident at all of the joints. Periostitis is present (*arrow*). The articular margins of the bones are eroded and small.

Approximately 70% of cases of juvenile idiopathic arthritis are Still disease, of which there are three clinical presentations. Classic systemic disease is usually seen before 5 years of age and is associated with severe systemic manifestations but mild or absent articular disease. Polyarticular disease may occur with systemic disease or may follow it. Sites of involvement are symmetric and may include the MCP and IP joints of the hand, the wrist,

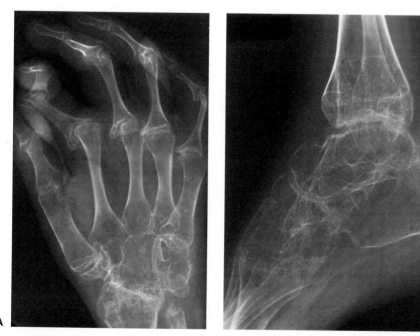

Figure 12.38 Sequelae of Still disease in a young adult. *A.* The hand has short bones whose growth plates fused prematurely. *B.* Intra-articular tarsal fusions are present; the bones are osteoporotic.

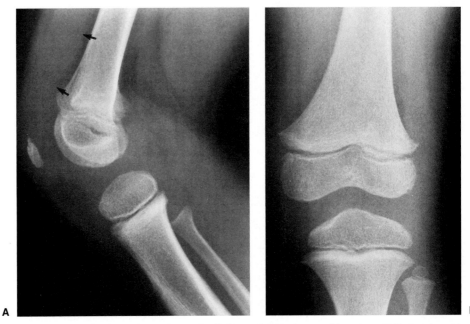

Figure 12.39 Juvenile idiopathic arthritis (Still disease) in a 4-year-old patient. Effusion is evident (*arrows*), but the disease is of too recent onset to have caused developmental effects. The appearance is nonspecific. *A.* Lateral radiograph. *B.* AP radiograph.

elbow, hip (Fig. 12.39), knee, ankle, foot, and cervical spine. The prognosis is generally poor. Pauciarticular or monarticular disease is the most common form of Still disease. It has a female predominance and is associated with iridocyclitis. Monarticular onset in a knee is the most common presentation (Fig. 12.40), but the ankle, elbow, and wrist are frequent sites. Joint contractures, muscle wasting, bony ankylosis, growth deformities, epiphyseal overgrowth, and early growth plate closure may follow the articular disease. In the hand, common findings include soft tissue swelling, osteoporosis, bony ankylosis, periostitis, growth disturbances, epiphyseal compression fractures, and joint subluxation.

The clinical and radiologic features of juvenile onset of adult-type seropositive rheumatoid arthritis and the seronegative spondyloarthropathies resemble their adult counterparts. However, in juvenile-onset rheumatoid arthritis, ankylosis and periostitis are

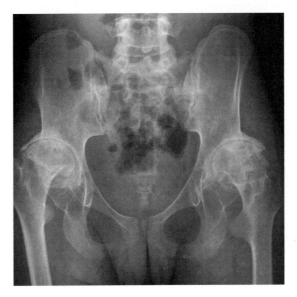

Figure 12.40 Juvenile idiopathic arthritis (Still disease) involving the hips. Radiograph shows diffuse joint space narrowing, secondary dysplasia, and superimposed degenerative changes.

prominent radiographic features, whereas erosions and joint space narrowing are not. Peripheral joint involvement occurs early in juvenile-onset ankylosing spondylitis.

SEPTIC ARTHRITIS

NONGONOCOCCAL ARTHRITIS

Septic arthritis is usually caused by nongonococcal bacteria in small children or elderly adults. Infections of joints usually follow hematogenous spread of organisms to the synovium from a preexisting infection in a remote site. Less commonly, adjacent osteomyelitis extends into a joint, or, rarely, a penetrating wound introduces organisms. The most common infecting organism in adults is *Staphylococcus aureus.* The most common organism in infants is β-hemolytic *Streptococcus,* and in preschool-aged children, *Haemophilus influenzae.* In patients with a chronic underlying disease such as diabetes or alcoholism, gram-negative bacteria are a common cause of septic arthritis in those with concurrent genitourinary tract infections, and *Streptococcus pneumoniae* is a common cause in those with concurrent lung infections. Other risk factors for septic arthritis include rheumatoid arthritis, SLE, total joint replacement, and old age.

> Septic arthritis is usually caused by hematogenous spread of organisms from a preexisting infection.

From the initial site of inflammation and microabscess formation in the synovium, the infection may spread to the joint space, bones, and soft tissues. Proteolytic enzymes released into the joint space by synovial cells and activated PMNs destroy the ground substance and then the collagen framework of the articular cartilage. Destruction of the joint takes only a few days. The usual clinical presentation is the abrupt onset of pain in a swollen, tender, inflamed joint. The nonspecific physical and laboratory signs of local and systemic infection may be present, but a preexisting source of infection is not always obvious. The diagnosis is made by arthrocentesis; injection of contrast medium under fluoroscopy can confirm intra-articular needle placement when necessary. The joint fluid is opaque, with a cell count of more than 100,000 WBC per mm^3, a differential with more than 85% PMNs, and a glucose level that is at least 50 mg per dL less than the concurrent serum level. Cultures of the fluid are almost always positive, and blood cultures are positive in 50% of cases. The knee is the most common site (Table 12.5). On radiographs, acute septic arthritis is evident as soft tissue swelling and effusion. Juxta-articular osteoporosis develops, and within 7 to 10 days, the articular cartilage is gone, and the joint space is narrowed. Findings in young children may be subtle, and sonography (to look for effusion) or MRI (to look for

Table 12.5: Frequency of Sites of Septic Arthritis (Nongonococcal)

	Site	Frequency (%)
Adults	Knee	55
	Hip	11
	Ankle	8
	Shoulder	8
	Wrist	7
	Elbow	6
	Other	5
Children	Knee	40
	Hip	28
	Ankle	14
	Elbow	11
	Other	7

From Kelley WN, Ruddy S, Harris ED Jr, et al., eds. *Textbook of rheumatology,* 5th ed. Philadelphia: WB Saunders, 1997:1450, with permission.

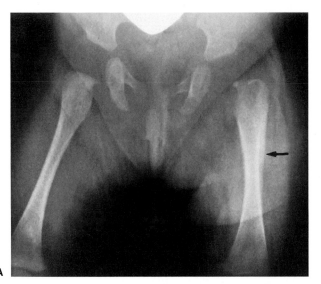

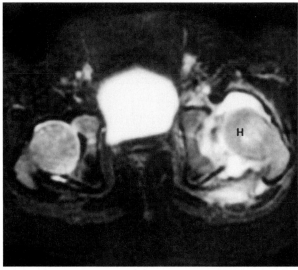

Figure 12.41 Septic arthritis on MRI in a child. *A*. Radiograph shows lateral subluxation of left hip and periosteal reaction in the femur (*arrow*). *B*. Axial T2-weighted MRI shows large left hip effusion distending the capsule and subluxating the femoral head (H).

effusion and osteomyelitis) may be helpful (Fig. 12.41). Prolonged antibiotic treatment and surgical drainage are often required, but the joint is usually destroyed despite treatment. Secondary degenerative changes ultimately develop.

GONOCOCCAL ARTHRITIS

Gonococcal arthritis occurs among sexually active young adults, especially women (80% of cases), and is the most common infectious arthritis in this age group. Preexisting HIV infection is a risk factor. Hematogenous dissemination of the organism causes fever and arthralgias, typically evident 2 weeks after the initial infection. Polyarticular and asymmetric involvement is usual, and there is a predilection for the knees, wrists, and ankles. Arthrocentesis fluid cultures are positive in fewer than 25%, but the response to antibiotics is rapid, and the outcome is good in nearly all cases. Radiographs may show only joint effusion and soft tissue swelling.

MISCELLANEOUS

GRANULOMATOUS SYNOVITIS

Granulomatous synovitis is a chronic, insidiously destructive process.

Tuberculosis, atypical mycobacteria, and fungi may spread to the joints, resulting in a granulomatous synovial infection that requires synovial biopsy or joint aspiration for diagnosis. These are chronic, insidiously destructive processes. In the usual situation, the underlying infection is in the lung, the process is monarticular, and there is osteomyelitis adjacent to the involved joint. On radiographs, osteopenia is prominent, and osteolysis with little or no reactive bone formation is characteristic (Fig. 12.42). A large joint effusion may be present. These infections have become progressively less rare in the United States since the beginning of the HIV epidemic (see Chapter 16).

VIRAL SYNOVITIS

Viral synovitis (toxic synovitis) is transient and self-limited in nearly all cases. The synovitis may be caused by direct viral infection of the synovium or by the deposition of immune com-

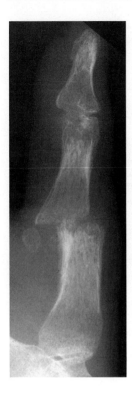

Figure 12.42 Tuberculous arthritis. Radiograph of the thumb shows destruction of the metacarpophalangeal joint with osteoporosis and minimal reactive bone formation.

plexes in the synovium as a systemic viremia is cleared. The viruses associated with arthritis include hepatitis B, rubella, enterovirus, adenovirus, varicella-zoster, Epstein-Barr, cytomegalovirus, and herpes simplex. No specific treatment is available or necessary, but aspiration of the joint may be indicated in children to exclude bacterial infection.

LYME DISEASE

Lyme disease is an inflammatory multisystem disease that follows infection by the spirochete *Borrelia burgdorferi*. The vector is the deer tick, an insect endemic to forested areas of the United States, Europe, and Australia. Clinical findings in the acute infection include a rash and flu-like syndrome. Months later, multisystem involvement may become apparent. In the musculoskeletal system, arthralgias of sudden onset and short duration appear, sometimes migratory and recurrent. One or more joints may be involved, most frequently the large joints, but also the temporomandibular and sacroiliac joints and the hands and feet. The radiographic appearance is nonspecific and may include peripheral enthesopathy and periostitis. Occasionally, a chronic inflammatory oligoarthritis that resembles rheumatoid arthritis develops, particularly in the knees.

SOURCES AND READINGS

Arnett FC, Edworthy SM, Bloch DA, et al. The American Rheumatism Association 1987 revised criteria for the classification of rheumatoid arthritis. *Arthritis Rheum* 1988;31:315–324.

Ball GV, Koopman WJ. *Clinical rheumatology*. Philadelphia: WB Saunders, 1998.

Blum U, Buitrago-Tellez C, Mundinger A, et al. Magnetic resonance imaging (MRI) for detection of active sacroiliitis—a prospective study comparing conventional radiography, scintigraphy, and contrast enhanced MRI. *J Rheumatol* 1996;23:2107–2115.

Brower AC. *Arthritis in black and white*, 2nd ed. Philadelphia: WB Saunders, 1997.

Forrester DM, Brown JC. *The radiology of joint disease*, 3rd ed. Philadelphia: WB Saunders, 1987.

Harrison BJ, Symmons DP, Barrett EM, et al. The performance of the 1987 ARA classification criteria for rheumatoid arthritis in a population based cohort of patients with early inflammatory polyarthritis. American Rheumatism Association. *J Rheumatol* 1998;25:2324–2330.

Klein MA, Winalski CS, Wax MR, et al. MR imaging of septic sacroiliitis. *J Comput Assist Tomogr* 1991;15:126–132.

McCarty DJ, Koopman WJ, eds. *Arthritis and allied conditions: a textbook of rheumatology*, 12th ed. Philadelphia: Lea & Febiger, 1993.

Murphey MD, Wetzel LH, Bramble JM, et al. Sacroiliitis: MR imaging findings. *Radiology* 1991;180:239–244.

Oostveen J, Prevo R, den Boer J, et al. Early detection of sacroiliitis on magnetic resonance imaging and subsequent development of sacroiliitis on plain radiography. A prospective, longitudinal study. *J Rheumatol* 1999;26:1953–1958.

Oostveen JC, van de Laar MA. Magnetic resonance imaging in rheumatic disorders of the spine and sacroiliac joints. *Semin Arthritis Rheum* 2000;30:52–69.

Resnick D, ed. *Diagnosis of bone and joint disorders*, 4th ed. Philadelphia: WB Saunders, 2002.

Ruddy S, Harris ED Jr, Sledge CB, eds. *Textbook of rheumatology*, 6th ed. Philadelphia: WB Saunders, 2001.

Sturzenbecher A, Braun J, Paris S, et al. MR imaging of septic sacroiliitis. *Skeletal Radiol* 2000;29:439–446.

Sugimoto H, Takeda A, Hyodoh K. Early-stage rheumatoid arthritis: prospective study of the effectiveness of MR imaging for diagnosis. *Radiology* 2000;216:569–575.

Yu W, Feng F, Dion E, et al. Comparison of radiography, computed tomography and magnetic resonance imaging in the detection of sacroiliitis accompanying ankylosing spondylitis. *Skeletal Radiol* 1998;27:311–320.

Zimmermann B, Mikolich DJ, Lally EV. Septic sacroiliitis. *Semin Arthritis Rheum* 1996;26:592–604.

NONINFLAMMATORY JOINT DISEASE

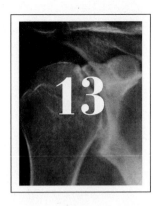

- Osteoarthritis (Degenerative Joint Disease)
- Neuropathic Osteoarthropathy (Charcot Joint)
- Crystal-Associated Diseases
- Metabolic Deposition Disease
- Miscellaneous Joint Conditions
- Degenerative Foot Conditions
- Degenerative Disc Disease
- Diffuse Idiopathic Skeletal Hyperostosis
- Baastrup Disease
- Sources and Readings

This chapter covers joint diseases that have predominantly noninflammatory features on radiographs.

OSTEOARTHRITIS (DEGENERATIVE JOINT DISEASE)

Osteoarthritis is a form of joint disease characterized by degenerative changes involving synovial joints. Osteoarthritis can be divided into primary and secondary types, but the division is artificial: The underlying cause is evident in secondary osteoarthritis but not in primary or idiopathic osteoarthritis. The distinction has some practical value in understanding the process and planning clinical management. Osteoarthritis is the most common form of arthritis. Its prevalence increases with age, so that osteoarthritis is nearly ubiquitous in patients older than 65 years of age. Up to 45 years of age, it is more prevalent in men; from 45 to 55 years of age, the prevalence is equal; and after 55 years of age, it is more prevalent in women. The most common presentation of osteoarthritis is joint pain and limitation of activity. Laboratory tests are used to eliminate other forms of arthritis as clinical possibilities.

Osteoarthritis is the most common form of arthritis.

PRIMARY OSTEOARTHRITIS

The early morphologic abnormality in primary osteoarthritis is fibrillation of the articular cartilage. The surface develops fibril-like projections and becomes irregular. Underlying this morphologic change is disruption at the molecular level of the superficial armor-plate layer and collagen framework, resulting in progressive loss of proteoglycans from the ground substance and collagen from the framework. Chondrocytes increase protein synthesis, presumably in response to the continuing loss of structural components. Progressive erosion and formation of fissures in the surface eventually expose the subchondral bone. The initial event

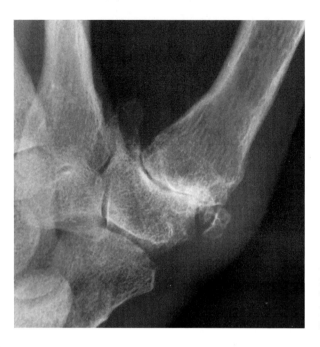

Figure 13.1 Osteoarthritis at the first carpometacarpal joint with narrowing of the articular space, osteophyte formation, subchondral sclerosis, and subluxation.

Primary osteoarthritis may result from an alteration in articular cartilage physiology.

Osteophytes tend to be largest in the plane of motion.

that incites fibrillation of the cartilage surface is unknown; some forms of primary osteoarthritis may result from an initial alteration in articular cartilage physiology.

Radiographic findings do not appear in osteoarthritis until articular cartilage loss results in secondary adaptive changes in bone. These findings include uneven loss of articular space, subchondral sclerosis, osteophytes, and subchondral cysts (Fig. 13.1); the absence of osteoporosis, ankylosis, and erosions is characteristic. Osteophytes tend to be largest in the plane of motion; therefore, osteophytes at the distal interphalangeal (DIP) and proximal interphalangeal (PIP) joints are best seen on the lateral view. In the hand and wrist, primary osteoarthritis typically affects the DIP and PIP joints and the basal joints of the thumb (Fig. 13.2). The basal joints of the thumb are composed of the first carpometacarpal (CMC) joint and the scaphoid-trapezium-trapezoid joints. Isolated degenerative involvement at this specific site is virtually diag-

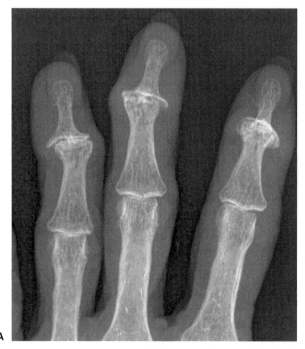
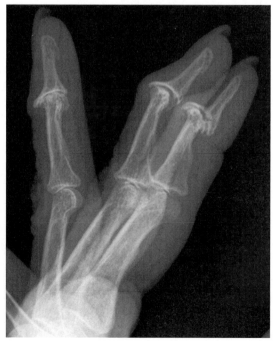

Figure 13.2 Osteoarthritis at the distal interphalangeal joints of the fingers. *A.* PA radiograph. *B.* Lateral radiograph.

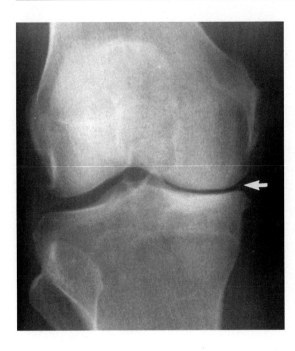

Figure 13.3 Osteoarthritis of the knee with medial compartment cartilage space narrowing (*arrow*) and varus deformity.

nostic of primary osteoarthritis. The first metatarsophalangeal (MTP) joint, hips and knees, and the cervical and lumbar spine are also common sites of involvement. The metacarpophalangeal (MCP) joints, wrist, elbow, shoulder, and ankle are typically spared. The severity of radiographic changes does not necessarily correlate with the severity of symptoms.

In the knee, the characteristic distribution of involvement is in the medial compartment and, to a less severe degree, the patellofemoral compartment. Joint space narrowing, subchondral sclerosis, osteophytes, and subchondral cysts are typical findings (Fig. 13.3). Occasionally, more severe involvement of the lateral or patellofemoral compartments occurs. Angular deformities and joint space narrowing are best demonstrated on standing views. Because the severity of involvement of the anterior and posterior portions of the femoral cartilage is typically uneven, the amount of joint space narrowing may vary between radiographs with the knee in extension and flexion. On MRI, early osteoarthritis is evident as abnormal high signal in articular cartilage on T2-weighted MRI. When isolated to the patella, this condition is called *chondromalacia patellae* (Fig. 13.4). Fibrillation of the cartilage surface, thin-

In the knee, angular deformities and joint space narrowing are best demonstrated on standing views.

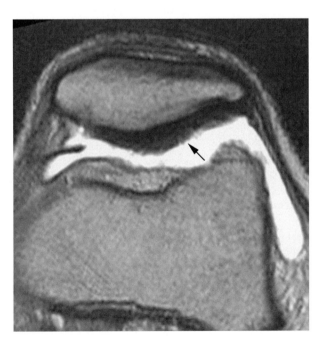

Figure 13.4 Chondromalacia patellae with effusion and fibrillated patellar cartilage (*arrow*) shown on axial T2-weighted MRI.

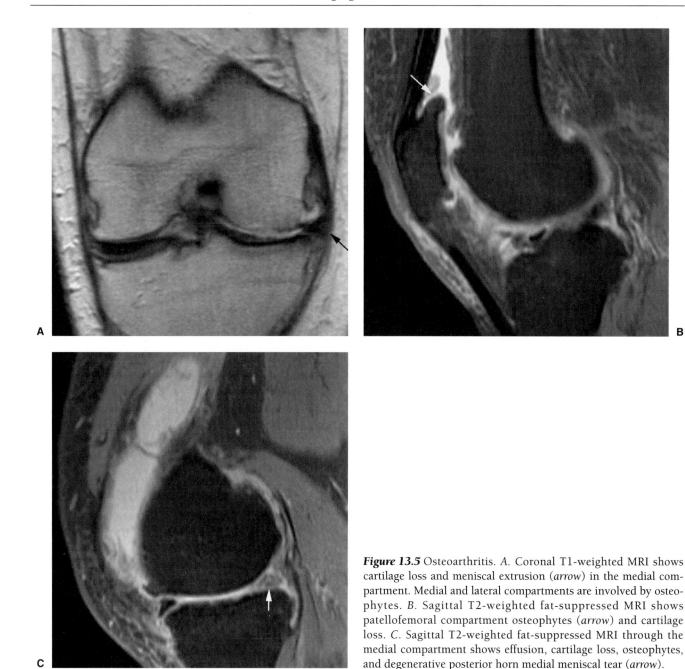

Figure 13.5 Osteoarthritis. *A.* Coronal T1-weighted MRI shows cartilage loss and meniscal extrusion (*arrow*) in the medial compartment. Medial and lateral compartments are involved by osteophytes. *B.* Sagittal T2-weighted fat-suppressed MRI shows patellofemoral compartment osteophytes (*arrow*) and cartilage loss. *C.* Sagittal T2-weighted fat-suppressed MRI through the medial compartment shows effusion, cartilage loss, osteophytes, and degenerative posterior horn medial meniscal tear (*arrow*).

ning of the cartilage, and frank loss of cartilage may be seen in progressively more severe cases. Subchondral bone edema at sites of cartilage loss, osteophyte formation, loose bodies, and effusions may be present in established osteoarthritis (Figs. 13.5 through 13.7).

In the hip, loss of articular space is usually found along the superior (horizontal) portion of the joint (Fig. 13.8). Less commonly, the medial joint space is narrowed. Osteophyte formation in the femoral head often forms a collar of bone around the femoral neck at the margin of the articular surface, usually seen best on frog lateral views. As with the knee, uneven involvement of the articular cartilage results in varying amounts of joint space narrowing from position to position. Mapping cartilage thickness with fluoroscopically positioned spot radiographs or cartilage-specific imaging parameters on MRI can be helpful in planning rotational osteotomies for treatment.

Osteoarthritis of the synovial joints of the spine may be the predominant feature of degenerative spine disease or may occur in association with other features such as degenera-

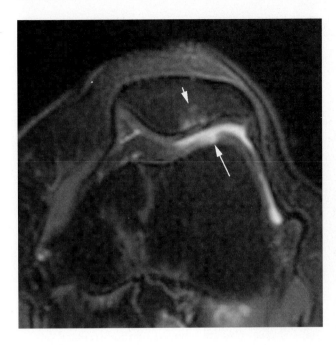

Figure 13.6 Patellofemoral osteo-arthritis. Axial T2-weighted MRI shows loss of cartilage from the lateral facet of the patella and the patellofemoral groove (*long arrow*) and subchondral marrow edema at the site of cartilage loss (*short arrow*). An effusion is present.

tive disc disease, previous trauma, scoliosis, kyphosis, or vertebral anomalies. The common sites of synovial joint osteoarthritis are the lower cervical and lower lumbar spine. The atlantoaxial joint is also synovial and may be affected. The pathologic process is identical to that of other synovial joints, leading to joint space narrowing, subchondral sclerosis, and osteophytes. Loss of articular cartilage may allow subluxation or excessive motion; bony hypertrophy may reduce motion. Osteophytes and ligamentous thickening may lead to nerve root involvement. These findings are best demonstrated by CT (Fig. 13.9).

Osteoarthritis of the acromioclavicular joint is a common finding on shoulder imaging. On radiographs, osteophytes may be seen. On MRI, osteophytes and hypertrophy of the joint

Synovial joint osteoarthritis is common in the lower cervical and lower lumbar spine.

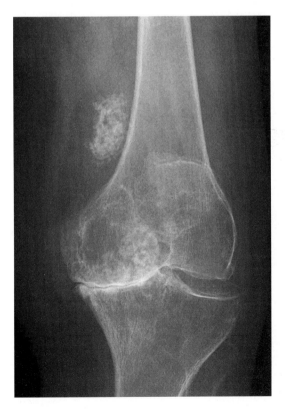

Figure 13.7 Osteoarthritis of the knee with calcified loose bodies.

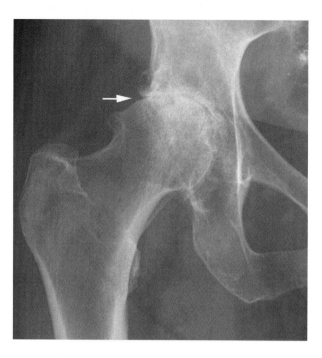

Figure 13.8 Osteoarthritis of the hip with advanced joint space narrowing superiorly (*arrow*).

are typical, often with subchondral edema in the distal clavicle and acromion and fluid in the joint (Fig. 13.10).

In inflammatory (erosive) osteoarthritis, inflammation rather than degeneration dominates the clinical presentation.

Inflammatory (erosive) osteoarthritis is a condition in which an acute synovitis accompanies primary osteoarthritis. Although joint degeneration always has some component of synovial inflammation because of the presence of joint debris and cartilage breakdown products, the inflammation dominates the clinical presentation in erosive osteoarthritis. Radiographs show the degenerative features and distribution of primary osteoarthritis, but the acute synovitis causes inflammatory erosions, uniform joint space narrowing, and sometimes ankylosis (Fig. 13.11). A characteristic "seagull" appearance may be seen on PA radiographs at the interphalangeal (IP) joints of the fingers, corresponding to central erosions and bony hypertrophy. The

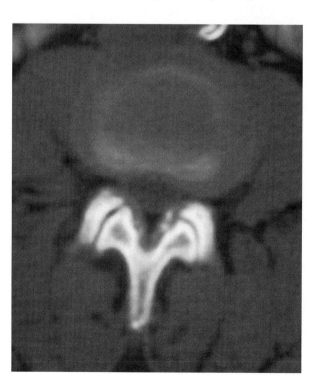

Figure 13.9 Lumbar facet osteoarthritis on CT scan.

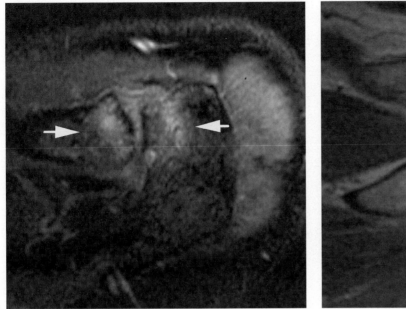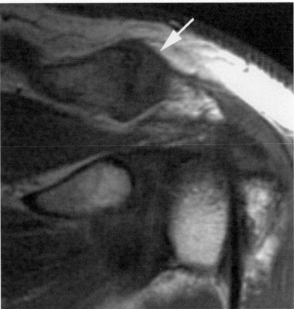

A · B

Figure 13.10 Osteoarthritis of the acromioclavicular joint. *A.* Axial T2-weighted fat-suppressed MRI shows subchondral edema in the clavicle and acromion (*arrows*). *B.* Oblique coronal T1-weighted MRI shows hypertrophy of the acromioclavicular joint (*arrow*) with mass effect on the supraspinatus muscle.

typical age at onset is in the fifth or sixth decade, and women are affected far more frequently than men. The inflammation usually subsides within a few months to a couple of years, leaving the degenerative changes. In the hand, erosive osteoarthritis characteristically affects the DIP and PIP joints and the basal joints of the thumb, as does nonerosive primary osteoarthritis.

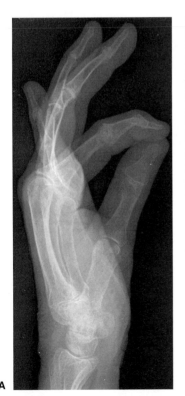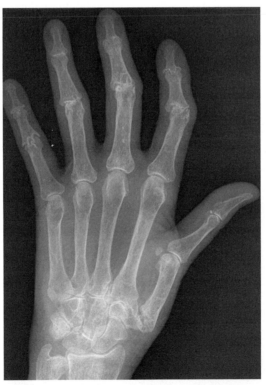

A · B

Figure 13.11 Inflammatory osteoarthritis with erosions and osteophytes at the proximal interphalangeal joints and the first carpometacarpal joint. *A.* Lateral radiograph. *B.* PA radiograph.

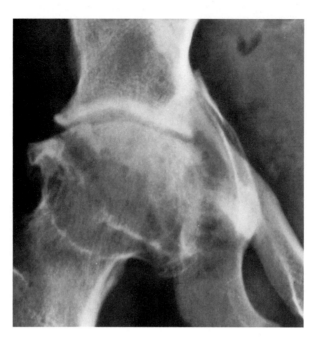

Figure 13.12 Posttraumatic osteoarthritis 12 years after acetabular fracture.

SECONDARY OSTEOARTHRITIS

Secondary degenerative changes in the joints result from three major factors: an abnormality of the articular cartilage, loss of subchondral bony support beneath normal articular cartilage, and abnormal alignment and mechanical stress. Any condition with one of these features may lead to permanent, progressive osteoarthritis. Secondary osteoarthritis may follow inflammatory arthritis if the inflammatory process has caused permanent cartilage damage and is quiescent long enough for the degenerative changes to develop. Mechanical trauma may injure the articular cartilage, which has a limited ability for repair. A fibrocartilage scar may replace damaged areas of hyaline cartilage. Joint debris, loose bodies, or displaced meniscal fragments within a joint may erode the articular cartilage. Osteochondral loose bodies derive nutrition from synovial fluid and may grow. Healthy cartilage wears prematurely when its

Osteochondral loose bodies derive nutrition from synovial fluid and may therefore grow.

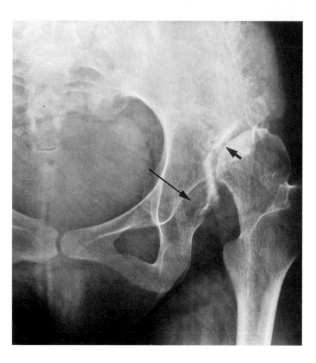

Figure 13.13 Secondary osteoarthritis in the left pseudoacetabulum (*short arrow*) in a 20-year-old woman with untreated developmental dysplasia of the hip. The native acetabulum (*long arrow*) is empty.

underlying bony support is lost. For example, collapse of the subchondral bone of the femoral head after osteonecrosis leads rapidly to secondary degeneration. Less obvious changes in the subchondral bone due to repetitive subclinical trauma may also lead to osteoarthritis. An abnormally aligned joint or a joint that is subject to mechanical disadvantage or abnormal stresses may wear prematurely. Posttraumatic osteoarthritis may follow malunion of long-bone fractures, imperfectly reduced intra-articular fractures (Fig. 13.12), or posttraumatic joint instability. Many forms of developmental and acquired bone and joint dysplasia lead to early osteoarthritis, including developmental dysplasia of the hip (Fig. 13.13), Legg-Calvé-Perthes disease, and multiple epiphyseal dysplasia. The premature wear resulting from the abnormal joint geometry worsens in a vicious cycle of progressive malalignment, mechanical disadvantage, and abnormal stress.

NEUROPATHIC OSTEOARTHROPATHY (CHARCOT JOINT)

Neuropathic joints have lost proprioception and deep pain sensation. With continued use of the joint, relaxation and hypotonia of the supporting structures lead to malalignment and recurrent injury. Rapidly progressive erosion of the articular cartilage, reactive subchondral sclerosis, fractures, and fragmentation of the subchondral bone result in a disorganized joint. The presence of joint debris induces synovitis and chronic effusion. The damage and derangement may occur over a period of days to weeks with relatively little symptomatology. Both lower motor neuron (peripheral) and upper motor neuron (central) lesions may result in neuropathic osteoarthropathy. Diabetic neuropathy is the most common lower motor neuron lesion causing neuropathic osteoarthropathy; other causes include alcoholism, tuberculosis, amyloidosis, leprosy, peripheral nerve trauma, steroids, and congenital indifference to pain. Syringomyelia is the most common upper motor neuron lesion; other causes include meningomyelocele, trauma, multiple sclerosis, tabes dorsalis (syphilis), and cord compression.

Neuropathic osteoarthropathy occurs in 0.1% of all diabetics and in 5.0% of those with diabetic neuropathy. Diabetic peripheral neuropathy causes loss of pain sensation and proprioception, leading to exceptional wear and tear without patient awareness of injury. The most frequent site of involvement is the foot (80%), especially the tarsometatarsal (TMT), intertarsal, and MTP joints; involvement may be unilateral or bilateral. Tarsal-metatarsal

> Neuropathic osteoarthropathy may develop over a period of days to weeks.

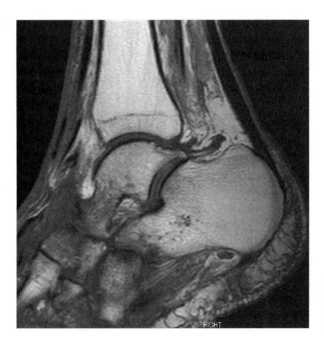

Figure 13.14 Neuropathic osteoarthropathy. Sagittal T1-weighted MRI of the foot shows swelling, disorganization, and edema of the midfoot.

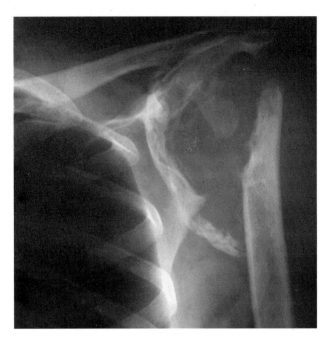

Figure 13.15 Neuropathic shoulder joint.

fracture-dislocation (Lisfranc fracture-dislocation) may occur spontaneously or with minimal trauma. Extensive sclerosis, osteophytosis, fractures, bony fragmentation, subluxation, dislocation, bony debris, effusion, and subchondral cysts are common findings. Chronic osteomyelitis is also relatively common in the diabetic foot, and the possible combination of neuropathic osteoarthropathy with infection can pose a diagnostic dilemma (Fig. 13.14). MRI with gadolinium enhancement may be helpful in this circumstance.

Neuropathic osteoarthropathy occurs in 25% of patients with syringomyelia. The joint changes are usually in the upper extremity (80%), and they may be atrophic rather than proliferative. Acute resorption of the articulating ends of the bone without evidence of repair, gross soft tissue swelling, and bony debris in the soft tissues are common findings. This process may mimic destruction from tumor or infection. The most commonly involved joint is the shoulder (Fig. 13.15).

CRYSTAL-ASSOCIATED DISEASES

Deposits of crystals shed into the joint space may cause acute crystal synovitis.

Crystal-associated joint diseases are pathologic conditions that occur in the presence of crystals. The crystals contribute to tissue damage, but the causal relationship between crystals and tissue damage is not well understood. Crystals precipitate from the extracellular fluid space into the articular tissues, where they accumulate. Deposits of crystals may then be shed episodically into the joint space. Clearance of crystals from the joint space and articular cartilage is poor because these structures are avascular, alymphatic, and largely devoid of scavenger cells. The presence of particles alters the mechanical properties of the tissues, tending to make them less elastic. Articular cartilage is particularly vulnerable to damage and ultimately undergoes degenerative changes. Large crystalline particles in the joint space can cause direct abrasive damage to the articular surfaces. Small particles can cause damage by biophysical and biochemical interactions with cell membranes and macromolecules and may also provoke an acute synovitis. Although the precise mechanisms mediating acute synovial inflammation are incompletely understood, different mechanisms appear to be activated by different crystals. These crystal-induced inflammatory reactions tend to have a sudden onset and a rapid, self-limited course. The sudden onset is probably related to the abrupt shedding of crystals into the joint space from a deposit in the articular tissues.

Crystal deposition diseases have three clinical presentations: (a) an asymptomatic state in which crystals can be detected, (b) an inflammatory arthritis, and (c) a chronic destructive

Table 13.1: Crystal Deposition Diseases of Joints

Crystal	Associated Clinical Conditions
Calcium pyrophosphate dihydrate	Chondrocalcinosis
	Pseudogout
	Pyrophosphate arthropathy
Calcium hydroxyapatite	Asymptomatic calcification
	Calcific tendonitis, bursitis, and periarthritis
	Chronic destructive joint disease
Monosodium urate monohydrate	Hyperuricemia
	Gouty arthritis
	Tophaceous gout

arthropathy. The particular diseases are defined by the presence of characteristic crystals within affected joints. Aspiration of the joint during an acute inflammatory episode may yield material in which the associated crystal can be demonstrated. The three types of crystals that are commonly associated with joint diseases are calcium pyrophosphate dihydrate (CPPD), calcium hydroxyapatite, and monosodium urate monohydrate (Table 13.1).

CALCIUM PYROPHOSPHATE DIHYDRATE CRYSTAL DEPOSITION DISEASE

CPPD crystal deposition disease is a polyarticular arthritis with deposition of CPPD crystals in articular tissues. Its initial presentation may be monoarticular. The definitive clinical diagnosis requires the identification of CPPD crystals from joint fluid, but the radiologic findings can be diagnostic. CPPD deposition disease has been associated with hyperparathyroidism, hemochromatosis, aging, and osteoarthritis. It has been weakly associated with hypothyroidism, ochronosis, Paget disease, Wilson disease, acromegaly, diabetes, and gout. CPPD crystal deposition disease has three manifestations: chondrocalcinosis, crystal-induced synovitis, and pyrophosphate arthropathy (Table 13.2).

CPPD crystals are generated locally in the articular tissues, where asymptomatic deposits may accumulate in cartilage, joint capsules, intervertebral discs, tendons, and ligaments. In cartilage, these deposits may be evident radiographically as chondrocalcinosis. Chondrocalcinosis is most common in the knees, wrists, elbows, and hips, and is found in both fibrocartilage and hyaline cartilage. Chondrocalcinosis in the menisci has high signal intensity that can mimic a meniscal tear on MRI. Chondrocalcinosis in the hyaline cartilage appears as linear or punctate areas of low signal intensity, which becomes more noticeable on gradient-recalled echo sequence because of the blooming artifact.

Shedding of crystals into the joint space after rupture of a deposit causes an acute, self-limited, crystal-induced synovitis. This acute synovitis is clinically similar to acute gouty arthritis and has been known as *pseudogout*. As with gouty arthritis, acute episodes of inflam-

Asymptomatic deposits of CPPD crystals may accumulate in cartilage, joint capsules, intervertebral discs, tendons, and ligaments.

Table 13.2: Clinical Syndromes of Calcium Pyrophosphate Dihydrate Crystal Deposition Disease

Asymptomatic chondrocalcinosis
Acute crystal synovitis
   Acute, intermittent (pseudogout)
   Subacute or chronic (resembles rheumatoid arthritis)
Pyrophosphate arthropathy (resembles osteoarthritis)
   Without attacks of pseudogout
   With intermittent attacks of pseudogout
   Neuropathic-like (resembles neuropathic osteoarthropathy)

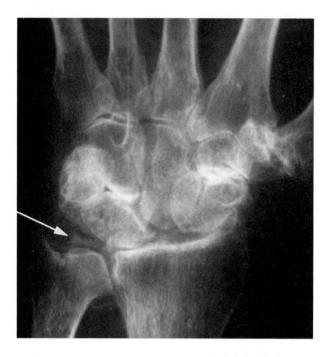

Figure 13.16 Pyrophosphate arthropathy with scapholunate advanced collapse wrist. Chondrocalcinosis involves the triangular fibrocartilage complex (*arrow*).

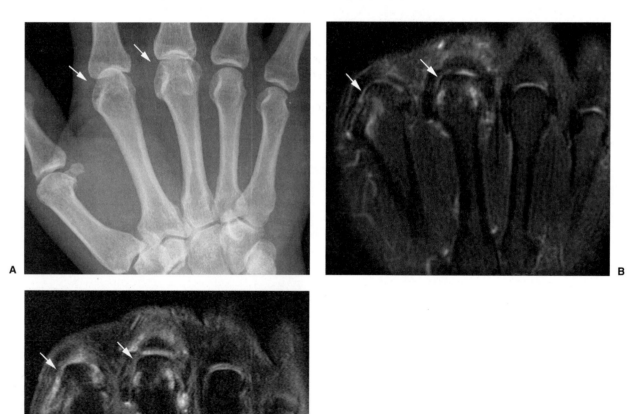

Figure 13.17 Calcium pyrophosphate dihydrate hand on MRI. *A.* PA radiograph shows joint space narrowing (*arrows*) at the index and middle metacarpophalangeal (MCP) joints. *B.* Coronal T2-weighted MRI with fat suppression shows high signal (*arrows*) at the index and middle MCP joints. *C.* Coronal T1-weighted MRI with fat suppression after injection of gadolinium shows enhancement (*arrows*) at the index and middle MCP joints.

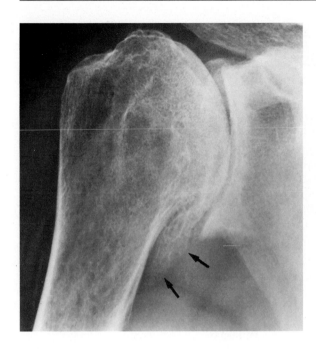

Figure 13.18 Pyrophosphate arthropathy of the shoulder with prominent osteophyte formation (*arrows*), loss of articular space, and superior subluxation.

matory synovitis may recur intermittently. During an acute episode, CPPD crystals can be recovered by joint aspiration and identified by polarized light microscopy or more definitive physical means. Uncommonly, these episodes can run together into a subacute or chronic crystal synovitis that resembles rheumatoid arthritis, except that the large joints of the limbs tend to be involved rather than the small ones of the hands and feet.

Pyrophosphate arthropathy is the degenerative result of structural joint damage caused by chronic CPPD crystal deposition and irreversible destruction of the articular cartilage. The degenerative changes can be identical to osteoarthritis, but the distribution of involvement is different. In the hand, the MCP joints are characteristically involved. In the wrist, the radiocarpal joint is characteristically involved. In severe cases, the process causes gross scapholunate dissociation in association with degenerative radiocarpal changes. The scaphoid and lunate separate, and the capitate migrates proximally into the resulting gap. This syndrome is called *scapholunate advanced collapse*, or *SLAC*, wrist (Figs. 13.16 and 13.17). The SLAC wrist usually includes pancompartmental degenerative involvement. The shoulder (glenohumeral), knee (especially patellofemoral), elbow, ankle, and foot (talonavicular) are the other common sites of involvement (Fig. 13.18). Chondrocalcinosis need not be present and is absent if there is no remaining cartilage. Isolated severe involvement of the patellofemoral compartment of the knee or selective radiocarpal involvement of the wrist is virtually diagnostic of pyrophosphate arthropathy. Pyrophosphate arthropathy is often, but not necessarily, combined with acute episodes of crystal-induced synovitis. Very severe degenerative changes may lead to an appearance that resembles neuropathic osteoarthropathy.

HYDROXYAPATITE DEPOSITION DISEASE

Hydroxyapatite deposition disease is a heterogeneous group of conditions that have in common the abnormal presence of amorphous hydroxyapatite (basic calcium phosphate) crystals in the soft tissues. Ion contaminants such as carbonate, magnesium, fluoride, and chloride are present. It is probably the result of multiple causes, and there may be more than one mechanism of deposition. The radiologic manifestations of hydroxyapatite deposition disease are similar to other crystal-associated conditions: asymptomatic deposits, acute crystal-induced synovitis, and chronic destructive arthropathy. Unlike CPPD deposition disease, hydroxyapatite deposition disease typically involves the tendons, ligaments, and joint capsules rather than the articular cartilage and subchondral bone.

Deposits of hydroxyapatite in the soft tissues appear on radiographs as dense, homogeneous, sharply marginated, and amorphous calcifications. They may have linear, angular, or

Hydroxyapatite deposition disease typically involves the tendons, ligaments, and joint capsules.

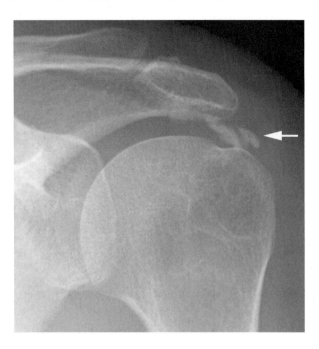

Figure 13.19 Calcium hydroxyapatite deposit in the supraspinatus tendon of the rotator cuff (*arrow*).

round shapes, and unlike chondrocalcinosis, the calcifications do not conform to hyaline or fibrocartilage structures. Occasionally, these deposits may mimic mineralized osteoid tumor matrix, which they may resemble. The soft tissue calcifications of immune-mediated connective tissue diseases such as scleroderma, polymyositis, and dermatomyositis are also in the form of hydroxyapatite, but the clinical condition of hydroxyapatite deposition disease is different from these. Hydroxyapatite deposition disease is thought to be a process of abnormal mineral metabolism, possibly systemic but perhaps localized only to the sites of tissue damage; the cause and pathogenesis are not understood. These deposits may occur in periarticular soft tissues as well as tendons, ligaments, capsules, entheses, and bursae (Figs. 13.19 through 13.22). A minority of patients with hydroxyapatite deposits have symptoms. Metastatic soft tissue deposits of hydroxyapatite around joints (periarticular calcinosis, tumoral calcinosis) may be found in patients on dialysis for chronic renal failure (Fig. 13.23). Because

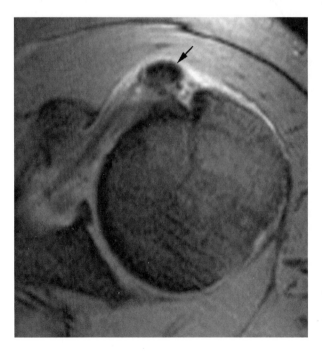

Figure 13.20 Hydroxyapatite deposit (*arrow*) in the rotator cuff shown on axial gradient-recalled echo MRI.

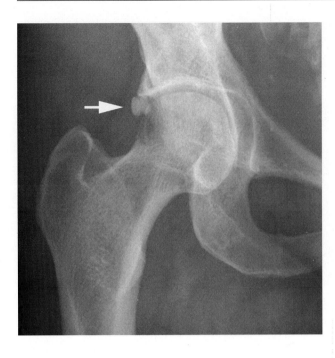

Figure 13.21 Hydroxyapatite deposition in the acetabular labrum (*arrow*).

the crystals are often aqueous suspensions (milk of calcium), CT and upright radiographs may demonstrate fluid-sediment levels. The calcification is difficult to detect on most MRI sequences, except for gradient-recalled echo sequences, because the calcified collections are of low signal and isointense to the involved tendons. MRI may show muscle and soft tissue edema associated with the calcifications.

Recurrent episodes of calcific tendonitis or calcific bursitis are commonly associated with hydroxyapatite deposits. Most patients are adults in their 40s and 50s and present with acute pain, swelling, and tenderness. Symptoms respond rapidly to a nonsteroidal anti-

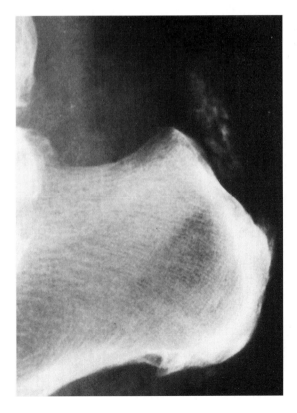

Figure 13.22 Calcific retrocalcaneal bursitis.

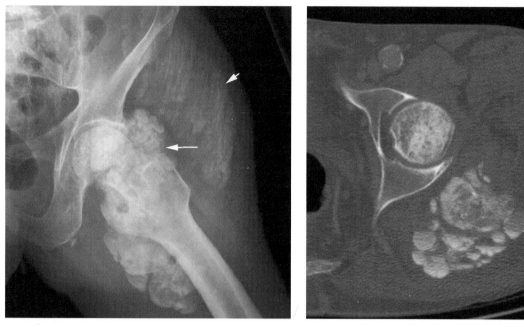

Figure 13.23 Periarticular calcinosis in patient on hemodialysis for chronic renal failure. *A.* Radiograph shows calcium deposits around the hip (*long arrow*) and gluteal musculature (*short arrow*). *B.* Axial CT scan shows fluid-fluid levels (*arrow*) within the calcium deposits.

inflammatory agent. The shoulder, commonly the supraspinatus tendon, is a common site of involvement. Tendons may atrophy and rupture, but it is unclear whether the deposits initially caused the local tissue damage or preexisting tissue damage allowed the deposits to accumulate. The deposits around the shoulder are bilateral in approximately half of cases and may migrate to contiguous structures. After clinical resolution, the deposits may disappear.

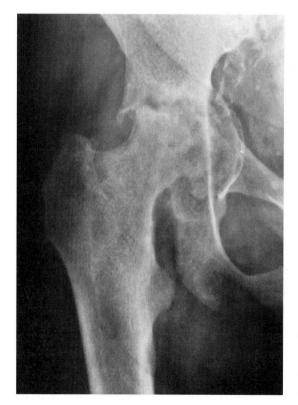

Figure 13.24 Hydroxyapatite arthropathy. Hip shows destructive changes in the femoral head and acetabulum. Note the medial acetabular protrusion (protrusio acetabuli).

The process is usually monarticular, but multiple joints may be involved at the same time or successively. Other common sites of involvement include the long head of the biceps tendon, the extensors of the wrist, the myotendinous attachments along the linea aspera (thigh adductors) and at the medial border of the proximal tibia (pes anserinus), the olecranon bursa, the trochanteric bursa, and the ischial bursa.

Hydroxyapatite crystals have been associated with a chronic destructive arthritis similar to osteoarthritis or CPPD deposition disease. This situation is relatively uncommon and most often occurs in the setting of renal failure and hyperparathyroidism (Fig. 13.24). Mixtures of crystals may be recovered from such joints, including CPPD and hydroxyapatite.

GOUT

Gout is defined by the presence of hyperuricemia (serum uric acid concentration greater than 7 mg per dL). Hyperuricemia may be idiopathic or secondary to known conditions, including excess ingestion (in protein), intrinsic overproduction, or reduced renal secretion. There is a familial incidence that appears to be controlled by multiple genes. Specific mutations with biochemical defects in purine metabolism leading to hyperuricemia have been found in a few cases. Gout is associated with obesity, diabetes, hyperlipidemia, hypertension, atherosclerosis, alcohol consumption, acute illness, and pregnancy. There is a negative association with rheumatoid arthritis. The prevalence of the symptomatic forms of gout, gouty arthritis, and tophaceous gout has declined dramatically with the increasing use of drugs that control hyperuricemia. Gouty arthritis is similar to other crystal-related joint diseases, whereas tophaceous gout has the radiology of a metabolic deposition disease (discussed in the section Metabolic Deposition Disease).

> There is a familial incidence of gout that appears to be controlled by multiple genes.

Gouty arthritis is the articular disease associated with monosodium urate monohydrate, the crystalline form in which uric acid is precipitated from solution into the soft tissues. The age of peak onset of gouty arthritis is 50 years, and it develops only after decades of sustained hyperuricemia. Gouty arthritis commonly presents as an acute crystal-induced synovitis that tends to be recurrent and episodic. Radiographs may show only fusiform soft tissue swelling unless there are concurrent features of tophaceous gout. Shedding of monosodium urate crystals into the synovial fluid or synovial tissues apparently causes the acute synovitis, provoking an inflammatory response. A chronic destructive arthropathy may also develop. Approximately 90% of cases occur in men. The manifestations of gouty arthritis are generally peripheral, in the hands or feet. Gouty arthritis has a predilection for the joints of the lower extremity, especially the first MTP joint (podagra), intertarsal joints, ankle, and knee. The first MTP joint is the most common site of initial involvement; the great toe is the site of 70% of attacks. Involvement of the hands, wrists, and elbows may occur later in the clinical course. The limb girdles and axial skeleton are typically spared. The acute episode usually responds quickly and dramatically to colchicine or a nonsteroidal anti-inflammatory agent.

> Approximately 90% of cases of gouty arthritis occur in men.

METABOLIC DEPOSITION DISEASE

Metabolic deposition diseases involving the joints, in which the body accumulates a substance it cannot excrete or metabolize, include tophaceous gout, multicentric reticulohistiocytosis, and amyloidosis. Except for gout, these types of joint disease are relatively uncommon. If focal, mass-like deposits are located in the musculoskeletal system, the result is a clinically indolent disease with randomly distributed, slowly enlarging, space-occupying deposits.

TOPHACEOUS GOUT

Unlike the other crystal-induced joint conditions, gout may present with the radiologic features of a metabolic deposition disease. Deposits of monosodium urate crystals are called *tophi*. The development of tophi requires decades of sustained hyperuricemia and is related

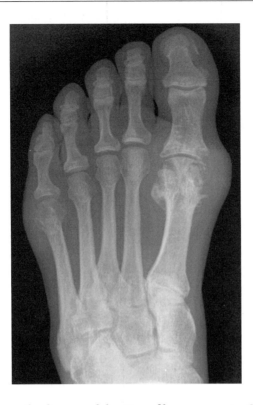

Figure 13.25 Tophaceous gout with overhanging edge and chronic erosions at the first metatarsophalangeal joint. The adjacent articular space is preserved.

Tophi cause a lumpy-bumpy appearance of the soft tissues.

to the degree and duration of hyperuricemia. Control of hyperuricemia by drugs has reduced the incidence of tophi in people with gout from more than 50% in the 1950s to approximately 3% currently. Deposits near the joints and tendons cause a lumpy-bumpy appearance. These localized areas of swelling may cause the slow development of pressure erosions on adjacent bone. Such erosions have well-defined sclerotic margins. A shell of new bone may attempt to encompass the deposit, leaving an overhanging edge (Figs. 13.25 through 13.28). The artic-

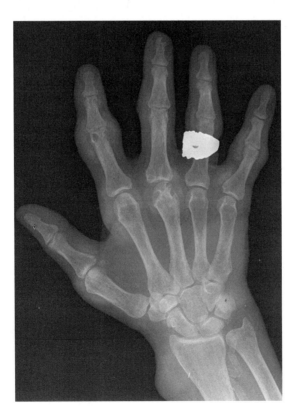

Figure 13.26 Tophaceous gout involving the hand. PA radiograph shows lumpy-bumpy soft tissue swelling and chronic focal bone erosions.

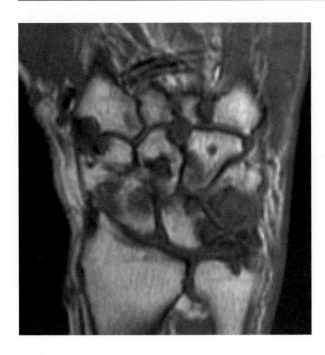

Figure 13.27 Tophaceous gout involving the carpus. Coronal T1-weighted MRI shows multiple low-signal masses eroding the carpal bones.

ular spaces may be preserved until late in the disease. Tophaceous gout may occur in combination with episodes of gouty arthritis.

MULTICENTRIC RETICULOHISTIOCYTOSIS

In the rare condition of multicentric reticulohistiocytosis, lipid-containing macrophages are deposited in the soft tissues around joints and tendons in random distribution. Skin nodules are common. As with gout and other metabolic deposition diseases, normal bone density and normal joint spaces are associated with intraosseous and juxta-articular accumulations. Bone erosions with sclerotic margins and overhanging edges are typical (Fig. 13.29), but sometimes a destructive arthritis ensues (arthritis mutilans). The origin of the abnormal lipid is unknown. In approximately 28% of cases, multicentric reticulohistiocytosis appears to be caused by a paraneoplastic disorder related to an underlying malignancy.

AMYLOID ARTHROPATHY

Amyloidosis is the result of several different underlying diseases in which a characteristic proteinaceous material accumulates in the body. The joint findings of amyloidosis in chronic renal dialysis patients have been well documented. Hemodialysis clears beta-immunoglobulins poorly from the blood. As these proteins accumulate in the body, they polymerize into

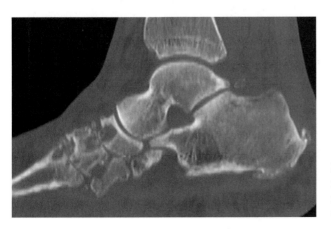

Figure 13.28 Tophaceous gout involving the midfoot. Sagittal CT-reformatted image shows multiple erosions with fragmentation.

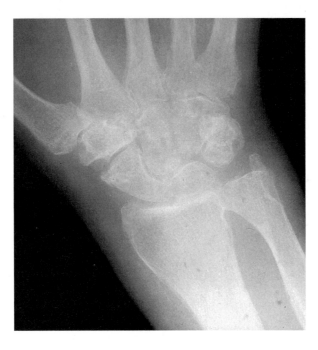

Figure 13.29 Multicentric reticulo-histiocytosis. The soft tissues are thickened, and there are chronic erosions with overhanging edges.

Amyloidosis may cause a chronic symmetric arthropathy.

beta-pleated sheets and become deposited in subcutaneous tissues, around joints, and occasionally in parenchymal organs. In addition to periarticular masses, a chronic symmetric arthropathy may also result, with clinical features similar to those of rheumatoid arthritis. Compression of the median nerve may result from deposition of amyloid in the carpal tunnel. Contractures and soft tissue swelling are common, and severe constitutional symptoms may be present. Amyloidosis has variable MRI appearance: low signal on both T1- and T2-weighted

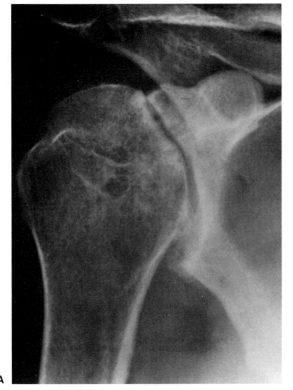

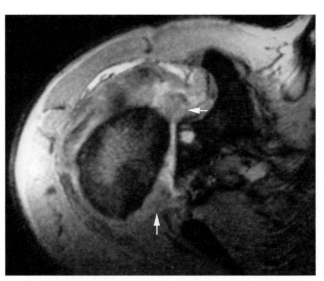

A   B

Figure 13.30 Amyloid arthropathy. *A.* Radiograph of the shoulder shows cartilage space loss and remodeling of the glenohumeral joint. *B.* Axial gradient-recalled echo MRI shows synovial masses (*arrows*) and degenerative changes.

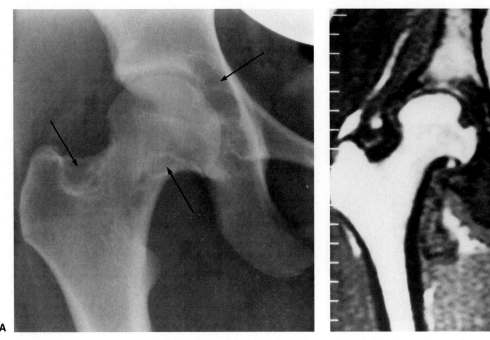

A   B

Figure 13.31 Diffuse pigmented villonodular synovitis of the hip. *A.* Radiograph shows chronic femoral neck erosions and medial acetabular erosions (*arrows*). *B.* Coronal T1-weighted MRI shows bulky low-signal masses in the synovium (*arrow*).

images (corresponding to fibrous tissue, amyloid deposits, or both), low signal on T1- with high signal on T2-weighted images (corresponding to fluid), and high signal on both T1- and T2-weighted images (corresponding to fatty component) (Fig. 13.30).

MISCELLANEOUS JOINT CONDITIONS

PIGMENTED VILLONODULAR SYNOVITIS

Pigmented villonodular synovitis (PVNS) is a benign neoplasm (rather than an inflammatory condition) of the synovium that usually presents as recurrent monarticular hemor-

PVNS may involve any synovial joint.

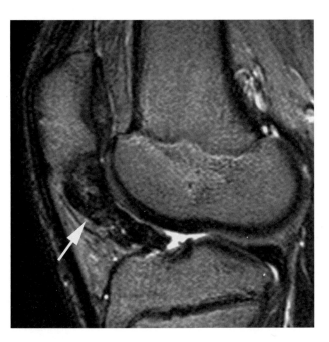

Figure 13.32 Focal pigmented villonodular synovitis of the knee. Sagittal T2-weighted fat-suppressed MRI shows dark signal within the mass (*arrow*).

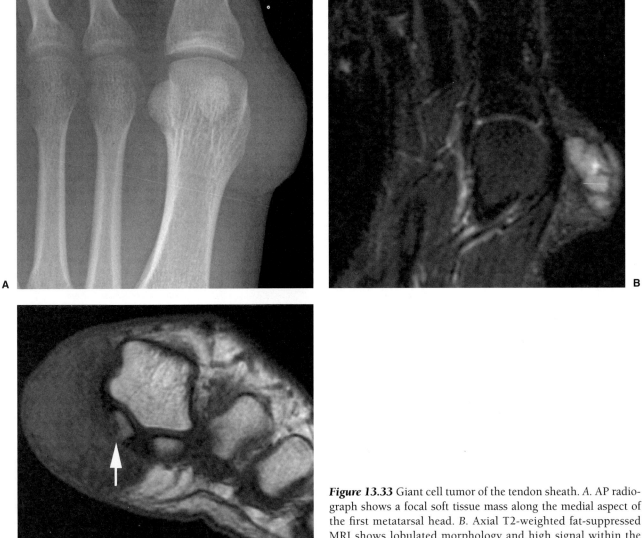

Figure 13.33 Giant cell tumor of the tendon sheath. *A*. AP radiograph shows a focal soft tissue mass along the medial aspect of the first metatarsal head. *B*. Axial T2-weighted fat-suppressed MRI shows lobulated morphology and high signal within the lesion. *C*. Coronal T1-weighted MRI shows low signal within the mass. The mass erodes the tibial sesamoid (*arrow*).

rhagic effusions in adults. It may have localized or diffuse involvement of the joint. The localized variety is typically represented by a focal nodular mass projecting into a joint. Common locations include the knee or hip, but any synovial tissue may be involved. Chronic, erosive changes from thickened, nodular synovial proliferation may be seen on radiographs. Localized osteoporosis is common. Arthritic changes such as joint space narrowing and osteophytes are generally absent. Arthrography shows multiple nodular filling defects. MRI shows effusion and multiple low-signal synovial masses (Figs. 13.31 and 13.32). The lesions are pigmented on gross examination because of hemosiderin deposition from repeated bleeding.

The extra-articular counterpart of PVNS, which is histologically identical, is called *giant cell tumor of the tendon sheath*. This lesion presents most commonly as a painless soft tissue mass in the hand, located along a tendon sheath. On radiographs, soft tissue swelling may be seen. On MRI, a soft tissue mass with low to intermediate signal intensity on T1-weighted images and heterogeneous high signal intensity on T2-weighted images is typical (Fig. 13.33). Enhancement after gadolinium injection may be seen on T1-weighted images. Giant cell tumor of the tendon sheath is not related to giant cell tumor of bone.

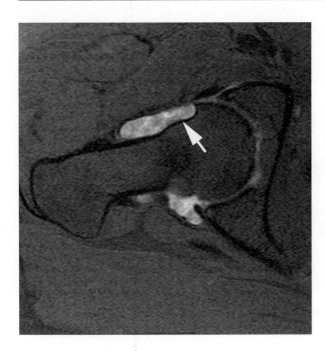

Figure 13.34 Synovial chondromatosis of the hip. Axial T1-weighted fat-suppressed MRI with intra-articular gadolinium injection shows erosions (*arrow*) of the femoral neck with synovial chondromas.

SYNOVIAL CHONDROMATOSIS

Synovial chondromatosis (synovial osteochondromatosis, synovial chondrometaplasia) is a condition characterized by the presence of multiple, benign cartilaginous nodules in the synovium. They may be loose within the joint or attached to the synovium. They may be calcified, ossified, or neither. When a synovial chondromatosis is not calcified, MRI examination shows a confluent soft tissue mass of high signal intensity on T2-weighted images within the joint. The mass may have foci of low signal on both T1- and T2-weighted images (Figs. 13.34 and 13.35). Synovial chondromatosis appears to be a reactive process rather than a neoplastic or degenerative one and can be distinguished histologically from secondary synovial chondrometaplasia, in which pieces of bone or cartilage from trauma or osteoarthritis become embedded in the synovium and stimulate a second-

Synovial chondromas may be calcified, ossified, or neither.

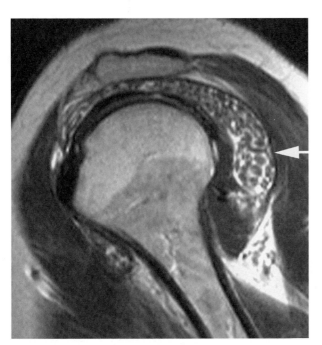

Figure 13.35 Synovial chondromatosis (*arrow*) of the shoulder. Oblique sagittal T2-weighted MRI shows multiple small synovial chondromas filling the subdeltoid subacromial bursa.

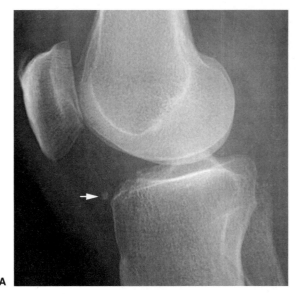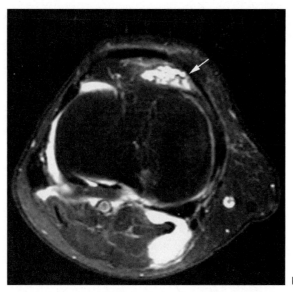

Figure 13.36 Synovial hemangioma. *A.* Lateral radiograph of knee shows a phlebolith (*arrow*) in infrapatellar fat pad. *B.* Axial T2-weighted MRI with fat suppression shows a high-signal-intensity lobulated mass (*arrow*) with septations. An incidental Baker cyst is present.

ary cartilaginous metaplasia. Because synovial chondromatosis may cause a mechanical destructive osteoarthritis, it may coexist with secondary synovial chondrometaplasia. Men are affected more than women by a ratio of 2:1, and the peak age of presentation is in the 40s.

SYNOVIAL HEMANGIOMATOSIS

Synovial hemangiomatosis is an unusual condition in which the joint capsule is involved by hemangiomas (Fig. 13.36). Hemangiomatosis results in intracapsular soft tissue masses that may cause extrinsic erosion of bone similar to those seen in PVNS or synovial chondromatosis. On radiographs, effusion, phleboliths, and erosions are seen. On arthrography or CT arthrography, synovial masses are seen. On MRI, the vascular nature of the lesion may be evident, with low signal on T1-weighted MRI, high signal on T2-weighted MRI, and enhancement on T1-weighted MRI after gadolinium injection. Repeated hemarthrosis is a potential complication.

BAKER CYST

A Baker cyst is a common synovial cyst that is located in the popliteal fossa. A Baker cyst results from distention of the gastrocnemius-semimembranosus bursa by fluid from the knee joint. The fluid enters through a slit-like communication with the posteromedial aspect of the knee capsule—just above the joint line—between the tendons of the medial head of the gastrocnemius and semimembranosus muscles. Baker cysts may be associated with any condition in which there is a knee effusion, including various forms of arthritis and various types of internal derangements. The most common complication of Baker cyst is rupture or dissection of fluid into the adjacent gastrocnemius muscle belly, often resulting in a pseudothrombophlebitis syndrome that mimics deep venous thrombosis of the calf. On MRI, a ruptured Baker cyst may be recognized by the presence of fluid extending from a Baker cyst or the site of a Baker cyst into the belly of the medial gastrocnemius muscle or the adjacent calf or thigh muscles (Fig. 13.37). A coexistent deep venous thrombosis may be present.

The most common complication of a Baker cyst is dissection of fluid into the adjacent gastrocnemius muscle belly.

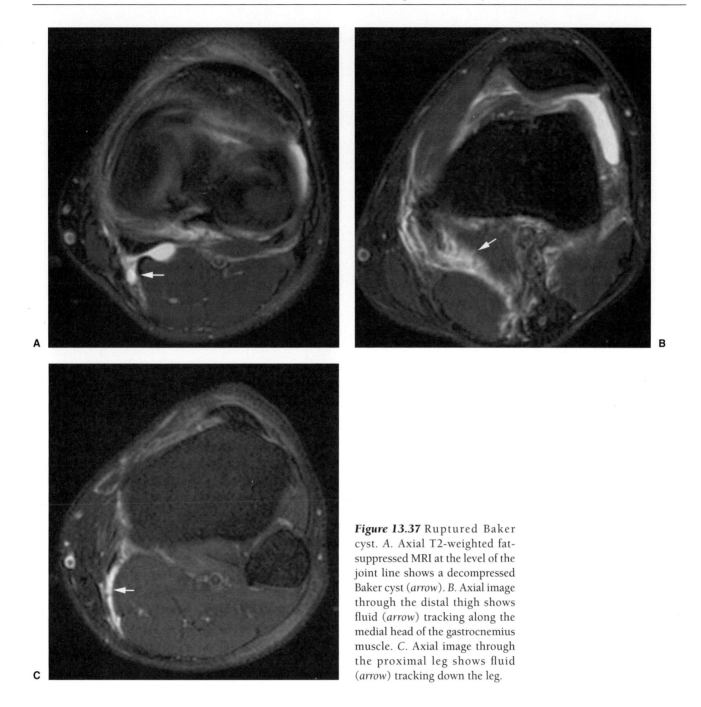

Figure 13.37 Ruptured Baker cyst. *A.* Axial T2-weighted fat-suppressed MRI at the level of the joint line shows a decompressed Baker cyst (*arrow*). *B.* Axial image through the distal thigh shows fluid (*arrow*) tracking along the medial head of the gastrocnemius muscle. *C.* Axial image through the proximal leg shows fluid (*arrow*) tracking down the leg.

POSTTRAUMATIC OSTEOLYSIS OF THE DISTAL CLAVICLE

Posttraumatic osteolysis of the distal clavicle is a painful condition that may result from previous acromioclavicular joint dislocation or repetitive microtrauma. On radiographs, posttraumatic osteolysis is evident as cortical irregularity of the distal clavicle with cyst-like erosions of subchondral bone, osteopenia, and soft tissue swelling (Fig. 13.38). Sometimes, aggressive osteolysis of the entire distal clavicle may be seen. On MRI, bone marrow edema in the distal clavicle without marrow edema in the acromion process is characteristic. Soft tissue swelling, periarticular erosions, and periostitis may also be present.

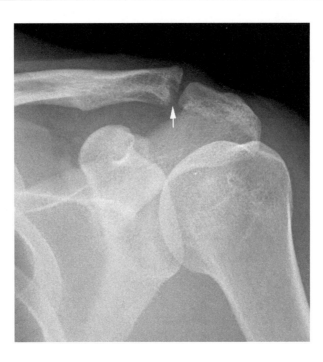

Figure 13.38 Osteolysis of the distal clavicle, with subchondral erosions (*arrow*).

DEGENERATIVE FOOT CONDITIONS

FLATFOOT (PES PLANUS)

Acquired flatfoot in adults (pes planus) is a common condition in which the medial longitudinal arch collapses during standing. The medial longitudinal arch consists of the bones along the medial side of the foot (calcaneus, talus, navicular, first cuneiform, first metatarsal) and the plantar fascia that helps maintain their position like a bowstring. The tibialis posterior muscle is a dynamic stabilizer of the arch that inserts on the navicular, the keystone of the arch. On the weight-bearing lateral radiograph, the talus, navicular, first cuneiform, and first metatarsal should be oriented in a straight line. Flatfoot is characterized by sagging of the midfoot below this hypothetical line at either the talonavicular joint (Fig. 13.39) or the navicular-cuneiform joint. An additional radiologic feature is superimposition of the metatarsal bases. On the weight-bearing AP radiograph, the metatarsals may appear splayed, and the talocalcaneal angle may be widened. If the medial longitudinal arch is restored to its normal alignment on non–weight-bearing radiographs, the flat foot is said to be flexible. The most common cause of flatfoot is hereditary, and the majority of the 15% to 20% of the adult U.S. population with flatfoot is asymptomatic. Patients with developmentally hypermobile joints—such as those with Marfan syndrome, Ehler-Danlos syndrome, or Down syndrome—often have flexible flatfoot. Flexible flatfoot is also common among those with acquired hypermobile joints in conditions such as systemic lupus erythematosus. Rigid flatfoot may result from conditions such as heel cord contractures and tarsal coalitions.

> Flatfoot is characterized by sagging of the midfoot at either the talonavicular or the navicular-cuneiform joints.

CALCANEUS

Calcaneal spurs are common enthesopathic changes involving the insertions of the plantar aponeurosis and the Achilles tendon. They may become symptomatic through pressure and inflammation of adjacent soft tissues and bursae. Posttraumatic ossification is also common at these sites.

A Haglund deformity is a prominence of the posterior superior margin of the calcaneus that becomes symptomatic because of impingement of improperly fitted footwear.

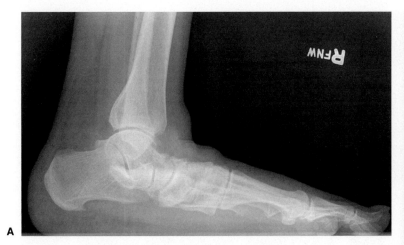

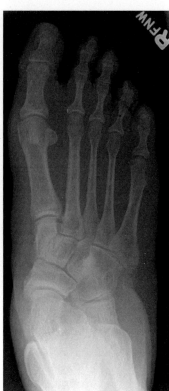

Figure 13.39 Flatfoot (pes planus). *A.* Weight-bearing lateral radiograph shows sagging of a hypothetical line drawn between the first metatarsal and the neck of the talus. The metatarsal bases are superimposed on each other. *B.* Weight-bearing AP radiograph shows mild splaying of the metatarsals with the metatarsal bases overlapping each other only slightly.

Plantar fasciitis is an inflammatory condition involving the calcaneal origin of the medial cord of the plantar aponeurosis. The sole of the foot is typically painful with weight-bearing or athletic activity. A bony spur may develop at the plantar aspect of the calcaneus. On MRI, the plantar aponeurosis may be thickened at its origin and show increased signal on both T1- and T2-weighted images (Fig. 13.40). Surrounding edema may also be present in the soft tissues and occasionally in the adjacent calcaneal tuberosity.

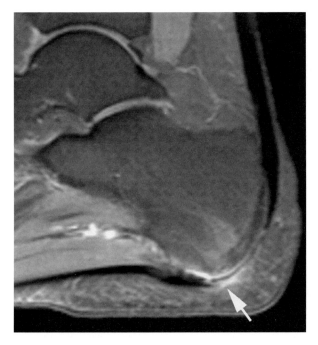

Figure 13.40 Plantar fasciitis. Sagittal T2-weighted fat-suppressed MRI shows high signal at the calcaneal origin of the medial cord of the plantar aponeurosis (*arrow*).

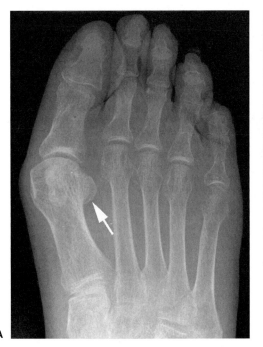
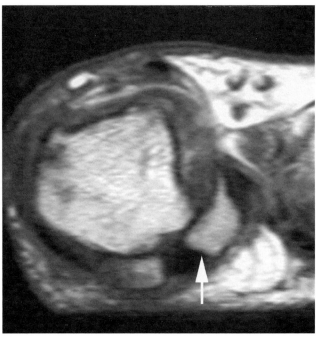

Figure 13.41 Bunion deformity (hallux valgus metatarsus primus varus). *A.* AP weight-bearing radiograph of the foot shows varus deformity of the first metatarsal combined with valgus deformity of the great toe. Note the overriding of the second toe over the great toe and lateral subluxation of the lateral sesamoid (*arrow*) relative to the head of the first metatarsal. *B.* Coronal T1-weighted MRI through the head of the first metatarsal shows lateral subluxation of the sesamoids (*arrow*) with degenerative change.

GREAT TOE

A bunion (hallux valgus metatarsus primus varus) is a symptomatic complex of deformities characterized by a bony prominence at the medial aspect of the first MTP joint. It consists of lateral deviation of the great toe (hallux valgus), medial deviation of the first metatarsal (metatarsus primus varus), soft tissue contractures of the great toe flexors, and secondary degenerative change at the first MTP joint. Progressive soft tissue contracture pulls like a bowstring to increase the deformity. A bunion can be recognized on weight-bearing AP radiographs of the foot by varus deviation of the first metatarsal and valgus deviation of the great toe. The degree of uncovering of the articular surface of the first metatarsal head by the proximal phalanx of the great toe depends on the severity of the hallux valgus. Together, these deformities result in lateral subluxation of the sesamoids relative to the head of the first metatarsal (Fig. 13.41). In severe cases, the second toe may override the great toe because of the hallux valgus.

Hallux rigidus and *hallux limitus* refer to osteoarthritis at the first MTP joint with stiffness and limitation of motion. There is typically a prominent dorsal osteophyte at the distal articular surface of the first metatarsal.

LESSER TOES

Deformities of the lesser toes are usually caused by contractures of the flexor or extensor tendons of the foot. A claw toe deformity is hyperextension of the MTP joint and flexion of the IP joints. A hammer toe deformity is flexion at the PIP joint, usually with hyperextension at the MTP joint (it may be identical to a claw toe deformity) (Fig. 13.42). A mallet toe deformity is DIP flexion. These various toe deformities are generally treated surgically with resection arthroplasty. Rather than lengthening the tendons, this procedure shortens the bones so that the tendons are at the correct relative length.

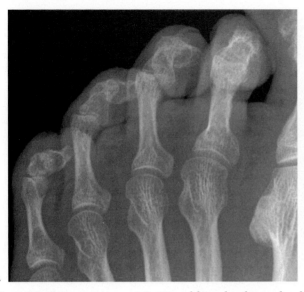
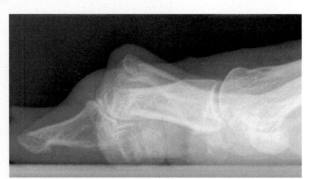

A   **B**

Figure 13.42 Hammer toes. *A,B.* AP and lateral radiographs show proximal interphalangeal joint flexion deformities of the lesser toes.

A bunionette deformity (also called a *tailor's bunion*) is a bony prominence on the lateral side of the fifth metatarsal head. When symptomatic, there may be overlying soft tissue swelling.

DEGENERATIVE DISC DISEASE

Degenerative disc disease commonly coexists with osteoarthritis of the synovial joints of the spine. The biomechanical loads on the spine are shared among the intervertebral disc joints, the various fibrous articulations, and the synovial joints, so that the integrity of each component is dependent on the others. There is some evidence that primary degeneration of the cartilaginous end plates, through which water diffuses to the disc, leads to dehydration of both the nucleus pulposus and the annulus fibrosus. Dehydration of the nucleus pulposus can be demonstrated by MRI in young adults and is perhaps an early consequence of aging. The normal nucleus pulposus has high signal on T2-weighted MRI; if it is dehydrated, it has low signal. Congenital factors as well as abnormalities such as scoliosis and spondylolysis may contribute. The loss of hydration results in decreased tissue resiliency and is greatest in the nucleus pulposus. The normal hydraulic distribution of stresses over the entire articular surface is lost, and secondary tears and degeneration of the annulus fibrosus may result. Adaptive changes eventually involve the bones. The radiographic result is moderate to severe loss of intervertebral disc height, gas in the intervertebral disc, and well-defined sclerosis of the adjacent vertebral body end plates (Fig. 13.43). This condition of disc degeneration is called *intervertebral osteochondrosis*. Breakdown of the attachment of the outer (Sharpey) fibers of the annulus fibrosus to the vertebral rim allows circumferential displacement (bulging) of the disc. Osteophytes grow at the attachments of the annulus fibrosus and the anterior longitudinal ligament to the vertebral body. This degenerative process with osteophyte formation is called *spondylosis deformans*. Tears through the annulus fibrosus allow fragments of the disc to protrude into the substance of the annulus and herniate through it. Herniated disc fragments may impinge on neural structures, often nerve roots, and cause symptoms. Circumferential disc bulges may narrow the spinal canal. CT and MRI may demonstrate degenerative changes and disc pathology (Fig. 13.44), but the correlation of radiologic findings with symptoms is not consistent. The facet and costovertebral joints may be secondarily involved from altered biomechanics caused by disc degeneration.

Senile kyphosis occurs in the thoracic spine of older patients. It is related to mechanical failure of the anterior aspect of the intervertebral disc, leading to loss of disc height anteriorly,

Spondylosis deformans is the degenerative process in which osteophytes form along the anterior vertebral bodies.

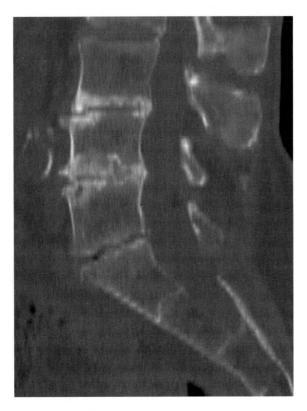

Figure 13.43 Discogenic sclerosis in the lower lumbar spine, with loss of disc height, shown on sagittal CT-reformatted image.

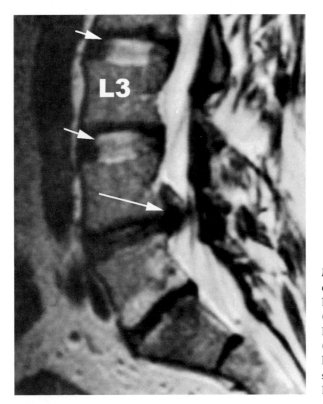

Figure 13.44 Degenerative lumbar disc herniation. Sagittal T2-weighted MRI shows degenerative disc disease (low signal) at L4-L5 and L5-S1. The L4-L5 disc has herniated posteriorly (*long arrow*). Note normal disc height and normal hydration (high signal) of the nucleus pulposus at L3-L4 and L2-L3 (*short arrows*).

secondary vertebral sclerosis, and sometimes ankylosis. Osteoporotic kyphosis is a different (but sometimes coexisting) process involving insufficiency fractures of the anterior aspects of osteoporotic vertebral bodies (see Chapter 15).

DIFFUSE IDIOPATHIC SKELETAL HYPEROSTOSIS

Diffuse idopathic skeletal hyperostosis (DISH) (ankylosing hyperostosis of the spine, Forestier disease) is a radiographically defined condition characterized by ossification of the soft tissues at the attachments of muscles, ligaments, and tendons to bone. DISH appears to represent an ossifying diathesis or bone-forming tendency of unknown etiology that increases in incidence with age.

DISH may lead to extra-articular bony ankylosis of the spine.

DISH is common in older adults, more frequently men, and the symptoms are often back stiffness and pain. The precise definition of DISH is still evolving. Resnick and Niwayama give the following criteria for spinal involvement in DISH: (a) flowing calcification and ossification along the anterolateral aspect of at least four contiguous vertebral bodies, (b) relative preservation of disc height in the involved vertebral body segments and absence of extensive radiographic changes of degenerative disc disease (gas in the disc space or vertebral body sclerosis), and (c) absence of facet joint ankylosis and sacroiliac (SI) joint erosion, sclerosis, or intra-articular osseous fusion. These criteria distinguish DISH from spondylosis deformans, intervertebral osteochondrosis, and ankylosing spondylitis. There are no associated laboratory abnormalities. Bone density remains normal. Extraspinal manifestations of DISH are exceedingly common in older patients. Ossification at the insertion of tendons may be seen throughout the extremities (Fig. 13.45). In the pelvis, whiskering bone proliferation is common along sites where muscles and ligaments attach. Para-articular bone growths correspond to ossification at the attachments of joint capsules. For practical purposes, the diagnosis of DISH can be made radiographically when there is excessive enthesal ossification in the absence of other conditions known to cause such ossification (e.g., spondyloarthropathy or previous trauma).

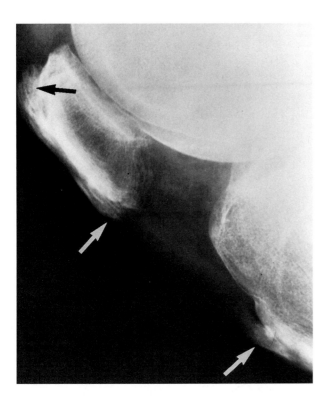

Figure 13.45 Diffuse idiopathic skeletal hyperostosis with ossified entheses at the quadriceps and infrapatellar tendons (*arrows*).

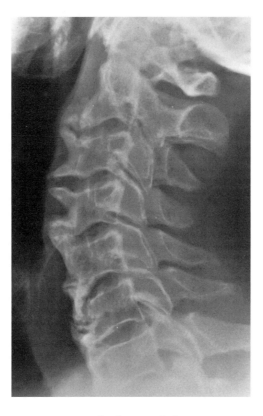

Figure 13.46 Diffuse idiopathic skeletal hyperostosis involving cervical spine.

Extra-articular bony ankylosis is very common in the thoracic spine and somewhat less common in the cervical and lumbar regions (Fig. 13.46). Extra-articular ankylosis of the spine makes the spine stiff. Despite the increase in bone mass, the spine may be more fragile biomechanically when subjected to trauma. The lack of motion and the loss of the

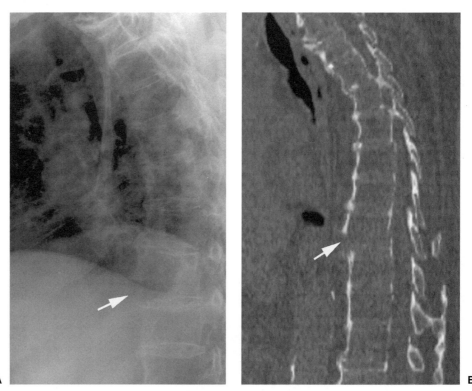

Figure 13.47 Fracture (*arrows*) at the thoracolumbar junction in a patient with diffuse idiopathic skeletal hyperostosis. *A.* Lateral radiograph. *B.* Sagittal CT-reformatted image.

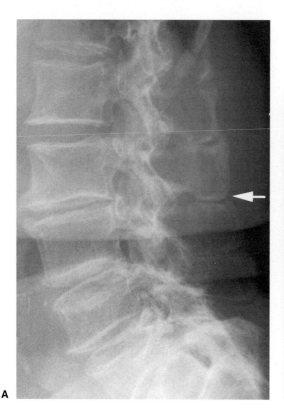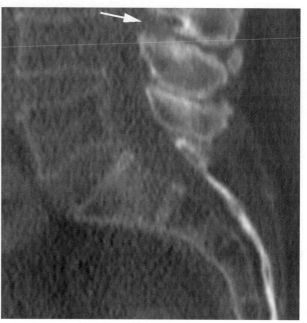

A   B

Figure 13.48 Baastrup disease (different patients). *A.* Lateral radiograph shows hyperostosis of the spinous processes with kissing spines (*arrow*). *B.* Sagittal CT reformation shows kissing spines (*arrow*).

energy-absorbing function of the intervertebral discs and ligaments contribute to its decreased ability to absorb loading. Fractures and fracture-dislocations of the spine may be catastrophic (Fig. 13.47).

BAASTRUP DISEASE

Baastrup disease (osteoarthrosis interspinalis) is a degenerative condition described in the lumbar spine in which there is hyperostosis of the spinous processes leading to remodeling and joint formation between adjacent spinous processes (Fig. 13.48). The condition has also been described as *kissing spines*. The relationship of Baastrup disease to chronic low back pain is uncertain.

SOURCES AND READINGS

Brandt KD, Doherty M, Lohmander LS, eds. *Osteoarthritis.* New York: Oxford University Press, 1998.

Brower AC. *Arthritis in black and white,* 2nd ed. Philadelphia: WB Saunders, 1997.

Burke BJ, Esobedo EM, Wilson AJ, et al. Chondrocalcinosis mimicking a meniscal tear on MR imaging. *AJR Am J Roentgenol* 1998;170:69–70.

Dieppe P, Calvert P. *Crystals and joint disease.* London: Chapman and Hall, 1983.

Forrester DM, Brown JC. *The radiology of joint disease,* 3rd ed. Philadelphia: WB Saunders, 1987.

Frediani B, Falsetti P, Storri L, et al. Quadricepital tendon enthesitis in psoriatic arthritis and rheumatoid arthritis: ultrasound examinations and clinical correlations. *J Rheumatol* 2001;28:2566–2568.

Groshar D, Rozenbaum M, Rosner I. Enthesopathies, inflammatory spondyloarthropathies and bone scintigraphy. *J Nucl Med* 1997;38:2003–2005.

Huskisson EC, Dudley Hart F. *Joint disease: all the arthropathies*, 4th ed. Bristol: Wright, 1987.

Kaplan PA, Helms CA, Dussault R, et al. *Musculoskeletal MRI.* Philadelphia: WB Saunders, 2001.

Kaushik S, Erickson JK, Palmer WE, et al. Effect on chondrocalcinosis on the MR imaging of knee menisci. *AJR Am J Roentgenol* 2001;177:905–909.

McCarty DJ, Koopman WJ, eds. *Arthritis and allied conditions: a textbook of rheumatology*, 12th ed. Philadelphia: Lea & Febiger, 1993.

McGonagle D, Gibbon W, Emery P. Classification of inflammatory arthritis by enthesitis. *Lancet* 1998;352:1137–1140.

Modic MT, Masaryk TJ, Ross JS. *Magnetic resonance imaging of the spine*, 2nd ed. St. Louis: Mosby, 1994.

Moskowitz RW, Howell DS, Altman RD, et al., eds. *Osteoarthritis: diagnosis and medical/surgical management.* Philadelphia: WB Saunders, 2001.

Olivieri I, Barozzi L, Padula A. Enthesiopathy: clinical manifestations, imaging and treatment. *Bailliere Clin Rheum* 1998;12:665–681.

Resnick D, ed. *Diagnosis of bone and joint disorders*, 4th ed. Philadelphia: WB Saunders, 2002.

Resnick D, Niwayama G. Entheses and enthesopathy. Anatomical, pathological, and radiological correlation. *Radiology* 1983;146:1–9.

Ruddy S, Harris ED Jr, Sledge CB, et al., eds. *Textbook of rheumatology*, 6th ed. Philadelphia: WB Saunders, 2001.

Salvarani C, Cantini F, Olivieri I, et al. Magnetic resonance imaging and polymyalgia rheumatica. *J Rheumatol* 2001;28:918–919.

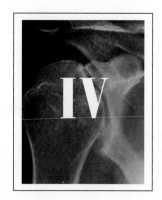

MISCELLANEOUS TOPICS

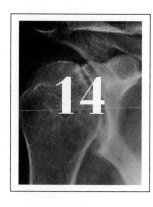

DEVELOPMENTAL AND CONGENITAL CONDITIONS

This chapter describes the radiology of many developmental and congenital conditions that affect the musculoskeletal system. Many of these conditions are heritable (Table 14.1).

SKELETAL MATURATION

The skeleton develops and matures with a consistent and irreversible sequence of changes in osseous size and contour. Particular features in the contours of developing bones are useful maturational landmarks in the sequence of ossification. These features are used to estimate skeletal age. The most practical method is to use the radiographic atlas of Greulich and Pyle.

This atlas contains radiographs of the left hand and wrist in boys and girls of different ages—correlated with their chronologic age—from the neonate to the skeletally mature. A radiograph of the left hand and wrist of the individual patient is compared to these standards, and a best match is found. Each chronologic age has a mean bone age and a standard deviation in bone age. The radiologic report of the bone age should include the bone age itself as well as the standard deviation in bone age for the patient's chronologic age.

OTHER DISORDERS

Greulich and Pyle's atlas is based on radiographs of healthy children of northern European ancestry from Cleveland, Ohio, whose families were incidentally above average in economic and educational status. These children were followed between 1931 and 1942 as

Table 14.1: Relatively Common Heritable Disorders of the Musculoskeletal System

Autosomal-dominant inheritance	Autosomal-recessive inheritance
Multiple hereditary exostoses	Congenital insensitivity to pain
Achondroplasia	Diastrophic dwarfism
Brachydactyly	Gaucher disease
Cleidocranial dysostosis	Hurler syndrome
Marfan syndrome	Morquio syndrome
Multiple epiphyseal dysplasia	Scheie syndrome
Nail patella syndrome	Hypophosphatasia
Neurofibromatosis	Osteogenesis imperfecta (severe forms)
Polydactyly	Osteopetrosis
Osteopathia striata	
Osteogenesis imperfecta (mild forms)	
Osteopetrosis	
X-linked inheritance	
X-linked dominant	
Vitamin D–resistant rickets	
X-linked recessive	
Hemophilia	
Pseudohypertrophic muscular dystrophy	

part of a longitudinal long-term investigation of human growth and development. This project produced atlases of skeletal development for the hand and wrist, the knee, and the foot and ankle. One limitation to the applicability of these atlases is the particular population that was studied, but such a study is unlikely ever to be duplicated.

HERITABLE CONNECTIVE TISSUE DISORDERS

OSTEOGENESIS IMPERFECTA

Osteogenesis imperfecta is a group of inborn connective tissue disorders characterized by radiographically decreased bone density. The underlying problem is one of abnormal collagen synthesis, in which a variety of different molecular defects in collagen produces a continuous spectrum of phenotypes. In the skeleton, the bone matrix is deficient, resulting in thin, osteoporotic, and fragile bones that are subject to repeated insufficiency fractures and consequent deformity (Fig. 14.1). The condition is heritable, but cases are often sporadic. In general, there are autosomal-recessive severe forms that present at birth and autosomal-dominant forms that present later and have a mild course. The condition ranges from severe, congenital involvement with multiple fractures in utero and perinatal death to mild, late manifestations in adulthood. The severe forms account for 10% of cases; the less severe forms account for the remaining 90%. The incidence of osteogenesis imperfecta is 1 per 20,000 to 60,000 live births. Associated clinical features—with variable expression—include blue sclerae (90%); thin, translucent skin; hypermobile, lax peripheral joints; abnormal teeth (dentinogenesis imperfecta); and deafness (fragile otic bones).

> Osteogenesis imperfecta is heritable, but cases are often sporadic.

OTHER DISORDERS

Marfan syndrome, homocystinuria, and Ehlers-Danlos syndrome are heterogeneous groups of heritable connective tissue disorders with musculoskeletal manifestations. Marfan syndrome is associated with excessive height, long spidery digits (arachnodactyly), hypermobile joints, and scoliosis (Fig. 14.2). Ocular and cardiovascular abnormalities dominate the clinical picture. Accumulation of amino acid metabolites in homocystinuria interferes with collagen cross linking, leading to fragile bones, scoliosis, and excessive

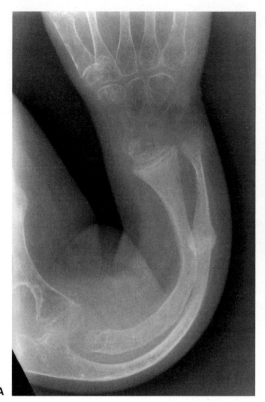 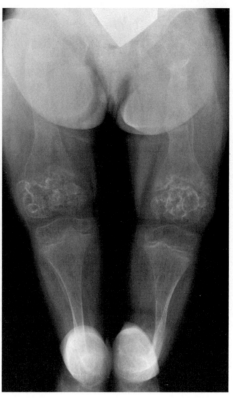

Figure 14.1 Osteogenesis imperfecta. *A.* Radiograph of forearm shows osteoporosis, bowing deformity, and healing-insufficiency fractures of different ages. *B.* Lower extremities show similar findings along with popcorn epiphyses.

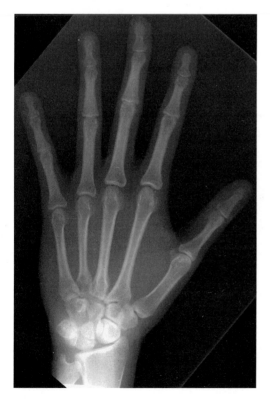

Figure 14.2 Marfan syndrome. Radiograph of the hand shows arachnodactyly. Hypermobility is present at the carpus, with overlap of the proximal and distal carpal rows.

length of long bones. Ehlers-Danlos syndrome is associated with fragile skin and hypermobile joints.

SCLEROSING DYSPLASIAS

The sclerosing skeletal dysplasias are a heterogeneous group of conditions characterized radiographically by dense bones.

OSTEOPETROSIS

Osteopetrosis is a group of heritable diseases characterized by reduced bone resorption from osteoclast failure. Many genetic defects may cause osteoclast failure, each having different underlying biochemical and histopathologic abnormalities. One form is associated with renal tubular acidosis and rickets. The final common effect is that bone remodels incompletely or not at all. There are three major clinical groups: infantile-malignant autosomal recessive, which is fatal within the first few years of life (in the absence of effective therapy); intermediate autosomal recessive, which appears during the first decade of life but does not follow a malignant course; and autosomal dominant (Albers-Schönberg disease or marble bones), which has a normal life expectancy but many orthopedic problems. The infantile variant has clinical manifestations that correlate with the lack of marrow development (anemia and thrombocytopenia) and the lack of enlargement of bony remodeling (small cranial foramina result in cranial nerve dysfunction, hydrocephalus, convulsions, and mental retardation). Radiographs show uniformly dense bones with no medullary space, broadened metaphyses (Erlenmeyer flask deformity), and bone-within-a-bone appearance at the tarsals, carpals, phalanges, vertebrae, and iliac wings (Fig. 14.3). Transverse insufficiency fractures occur

> Osteopetrotic bone is fragile and remodels poorly in response to stress.

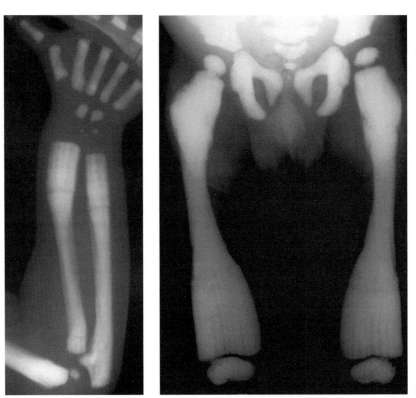

Figure 14.3 Osteopetrosis, autosomal-dominant type (Albers-Schönberg disease). *A.* Radiograph of the arm shows dense bones lacking a medullary space. *B.* Radiograph of femurs shows club-shaped metaphyses.

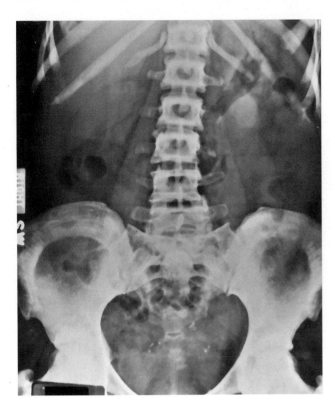

Figure 14.4 Osteopetrosis, incidental adult presentation.

often. Medical treatments involve high-dose calcitriol to stimulate osteoclast differentiation and bone marrow transplantation to provide monocytic osteoclast precursors. The intermediate and autosomal-dominant forms have mild manifestations that include anemia, cranial nerve palsies, and orthopedic problems. The fragility of osteopetrotic bone and its inability to remodel in response to stress result in repeated insufficiency fractures. Coxa vara, long-bone bowing, hip and knee degenerative arthritis, and mandibular and long-bone osteomyelitis may also occur. Even milder forms of osteopetrosis may be asymptomatic and discovered incidentally on radiographs (Fig. 14.4).

OSTEOPOIKILOSIS

Osteopoikilosis (spotted bones, osteopathia condensans disseminata) is an uncommon osteosclerotic dysplasia with sporadic and familial occurrence. Symptoms are generally absent or mild, and its discovery is frequently incidental. The condition is defined by the presence of numerous small, well-defined, homogeneous ovoid or circular foci of increased radiodensity clustered in periarticular osseous regions. The distribution is symmetric, typically involving the epiphyses and metaphyses of long bones, as well as the carpus, tarsus, scapula, and pelvis (Fig. 14.5). The lesions may increase or decrease in size or number. They are histologically identical to bone islands but have no clinical significance unless mistaken for other lesions.

OSTEOPATHIA STRIATA

Osteopathia striata (Voorhoeve disease) is a rare condition whose transmission is probably autosomal dominant. The condition is defined by the presence of linear, regular bands of increased radiodensity extending from the metaphyses to the diaphyses of tubular bones and the pelvis (Fig. 14.6). Osteopathia striata is usually bilateral, and it is unusual for it to involve the small bones of hands or feet, skull or face, or spine. The cause and pathogenesis are unknown. Clinical manifestations are usually absent, although facial deformity has been described. Discovery is usually incidental.

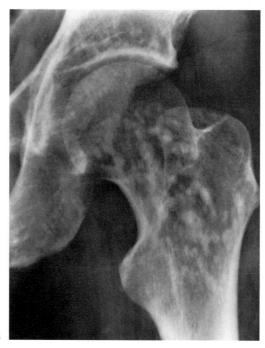

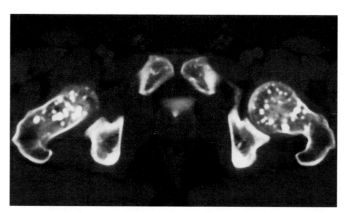

Figure 14.5 Osteopoikilosis. *A.* AP radiograph. *B.* CT scan.

MELORHEOSTOSIS

Melorheostosis is a rare, nonhereditary condition that presents in childhood with extremity pain, limitation of motion, and intermittent joint swelling. Growth disturbances, soft tissue involvement, and increasing muscle contractures due to tendon and ligament shortening may result in considerable deformity and disability. The condition

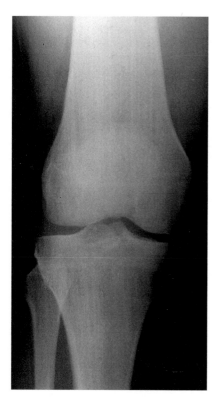

Figure 14.6 Osteopathia striata.

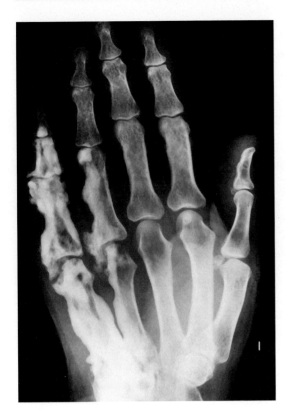

Figure 14.7 Melorheostosis involving the fourth and fifth rays of the hand.

is commonly limited to a single limb, usually lower. Radiologically, there is extensive periosteal or endosteal cortical hyperostosis with bony excrescences extending along the length of the bone, giving it a wavy contour that has been likened to wax dripping down a candle (Figs. 14.7 and 14.8). Endosteal hyperostosis may fill the medullary cavity, but periosteal and endosteal hyperostosis usually do not occur together. The radiologic appearance is characteristic. The cause and pathogenesis are unknown; the bony excrescences are histologically normal bone.

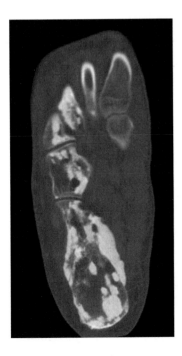

Figure 14.8 Melorheostosis involving the foot shown on axial CT scan.

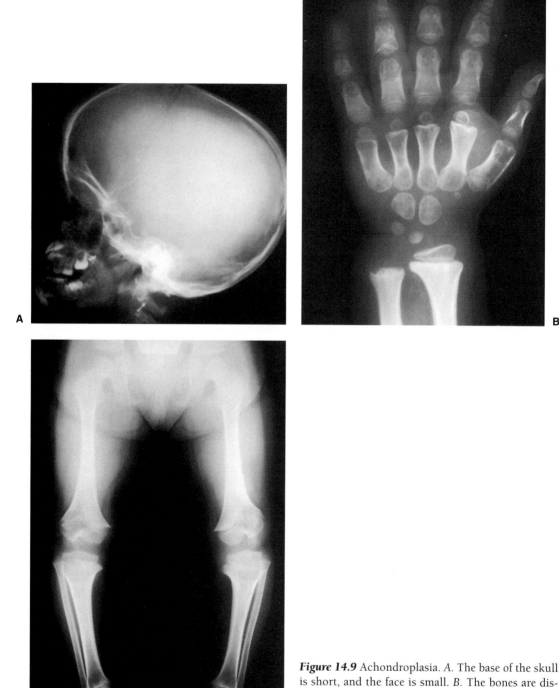

Figure 14.9 Achondroplasia. *A.* The base of the skull is short, and the face is small. *B.* The bones are disproportionately short, and the fingers appear stubby. *C.* The femurs are short and thick.

CONGENITAL DWARFISM

Dwarfism is the condition of being disproportionately undersized. Skeletal dysplasias with dwarfism are legion. Dozens of specific types are listed in the International Nomenclature of Constitutional Diseases of Bone as revised in 1983 by the European Society of Pediatric Radiology. For most of these conditions, there are only a handful of reported cases. Many conditions are lethal, none are reversible, and most are not defined on a radiologic basis. The distinction among the dysplasias with dwarfism often requires detailed genetic, biochemical, histochemical, and histopathologic analysis.

ACHONDROPLASIA

Achondroplasia is the most common type of dwarfism and has a classic radiologic appearance. Achondroplasia is the result of a generalized defect in enchondral bone formation, leading to underdevelopment of the portions of bones that grow by this mechanism. The result is a symmetric short-limbed dwarfism in which the proximal segments of the extremities are disproportionately short (rhizomelic micromelia). Because periosteal bone growth is unaffected, the shafts of the long bones are of normal diameter. The fingers are short and stubby. The skull base, formed by enchondral bone formation, is abnormally short and has a small foramen magnum. The calvaria, formed by intramembranous bone formation, is appropriately large for the intracranial contents, giving the head a characteristic brachycephaly with frontal bossing and a small face (Fig. 14.9). The spinal canal is narrow in both anteroposterior and lateral dimensions, but the trunk length is nearly normal. There is an exaggerated lumbar lordosis with prominent buttocks. These abnormalities are usually evident at birth and become more apparent with age. Achondroplasia has autosomal-dominant genetic transmission, but most cases are sporadic. The classic form is heterozygous, has no associated congenital defects, and is compatible with a normal life span. Complications of congenital spinal stenosis are common in adulthood (Fig. 14.10). The homozygous condition is lethal in infancy and has a radiologic appearance identical to thanatophoric dwarfism. Thanatophoric ("death-bringing") dwarfism is the most common lethal bone dysplasia.

The long bones have normal shaft widths in achondroplasia.

OTHER TYPES

Other types of dwarfism may be characterized and classified by the predominant location of disproportionate shortening. Mesomelic micromelia refers to shortening of the forearms

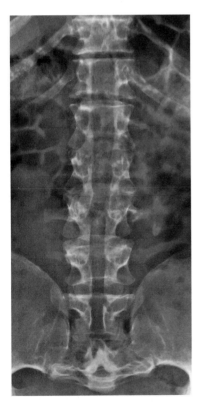

Figure 14.10 Achondroplasia in an adult with spinal stenosis in the lumbar region. Laminectomy has been performed at all levels.

and lower legs. Examples of mesomelic dwarfism include camptomelic dwarfism and dyschondrosteosis of the Nievergett and Langer types. Acromelic micromelia refers to shortening of the hands and feet. Examples of acromelic dwarfism include asphyxiating thoracic dystrophy (Jeune syndrome), chondroectodermal dysplasia (Ellis-van Creveld syndrome), and pyknodysostosis. Many of these dysplasias are amenable to prenatal diagnosis with obstetric sonography, reducing even further the role of radiography.

MISCELLANEOUS GENERALIZED CONDITIONS

NEUROFIBROMATOSIS

Neurofibromatosis is one of the heritable phakomatoses, characterized by multisystem involvement of hamartomas involving all three germ cell layers. Neurofibromatosis has autosomal-dominant transmission. There are multiple subtypes. Major musculoskeletal manifestations include scoliosis, mesodermal dysplasia, and neurofibromas. Although the scoliosis may be gently curving and identical to idiopathic scoliosis, occasionally a sharply angulated dysplastic thoracic kyphoscoliosis is present and virtually diagnostic. Mesodermal dysplasia may result in focally abnormal or deficient bone formation, often manifested by the presence of multiple nonossifying fibromas (Fig. 14.11). Orthopedic complications in neurofibromatosis include bowing, pathologic fracture, pseudoarthrosis, and defective fracture healing (Fig. 14.12). The tibia is a characteristic site for pseudoarthrosis; repeated failures to heal after treatment often lead to amputation. Neurofibromas may erode adjacent bones and present as soft tissue masses.

> A sharply angulated dysplastic thoracic kyphoscoliosis is virtually diagnostic of neurofibromatosis.

MULTIPLE EPIPHYSEAL DYSPLASIA

Multiple epiphyseal dysplasia (dysplasia epiphysealis multiplex, Fairbank disease) is the most common of a heterogeneous group of disorders characterized by abnormal growth and development of epiphyses at multiple sites. Multiple epiphyseal dysplasia has autosomal-

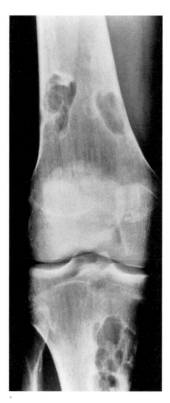

Figure 14.11 Multiple nonossifying fibromatosis at the knee in neurofibromatosis.

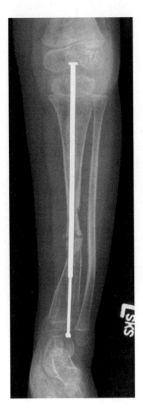

Figure 14.12 Pseudoarthrosis of the tibia in neurofibromatosis. A telescoping rod has been placed for mechanical support.

dominant transmission. The primary defect involves an abnormality in the biochemical composition of the ground substance produced by the epiphyseal chondrocytes, resulting in delayed and disorderly ossification, joint incongruity, and secondary degenerative change. After onset in early childhood, the variable clinical manifestations include articular pain, gait disturbances, short stature, and involvement of multiple sites. Radiographically, the secondary ossification centers occur late and are irregular in morphology. After skeletal maturity, the epiphyses remain irregular and abnormal in shape, tending to be flattened and squared off (Fig. 14.13). Early osteoarthritis is a common sequela.

CEREBRAL PALSY

Cerebral palsy can result in generalized or focal neuromuscular disease in which secondary bone changes and complications are seen. These changes are the result of abnormal stresses

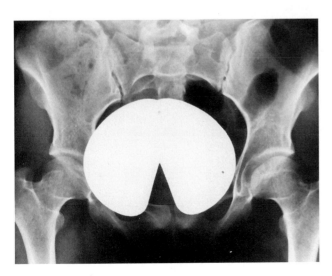

Figure 14.13 Multiple epiphyseal dysplasia (dysplasia epiphysealis multiplex).

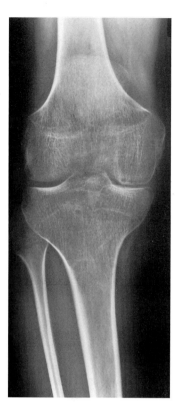

Figure 14.14 Cerebral palsy in a young adult. The epiphyses at the knee are large and dysplastic.

on the growing skeleton from muscular spasm, weakness, atrophy, and imbalance (Fig. 14.14). When the normal skeleton remodels in response to abnormal stress, dysplastic changes in the bones and joints may result. Long bones often appear overtubulated (narrow shaft, broad epiphysis). Hip dysplasia secondary to chronic, spastic dislocation is common. Spasm of the thigh adductor muscles positions the femoral head on the lateral acetabular rim, resulting in deformity, subluxation, and, ultimately, hip dislocation (Fig. 14.15).

Scoliosis, soft tissue atrophy, and flexion or extension contractures may be found. Foot deformities of various kinds are common. Similar developmental changes are seen in

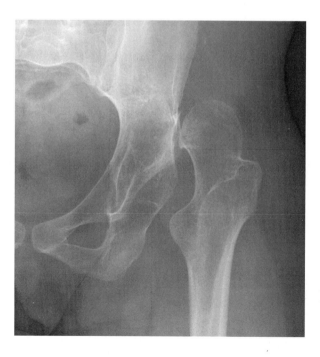

Figure 14.15 Adult with developmental dysplasia of the hip resulting from cerebral palsy and chronic hip dislocation without weight bearing.

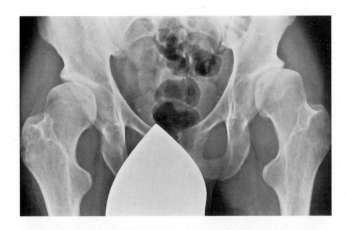

Figure 14.16 Muscular dystrophy in a young adult. The hips are shallow, and the femoral neck angles are nearly straight.

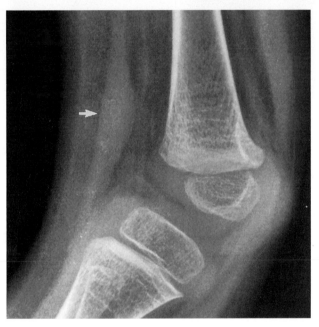

Figure 14.17 Arthrogryposis with poor muscle development and recurvatum deformity (anterior to left; arrow points to cartilaginous patella).

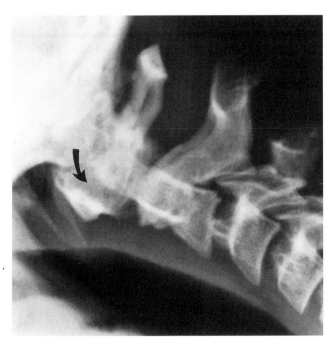

Figure 14.18 Down syndrome with atlantoaxial subluxation (*arrow*).

conditions such as arthrogryposis, muscular dystrophy (Fig. 14.16), peripheral nerve palsy, and polio.

ARTHROGRYPOSIS MULTIPLEX CONGENITA

Arthrogryposis multiplex congenita is an uncommon nonhereditary congenital disorder that manifests with deformed joints, dislocations, and muscle wasting (Fig. 14.17). The deformities are widespread and bilateral and usually cause severe disabilities, but the patient's life span is often normal. Frequent deformities include clubfoot (talipes equinovarus, present in 75% of cases), flexion deformity of the knee (60%), flexion deformity of the hip (40%), and dislocation of the hip with resultant dysplasia (40%).

DOWN SYNDROME

Generalized ligamentous laxity in Down syndrome (trisomy 21) may be manifested by atlantoaxial (C1-C2) subluxation (Fig. 14.18), recurrent patellar dislocation, pes planus (flatfoot deformity), and voluntary, painless hip dislocation. The iliac wings may have a flared appearance. The significance of atlantoaxial subluxation with respect to participation in sports is controversial.

MISCELLANEOUS LOCALIZED CONDITIONS

CLEIDOCRANIAL DYSPLASIA

The cardinal features of cleidocranial dysplasia (cleidocranial dysostosis) are absence of a portion of the clavicles and poor ossification of the skull with wormian bones and hypoplastic paranasal and mastoid sinuses. Sometimes, there may be total absence of the clavicles (Fig. 14.19). Other dysplastic features may be present throughout the skeleton, including hypoplastic limb girdles, dysplastic long bones with narrow diaphyses and expanded ends, and spina bifida occulta at multiple levels. Cleidocranial dysplasia is an autosomal-dominant condition with high penetrance.

RADIOULNAR SYNOSTOSIS

Radioulnar synostosis is an anomaly of longitudinal segmentation in which the proximal radioulnar joint space fails to form (Fig. 14.20). It occurs both sporadically and familially and is bilateral in approximately 60% of cases. It may also be seen in a variety of other

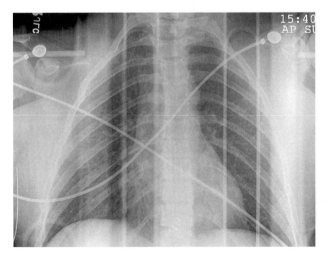

Figure 14.19 Cleidocranial dysplasia. AP radiograph obtained because of trauma incidentally shows complete absence of both clavicles.

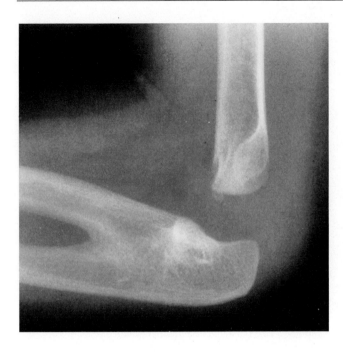

Figure 14.20 Radioulnar synostosis.

developmental syndromes and can be acquired from conditions such as infantile cortical hyperostosis or infection. Patients have functional impairment from inability to pronate and supinate the forearm.

Proximal Focal Femoral Deficiency

Proximal focal femoral deficiency is a spectrum of bony deficiencies of the proximal femur, ranging from shortening and varus deformity of the shaft to aplasia of the femoral head, neck, and proximal shaft. Dysplastic changes in the acetabulum correlate with the degree of femoral head deformity or hypoplasia. It is congenital but not heritable; the cause is unknown. The condition can be bilateral (Fig. 14.21).

Tibia Vara

Tibia vara (also called *Blount disease*) is a growth disorder of the medial portion of the proximal tibial growth plate that results in a varus deformity. The causes of tibia vara are

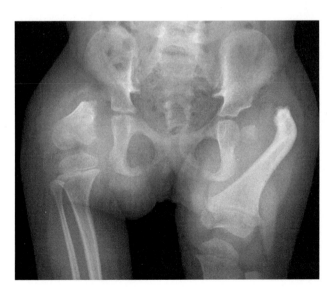

Figure 14.21 Bilateral proximal focal femoral deficiency.

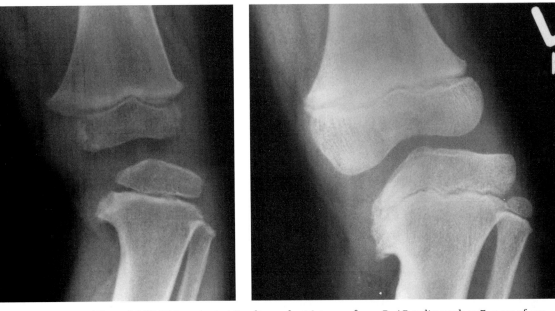

Figure 14.22 Tibia vara. *A.* AP radiograph at 3 years of age. *B.* AP radiograph at 7 years of age.

thought to be multifactorial, but the end result appears to be an injury to the medial growth plate, slowing its growth, leading to the varus deformity from continued normal growth on the lateral side of the growth plate. On radiographs, beaking, irregularity, and distortion of the metaphysis are seen along with the varus deformity at the growth plate (Fig. 14.22).

DIGITAL ANOMALIES

Anomalies of the fingers or toes may be sporadic or inherited and may be either isolated or associated with a congenital syndrome. Syndactyly is congenital fusion of two or more digits. The fusion may be soft tissue or osseous and either partial or complete. The most common situation is a soft tissue web between two fingers. Polydactyly is the presence of supernumerary digits, either partial (Fig. 14.23) or complete (Fig. 14.24). Symphalangia is

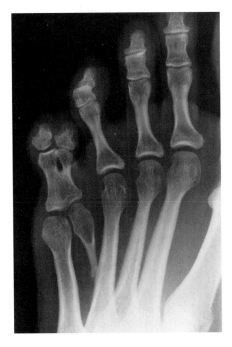

Figure 14.23 Partial supernumerary digit between fourth and fifth rays.

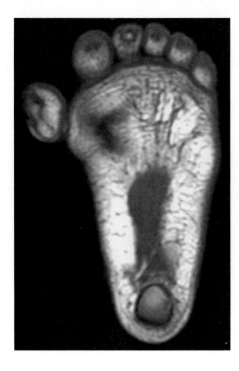

Figure 14.24 Polydactyly of the foot shown on T1-weighted MRI.

congenital fusion of one phalanx to another in the same digit, presumably from failure of the intervening joint to develop. Although other deformities of the appendage may be present, symphalangia is common in the small toes and generally has no significance. Hyperphalangia is the presence of extra phalanges in the longitudinal axis of a digit. It is seen almost exclusively as a triphalangeal thumb.

CARPAL COALITION

Carpal coalitions are relatively common anomalies in which two or more carpal bones fail to segment during development, resulting in a congenital fusion (Fig. 14.25). The fusion

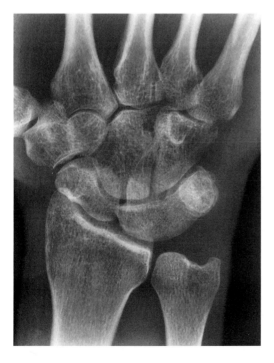

Figure 14.25 Carpal coalition (lunate and triquetrum).

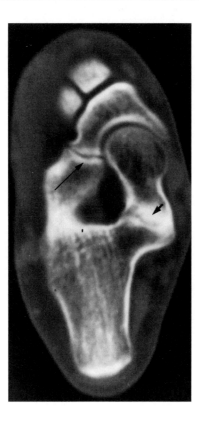

Figure 14.26 Tarsal coalition. Axial CT scan shows calcaneonavicular (*long arrow*) and middle subtalar facet (*short arrow*) coalitions.

can be bony, cartilaginous, or fibrous. Carpal coalitions are usually isolated anomalies that involve bones of the same row. The most common coalition is between the lunate and triquetrum. These coalitions are often of no clinical significance, although some patients with carpal coalition may complain of pain.

TARSAL COALITION

Tarsal coalition is an abnormal bony or fibrous articulation between two tarsal bones. The condition is congenital and appears to result from lack of segmentation rather than from fusion of a fully developed joint. Most coalitions are either between the calcaneus and the navicular or between the calcaneus and the talus. Calcaneal-talar coalitions usually involve the middle facet. Coalitions are bilateral in approximately 20% of cases. Coalitions cause the foot to lose some of its normal mobility, leading to a painful flatfoot. The coalition may be fibrous, cartilaginous, or osseous. Typically, the coalition is cartilaginous but becomes ossified as the skeleton matures; with ossification come rigidity and the onset of symptoms. Special views and conventional tomography or CT may be necessary to identify the presence and precise site of coalition. An indirect sign of a coalition between the calcaneus and the talus is talar beaking. A talar beak is a bony spur from the anterior superior aspect of the talus consequent to limited subtalar motion, hypoplasia of the head of the talus, and dorsal subluxation of the navicular bone. A talar beak may occur in any condition that causes abnormal talonavicular motion. The C-sign may be evident on lateral views when a middle facet coalition is present. The dome of the talus forms the top of the C, the coalition forms the middle, and the sustentaculum forms the bottom (Fig. 14.26). CT is an excellent method for identifying and characterizing tarsal coalitions. CT is most accurate when scanning or image reformations are obtained in axial, coronal, and sagittal planes (Fig. 14.27). MRI is also an excellent method for diagnosing tarsal coalitions (Fig. 14.28) and can demonstrate coalitions before they are ossified.

Tarsal coalitions are bilateral in approximately 20% of cases.

A talar beak may occur in any condition that causes abnormal talonavicular motion.

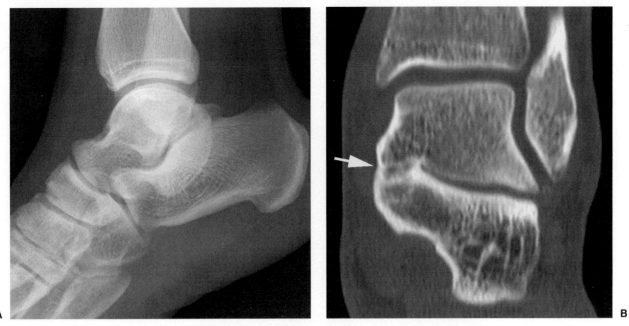

A

B

Figure 14.27 Tarsal coalition. *A.* Lateral radiograph shows C-sign of talocalcaneal coalition. *B.* Coronal CT reconstruction shows fusion of the middle subtalar facet (*arrow*).

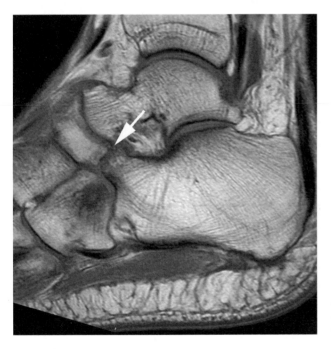

Figure 14.28 Calcaneonavicular coalition (*arrow*) on sagittal T1-weighted MRI.

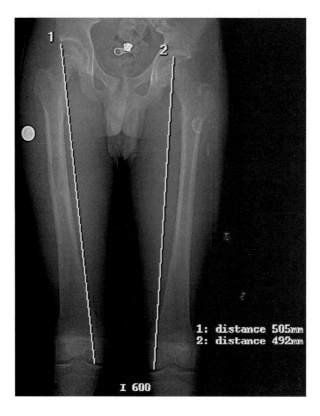

Figure 14.29 Scanogram for limb length discrepancy shows a healed fracture of the right femoral shaft with 13-mm length discrepancy.

LIMB LENGTH DISCREPANCY

Limb length discrepancy (also called *anisomelia*) is a clinical problem only in the lower limbs, where it may result in abnormal gait and scoliosis. Lower-limb length discrepancy is often the result of undergrowth of one limb due to trauma (especially trauma to the growth plate) or disease. Angular deformity of the limb also results in shortening. Overgrowth of a limb is common in hyperemic states such as those accompanying fractures or inflammatory bone or joint disease. The presence and amount of leg length discrepancy can be assessed by a scanogram. The radiographic scanogram is a view of both ankles, knees, and hips taken in separate exposures with the x-ray tube centered at the level of the joints; a radiopaque measuring stick is radiographed with the limbs. This allows the length of each femur and tibia to be measured. The computed scanogram using CT is more precise than the radiographic scanogram because it eliminates the effects of magnification and geometric distortion inherent in standard radiographic techniques and allows precise measurements on the workstation (Fig. 14.29). The usual landmarks for measurement in children are the top of the femoral head, the bottom of the medial femoral condyle, and the tibial plafond.

> Overgrowth of a limb is common in hyperemic states such as those accompanying fractures or inflammatory bone or joint disease.

HIP CONDITIONS

Three distinct chronic conditions of the hip occur in children; each affects a different age group (Table 14.2).

DEVELOPMENTAL DYSPLASIA OF THE HIP

In developmental dysplasia of the hip (DDH), an abnormally lax joint capsule allows the femoral head to fall out of the acetabulum shortly before or after birth, leading to congenital or postnatal deformation of an initially normal structure. The causes of this condition are multifactorial and appear to be related to the effects of restricted movement in the

Table 14.2: Pediatric Hip Disease

Disease	Peak Age of Diagnosis	Sex Predominance	Bilaterality
Developmental dysplasia of the hip	Neonates	Girls (6:1)	25%
Legg-Calvé-Perthes disease	7 yr	Boys (5:1)	10–20%
Slipped capital femoral epiphysis	Girls 11 yr; boys 14 yr	Boys (2.5:1.0)	20–35%
Toxic synovitis	—	—	—

womb and of maternal hormones on the fetus. Restricted fetal movement during the third trimester resulting from conditions such as breech presentation or oligohydramnios may partially or completely dislocate the hip. The maternal hormones (e.g., estrogen) that relax the ligaments of the pelvis and facilitate childbirth also affect the fetus by increasing the laxity of the ligaments and joint capsules. This effect is particularly evident in female fetuses and may account for the 6:1 female preponderance of DDH. This condition has a familial tendency perhaps related to an inherited abnormality in estrogen metabolism.

There is a 6:1 female preponderance of DDH.

Both the femoral head and the acetabulum must be present and articulating with each other for a normal hip to form. If contact is absent, adaptive changes occur in both structures. DDH is the result of abnormal mechanical stresses caused by abnormal position of the femoral head. If the hip dislocates, the pressure of the femoral head on the rapidly growing, pliable chondro-osseous pelvis produces a false acetabulum (pseudoacetabulum). The native acetabulum becomes flattened and dish shaped—rather than cup shaped—and fills with fibrofatty debris. The earlier in life the dislocation occurs, the greater the adaptive abnormalities are. If the hip subluxates, the pressure of the femoral head against the acetabular labrum causes the labrum to deform. The labrum can become completely inverted into the acetabulum; in this situation, it is called a *limbus*. Remodeling of the ilium as growth proceeds in the presence of subluxation is seen radiographically as a shallow, steep acetabulum. A pseudoacetabulum may eventually form. The abnormal position of the femur may cause secondary changes in the capsule and iliopsoas mechanism. The longer the abnormal position persists, the more fixed the abnormalities become. If the femoral head can be relocated and held in the normal position, normal development is often reestablished.

DDH is best diagnosed clinically in the neonatal period. The capsule and iliopsoas mechanism are lax enough for the hip to be easily dislocated and relocated; this is felt as a characteristic click or clunk by the examiner. Clinical examination becomes more difficult as the baby grows older because contractures and progressive deformity make it difficult to relocate a partially or completely dislocated hip.

Sonography is useful and has the advantage of immediate correlation with physical examination (Fig. 14.30). Most sonographers image the infant hip in the coronal plane, the so-called standard imaging plane of Graf. The key features to observe on this image are the location of the femoral head relative to the acetabulum, the shape of the femoral head (round), the size and ossification of the femoral head (Is one side lagging in development?), the bony acetabulum, and the coverage of the femoral head by the bony acetabulum. The bony acetabulum is assessed by measurement of the alpha angle, the angle between the lateral cortex of the ilium and the acetabular roof (60 degrees or greater is normal). The bony coverage of the femoral head is expressed as a percentage but can also be described by qualitative terms such as "good," "adequate," or "deficient."

In the neonate, radiographs in suspected DDH are unreliable because of the paucity of skeletal ossification. After 1 month of age, the AP radiograph becomes more reliable (Fig. 14.31). Each hip is divided into quadrants by drawing a horizontal baseline through the triradiate cartilages (Hilgenreiner's horizontal line) and a perpendicular line through the most lateral ossified margin of the roof of the acetabulum (Perkins' line) (Fig. 14.32). The

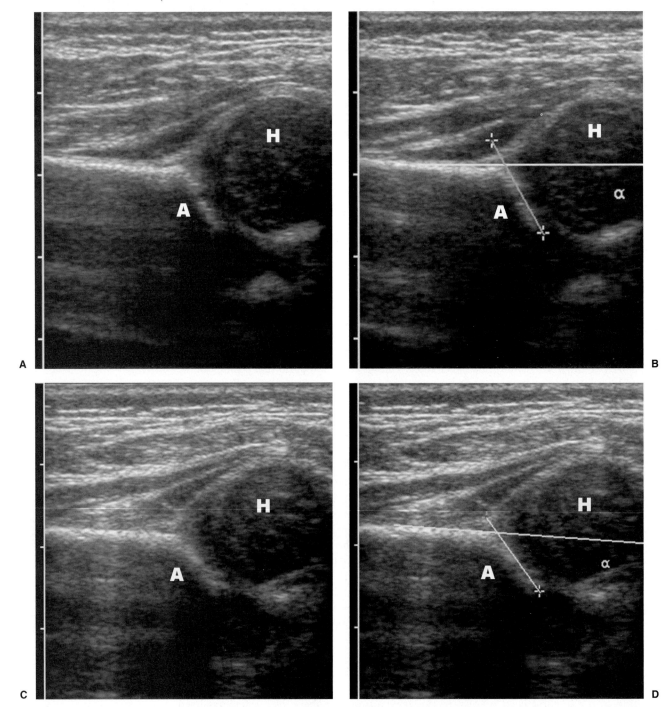

Figure 14.30 Neonatal hip at 3 weeks of age (head to left, feet to right). *A,B.* Sonogram of the right hip is normal. The femoral head (H) is normally located, and there is greater than 50% bony coverage of the head. The alpha angle (α) was measured at 61 degrees. *C,D.* Sonogram of the left hip shows acetabular dysplasia. The femoral head is normally located, but there is only 33% bony coverage of the head. The alpha angle was measured at 50 degrees. A, acetabular roof.

On radiographs, the normal location of the femoral head is in the lower inner quadrant of the hip (down and in).

normal location of the femoral head is in the lower inner quadrant (down and in). A dislocated femoral head is in the upper outer quadrant (up and out), and a subluxated femoral head is in the lower outer quadrant (down and out). The angle between the acetabulum and the horizontal baseline should be less than 40 degrees in a newborn, 33 degrees in a 6-month-old child, and 30 degrees in a 1-year-old child. In the normal hip, a smooth curve

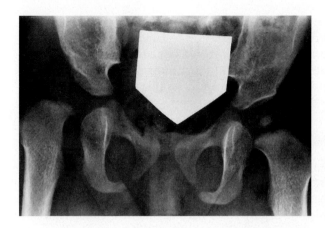

Figure 14.31 Developmental dysplasia of the hip in a 12-month-old infant. The right hip is dislocated; the left hip is normal. Note the short, steep acetabulum and delayed ossification of the right femoral head.

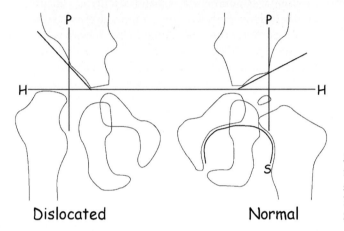

Figure 14.32 Radiologic diagnosis of developmental dysplasia of the hip. H, Hilgenreiner's horizontal line; P, Perkins' line; S, Shenton's line.

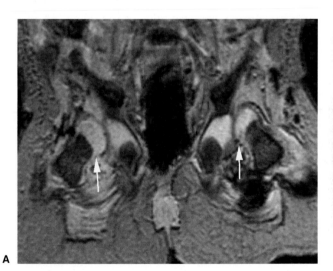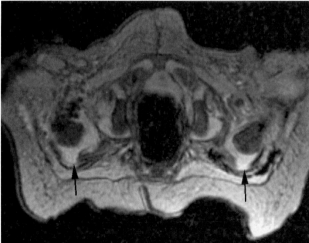

Figure 14.33 MRI of developmental dysplasia of the hip. *A.* Coronal gradient-recalled echo MRI shows bilateral superior dislocation of the femoral heads (*arrows*). *B.* Axial gradient-recalled echo MRI shows bilateral posterior dislocation of the femoral heads (*arrows*).

can be drawn along the inferior margin of the superior pubic ramus and the medial femoral cortex (Shenton's line). Other findings include a shallow acetabulum, development of a false acetabulum, and delayed ossification of the involved capital femoral epiphysis. CT may be necessary to confirm anatomic relocation of the hips once the patient has been placed in a cast. MRI may be used to evaluate problematic cases (Fig. 14.33). The long-term sequela of untreated DDH is early degenerative arthritis.

Legg-Calvé-Perthes Disease

Legg-Calvé-Perthes disease is idiopathic osteonecrosis of the capital femoral epiphysis in a skeletally immature child. Boys are affected more often than girls by a 4:1 ratio. The mean age of onset is 7 years, and the range is 2 to 13 years. In 20% of cases, the condition is bilateral. The bone age of affected children is usually 1 to 3 years behind their chronologic age. Interruption of the blood supply to the femoral head leads to partial or total osteonecrosis. Both enchondral ossification of the capital femoral epiphysis and activity at the growth plate stop. The articular cartilage, nourished by synovial fluid, continues to grow. If the disease is detected at this stage, the ossific nucleus of the capital femoral epiphysis is smaller than normal, and overgrowth of the articular cartilage is apparent as joint space widening. The patient may be asymptomatic. Revascularization of the femoral head leads to centripetal ossification, usually from multiple sites that are not contiguous with the original ossific nucleus. This results in an appearance often described as *fragmentation of ossification*. Apposition of new bone to the dead bone may increase the radiographic density of the head (Fig. 14.34). Resorption of subchondral bone may lead to subchondral fracture and the onset of clinical symptoms: hip pain and limp. MRI appears to be more sensitive in the detection of early changes of Legg-Calvé-Perthes disease. In addition to the morphologic changes that may be seen on radiographs, MRI may show marrow changes in the femoral head (Fig. 14.35). Several entities should be considered in the differential diagnosis of this entity. The severity of the clinical findings is highly variable and does not necessarily correlate with the radiographic findings. The end result is a short, thick femoral neck and an enlarged femoral head (coxa magna). Premature closure of the growth plate accentuates the deformity. Secondary osteoarthritis is a late complication.

The goal of therapy is to prevent the development of femoral head deformity and subsequent osteoarthritis. Centering of the femoral head within the acetabulum during the revascularization and reossification stages of healing presumably allows the acetabulum to act as a mold for the healing femoral head, averting the development of deformity. Acetabular coverage for the femoral head may be obtained by abduction of the femoral head relative to the acetabulum with a brace, varus osteotomy of the proximal femur, or osteotomy of the pelvis. Arthrography or MRI of the hip may be required to delineate the morphology of the unossified portion of the femoral head for surgical planning.

Osteonecrosis of the femoral head and other growing epiphyses may occur as a result of trauma or other disease. The pathophysiology and the gamut of radiologic findings are similar to those of Legg-Calvé-Perthes disease.

Slipped Capital Femoral Epiphysis

A slipped capital femoral epiphysis (SCFE) is displacement of the femoral head relative to the femoral neck through the open growth plate in an adolescent. The head remains in the acetabulum as the neck progressively displaces anteriorly and superiorly (the head goes inferiorly and posteriorly). SCFE occurs in boys and girls of approximately the same skeletal age shortly before closure of the growth plate (chronologic age of approximately 11 years in girls and 14 years in boys). Boys are affected more often than girls by a ratio of 2.5:1.0. Many patients are overweight and have mildly delayed skeletal ages. Bilateral involvement is present in approximately half of the patients. The etiology is not known; the pathophysiology may be related to an endocrine process or a biomechanical problem. The slippage between the femoral head and neck occurs between the proliferative and

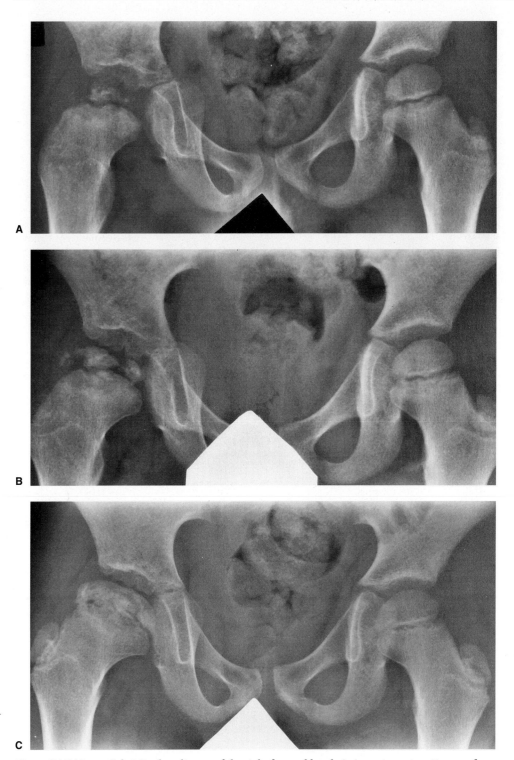

Figure 14.34 Legg-Calvé-Perthes disease of the right femoral head. *A.* At presentation, 5 years of age, the right femoral head is large and misshapen. The femoral neck is short and broad. *B.* At 6 years of age, the cartilaginous portion of the epiphysis is ossifying from multiple foci. *C.* At 8 years of age, ossification of the epiphysis is complete; the head no longer fits into the acetabulum.

hypertrophic zones of the growth cartilage. This is different from a Salter type I fracture, which occurs between the hypertrophic and provisional calcification zones of the cartilage. SCFE may be a chronic, slow process that allows bony remodeling of both head and neck as the deformity progresses (Fig. 14.36), or it may be a relatively acute process (usually

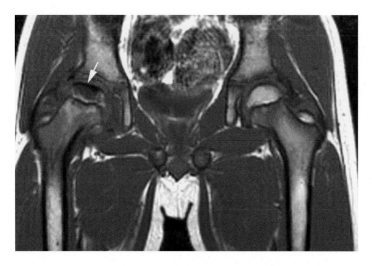

Figure 14.35 Legg-Calvé-Perthes disease. Coronal T1-weighted MRI shows abnormal signal and collapse of the right femoral epiphysis (*arrow*).

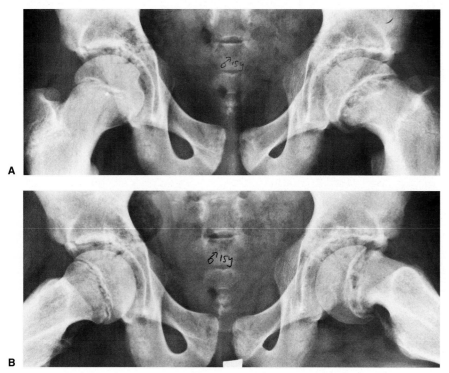

Figure 14.36 Chronic slipped capital femoral epiphysis. *A.* AP radiograph shows abnormal left proximal femur. *B.* Frog-leg lateral radiograph.

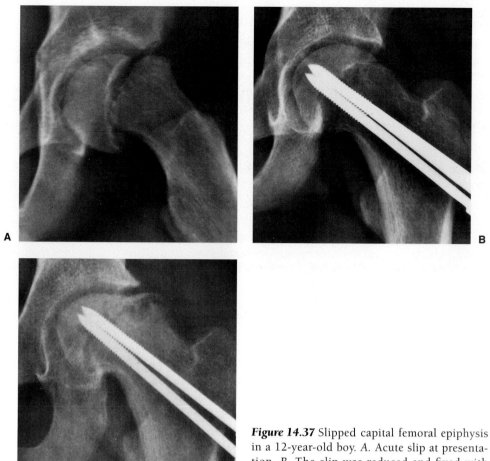

Figure 14.37 Slipped capital femoral epiphysis in a 12-year-old boy. *A.* Acute slip at presentation. *B.* The slip was reduced and fixed with Knowles pins. *C.* Osteonecrosis with early collapse of the femoral head 6 months after presentation.

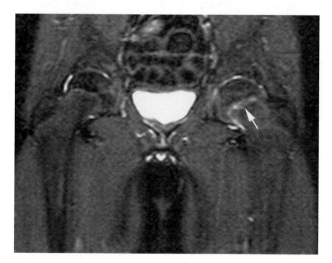

Figure 14.38 Slipped capital femoral epiphysis. Coronal T2-weighted fat-suppressed MRI demonstrates slippage of the epiphysis on the left with increased signal (*arrow*) at the femoral growth plate.

lasting less than 3 weeks), the presentation of which is not unlike that of a stress fracture (Fig. 14.37). Mild cases may go undetected, but MRI appears to be more sensitive than radiographs for detecting SCFE. On MRI, abnormally increased signal within the region of the growth plate may be present on T2-weighted MRI (Fig. 14.38). SCFE is treated by stabilization of the head without attempt at anatomic reduction. Multiple pins fix the position of the head and promote closure of the growth plate. Dysplasia of the hip and early osteoarthritis may develop; osteonecrosis is a devastating complication that is more common in acute slips.

PREMATURE PHYSEAL CLOSURE

Premature closure of a growth plate results in an angular deformity if the closure is partial and growth arrest if the closure is complete. Conditions that may cause premature closure include disuse, radiation, infection, tumor, vascular impairment, neural involvement, metabolic abnormality, frostbite, developmental, and iatrogenic. Disuse results in atrophy of muscle and other soft tissues and, if prolonged, of bone as well. Growth arrest lines are not uncommon (Fig. 14.39) and represent bone formation at the physis during a period of growth arrest. Rarely, the physis may close. Therapeutic radiation may inhibit or destroy physeal cartilage, resulting in closure; diagnostic radiation does not. Osteomyelitis involving the metaphysis may extend through the growth plate into the epiphysis, leading to closure. Benign tumors that involve the physis may lead to closure. Disruption of the epiphyseal blood supply may lead to closure. Neuromuscular conditions such as poliomyelitis, cerebral palsy, and congenital insensitivity to pain are associated with premature physeal closure; the mechanism is unknown. Metabolic abnormalities, including vitamin A toxicity and scurvy, may be associated with premature physeal closure. Cold injury may

> Osteomyelitis involving the metaphysis may extend through the growth plate into the epiphysis, leading to premature closure or tethering.

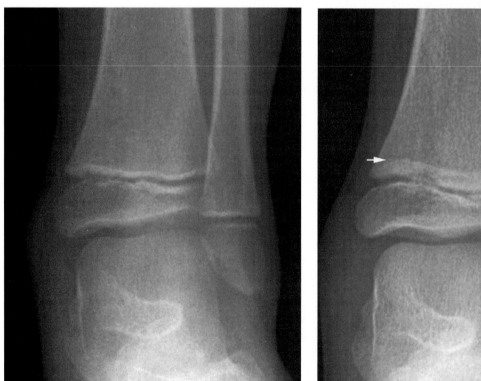

A   B

Figure 14.39 Growth arrest lines at the ankle in a patient with osteomyelitis of the proximal tibia. *A.* Ankle radiograph at presentation is normal. *B.* Ankle radiograph 3 months after surgery shows a growth arrest line (*arrow*) parallel to the distal tibial physis.

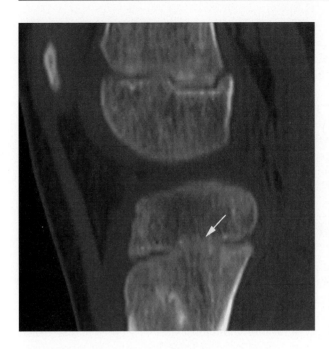

Figure 14.40 Premature closure of the growth plate after osteomyelitis. Sagittal reformatted CT images show a defect in the anterior tibial metaphysis where surgical drainage for osteomyelitis had been performed. A well-developed bridge of bone (*arrow*) traverses the central portion of the physis.

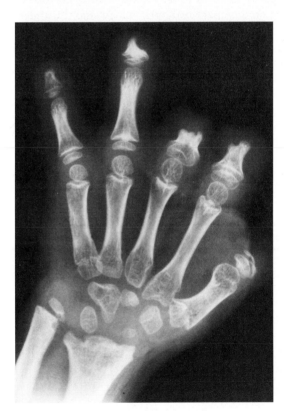

Figure 14.41 Multiple finger amputations and coned epiphyses in the hand from meningococcemia in infancy.

result in premature physeal closure, especially in the phalanges, from either direct injury to the chondrocytes or ischemic vascular changes. Surgery involving the growth plate may result in closure, including the placement of pins for fracture stabilization, curettage for nearby tumors, and débridement for infection. Immunosuppressive drugs may cause premature closure.

On radiographs, the growth plate is initially normal at the time of injury and only becomes abnormal in appearance as premature closure proceeds. If the closure involves the entire growth plate, then the growth plate disappears, and the bone begins to remodel, leaving a short bone. If the closure is partial and asymmetric, continued growth in the open portion of the physis may lead to a progressive angular deformity as well as a short bone (Fig. 14.40). If the closure is partial and central, a coned epiphysis develops (Fig. 14.41).

OSTEOCHONDROSES

The osteochondroses are a varied group of acquired, localized conditions of childhood in which a disease process is superimposed on the growth process. Grouped together initially because of their radiographic appearance, these lesions are characterized by fragmentation and sclerosis of an epiphyseal or apophyseal ossification center in a child. These conditions have been described in a wide variety of locations, and most sites have eponyms associated with them. The eponyms in common usage are listed in Table 14.3. Avascular necrosis of the growing epiphysis is thought to be the predominant pathophysiology, and the underlying cause is thought to be repetitive microtrauma at a site with a tenuous blood supply. Fragmentation and collapse are followed by reossification as the blood supply is reestablished. On radiographs, the ossification center of the apophysis or epiphysis becomes dense and undergoes fragmentation, then reossification. Dysplastic change in the shape of the bone sometimes occurs, although it may reconstitute itself. This process can be difficult to distinguish from the normal developmental variation in ossification of epiphyses and apophyses. The presence of pain in the appropriate age group and at the appropriate location should be established before making the diagnosis. Because healing is spontaneous in most cases, treatment is management of symptoms and modification of the aggravating activity.

OSTEOCHONDRITIS DISSECANS (KNEE)

Osteochondritis dissecans is an osteochondrosis involving the knee, typically the non–weight-bearing lateral aspect of the medial femoral condyle in adolescents. (Osteochondrosis of the talar dome—a different condition—may also be called *osteochondritis dissecans*.) There is a male predominance of 3:1. The mechanism of injury is thought to be repetitive trauma transmitted to the subchondral bone through the articular cartilage that results in osteonecrosis and healing. The articular cartilage may be intact over the surface of the lesion, but if it is not, the fragment may become a loose body within the joint. On radio-

---

Table 14.3: Common Osteochondroses

Legg-Calvé-Perthes disease	Capital femoral epiphysis
Köhler disease	Tarsal navicular
Kienbock disease	Lunate
Osgood-Schlatter disease	Tibial tuberosity
Scheuermann disease	Vertebral ring apophyses
Freiberg infraction	Metatarsal head
Osteochondritis dissecans	Medial femoral condyle, talar dome
Panner disease	Capitellum
Seiver disease	Calcaneal apophysis

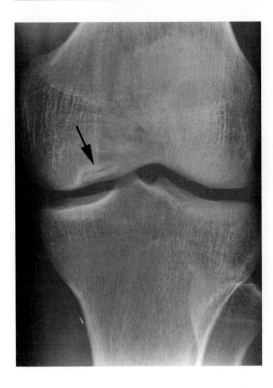

Figure 14.42 Osteochondritis dissecans of the knee (*arrow*).

graphs, osteochondritis dissecans may be recognized by the presence of a sclerotic lesion in the subchondral bone at the lateral surface of the medial femoral condyle (Fig. 14.42). If the osteochondral fragment has become displaced, a defect in the subchondral bone is seen. Depending on the severity of the lesion, MRI may show abnormal signal in the articular cartilage, abnormal signal in the marrow, or both. If a well-defined fragment is present, MRI may demonstrate whether the overlying cartilage is intact. Fluid signal surrounding the fragment on T2-weighted images indicates that it has become detached, although not necessarily displaced (Fig. 14.43). In addition to the medial femoral condyle, other por-

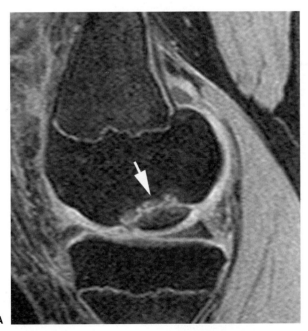

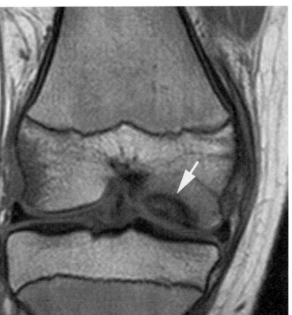

A   B

Figure 14.43 Osteochondritis dissecans of the knee (*arrows*). *A.* Sagittal STIR MRI. *B.* Coronal T1-weighted MRI.

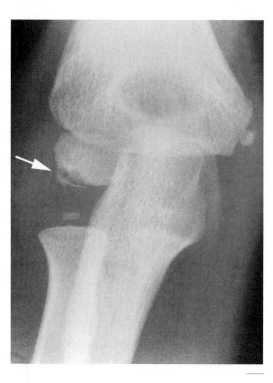

Figure 14.44 Osteochondrosis of the capitellum (Panner disease) (*arrow*).

tions of the knee may be involved, including the lateral femoral condyle and the patella. Multiple sites may be involved in the same knee, and bilateral disease may be present in up to 25% of cases.

PANNER DISEASE (CAPITELLUM)

Panner disease is osteochondrosis of the capitellum. Repetitive trauma is often the result of participation in throwing sports, such as baseball pitching. On radiographs, the condition is manifest by focal sclerosis and collapse in the capitellar ossification center (Fig. 14.44). The abnormality may be more conspicuous on MRI (Fig. 14.45).

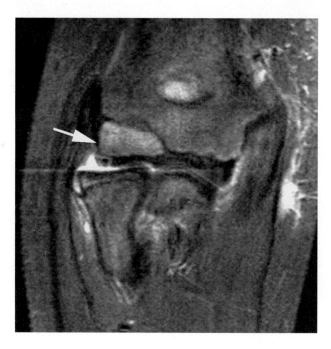

Figure 14.45 Osteochondrosis of the capitellum (Panner disease) (*arrow*) shown on coronal STIR MRI.

OSGOOD-SCHLATTER DISEASE (TIBIAL TUBERCLE)

Osgood-Schlatter disease is osteochondrosis of the tibial tubercle from repetitive microtrauma, commonly jumping sports such as basketball. On radiographs, there is separation of small bone fragments from the developing ossification of the tibial tuberosity, with overlying soft tissue swelling. After the acute stage, the soft tissue swelling subsides, and the fragments may remodel and coalesce to form a normal tibial tubercle, or ossific fragments may persist at the site.

SINDING-LARSEN-JOHANSSON DISEASE (PATELLA)

Sinding-Larsen-Johansson disease is osteochondrosis of the distal pole of the patella that is similar to Osgood-Schlatter disease in that it also is thought to result from repetitive microtrauma, commonly jumping sports. It is sometimes called *jumper's knee* and has similar radiographic features, except that they occur at the inferior pole of the patella where the infrapatellar tendon attaches.

KÖHLER DISEASE (TARSAL NAVICULAR)

Köhler disease is osteochondrosis of the tarsal navicular. It occurs in boys between 3 and 5 years of age and in girls between 2 and 4 years of age. Radiographs show collapse and increased density of the ossification center of the tarsal navicular, followed by patchy deossification and reossification. Localized inflammation, tenderness, and limpness characterize the clinical presentation. After reconstitution, sclerosis, dysplasia, and fragmentation of the tarsal navicular may persist (Fig. 14.46), and secondary degenerative changes may follow.

FREIBERG INFRACTION (METATARSAL HEAD)

Freiberg infraction is osteochondrosis of the metatarsal head, usually the second metatarsal. The condition most commonly affects adolescent girls. After reconstitution, residual overgrowth and articular irregularity may lead to secondary osteoarthritis.

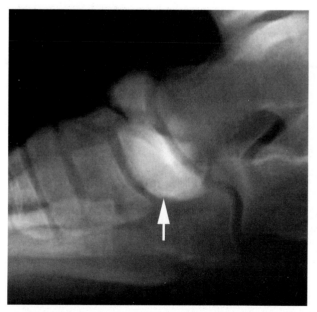 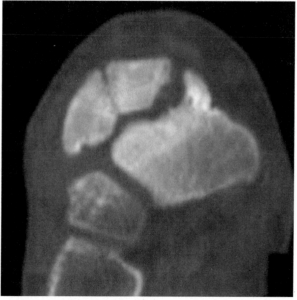

A   B

Figure 14.46 Residual features of Köhler disease in a teenager. *A.* Lateral radiograph shows sclerosis and dysplasia of the navicular (*arrow*). *B.* Coronal CT reformation shows sclerosis and fragmentation of the navicular.

CONGENITAL FOOT DEFORMITIES

Weight-bearing lateral and AP views should be obtained for the radiologic diagnosis of congenital foot deformities.

Most clinically evident deformities of the foot in the infant and child are flexible and mild and correct with growth or cause little or no handicap in adult life. The diagnosis of congenital foot deformities is accomplished principally by radiographs. Lateral and AP views should be obtained while weight bearing or, in the case of infants, with dorsiflexion stress simulating weight bearing. The hindfoot is comprised of the talus and calcaneus. In the normal foot, until approximately 2 years of age, the long axis of the talus and the long axis of the calcaneus form an angle (talocalcaneal angle) that is approximately 40 degrees on both lateral and AP radiographs (Fig. 14.47). If one considers the talus to be fixed in the ankle mortise, then abnormal varus (medial) alignment of the calcaneus relative to the talus reduces the talocalcaneal angle in the AP projection, and abnormal valgus (lateral) alignment increases it. Because of the geometric and ligamentous linkage between the talus and the calcaneus, changes in the talocalcaneal angles are approximately equal on both AP and lateral radiographs. Thus, on AP and lateral radiographs, a small talocalcaneal angle (close to parallel, approximately 10 degrees or less) is called *hindfoot varus*, and a large talo-

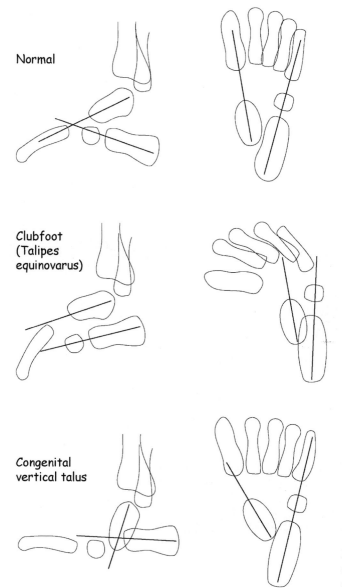

Normal

Clubfoot
(Talipes
equinovarus)

Congenital
vertical talus

Figure 14.47 Radiographic diagnosis of congenital foot deformities.

calcaneal angle (approximately 70 degrees or more) is called *hindfoot valgus*. On AP radiographs, the first metatarsal should be aligned with the talus, and the fourth or fifth metatarsal should be aligned with the calcaneus. On lateral radiographs, the first metatarsal should be aligned with the talus. If the first metatarsal is angled plantar relative to the talus, the plantar arch is elevated, and the deformity is called a *cavus arch* or *cavus foot*. If the first metatarsal is angled dorsally relative to the talus, the plantar arch is flattened, and the deformity is called *pes planus* or *flatfoot*. There is a wide range of normal variation in the alignment of the bones of the foot, and actually drawing and measuring any of these angles may give a misleading sense of accuracy and precision.

TALIPES EQUINOVARUS

Talipes equinovarus, or congenital clubfoot, is a common abnormality with an incidence of 1 per 1,000 live births. The condition is bilateral in approximately half the cases and is three times more common in boys than in girls. When unilateral, it is usually the left foot that is abnormal. The deformity is believed to be caused by a combination of intrauterine and genetic factors. Clubfoot may also occur in association with arthrogryposis or meningomyelocele. The key radiologic finding is hindfoot varus (decreased talocalcaneal angle) combined with medial deviation and inversion of the forefoot (Fig. 14.48). The plantar arch is elevated. Clubfoot may be treated by serial manipulation and casting or by surgical release of the soft tissues and realignment of the foot.

METATARSUS ADDUCTUS

Metatarsus adductus refers to a group of related foot deformities that produce incurvation of the forefoot. The incidence is approximately 1 per 1,000 live births. The most common of these is simple medial deviation of the forefoot relative to the hindfoot, without hindfoot

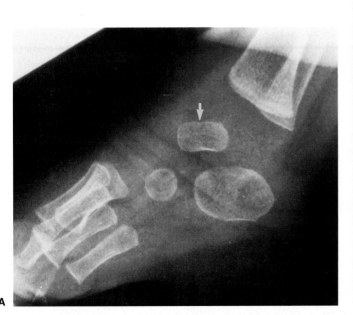
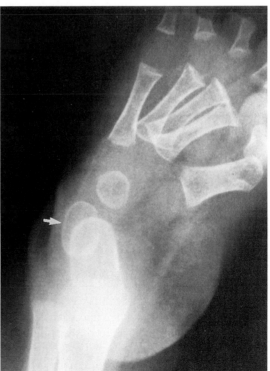

A

B

Figure 14.48 Talipes equinovarus. *A,B.* Lateral and AP radiographs show a narrow talocalcaneal angle (arrows indicate talus).

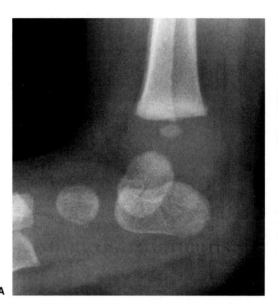
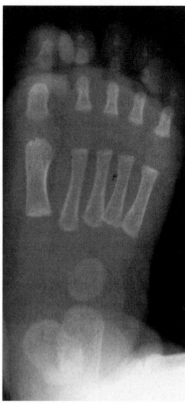

Figure 14.49 Congenital vertical talus. *A.* Lateral radiograph. *B.* AP radiograph.

abnormality. Less common varieties include inversion of the forefoot or combinations of medial deviation, inversion, and hindfoot valgus. Most cases are mild, supple deformities that resolve spontaneously; severe deformities may be rigid and require treatment. The condition is bilateral in 50% of cases.

CONGENITAL VERTICAL TALUS

Congenital vertical talus is an unusual deformity characterized by hindfoot valgus (increased talocalcaneal angle) and dorsal dislocation of the navicular on the talus (Fig. 14.49). The plantar arch is flattened, and in severe cases, a rocker-bottom deformity (convex plantar surface of the foot) may result. Congenital vertical talus may occur in isolation or in association with neurofibromatosis, arthrogryposis, meningomyelocele, and other central nervous system and genetic syndromes.

SPINE CONDITIONS

IDIOPATHIC SCOLIOSIS

Scoliosis is lateral spinal curvature in the coronal plane. By convention, it is named for the side that is convex so that right scoliosis is convex to the right. Known causes of scoliosis include congenital architectural imbalance; growth asymmetry; neoplastic, traumatic, or infectious damage; therapeutic irradiation; bone dysplasia; asymmetric neuromuscular control; leg length discrepancy; and reflexive splinting due to pain or nerve irritation. Approximately 85% to 90% of scoliosis cases are idiopathic. Idiopathic scoliosis is thought to have a genetic basis. In the United States, idiopathic scoliosis is usually found in children between 11 and 14 years of age during mandatory visual

Table 14.4: Prevalence of Idiopathic Scoliosis in the United States

Magnitude of Curve (degrees)	Prevalence (per 1,000)
= 10	25.0
= 20	5.0
= 30	1.5

Adapted from Kane WJ. Scoliosis prevalence: a call for a statement of terms. *Clin Orthop* 1977;126:43–46.

screening in schools. The prevalence of scoliosis is related to the severity of the curve (Table 14.4). Girls are much more likely to have severe or progressive curves. The classic curve is a painless, S-shaped curve that is convex to the right in the thoracic region between T5 and T12 (Fig. 14.50). In addition to the more obvious abnormality of alignment of the entire spine in which the relations between vertebrae are abnormal, each individual vertebra in the region of the curves has an abnormal shape. A painful curve raises suspicion of an underlying lesion. Radiography is used to confirm the presence of scoliosis, to document its magnitude and extent, and to detect or exclude congenital or other abnormalities. Radiographs are made with the patient standing without shoes and should include the entire spine on a single long (3-ft) film; spot films and additional imaging modalities are used as needed. The standard of measurement is the Cobb method, but the variability of the method is 5 to 10 degrees. It is important to protect the breasts from radiation, particularly in girls, because the average patient followed for idiopathic scoliosis will have many examinations. Severe curves in the thoracic region interfere with the mechanics of respiration. The primary goal of treatment is the ultimate preservation of lung function. Scoliotic curves of 20 degrees or less are usually not treated. Modalities of treatment include rigid braces, electrical stimulation, and spinal fusion (see Chapter 17 for methods of surgical fusion).

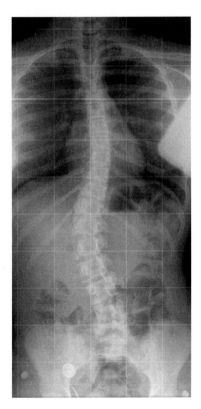

Figure 14.50 Idiopathic scoliosis in a 14-year-old girl. The curves may be measured directly on the digital image using tools on the workstation.

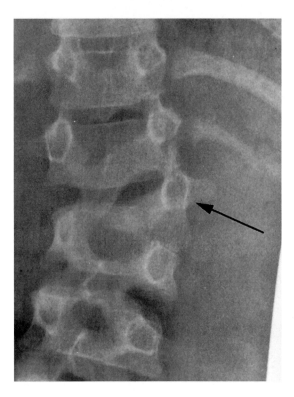

Figure 14.51 Congenital scoliosis with a hemivertebra (*arrow*) at the thoracolumbar junction.

CONGENITAL SCOLIOSIS

The obvious causes of congenital scoliosis relate to failure of normal formation of individual vertebrae. During the embryonic conversion of mesenchymal vertebrae to cartilaginous vertebrae before week 9 of development, each vertebral body becomes chondrified from two centers of chondrification on either side of the midline. If chondrification fails on only one side, an isolated hemivertebra results. If the centers of chondrification do not fuse at the same level (as they should) but fuse across levels instead, a trapezoidal vertebra results (Figs. 14.51 and 14.52). Each side of the neural arch also has its own center of chondrification, and similar

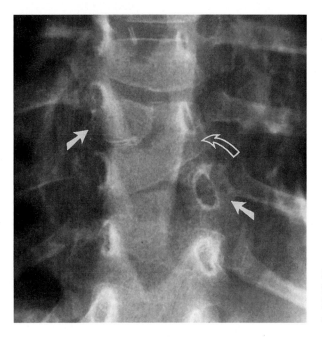

Figure 14.52 Vertebral anomalies in a 3-year-old girl with hemivertebrae (*solid arrows*) and a trapezoidal vertebra (*curved arrow*).

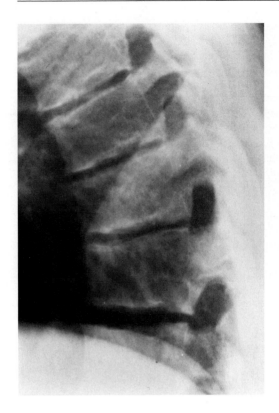

Figure 14.53 Scheuermann disease (juvenile kyphosis).

failures of development or abnormal fusion result in anomalies. The most common vertebral anomalies causing congenital scoliosis include hemivertebrae, trapezoidal vertebrae, and unilateral neural arch fusions. Combinations of anomalies and multilevel involvement are frequent. Congenital scoliosis may also result from differences in growth potential between vertebrae and from congenital neurologic conditions that result in neuromuscular imbalance.

JUVENILE KYPHOSIS

Juvenile kyphosis is a term that is used to describe thoracic kyphosis exceeding 40 degrees in adolescents, as measured from the superior end plate of T3 or T4 to the inferior end plate of T12. Most cases are considered postural kyphosis and may simply represent the extremes of normal variation. Kyphosis is the only clinical and radiographic finding. Scheuermann disease (juvenile thoracic kyphosis) is diagnosed on radiographs by decreased disc space heights, increased AP diameter of the involved vertebral bodies, and irregularity of the end plates (Fig. 14.53). Anterior wedging of at least 5 degrees typically involves three or more consecutive vertebrae. The process is thought to result from fissures developing in the cartilaginous vertebral end plates through which material from the nucleus pulposus herniates. Fibrosis and reactive sclerosis outline these pockets (individually called *Schmorl nodes*). The loss of disc material results in kyphosis. Increased stress on the anterior portion of the vertebral bodies results in growth abnormality, leading to the wedge shape and the increased AP dimension. These are not compression fractures. An alternative explanation for Scheuermann disease is that the condition is an osteochondrosis of the vertebral ring apophyses.

SOURCES AND READINGS

Armstrong DG, Newfield JT, Gillespie R. Orthopedic management of osteopetrosis: results of a survey and review of the literature. *J Pediatr Orthoped* 1999;19:122–132.

Beighton P, ed. *McKusick's heritable disorders of connective tissue*, 5th ed. St. Louis: Mosby–Year Book, 1993.

Carey J, Spence L, Blickman H, et al. MRI of pediatric growth plate injury: correlation with plain film radiographs and clinical outcome. *Skeletal Radiol* 1998;27:250–255.

Davis LA, Hatt WS. Congenital abnormalities of the foot. *Radiology* 1955;64:818–825.

Fasth A, Porras O. Human malignant osteopetrosis: pathophysiology, management and the role of bone marrow transplantation. *Pediatr Transplant* 1999;3[Suppl 1]:102–107.

Gilmore A, Thompson GH. Radiographic evaluation of children and adolescents with a spinal deformity. *Sem Musculoskelet Radiol* 2000;4:349–359.

Goh S, Price RI, Leedman PJ, et al. A comparison of three methods for measuring thoracic kyphosis: implications for clinical studies. *Rheumatology* 2000;39:310–315.

Goh S, Price RI, Song S, et al. Magnetic resonance-based vertebral morphometry of the thoracic spine: age, gender, and level-specific influences. *Clin Biomech* 2000;15:417–425.

Greiner KA. Adolescent idiopathic scoliosis: radiologic decision-making. *Am Fam Physician* 2002;65:1817–1822.

Greulich WW, Pyle SI. *Radiographic atlas of skeletal development of the hand and wrist*, 2nd ed. Stanford: Stanford University Press, 1959.

Harty MP, Hubbard AM. MR imaging of pediatric abnormalities in the ankle and foot. *Magn Reson Imaging Clin N Am* 2001;9:579–602.

Hoerr NL, Pyle SI, Francis CC. *Radiographic atlas of skeletal development of the foot and ankle. A standard of reference*. Springfield, IL: Charles C Thomas, 1962.

Jones KL, Smith DW, Fletcher J, eds. *Smith's recognizable patterns of human malformation*. Philadelphia: WB Saunders, 1996.

Kane WJ. Scoliosis prevalence: a call for a statement of terms. *Clin Orthop* 1977;126:43–46.

Keats TE, Anderson MW. *Atlas of normal roentgen variants that may simulate disease*. St. Louis: Mosby, 2001.

Keats TE, Sistrom C. *Atlas of radiologic measurement*, 7th ed. St. Louis: Mosby, 2001.

Kozlowski K, Beighton P. *Gamut index of skeletal dysplasias: an aid to radiodiagnosis, 3rd ed*. New York: Springer-Verlag New York, 2001.

Kuhn JP, Slovis TL, Haller JO, eds. *Caffey's pediatric diagnostic imaging*, 10th ed. St. Louis: Mosby, 2002.

Lachman RS. International nomenclature and classification of the osteochondrodysplasias. *Pediatr Radiol* 1998;28:737–744.

Lazner F, Gowen M, Pavasovic D, et al. Osteopetrosis and osteoporosis: two sides of the same coin. *Hum Mol Genet* 1999;8:1839–1846.

Lohman M, Kivisaari A, Vehmas T, et al. MRI in the assessment of growth arrest. *Pediatr Radiol* 2002;32:41–45.

Lonstein JE, Bradford DS, Winter RB, eds. *Moe's textbook of scoliosis and other spinal deformities*, 3rd ed. Philadelphia: WB Saunders, 1995.

Lovell WW, Morrissy BT, Winter RB, eds. *Lovell and Winter's pediatric orthopaedics*, 5th ed. Philadelphia: Lippincott Williams & Wilkins, 2001.

McAlister WH, Shackelford GD. Measurement of spinal curvatures. *Radiol Clin North Am* 1975;13:113–121.

McMaster MJ, Singh H. Natural history of congenital kyphosis and kyphoscoliosis. A study of one hundred and twelve patients. *J Bone Joint Surg Am* 1999;81:1367–1383.

Murray PM, Weinstein SL, Spratt KF. The natural history and long-term follow-up of Scheuermann kyphosis. *J Bone Joint Surg Am* 1993;75A:236–248.

Ozonoff MB. *Pediatric orthopaedic radiology*, 2nd ed. Philadelphia, WB Saunders, 1992.

Poznanski AK. *The hand in radiologic diagnosis*, 2nd ed. Philadelphia: WB Saunders, 1984.

Pyle ST, Hoerr NL. *Radiographic atlas of skeletal development of the knee*. Springfield, IL: Charles C Thomas Publisher, 1955.

Rockwood CA, Kasser JR, Wilkins K, eds. *Rockwood and Wilkins' fractures in children*. Philadelphia: Lippincott Williams & Wilkins, 2001.

Schmidt H, Freyschmidt J. *Köhler/Zimmer Borderlands of the normal and early pathologic findings in skeletal radiography*, 4th ed. Stuttgart: Thieme Medical Publishers, 1993.

Shapiro F. Epiphyseal disorders. *N Engl J Med* 1987;317:1702–1710.

Shapiro F. Osteopetrosis. Current clinical considerations. *Clin Orthop* 1993;294:34–44.

Soucacos PN, Zacharis K, Soultanis K, et al. Risk factors for idiopathic scoliosis: review of a 6-year prospective study. *Orthopedics* 2000;23:833–838.

Taybi H, Lachman RS. *Radiology of syndromes, metabolic disorders, and skeletal dysplasias*, 4th ed. St. Louis: Mosby–Year Book, 1996.

Vande Berg BC, Malghem J, Lecouvet FE, et al. Magnetic resonance imaging and differential diagnosis of epiphyseal osteonecrosis. *Semin Musculoskelet Radiol* 2001;5:57–67.

Vande Berg BC, Malghem J, Lecouvet FE, et al. MR imaging of bone infarction and epiphyseal osteonecrosis. *J Belg Radiol* 1997;80:243–250.

Wilson CJ, Vellodi A. Autosomal recessive osteopetrosis: diagnosis, management, and outcome. *Arch Dis Child* 2000;83:449–452.

Wright N. Imaging in scoliosis. *Arch Dis Child* 2000;82:38–40.

Wynne-Davies R, Hall CM, Apley AG. *Atlas of skeletal dysplasias.* Edinburgh: Churchill Livingstone, 1985.

METABOLIC, ENDOCRINE, AND NUTRITIONAL CONDITIONS

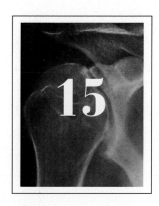

15

This chapter describes the radiology of many systemic, metabolic, and endocrine conditions that have bone or soft tissue manifestations.

OSTEOPOROSIS

Osteoporosis is the most common metabolic bone disease. Osteoporosis is characterized by generalized loss of mass from otherwise normal bone. This loss of bone substance results in microarchitectural deterioration of the trabecular structure, increased bone fragility, and increased risk of fracture. Osteoporosis may be considered to be primary or secondary. Primary osteoporosis, also called *involutional osteoporosis*, is idiopathic in etiology. Secondary osteoporosis has a known, underlying etiology.

PRIMARY OSTEOPOROSIS (INVOLUTIONAL OSTEOPOROSIS)

More than 95% of adults with osteoporosis have involutional osteoporosis (also called *idiopathic* or *primary osteoporosis*). There are two main clinical types: postmenopausal (also called *type I*) and senile or age-related (type II). Type I involutional osteoporosis is characterized by accelerated bone loss, mainly trabecular, and is caused by factors related to

The pathogenesis of osteoporosis seems to involve both excessive bone resorption as well as impaired bone formation.

menopause. Type II involutional osteoporosis is characterized by slowly progressive trabecular and cortical bone loss and is caused by factors related to aging. The pathogenesis of osteoporosis is incompletely understood; it seems to involve not only excessive bone resorption but also impaired bone formation. Deteriorating bone strength results in increased vulnerability to traumatic and fatigue fractures. Most fractures of the spine, proximal femur, and distal radius in adults older than 50 years of age are associated with osteoporosis (see Chapter 1). In type I involutional osteoporosis, vertebral crush fractures and distal radius fractures are the most common; in type II involutional osteoporosis, multiple vertebral wedge fractures and hip fractures are the most common. Fractures are the major cause of morbidity and mortality in osteoporosis.

The prevalence of involutional osteoporosis in the United States is estimated at 28 million, or approximately 10% of the entire population. Risk factors for developing involutional osteoporosis include advancing age; female gender; white or Asian race; family history; thin, small bones; menopause; low dietary calcium; low dietary vitamin D; excessive alcohol, caffeine, and salt; smoking; and sedentary lifestyle. As the proportion and absolute numbers of the population in the United States older than 50 years of age increase, the prevalence of involutional osteoporosis may be expected to increase substantially.

Osteopenia, the radiographic hallmark of osteoporosis, may not be recognizable on radiographs until 30% to 50% of the bone mineral has been lost.

The radiographic hallmark of osteoporosis is osteopenia, the increased radiolucency of bone. Osteopenia may not be recognizable on plain films until 30% to 50% of the bone mineral has been lost. A coarsened trabecular pattern results from the loss of smaller trabeculae, making the remaining ones more prominent. Linear, band-like, or spotty radiolucent areas may also be seen. Cortical thinning can be a generalized, uniform, slowly progressive process (Fig. 15.1). Cortical bone loss may also be manifested by scalloped, endosteal erosions, intracortical radiolucent areas or striations (intracortical tunneling), or subperiosteal erosions. Vertebral deformities are related to insufficiency fractures of the end plates. These can have the form of biconcave depressions of contiguous superior and inferior end plates (so-called fish or codfish vertebrae, named for their resemblance to vertebrae in codfish), anterior wedge fractures, crush fractures of entire vertebral bodies, and increased thoracic kyphosis (dowager's hump) (Figs. 15.2 and 15.3). The net result is progressive loss of stature.

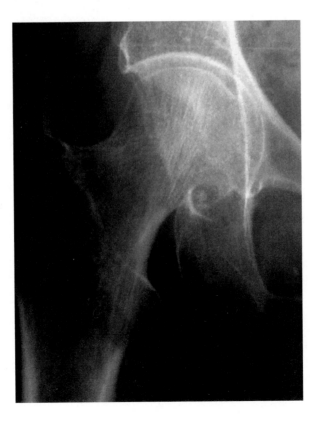

Figure 15.1 Osteoporosis of the hip with thin cortex and loss of trabecular bone in the neck.

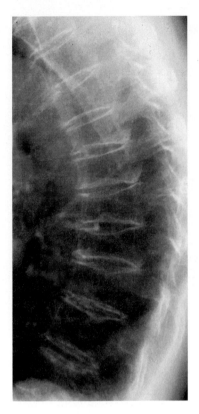

Figure 15.2 Osteoporosis in the spine with central end-plate depressions of the vertebral bodies at multiple levels.

BONE MINERAL DENSITOMETRY

Bone mineral densitometry (BMD) is the best noninvasive method for the diagnosis of osteoporosis in asymptomatic patients. BMD can also be used to estimate the risk of fracture and monitor patients receiving therapy for osteoporosis. The availability of effective therapies for osteoporosis—including estrogen, bisphosphonates, and other pharmacologic agents—has

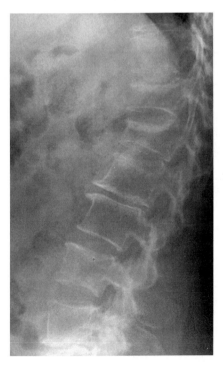

Figure 15.3 Osteoporosis with multiple anterior wedge fractures in the thoracic spine.

> ### *Table 15.1: Clinical Indications for Bone Mineral Densitometry*
>
> National Osteoporosis Foundation
>   Postmenopausal women younger than 65 years of age who have one or more additional
>   risk factors for osteoporosis
>   Women 65 years of age and older regardless of additional risk factors
> U.S. federal government (Department of Health and Human Services)
>   Estrogen-deficient women at clinical risk for osteoporosis
>   Individuals with vertebral abnormalities
>   Individuals receiving long-term glucocorticoid therapy
>   Individuals with primary hyperparathyrodism
>   Individuals being monitored on osteoporosis therapy
>
> Adapted from National Osteoporosis Foundation. *Federal Register* 1998;63:34320.

The absolute amount of bone mineral is predictive of fracture risk.

increased the usefulness of screening patients with various risk factors (Table 15.1). The absolute amount of bone mineral is predictive of fracture risk. Radiographic measurement of BMD accurately and precisely assesses bone mineral content. Dual-photon absorptiometry (DPA) and dual-energy x-ray absorptiometry (DXA) use a dual-energy radionuclide or x-ray source, respectively, to measure the bone density of the lumbar spine or hip. DPA and DXA measure the absorption of photons by bone and provide a combined measurement of cortical and trabecular bone density. Quantitative CT measures the trabecular bone density in lumbar vertebral bodies by comparing the CT numbers of trabecular bone with the CT numbers of standardized solutions of calcium suspensions. Quantitative ultrasound measures the sound conduction in bone as a correlate of BMD. Broadband ultrasound attenuation has also been correlated with BMD as another method of quantitative ultrasound. Measures of BMD can be compared to age- and sex-matched populations to establish criteria for normality and abnormality. The relative risk of an osteoporotic fracture can also be estimated for various levels of BMD by comparing the incidence of fractures in large populations with BMD measurements. Because cortical and trabecular bone may not be involved to the same extent, methods that measure one or the other, or both, may not yield identical results.

DXA works on the physical principle that bone mineral (predominantly calcium) and soft tissue (predominantly fat and water) attenuate x-rays of high and low energy to different degrees. By measuring the differential absorption of x-rays of high and low energy, the absorption due to bone mineral alone can be determined, and from that, the absolute amount of bone mineral in the path of the x-rays can be calculated. Use of a single x-ray energy for measuring BMD is less accurate than using dual x-ray energy. Measuring BMD at the spine and proximal femur (central measurement) is considered more useful clinically than measuring BMD in the extremities (peripheral measurement). DXA provides measurements that reflect the BMD of trabecular and cortical bone together.

Clinical interpretation of the results of DXA is based on population statistics. An individual's BMD measurement from DXA is compared with those of normal populations. The consensus criteria used for clinical diagnosis are those of the World Health Organization (WHO)

> ### *Table 15.2: World Health Organization Diagnostic Criteria for Involutional Osteoporosis*
>
> | Diagnosis | T-score |
> |---|---|
> | Normal | −1.0 or higher |
> | Osteopenia | <−1.0 but >−2.5 |
> | Osteoporosis | <−2.5 but without fractures |
> | Established osteoporosis | <−2.5 with fractures |
>
> T-score, number of standard deviations from the mean relative to a normal young adult population.

(Table 15.2). According to WHO criteria, an individual's BMD is compared with those of a population of normal, young adults to derive a "T-score." The T-score is related to the number of standard deviations from the young, normal population mean the individual's measurement falls, so that a T-score of –2.0 would be 2 standard deviations below the mean of the young, normal population. Particular levels of bone mineral have been established as corresponding to disease. A T-score of less than –1.0 but greater than –2.5 corresponds to a diagnosis of *osteopenia*. A T-score of less than –2.5 corresponds to a diagnosis of *osteoporosis*. If fractures are present in a patient with a T-score of less than –2.5, the diagnosis is *established osteoporosis*. The comparison of an individual's BMD to an age-matched population (the Z-score) is not used in WHO criteria. There is significant controversy regarding the particular normal, young adult populations on whom the T-scores are based with regard to sample size, gender, and race. The use of the terms *osteopenia* and *osteoporosis* may also lead to confusion unless the context is clear; when these terms are used in conjunction with DXA, they should only refer to diagnoses according to WHO criteria.

In current practice, the DXA diagnosis of osteopenia and osteoporosis is based on BMD measurements of the lumbar spine and the proximal femur. In the spine, the frontal projection is used, and, ideally, an average of L1 through L4 is used to obtain the T-score (Fig. 15.4). If it is not possible to use L1 through L4, any two or three consecutive L1 through L4 vertebrae can be used. Use of a single vertebra is considered unreliable. In the hip, a region of the femoral neck is used (Fig. 15.5). The DXA report should include, as a minimum, a description of the basis of the measurement, the T-score, the relative fracture risk associated with the T-score, and the diagnosis according to WHO criteria.

Because DXA is a projection technique that measures the sum of the bone mineral between the x-ray source and the detector, disease or post-surgical conditions that increase or decrease the attenuation of the x-rays may compromise accuracy (Fig. 15.6). The most common condition leading to spurious BMD measurements (Table 15.3) is degenerative spine disease, in which sclerosis and osteophytes increase the BMD measurement. Similarly, diffuse idiopathic skeletal hyperostosis (DISH) may increase BMD measurement. Other common conditions that affect DXA measurements include compression fractures, laminectomy, metal artifacts and bone graft from spine fusion, focal sclerotic lesions such

> A T-score of less than –2.5 on DXA corresponds to a diagnosis of osteoporosis, according to the WHO criteria.

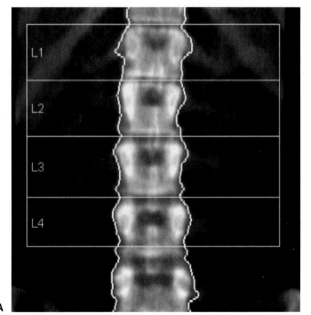
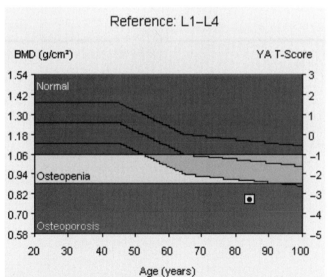

A **B**

Figure 15.4 Dual x-ray absorptiometry of the lumbar spine showing osteoporosis. *A*. Image shows regions of interest. *B*. Graphic shows bone mineral density (BMD) relative to young adult (YA)- and age-matched reference populations. The T-score was –3.3, diagnostic of osteoporosis.

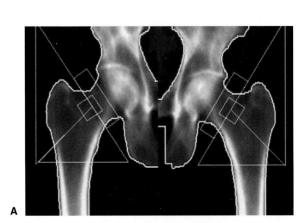
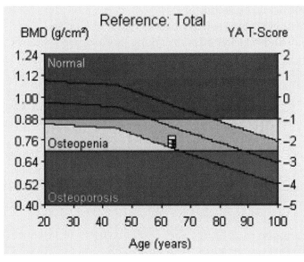

Figure 15.5 Dual x-ray absorptiometry of the hips showing osteopenia. *A.* Image shows regions of interest. *B.* Graphic shows bone mineral density (BMD) relative to young adult (YA)- and age-matched reference populations. The T-score on the right was –2.0, and the T-score on the left was –2.2, both diagnostic of osteopenia.

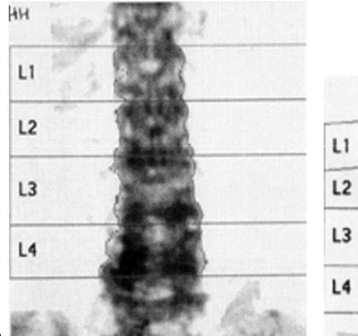
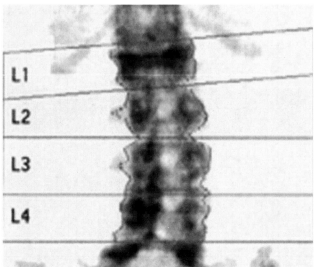

Figure 15.6 Dual x-ray absorptiometry artifacts. *A.* Degenerative spine disease with end-plate sclerosis and osteophytosis. *B.* Compression fracture at L1 and degenerative changes at L4. (*continued*)

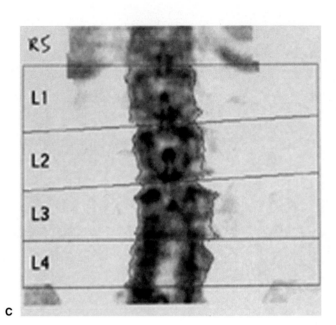
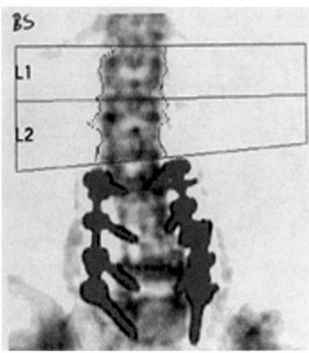

C **D**

Figure 15.6 (continued) C. Laminectomy and posterolateral fusion at L4. *D.* Lumbar spine fusion with hardware. Vertebral levels with artifacts are excluded from the analysis.

as blastic metastases or Paget disease, and focal lytic lesions such as lytic metastases or multiple myeloma. Similar conditions may affect DXA measurements of BMD at the hip.

SECONDARY OSTEOPOROSIS

Secondary osteoporosis is the loss of bone mass from otherwise normal bone as a result of a known cause. Secondary osteoporosis may manifest acutely or chronically, in a regional or systemic distribution. DXA and other methods for determining BMD may be applied to patients with chronic, systemic, secondary osteoporosis. DXA may be used to establish the diagnosis and to follow therapy. Common causes of secondary osteoporosis are listed in Table 15.4. More detailed descriptions of these conditions may be found in the appropriate portions of this book.

Table 15.3: Potential Causes of Spurious Bone Mineral Density (BMD) Measurements in the Spine

Spuriously increased BMD measurement
Degenerative joint disease
Diffuse idiopathic skeletal hyperostosis
Spinal fusion
Orthopedic hardware
Compression fracture
Blastic metastases
Paget disease
Spuriously decreased BMD measurement
Laminectomy
Lytic metastases
Multiple myeloma

Table 15.4: Some Causes of Secondary Osteoporosis in Adults

Inherited
  Osteogenesis imperfecta
  Homocystinuria
  Marfan syndrome
Nutritional
  Malabsorption syndromes
  Chronic liver disease
  Alcoholism
  Calcium deficiency
Endocrine
  Hypogonadism
  Thyrotoxicosis
  Hypercortisolism
  Hyperparathyroidism
Drugs
  Corticosteroids
  Phenobarbital
  Synthroid
  Dilantin
Other
  Multiple myeloma
  Rheumatoid arthritis
  Acromegaly
  Mastocytosis

ACUTE, TRANSIENT, REGIONAL, AND MIGRATORY OSTEOPOROSIS

Acute osteoporosis accompanies fracture healing as a normal physiologic response to hyperemia. It may also accompany immobilization and disuse, both common features of healing fractures, as well as conditions such as reflex sympathetic dystrophy (also called *complex regional pain syndrome*). On radiographs, acute osteoporosis may be recognized in cancellous bone by subcortical resorption of trabeculae, resulting in subcortical lucency that parallels the cortical surface (Fig. 15.7). On CT, the bone resorption tends to appear patchier (Fig. 15.8).

On radiographs, acute osteoporosis may be recognized in cancellous bone by subcortical resorption of trabeculae.

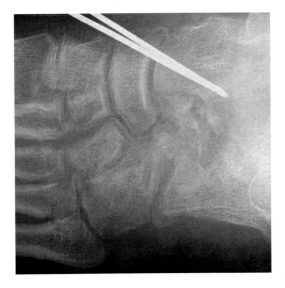

Figure 15.7 Acute osteoporosis of the foot.

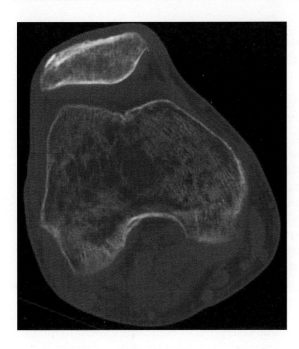

Figure 15.8 Acute osteoporosis associated with healing fractures demonstrated on CT scan.

Transient regional osteoporosis typically presents with monoarticular joint symptoms. It is characterized by a rapidly developing osteoporosis affecting periarticular bone that is self-limited and reversible and has no definite inciting event. There are two clinical syndromes that occur in adults, both more common in men. The first clinical syndrome is transient osteoporosis of the hip. This presents with the rapid onset of severe hip pain without a precipitating event. It is usually unilateral, involving either the right or left hip in men, or usually the left hip in women. The pain is self-limited but aggravated by activity and regresses in 2 to 6 months without permanent sequelae. Imaging may show a rapidly developing periarticular osteoporosis, particularly in the femoral head, that returns to normal after the resolution of symptoms. MRI shows diffuse edema and hip effusion but no infarction. Bone scans show increased activity consistent with the osteoporosis. The condition is thought to have a neurogenic origin, possibly related to reflex sympathetic dystrophy. The second clinical syndrome is regional migratory osteoporosis (Fig. 15.9). This usually involves the lower extremities of adults. Local pain and swelling develop rapidly, last up to 9 months, and

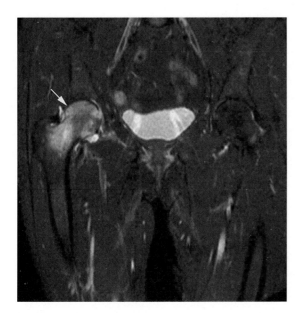

Figure 15.9 Transient osteoporosis of the hip. Coronal T2-weighted MRI with fat suppression shows amorphous bone marrow edema (*arrow*) in the right proximal femur.

then disappear only to be followed by involvement of other regions months to years later. Within weeks of the onset of each episode, periarticular osteoporosis is evident. This condition may begin as transient osteoporosis of the hip.

DISEASES OF MINERAL METABOLISM

The skeleton is a metabolically active reservoir of calcium and phosphorus in the extracellular space. These minerals are maintained in tiny hydroxyapatite crystals that have in aggregate a vast surface area and are rapidly and freely exchanged into the extracellular fluid space. When necessary, the skeleton gives up calcium to maintain the correct serum levels. The ionic concentration of calcium is generally determined by the renal glomerular filtration rate, tubular reabsorption of calcium, and the formation and resorption of bone. The serum calcium level is tightly controlled by parathyroid hormone and 1,25-dihydroxyvitamin D. Calcium can be directly released from the hydroxyapatite crystal or liberated by osteoclastic destruction of bone. Bone formation and destruction are closely coupled in the healthy person.

HYPERPARATHYROIDISM

Hyperparathyroidism stimulates osteoclastic resorption of bone. The excess parathyroid hormone can be a result of primary or secondary hyperparathyroidism. Primary hyperparathyroidism results in hypercalcemia and is caused by excess parathyroid hormone production from diffuse parathyroid hyperplasia or autonomously functioning parathyroid adenomas (single or multiple). Secondary hyperparathyroidism is a response to sustained hypocalcemia that is typically caused by chronic renal failure or gastrointestinal malabsorption. Patients with long-standing secondary hyperparathyroidism may develop relatively autonomous parathyroid function or tertiary hyperparathyroidism. Diagnosis of these disorders is made by clinical and laboratory findings, including direct measurement of serum calcium and parathyroid hormone levels.

The radiographic changes of hyperparathyroidism are best detected and monitored in the hands.

Although radiographic changes may occur at many sites, they are best detected and monitored in the hands. Skeletal surveys of the whole body are generally unnecessary. Radiologic signs of hyperparathyroidism include bone resorption, brown tumors, bone sclerosis, and chondrocalcinosis. Bone resorption occurs at all surfaces, including subperiosteal, intracortical (along haversian systems), endosteal, trabecular, subchondral, and subligamentous locations. Subperiosteal bone resorption is virtually diagnostic of hyperparathyroidism. Seen best and most frequently along the radial aspect of the phalanges of the hands, especially the middle phalanges of the index and middle fingers, subperiosteal bone resorption may also be evident at the phalangeal tufts (Fig. 15.10). Bone resorption at other surfaces is nonspecific. Subchondral bone resorption may lead to articular disease (Fig. 15.11). Brown tumors are focal areas of bone resorption where the bone has been replaced by fibrous tissue and osteoclasts (Fig. 15.12). Brown tumors may have the appearance of aggressive, focally destructive bone lesions such as metastases, but the associated presence of other radiographic changes of hyperparathyroid bone disease should clarify the situation. Brown tumors may be single or multiple in number and central, eccentric, or cortical in location (Figs. 15.13 and 15.14). Brown tumors heal by ossification (Fig. 15.15). Widespread sclerosis of bone in hyperparathyroidism occurs by an uncertain mechanism and may be prominent in the axial skeleton, especially the skull and spine. Widespread sclerosis is common in secondary hyperparathyroidism. When the spine is involved, horizontal bands of sclerosis in the vertebral bodies adjacent to the vertebral end plates may result in a rugger jersey appearance (Fig. 15.16). Chondrocalcinosis, or calcification of cartilage, is associated with the combination of primary hyperparathyroidism and calcium pyrophosphate dihydrate (CPPD) crystal deposition disease (see Chapter 13). This combination is found in 18% to 40% of primary hyperparathyroidism cases.

Widespread sclerosis is common in secondary hyperparathyroidism.

Sometimes, the distinction between primary and secondary hyperparathyroidism can be suggested. The following combination of findings is highly suggestive of primary hyper-

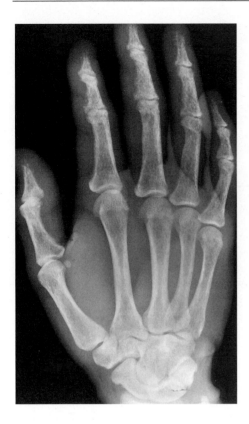

Figure 15.10 Secondary hyperparathyroidism. Subperiosteal bone resorption is evident throughout the hand and more advanced on the radial aspect.

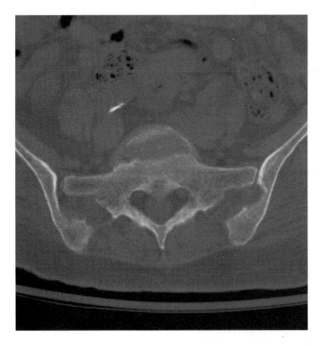

Figure 15.11 Hyperparathyroidism with sacroiliac joint bone resorption. Axial CT scan shows subchondral bone resorption and widening of the sacroiliac joints.

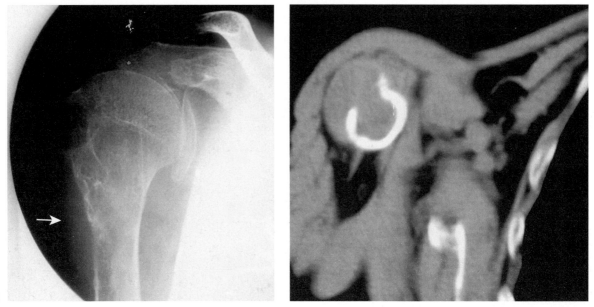

Figure 15.12 Brown tumor in hyperparathyroidism. *A.* AP radiograph shows osteoporosis and destructive lesion in proximal humerus (*arrow*). *B.* CT shows mass destroying cortex.

parathyroidism: subperiosteal bone resorption, bone resorption at other sites, bony sclerosis, and chondrocalcinosis. In secondary hyperparathyroidism, there is an increased frequency of vascular and soft tissue calcification, more commonly and more widespread bone sclerosis, and a decreased frequency of chondrocalcinosis. Secondary hyperparathyroidism is common; primary hyperparathyroidism is uncommon.

RICKETS, OSTEOMALACIA, AND RENAL OSTEODYSTROPHY

Rickets and osteomalacia are childhood and adult manifestations, respectively, of a systemic disease in which the calcification of osteoid is deficient. The final common pathway in both conditions is the lack of available calcium or phosphorus (or both) for mineralization of osteoid. In rickets, the predominant effect is on the growth plates; in osteomalacia, the predominant effect is on remodeling of mature bone. When rickets or osteomalacia occur in conjunction with chronic renal failure, the condition is called *renal osteodystrophy*.

Dietary deficiency of vitamin D, usually coupled with inadequate exposure to sunlight so that photochemical synthesis of vitamin D in the skin does not occur, results in reduced gastrointestinal calcium absorption, hypocalcemia, and secondary hyperparathyroidism to

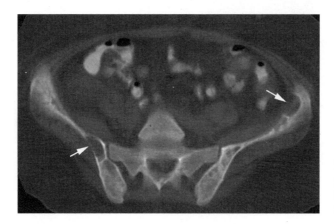

Figure 15.13 Secondary hyperparathyroidism with brown tumors (*arrows*) and bone resorption on CT.

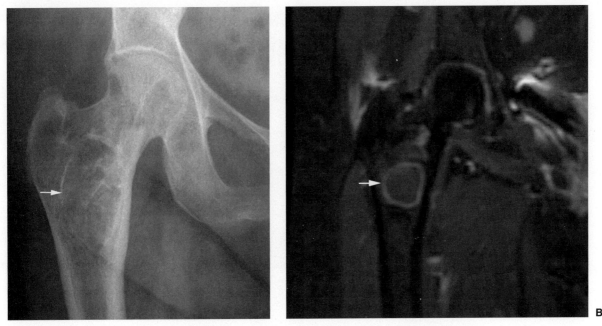

Figure 15.14 Brown tumor of the proximal femur. *A.* AP radiograph shows a lytic lesion (*arrow*) in the intertrochanteric region of the proximal femur. *B.* Axial T1-weighted MRI with fat suppression after gadolinium injection shows rim enhancement (*arrow*) in this cystic lesion.

mobilize calcium from the skeleton. Pure vitamin D deficiency–induced rickets and osteo-malacia are relatively rare in the United States except among immigrants, food faddists, the institutionalized elderly, and patients on total parenteral nutrition. Other causes include failure of enzymatic conversion of 25-hydroxyvitamin D to its physiologically more active metabolite 1,25-dihydroxyvitamin D, end-organ insensitivity to 1,25-dihydroxyvitamin D,

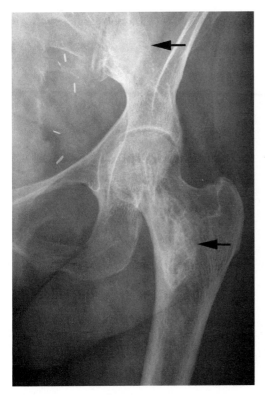

Figure 15.15 Healing brown tumors involving the pelvis and proximal femurs (*arrows*).

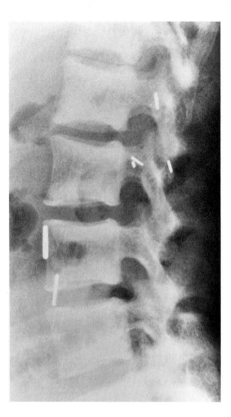

Figure 15.16 Secondary hyperparathyroidism. Osteosclerosis with greater density at the end plates (rugger jersey spine).

Gastrointestinal malabsorption is the most common cause of rickets and osteomalacia in the United States.

genetic and acquired renal tubular reabsorptive defects, and gastrointestinal malabsorption of dietary calcium or phosphorus. In the United States, gastrointestinal malabsorption from a variety of etiologies is the most common cause of rickets and osteomalacia. Rickets and osteomalacia may occur in association with polyostotic fibrous dysplasia and neurofibromatosis and may also be caused by chronic use of anticonvulsant medications or aluminum-containing antacids.

In rickets, there is widening of the growth plate because of continued cartilage growth in the absence of normal mineralization and ossification (Fig. 15.17). Radio-

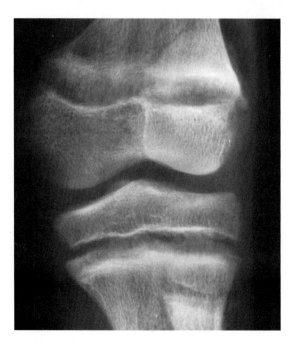

Figure 15.17 Renal osteodystrophy with thickened growth plates and irregular ossification at the interface with the metaphysis.

graphic findings are most apparent in the most active regions of growth, and the uncalcified cartilage may become quite bulky. Frequent sites of radiographic abnormalities include the costochondral junctions of ribs, the distal femur, both ends of the tibia, the proximal humerus, the distal radius, and the ulna. Irregular, disorganized mineralization of the zone of provisional calcification creates a frayed appearance. Mechanical stress on the thickened growth plate may lead to widening, cupping, and bowing deformities. Bone texture (trabecular pattern) appears coarsened, and there is delayed appearance of ossification centers. Rachitic bone is less resistant to bending and shearing loads, and stress fractures and bowing deformities are common. Transverse zones of lucency on the concave side of long bones, called *Milkman pseudofractures* or *Looser zones*, are focal collections of nonmineralized osteoid; they probably do not represent insufficiency injuries. After the initiation of successful treatment of rickets, the uncalcified osteoid calcifies, so that the zone of provisional calcification appears as a wide band that narrows the growth plate to its normal thickness (Fig. 15.18). Ossification of nonmineralized subperiosteal osteoid is apparent as new periosteal bone.

In osteomalacia, the radiologic findings are more subtle than rickets because the adult skeleton is less metabolically active. Osteopenia is the predominant appearance, and it may be indistinguishable from osteoporosis unless Looser zones or bowing deformities are present (Fig. 15.19). Occasionally, the bone texture may be recognized as subtly coarsened. As in osteoporosis, the risk of fractures from falls escalates with deteriorating bone strength.

In renal osteodystrophy, the skeletal abnormalities include the findings of rickets or osteomalacia, secondary hyperparathyroidism, osteoporosis, and soft tissue and vascular calcifications (Fig. 15.20). In children, slipped capital femoral epiphysis is common. The extent of the abnormalities depends on the severity and duration of disease. Advanced changes have become uncommon as the management of renal failure has improved.

Articular conditions that are related to chronic renal failure include amyloidosis, periarticular calcinosis (hemodialysis-related tumoral calcinosis), and hydroxyapatite crystal synovitis. These conditions are detailed in Chapter 13.

> Frequent sites of radiographic abnormalities in rickets include the costochondral junctions of the ribs, the distal femur, both ends of the tibia, the proximal humerus, the distal radius, and the ulna.

> Slipped capital femoral epiphysis is common in children with renal osteodystrophy.

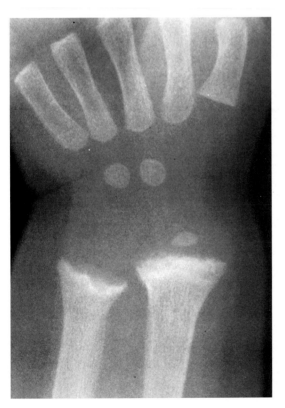

Figure 15.18 Healing rickets.

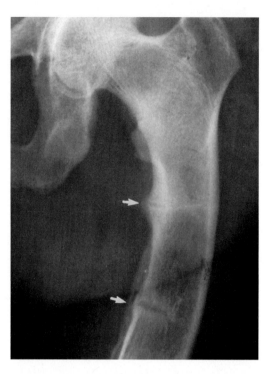

Figure 15.19 Osteomalacia with bowing deformity and Looser zones (*arrows*).

IDIOPATHIC TUMORAL CALCINOSIS

Idiopathic tumoral calcinosis is an uncommon disorder characterized by accumulations of calcium hydroxyapatite crystals in the periarticular soft tissues with granulomatous reaction. An inborn error in phosphorus metabolism is thought to be the cause of these non-neoplastic lesions; approximately one-third of reported cases are familial. The masses tend

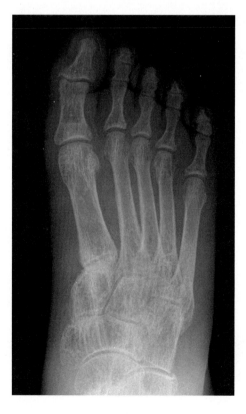

Figure 15.20 Renal osteodystrophy. AP radiograph of the foot shows a coarsened trabecular bone pattern, cortical thinning, osteopenia, and vascular calcification.

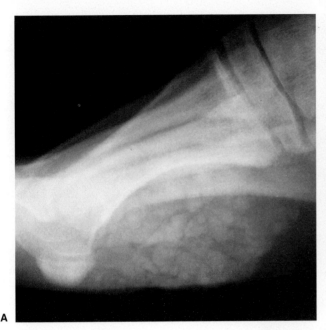 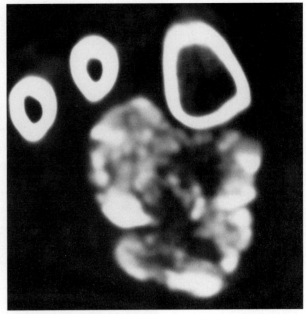

A   B

Figure 15.21 Idiopathic tumoral calcinosis. *A.* Lateral radiograph shows amorphous calcification in the plantar soft tissues. *B.* Axial CT shows calcifications with occasional fluid levels.

to grow slowly over many years to a large size; symptoms may be caused by their physical bulk. Most are discovered in the first or second decade of life. These accumulations are comprised of multiple globules of calcification separated by radiolucent bands. Fluid levels are usually present but may not be evident except on CT (Fig. 15.21). The lesions are frequently found in the normal location of bursae. The treatment is surgical, but local recurrences are not uncommon.

ENDOCRINE BONE DISEASE

HYPERCORTISOLISM

Hypercortisolism, or Cushing syndrome, is the clinical manifestation of excessive amounts of glucocorticoids. *Cushing disease* refers to endogenous, spontaneous hypercortisolism caused by an autonomously functioning pituitary or adrenal lesion or by nonendocrine adrenocorticotropic hormone–producing tumors. More commonly, hypercortisolism results from treatment with high doses of synthetic cortisol-like corticosteroids such as prednisone. Hypercortisolism has three major effects on the musculoskeletal system: osteoporosis, osteonecrosis, and muscle wasting. The combination of osteoporosis of the axial skeleton and multifocal osteonecrosis of the appendicular skeleton is typical of hypercortisolism. However, both osteoporosis and osteonecrosis may have other causes.

Demineralization of bone is almost always present if hypercortisolism has been present for a sufficient period. Glucocorticoids inhibit the absorption of calcium from the intestine and increase renal calcium loss, leading to secondary hyperparathyroidism. Glucocorticoids also exert a direct stimulatory effect on osteoclasts. At the same time, glucocorticoids inhibit osteoblastic activity by suppressing the collagen synthesis necessary for the formation of osseous matrix. The net result is continued generalized loss of bone that is prominent in the spine, pelvis, ribs, and cranial vault. In addition to osteopenia, there may be thinning of the cortex, loss of trabecular structure, intracortical tunneling, vertebral central end-plate depressions, and insufficiency fractures. Insufficiency fractures characteristically heal with exuberant callus formation. The vertebral end plates may have a sclerotic appearance that

Insufficiency fractures in hypercortisolism characteristically heal with exuberant callus formation.

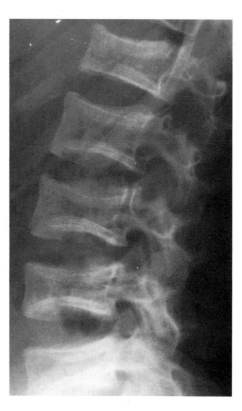

Figure 15.22 Hypercortisolism. Osteoporotic spine with advanced insufficiency fractures of all the vertebral bodies.

results from a combination of insufficiency compressive microfractures and subsequent healing (Fig. 15.22). The osteoporosis of hypercortisolism is virtually indistinguishable from involutional osteoporosis. Osteoporosis may persist long after cortisol metabolism has been restored to normal or synthetic corticosteroid treatment has ended.

Focal regions of osteonecrosis may result from hypercortisolism, particularly when the hypercortisolism results from exogenous corticosteroids. The classic sites of involvement have been reported as the femoral and humeral heads, but radiographically occult infarctions of the marrow in the shafts of long bones are also common. The manifestations of corticosteroid-associated osteonecrosis may be delayed, possibly appearing months or years after the treatment has begun or ended (see Chapter 16). The mechanisms through which corticosteroid treatment results in focal osteonecrosis are unknown. Severe secondary arthropathy may occur as a consequence of osteonecrosis and mechanical collapse of subchondral bone; the resulting loss of the bony support of the articular cartilage leads to excessive wear and osteoarthropathy. This is a particularly common problem in the femoral head.

Muscle wasting is frequent in hypercortisolism but may vary in severity from mild and virtually imperceptible to profound and obvious. In pronounced cases, it may simulate muscular dystrophy.

Hypercortisolism during skeletal immaturity suppresses growth, resulting in a short child with osteoporosis, truncal obesity, and delayed bone age. Growth resumes when the hypercortisolism is corrected, but permanent stunting may occur (Table 15.5). Osteonecrosis of a growing epiphyses may lead to abnormal development at the ends of bones and eventually results in the early development of degenerative osteoarthropathy.

Muscle wasting in hypercortisolism may simulate muscular dystrophy.

ACROMEGALY AND GIGANTISM

Clinical acromegaly is caused by excess growth hormone in adults. The underlying cause in the majority of cases is a pituitary adenoma that produces growth hormone autonomously; however, extrapituitary growth hormone–secreting tumors as well as central

Table 15.5: Some Endocrine Disorders Causing Abnormal Stature in Children

Tall stature
    Gigantism
    Hypergonadism (tall child, short adult)
    Hyperthyroidism
    Hyperinsulinemic states
Short stature
    Hypopituitarism
    Hypothyroidism
    Diabetes mellitus
    Hypercortisolism
    Somatomedin deficiency

and peripheral tumors that secrete growth hormone–releasing hormone may also cause acromegaly. Acromegaly has an equal incidence in men and women and has a mean age of diagnosis of 40 and 45 years, respectively. In younger patients, the onset tends to be rapid and often correlates with an aggressive tumor; in older patients, the onset may be slow and insidious with subtle changes occurring over a 5- to 10-year period. The clinical features of acromegaly are distinctive and include acromegalic facies, enlargement of the hands and feet, prognathism, and oily skin. Carpal tunnel syndrome, degenerative joint disease, hypertension, Raynaud phenomenon, and diabetes mellitus are commonly associated conditions. Many patients present with the signs and symptoms of a pituitary or hypothalamic mass rather than that of growth hormone excess. Definitive diagnosis is made by direct serum measurements of hormone levels.

> Definitive diagnosis of acromegaly is made by direct serum measurements of growth hormone levels.

Growth hormone activates sites of bone remodeling and may increase bone formation more than bone resorption. As a consequence, the bone mass may actually be elevated, with thickened cortex and increased trabecular bone volume. Periosteal bone formation at the insertions of tendons and ligaments and periarticular hypertrophy at the insertions of joint capsules contribute to the increase in skeletal mass.

Growth hormone increases chondrocytic activity and leads to hypertrophy of the hyaline articular cartilage. This thickened cartilage lacks the normal biomechanical characteristics of articular cartilage and is vulnerable to fissuring, ulceration, denudation, and degeneration of the articular surface. Disordered joint mechanics and a brisk reparative process lead to widespread osteophytic growths, subchondral cyst formation, and eventually to acromegalic arthropathy. Superficially, the appearance of acromegalic arthropathy is similar to osteoarthritis, but the joint spaces tend to be widened rather than narrowed (Fig. 15.23). When the process is so advanced that the cartilage has completely disintegrated, the joint spaces are narrowed. The distribution of involvement usually includes the large joints and the lumbosacral spine, including sites normally spared by osteoarthritis such as the ankle and glenohumeral joint. Calcinosis, skin hypertrophy, and nonspecific synovitis may be associated.

> On radiographs of the hand in acromegaly, the joint spaces tend to be widened.

Radiologic features of acromegaly include soft tissue thickening; enlarged sella with destructive changes; prominent facial bones and occipital protuberance; enlarged, excessively pneumatized sinuses; increased vertebral body and intervertebral disc height; posterior vertebral scalloping; exaggerated thoracic kyphosis; hand and foot changes; and bony proliferation at entheses. Osteoporosis may occur late in the clinical course.

The rare condition of growth hormone excess during skeletal development causes gigantism. Growth hormone stimulates bone growth and leads to proportional enlargement. The most striking feature is extreme height with normal body proportions, but because the sites of bone and cartilage formation that are stimulated in acromegaly (when the growth plates are closed) are also stimulated when the growth plates are open, features of acromegaly may be present. As with acromegaly, the most common cause of gigantism

> The most common cause of gigantism is an autonomously functioning pituitary adenoma.

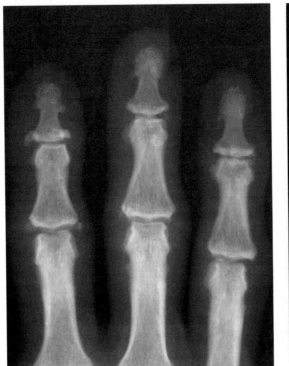
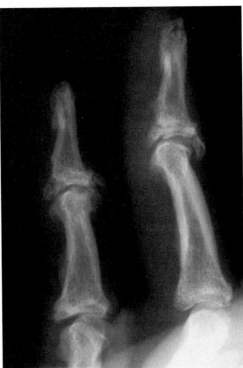

Figure 15.23 Acromegaly. *A,B.* There is mature proliferative bone at the phalangeal tufts and the insertions of the joint capsules. The soft tissues are thick, and the joint spaces are wide.

is an autonomously functioning pituitary adenoma. Unless treated, patients with gigantism develop progressively more striking features of acromegaly because the growth hormone excess continues after closure of the growth plates.

THYROID DISORDERS

Deficiency of thyroid hormone in the neonate results in mental retardation and developmental abnormalities. Bone maturation nearly stops, and dental development is delayed. Mass screening programs at birth for T4 and/or thyroid-stimulating hormone levels have made untreated congenital hypothyroidism rare. Knee films rather than hand films are more useful for bone age. In adult hypothyroidism, skeletal manifestations are mild, and typically, no radiographic features are evident.

Hyperthyroidism causes catabolism of protein and loss of connective tissue. Accelerated skeletal maturation occurs in children. In adults, increased bone turnover and remodeling lead to changes in bone mass and a rapidly progressive, generalized osteoporosis. Hypercalcemia, hypercalciuria, and elevated serum alkaline phosphatase levels may also be seen.

Reestablishment of a euthyroid state is accompanied by partial recovery of bone mineral content. Myopathy is a common clinical feature of hyperthyroidism, and symptoms may simulate those of arthritis. Muscle wasting, especially in the proximal muscle groups, is common.

GONADAL DISORDERS

Gonadal disorders may affect the skeleton through excessive or deficient levels of sex steroids. There are also syndromes that include both gonadal disorders and musculoskeletal dysmorphisms, not necessarily related. Albright syndrome, for example, occurs predominantly in females and consists of precocious puberty, fibrous dysplasia of bone, and café-au-lait spots, but the fibrous dysplasia is not believed to have an endocrine basis. The skeletal manifestation

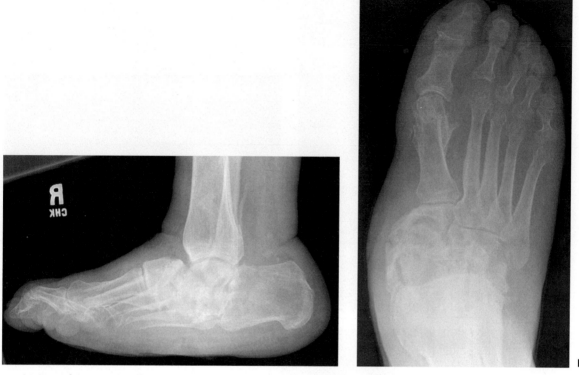

Figure 15.24 Diabetic neuropathic arthropathy with rocker-bottom deformity. *A.* Lateral radiograph. *B.* AP radiograph.

of hypergonadism in the child is precocious growth and maturation. The epiphyseal ossification centers appear early, the long bones grow rapidly, and the growth plates close early. Although there is an initial precocious growth spurt, the early closure of the growth plates has the ultimate result of short stature, with a tall child becoming a short adult (Table 15.5). The morphology of the skeleton is normal.

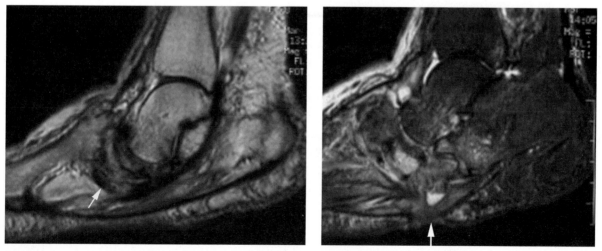

Figure 15.25 Diabetic neuropathic arthropathy. *A.* Sagittal T1-weighted MRI shows dorsal subluxation of the midfoot with fragmentation of tarsal bones (*arrow*). *B.* Sagittal T2-weighted MRI shows edema in the bones involved with the neuropathic joint as well as in the adjacent soft tissues. A plantar ulceration is present with adjacent inflammatory change (*arrow*).

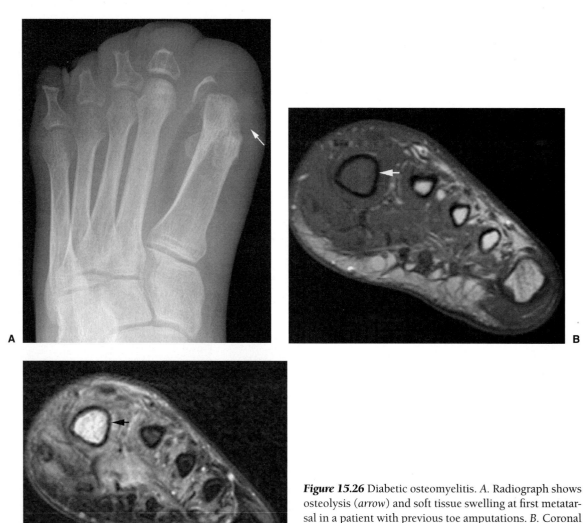

Figure 15.26 Diabetic osteomyelitis. *A.* Radiograph shows osteolysis (*arrow*) and soft tissue swelling at first metatarsal in a patient with previous toe amputations. *B.* Coronal T1-weighted MRI shows dark signal replacing the normal subcutaneous fat and marrow signal (*arrow*). *C.* Coronal T1-weighted fat-suppressed postgadolinium MRI shows enhancement in the first metatarsal (*arrow*) and surrounding soft tissues.

Hypogonadism in the prepubertal child results in delayed adolescence and delayed skeletal maturation. Delayed closure of the epiphyses has the effect of prolonging longitudinal growth and results in unusually long and slender tubular bones of the extremities. There may be generalized osteoporosis and a lack of normal muscular development. In the adult, hypogonadism may be associated with osteoporosis and its complications.

DIABETES MELLITUS

Calcification of the interdigital arteries of the foot is common in diabetics and uncommon in other conditions.

Insulin deficiency in childhood results in decreased growth, often with generalized osteoporosis and short stature. Insulin-dependent diabetes mellitus in the adult may be accompanied by generalized osteoporosis, but only if obesity is absent. Calcification of the interdigital arteries of the foot is common in diabetics and uncommon in other conditions. Additional skeletal manifestations relate to complications. Diabetic foot disease, the condition of chronic ulceration and infection, is the result of peripheral neuropathy and vascular insufficiency. Sensory loss leads to unrecognized trauma, often minor but chronic and repetitive. Motor defects result in foot deformities that lead to unusual pressure points and weight-bearing areas. Gradual derangement of the normal foot architecture progresses in a

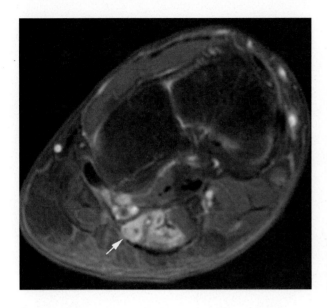

Figure 15.27 Diabetic myonecrosis. Coronal T2-weighted fat-suppressed MRI shows high signal in regions of myonecrosis (*arrow*).

vicious cycle (Fig. 15.24). Autonomic deficits and vascular disease contribute to impaired host defenses against infection. Trophic ulcers with secondary infection and cellulitis are common. The initial soft tissue lesions typically occur at the first and fifth metatarsophalangeal joints and at the calcaneus. On radiographs, one may find defects in soft tissue contour, loss of definition of tissue planes, and swelling. Contamination of bones and joints may lead to septic arthritis and osteomyelitis (Figs. 15.25 and 15.26). The typical findings of osteomyelitis may be absent in the diabetic foot because the blood supply is often inadequate for reactive bone formation and osteoporosis; therefore, great reliance may be placed on MRI for diagnosis. Peripheral arteriovenous fistulae may cause marked focal osteopenia or lysis of bone. In a small proportion of cases, frank neuropathic osteoarthropathy (Charcot joint) develops (see Chapter 13). Diabetes is the most common cause of neuropathic osteoarthropathy. Certain soft tissue conditions occur frequently in diabetics, including frozen shoulder, calcific tendinitis or bursitis, Dupuytren contracture, flexor tenosynovitis (trigger finger), and carpal tunnel syndrome. Skeletal muscle infarction may occur as a result of vascular insufficiency, particularly in the lower extremities. Acute muscle infarction may present as pain, tenderness, or swelling, similar to infection. On MRI, the condition is evident as diffuse enlargement and high signal on T2-weighted images in the regions of involvement (Fig. 15.27); these findings are not specific.

PAGET DISEASE

Paget disease (osteitis deformans) is a bone disease seen in middle-aged and elderly individuals. It is characterized by excessive and abnormal remodeling of bone. Usually asymptomatic, Paget disease has a prevalence of 3% in the adult population older than 40 years of age. In most cases, involvement is polyostotic. Although any bone may be involved, the preponderance of cases involves the pelvis, spine, skull, femur, or tibia.

Current evidence suggests that Paget disease is a slowly developing viral infection of osteoclasts. The disease has active and quiescent (inactive) phases. The active phase begins with a focus of excessive osteoclastic activity that results in a localized area of osteolysis, where bone is replaced by nonossified fibrovascular tissue. The demarcation between normal uninvolved bone and the area of osteolysis is typically quite sharp. Subsequently, the areas of osteolysis are filled in with pagetoid bone, even as the osteoclastic activity continues. Pagetoid bone consists of layers of disorganized woven bone separated by resorption cavities and nonossified fibrovascular tissue. Bone is formed both endosteally and peri-

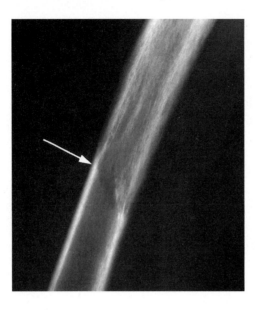

Figure 15.28 Paget disease in a femur showing the lucent zone of osteolysis (*arrow*) advancing distally into normal bone.

osteally. The combination of osteoclastic and osteoblastic activity results in rapid remodeling and turnover of bone. Eventually, for unknown reasons, the osteoclastic activity moderates, and after the osteolytic areas have filled with bone, the rate of bone turnover decreases. With the decrease in turnover, the bone enters the quiescent phase of Paget disease. Focal areas of pagetoid bone may be replaced by islands of lamellar bone, but haversian systems and remodeling along lines of stress do not occur. Slow endosteal and periosteal apposition of bone may continue to thicken the cortex and enlarge the bone, sometimes obscuring the marrow space on radiographs. The juxtaposition of lamellar and woven bone yields a mosaic appearance on microscopy that is diagnostic of Paget disease.

The progression of disease may be seen radiographically in a long bone (Fig. 15.28). The disease begins typically at an epiphysis and slowly advances at the rate of a few millimeters per year to involve the entire bone. The advancing edge of osteolysis is radiolucent, with a sharp transition between normal uninvolved bone and osteolysis. Behind the advancing osteolysis, pagetoid bone is found. Pagetoid bone has a coarsened trabecular appearance with diminished cortical density. In the quiescent phase, the bone may become extremely dense, and the overall size may be enlarged (Fig. 15.29). Because remodeling along lines of stress does not occur, insufficiency fractures and deformity are not uncommon. On MRI, the thickening of cortex and trabeculae may be seen (Fig. 15.30); however, the marrow space remains normal.

> Paget disease involves bone but not the marrow space.

In vertebral bodies, the periphery (cortex) is involved first, widening the body into a picture-frame appearance (Fig. 15.31). Continued endosteal progression results in a dense, sclerotic body. Characteristically, Paget disease involves the entire vertebra, including the posterior elements (Fig. 15.32).

In the skull, the common region of involvement is the cranial vault. The osteolytic phase is called *osteoporosis circumscripta* and appears as a geographic, well-demarcated region of bone resorption that may be mistaken for a metastasis. Focal radiodensities occur as pagetoid bone is formed. In the quiescent phase, there is a radiodense cotton-wool appearance with a thickened vault (typically 2 to 3 cm thick but often thicker). Basilar invagination of the skull may follow because, despite its thickness, pagetoid bone is weak.

The radionuclide bone scan can be used to identify all sites of involvement (Fig. 15.29). Clinical monitoring is accomplished by measuring serum alkaline phosphatase levels and urinary hydroxyproline levels, both of which are increased by osteoclastic activity. Although plain films can establish the initial diagnosis, they change too slowly and are too insensitive for clinical monitoring unless there is suspicion of a complication.

Paget disease can be treated with agents that arrest the osteolytic process: calcitonin, which is a potent inhibitor of bone resorption; diphosphonates (e.g., disodium etidronate),

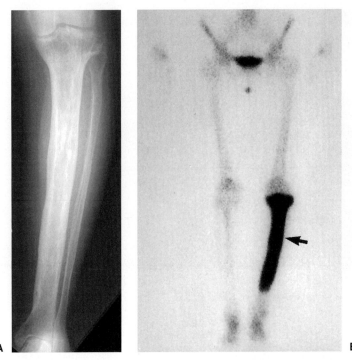

Figure 15.29 Paget disease in the tibia. *A.* AP radiograph shows typical changes of Paget disease in the tibia. *B.* Bone scan shows intense activity in the regions involved by Paget disease (*arrow*).

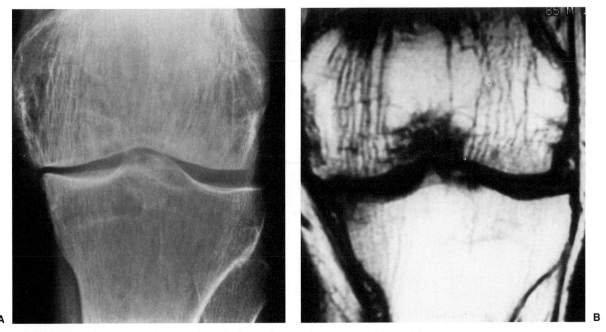

Figure 15.30 Paget disease at the knee. *A.* AP radiograph shows enlargement of the distal femoral cortex with thick trabeculae. *B.* Coronal T1-weighted MRI shows enlargement and the thick trabeculae.

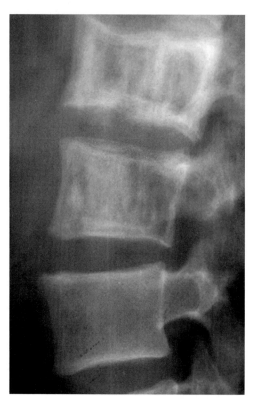

Figure 15.31 Paget disease with picture-frame vertebra appearance.

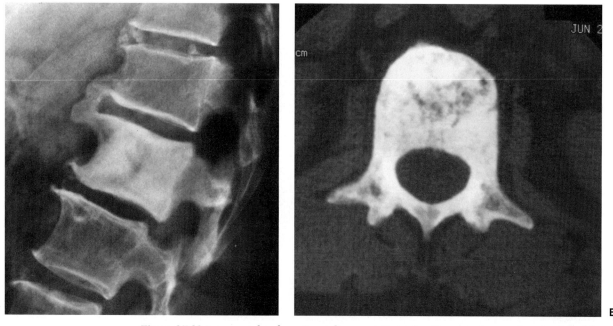

Figure 15.32 Ivory vertebra from Paget disease. *A.* Lateral radiograph shows sclerosis of the L1 vertebral body, obliterating the normal cortex and trabecular bone pattern. The process extends from the vertebral body into the pedicles. *B.* Axial CT shows increased density of the L1 vertebra with a disordered pattern of bone deposition.

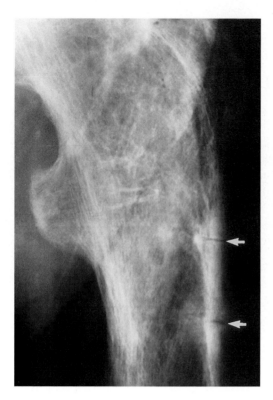

Figure 15.33 Insufficiency fractures (*arrows*) in Paget disease.

which inhibit demineralization from the hydroxyapatite crystal; and mithramycin, which is an antibiotic with cytotoxic activity.

Complications include insufficiency fractures and sarcomatous degeneration. Unless there is trauma, the insufficiency fractures are typically incomplete (Fig. 15.33). A complete fracture in the absence of trauma should raise suspicion of an underlying sarcoma. Sarcomatous degeneration of pagetoid bone occurs rarely but is more likely in patients with extensive disease. Osteolysis is the dominant radiographic feature (Fig. 15.34).

The most important differential diagnosis for Paget disease is metastatic disease. Metastatic disease may bear a superficial resemblance to Paget disease but does not have the characteristic appearance of pagetoid bone or the specific organization of active and quiescent phases in the long bones. Sometimes, the distinction is difficult to make. Although the distribution in the skeleton of Paget disease is similar to the distribution of metastatic dis-

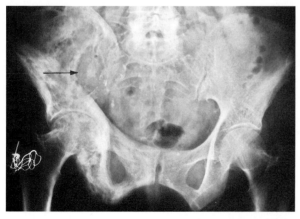
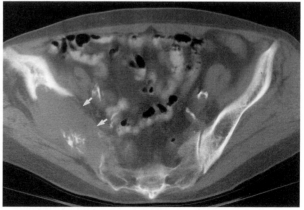

Figure 15.34 Paget sarcoma arising in the pelvis. *A.* Radiograph shows typical findings of Paget disease in the right hemipelvis and hip, with a medial region of destruction (*arrow*). *B.* CT shows destructive mass (*arrows*) and typical pagetoid changes in the remaining portion of the ilium.

ease, involvement of the ribs is rare in Paget disease and common in metastases. Discovery of a metastasis within pagetoid bone is a rare event.

NUTRITIONAL CONDITIONS

SCURVY

Dietary vitamin C deficiency impairs the ability of connective tissue to produce and maintain collagen. In a growing child, bone formation and cartilage proliferation cease, but mineralization and ossification of preexisting cartilage proceed. Generalized osteoporosis and a ground-glass bone texture with cortical thinning are seen (Fig. 15.35). There is widening and increased density of the zone of provisional calcification. Large subperiosteal hemorrhages may occur, elevating the periosteum. Nutritional scurvy is quite rare in the United States.

METAL TOXICITY

Chronic lead poisoning in children results in dense transverse lines across the growing metaphysis (Fig. 15.36). Lead interferes with the resorption of the primary spongiosa during growth. New bone is laid down on top of the primary spongiosa, but because normal resorption of the primary spongiosa does not occur during the period of exposure, a dense line becomes evident on radiographs; lead is present in only minute amounts. Lead lines are a late manifestation of chronic lead poisoning and are best seen at the knee or distal radius, where growth is the most rapid. Lead toxicity has been reported after retention of lead fragments after gunshot wounds. Chronic exposure to other heavy metals during growth, including phosphorus and bismuth, may result in transverse lines similar to those seen with chronic lead poisoning.

Fluorosis occurs after chronic ingestion of drinking water with endemic, excessive levels of fluoride (4 parts per million or greater), which are related to occupational expo-

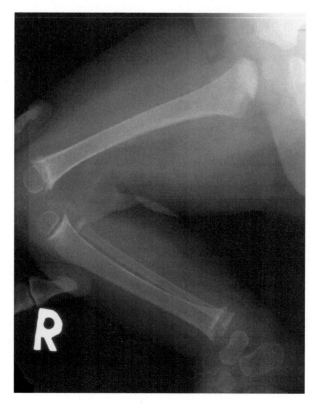

Figure 15.35 Scurvy manifested by osteopenia and cortical thinning shown on radiograph of the lower limb.

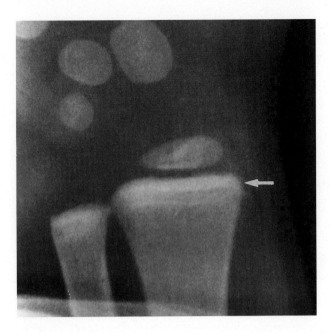

Figure 15.36 Lead poisoning with characteristic dense transverse metaphyseal lines (*arrow*).

sure or to fluoride-containing medication. Radiographic findings include osteosclerosis and hyperostosis involving the axial skeleton, periostitis and enthesopathy in the appendicular skeleton, and dental abnormalities (Fig. 15.37).

Aluminum toxicity may occur in the setting of dialysis for chronic renal failure. The clinical presentation is encephalopathy, myopathy, and bone pain. Radiographs may show rachitic or osteomalacic changes, but these may be impossible to distinguish from coexistent renal osteodystrophy.

DRUG TOXICITY

Drugs with teratogenic effects on the musculoskeletal system include thalidomide, anticonvulsants, vitamin A and synthetic retinoids, alcohol, and folic acid antagonists.

Many drugs may have nonteratogenic effects on the musculoskeletal system. Prostaglandin E, used in infants with ductus-dependent cyanotic congenital heart disease, is asso-

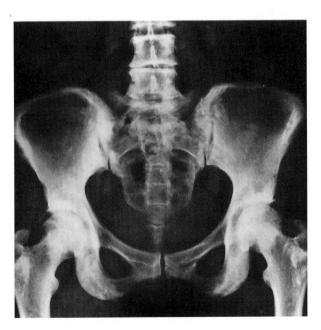

Figure 15.37 Skeletal fluorosis.

ciated with cortical hyperostosis. Methotrexate in the setting of chemotherapy may cause osteoporosis and scurvy-like changes in bone. Phenytoin and other anticonvulsants are associated with rachitic or osteomalacic changes in bone. High doses of vitamin D, sometimes used in the treatment of renal failure, are associated with metastatic calcification, osteoporosis, and osteosclerosis. The calcifications are often periarticular and may have a lobular morphology with fluid-fluid levels. Because similar findings are caused by renal osteodystrophy, hypervitaminosis D is usually not suspected until the clinical condition improves without corresponding radiographic improvement. Hypervitaminosis A, typically caused by excessive vitamin supplementation in infants and young children, causes soft tissue swelling and cortical hyperostosis. Retinoids are commonly used to treat skin diseases. In patients in whom high doses are chronically administered, bone proliferation at joints and entheses may occur. These may cause orthopedic complications and may be associated with musculoskeletal pain.

SOURCES AND READINGS

Chason DP, Fleckenstein JL, Burns DK, et al. Diabetic muscle infarction: radiologic evaluation. *Skeletal Radiol* 1996;25:127–132.

Chew FS. Radiologic manifestations in the musculoskeletal system of miscellaneous endocrine disorders. *Radiol Clin North Am* 1991;29:135–147.

Cummings SR, Melton LJ. Osteoporosis. I: Epidemiology and outcomes of osteoporotic fractures. *Lancet* 2002;359(9319):1761–1767.

Curtiss PH, Clark WS, Herndon CH. Vertebral fractures resulting from prolonged cortisone and corticotropin therapy. *JAMA* 1954;156:467–469.

Greenblatt RB, Nieburgs HW. Some endocrinologic aspects of retarded growth and dwarfism. *Med Clin North Am* 1947;31:712–730.

Hudson TM. *Radiologic-pathologic correlation of musculoskeletal lesions.* Baltimore: Williams & Wilkins, 1987:491–504.

Lawson JP. Drug-induced lesions of the musculoskeletal system. *Radiol Clin North Am* 1990;28:233–246.

Melmed S, Jackson I, Kleinberg D, et al. Current treatment guidelines for acromegaly. *J Clin Endocr Metab* 1998;83:2646–2652.

Morrison WB, Ledermann HP, Schweitzer ME. MR imaging of the diabetic foot. *Magn Reson Imaging Clin North Am* 2001;9(3):603–613.

Naganathan V, Jones G, Nash P, et al. Vertebral fracture risk with long-term corticosteroid therapy: prevalence and relation to age, bone density, and corticosteroid use. *Arch Intern Med* 2000;160:2917–2922.

Neustadter LM, Weiss M. Medication-induced changes of bone. *Semin Roentgenol* 1995;30:88–95.

Oda K, Shibayama Y, Abe M, et al. Morphogenesis of vertebral deformities in involutional osteoporosis. Age-related, three-dimensional trabecular structure. *Spine* 1998;23:1050–1055.

Resnick D. Disorders due to medications and other chemical agents. In: Resnick D, ed. *Diagnosis of bone and joint disorders*, 4th ed. Philadelphia: WB Saunders, 2002:3423–3455.

Riggs BL, Khosla S, Melton LJ 3rd. A unitary model for involutional osteoporosis: estrogen deficiency causes both type I and type II osteoporosis in postmenopausal women and contributes to bone loss in aging men. *J Bone Miner Res* 1998;13:763–773.

Siris ES, Miller PD, Barrett-Connor E, et al. Identification and fracture outcomes of undiagnosed low bone mineral density in postmenopausal women: results from the National Osteoporosis Risk Assessment. *JAMA* 2001;286:2815–2822.

States LJ. Imaging of metabolic bone disease and marrow disorders in children. *Radiol Clin North Am* 2001;39(4):749–772.

Swislocki ALM, Barnett CA, Darnell P, et al. Hyperthyroidism: an underappreciated cause of diffuse bone disease. *Clin Nucl Med* 1998;23:241–243.

Theodorou DJ, Theodorou SJ. Dual-energy x-ray absorptiometry in clinical practice: application and interpretation of scans beyond the numbers. *Clin Imaging* 2002;26(1):43–49.

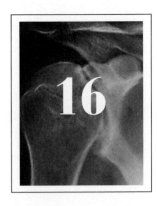

INFECTION AND MARROW DISEASE

This chapter describes the radiology of musculoskeletal infections, osteonecrosis and other marrow space disorders, and a few other skeletal conditions not covered elsewhere in this text.

ACUTE OSTEOMYELITIS

Acute osteomyelitis is a pyogenic infection of bone that typically occurs in a child who presents with an acute, systemic febrile illness. The infection is usually carried into the bone by the nutrient artery from a preexisting remote site of infection. Branches of the nutrient artery extend into the metaphysis, where they loop back and enter large sinusoidal veins. Slowing of blood flow in these sinusoidal veins permits bacterial colonies to grow and spread into the adjacent marrow, where small abscesses form. Thrombosis from minor mechanical trauma may be an associated factor. From the initial focus in the metaphysis, the acute suppurative inflammatory process may extend throughout the medullary cavity. Edema and the collection of pus increase the pressure within the closed space of the medullary cavity, leading to decreased blood flow, thrombosis, and necrosis. Osteoclasts separate dead bone from living bone. Enzymes elaborated by inflammatory cells dissolve the necrotic bone. Under pressure, pus exudes through the cortex into the subperiosteal space by way of haversian and Volkmann canals. The periosteum becomes elevated by pus, stripping away the periosteal blood supply and leading to cortical osteonecrosis. Infection may penetrate the periosteum and extend into the soft tissues (Figs. 16.1 through 16.4). Where there is capsular investment of the metaphyseal cortex, the joint may become infected. Reactive periosteal bone forms a shell around the infection, called the *involucrum* (Fig. 16.5). The central, devitalized bone is called the *sequestrum*. Defects in the involucrum, called *cloaca*, may permit drainage of pus or extrusion of sequestra through fistulas. Hyperemia causes osteoporosis in the limb. Because the metaphyseal arteries do not penetrate the growth plate, the epiphysis is initially spared, but infection may extend contiguously into the epiphysis, damaging the growth plate in the process. A solitary bone lesion that crosses the epiphyseal plate from the metaphyseal side is usually osteomyelitis. The common causative organism is *Staphylococcus aureus*.

Multifocal osteomyelitis is rare except in neonates. Because the nutrient vessels penetrate the epiphysis in neonates, early involvement of the epiphysis and growth plate is com-

Thrombosis from minor mechanical trauma may be an associated factor in the pathogenesis of acute osteomyelitis.

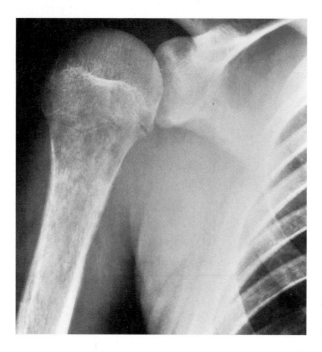

Figure 16.1 Acute osteomyelitis in the humeral metaphysis with permeated destruction.

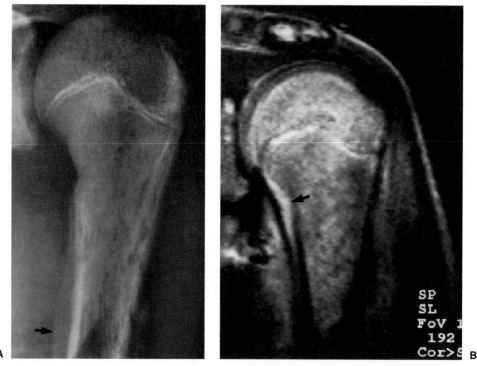

Figure 16.2 Acute osteomyelitis in the humeral metaphysis. *A.* Radiograph shows destruction and involucrum (*arrow*). *B.* Coronal T2-weighted MRI shows marrow edema and subperiosteal pus (*arrow*).

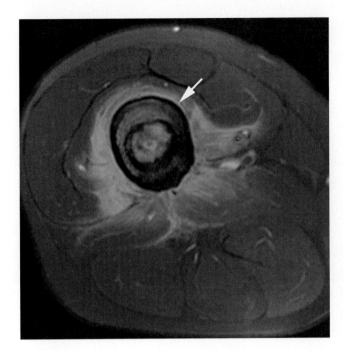

Figure 16.3 Osteomyelitis in the femur. Axial T1-weighted fat-suppressed postgadolinium MRI shows enhancement in the marrow and surrounding soft tissues, with a layer of periosteal reaction (involucrum) (*arrow*).

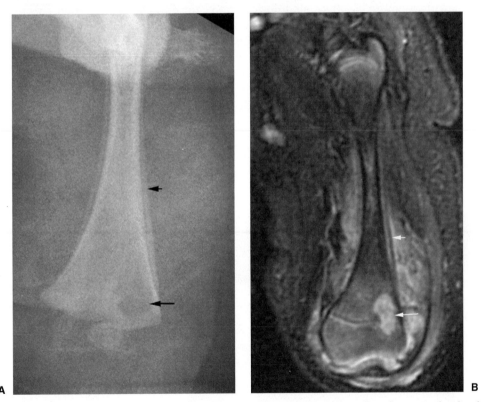

A   B

Figure 16.4 Osteomyelitis in a child. *A.* Radiograph of the femur shows a lytic lesion in the distal metaphysis (*long arrow*). Periosteal reactive bone surrounds the femur (*short arrow*). *B.* Coronal T2-weighted MRI shows high signal within the lesion (*long arrow*), periosteal reactive bone (*short arrow*), and extensive surrounding soft tissue edema. Soft tissue extension of the infection is present.

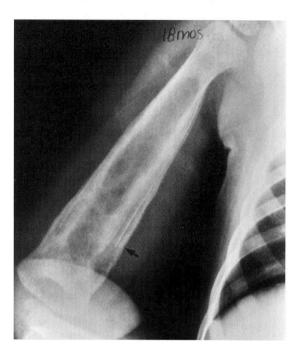

Figure 16.5 Osteomyelitis with layers of involucrum (*arrow*).

mon, with extension into the joint. Effusion may be the only early radiographic clue to the presence of infection. Subsequent bony reaction is exuberant, with periosteal reaction often involving the entire bone. Fistula formation is rare. The organisms that commonly cause multifocal osteomyelitis in neonates are β-hemolytic *Streptococcus* and *Escherichia coli*. When infection is monostotic, *S. aureus* may also be a causative organism.

Adults at risk for hematogenous osteomyelitis include patients who are debilitated or immunocompromised, elderly patients with genitourinary tract infections, patients with peripheral vascular insufficiency (especially diabetes), and intravenous drug abusers. Pathogens may also be implanted directly into the bone during trauma or surgery. Osteomyelitis does not occur in otherwise healthy adults. An antecedent history of trauma is common, and the bones of the hands and feet are commonly involved (Figs. 16.6 and 16.7). The feet are

The feet are particularly vulnerable to infection as a complication of peripheral vascular disease.

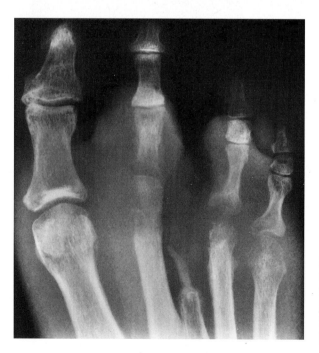

Figure 16.6 Osteomyelitis and septic arthritis involving the second and fourth metatarsophalangeal (MTP) joints in an adult diabetic. The third toe and MTP joint were amputated previously.

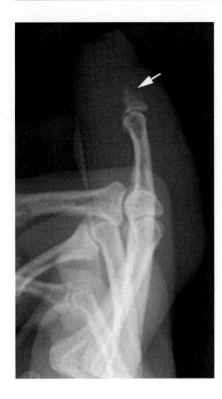

Figure 16.7 Diabetic osteomyelitis in the finger (*arrow*).

particularly vulnerable to infection as a complication of peripheral vascular disease. In adults, the initial location of infection is epiphyseal and subchondral because the nutrient artery loops into the sinusoidal veins at the ends of the bones. The common organism is *Staphylococcus*, unless the patient is immunocompromised. Contiguous spread of infection may involve the diaphysis, adjacent soft tissues, and joints. Fistula formation is frequent. Periosteal reaction may be minimal, especially in the feet. Because the periosteum is tightly applied, penetration of pus into the soft tissues is common, but subperiosteal collections are not. Multiple foci of infection do not occur.

Radiographic changes occur relatively late in acute osteomyelitis. Soft tissue swelling with obliteration of fat planes may be seen 3 days after onset, at which time pus has already penetrated the cortex. Periosteal reaction and osteolysis may not be evident on radiographs until 5 to 7 days in children and 10 to 14 days in adults. If the suspected site contains fatty marrow, CT can reveal marrow infiltration by fluid and pus early in the course of osteomyelitis, before bone destruction is detectable. CT extends the radiographic ability to define sequestra, soft tissue abscesses, sinus tracts, intramedullary and soft tissue gas, bone destruction, and reactive bone.

MRI is highly sensitive and specific in distinguishing between osteomyelitis and adjacent soft tissue infection, even in the presence of previous surgery, fracture, or chronic osteomyelitis. Early marrow edema is evident well before other imaging studies become abnormal, and subperiosteal or soft tissue collections of pus can be identified early. The key finding on MRI is abnormal signal within the marrow, low signal on T1-weighted images, and high signal on T2-weighted images. Enhancement is generally seen after gadolinium injection on T1-weighted images. Abscesses have high signal on T2-weighted images with rim enhancement after gadolinium injection on T1-weighted images.

The radionuclide bone scan is typically positive within 24 hours of onset, and a normal bone scan at this time eliminates osteomyelitis as a diagnostic possibility. Foci of acute osteomyelitis appear as areas of intense activity because of the hyperemia and reactive osteoblastic activity. Reactive hyperemia and osteoblastic activity are more extensive than the actual infected area. Devitalized, avascular areas of bone may appear as focal areas of decreased or absent activity, but the surrounding bone always has increased tracer uptake. Previous surgery, trauma, and other bone disease may complicate the interpretation of positive bone scans.

Additional problem-solving imaging tools in suspected osteomyelitis are nuclear scans with labeled leukocytes or with gallium. Both of these radiopharmaceuticals localize at sites of WBC aggregation, such as collections of pus, but both may require delayed imaging 24 to 72 hours after injection. The gallium scan may be particularly useful in following the course of treatment to confirm healing and obviate concern about possible chronic osteomyelitis.

Treatment of bacterial osteomyelitis with systemic antibiotics is effective when begun early. If there is pus formation and bone necrosis, the pus must be drained and the necrotic bone removed. Acute osteomyelitis may be complicated by chronic osteomyelitis.

CHRONIC OSTEOMYELITIS

Chronic osteomyelitis may exist many years after acute osteomyelitis, even if the acute infection was treated appropriately. Systemic antibiotics are ineffective against organisms sequestered in necrotic bone. Blood cultures are almost always negative, and cultures of the lesion are often negative as well. A rare complication of long-standing, chronic, draining osteomyelitis is development of malignancy—mostly squamous carcinomas—along the sinus tract. In chronic osteomyelitis, foci of bacteria persist within bone cavities that are filled with granulation tissue. Dense bone surrounds the site, and the cortex may be thickened as a result of long-term deposition of reactive medullary and periosteal bone (Fig. 16.8). Serpiginous sinus tracts may extend to the skin surface. Abscesses, sinus tracts, and sequestra may be obscured by the dense reactive bone, so that CT or MRI may be required. The radionuclide bone scan shows areas of increased uptake. Scans with gallium or labeled leukocytes should also be positive.

A Brodie abscess is a local, subacute bone abscess that is a fairly common cause of a solitary bone lesion. Symptoms of recurrent pain and local tenderness with swelling and erythema may be present for months or years. Most cases occur in adolescents and young adults, but the reported age range is 6 to 61 years. Men are affected more often than women (by 2:1). The typical location is the metaphysis or diaphysis of the femur or tibia. A Brodie abscess may begin de novo, develop in the same site as a preceding

> In chronic osteomyelitis, cultures of the lesion are often negative.

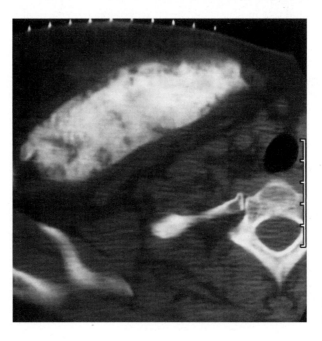

Figure 16.8 CT scan of chronic sclerosing osteomyelitis of the clavicle.

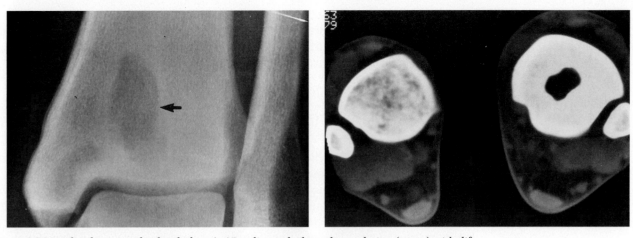

Figure 16.9 Brodie abscess in the distal tibia. *A.* AP radiograph shows lucent lesion (*arrow*) with diffuse surrounding sclerosis. *B.* CT shows the lucent lesion and the surrounding reactive bone.

episode of acute osteomyelitis, or follow an acute episode of osteomyelitis at another site. *S. aureus* appears to be the offending organism.

Radiographically, a Brodie abscess appears as a well-defined lucent area in cancellous bone with smooth, rounded geographic margins and a thick sclerotic rind that may merge imperceptibly with the surrounding bone (Figs. 16.9 and 16.10). The lesion may appear lobulated with lucent, serpentine tracts extending along the bone. CT is valuable for defining the reactive sclerosis and can permit identification of tracts in the bone. The corresponding pathology is an avascular cavity, typically 1 to 4 cm in size, lined with granulation tissue and filled with fluid but not frank pus. Thickening of trabeculae adjacent to the lesion by reactive endosteal bone formation may form the sclerotic rind around the cavity.

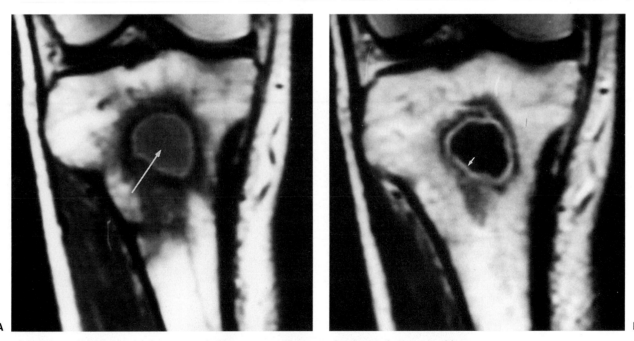

Figure 16.10 Brodie abscess in the proximal tibia. *A.* Coronal T1-weighted MRI shows central lesion (*arrow*) with surrounding sclerosis. *B.* Coronal T1-weighted gadolinium-enhanced MRI shows enhancement of the periphery of the lesion (*arrow*) but not the center.

The key radiologic feature of a Brodie abscess is the extensive reactive bone formation that has a sharp interface with the lesion but merges gradually with surrounding normal bone.

Although Brodie abscesses have a characteristic appearance, they may be confused with other focal bone lesions, including tumors. The key radiologic feature of a Brodie abscess is the extensive reactive bone formation that has a sharp interface with the lesion but merges gradually with surrounding normal bone.

SPINE INFECTIONS

Pyogenic vertebral osteomyelitis occurs in elderly adults with genitourinary tract infections, patients who are immunocompromised, and intravenous drug abusers.

Organisms from genitourinary tract infections ascend the vertebral column by way of the vertebral plexus of Batson, a valveless, venous bed that allows retrograde blood flow. The initial site of infection is the subcortical bone of the vertebral body adjacent to the intervertebral disc. The infection typically extends through the end plate, involving the disc and the adjacent vertebral body. Multiple levels of involvement are not uncommon, and the levels may be contiguous or noncontiguous. Lateral extension causes a paraspinal abscess; posterior extension can result in epidural abscess, cord compression, and meningitis.

Multiple contiguous or noncontiguous levels may be involved in spondylodiscitis.

The radiographic finding is disc space narrowing with destruction of the facing vertebral end plates. As the process evolves, increasing reactive bone production and sclerosis occur in the affected vertebral bodies on both sides of the involved disc space, often making it appear widened (Figs. 16.11 through 16.13). Bony ankylosis is one eventual outcome of this process. Paravertebral soft tissue swelling may indicate extension into the soft tissues. CT and MRI can delineate the anatomic extent of involvement.

The clinical presentation is fever, back pain, and stiffness. Diagnosis is often delayed; radiographic findings may not be apparent until 2 to 8 weeks after onset. In 60% of cases, the recovered organisms are *S. aureus*; in 30% of cases, the organisms are species of *Enterobacteriaceae*. In 40% of cases, a remote source of infection is known (usually genitourinary tract, skin, or respiratory tract).

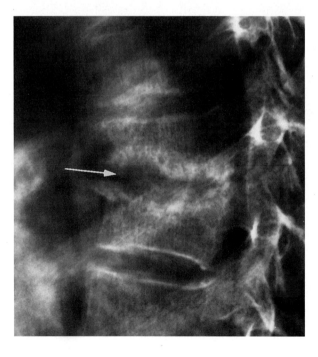

Figure 16.11 Vertebral discitis and osteomyelitis with destruction of the adjacent inferior and superior end plates (*arrow*).

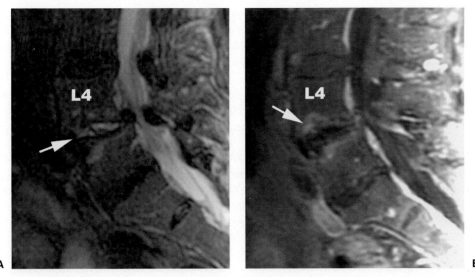

Figure 16.12 Lumbar vertebral discitis. *A.* Sagittal STIR MRI shows fluid at the L4-L5 disc space (*arrow*) and edema of adjacent vertebral body end plates. *B.* Sagittal T1-weighted fat-suppressed post-gadolinium MRI shows enhancement (*arrow*) around the L4-L5 disc space.

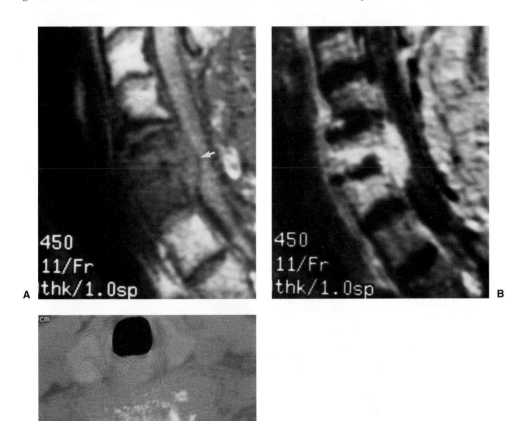

Figure 16.13 Vertebral discitis, osteomyelitis, and epidural abscess. *A.* Sagittal T1-weighted MRI shows infection of the C6-C7 level with epidural mass (*arrow*). *B.* Sagittal T1-weighted gadolinium-enhanced MRI shows an enhancing inflammatory mass with a low signal in the center. *C.* Axial CT scan at C6 shows vertebral body destruction.

MISCELLANEOUS INFECTIONS

TUBERCULOSIS

Tuberculosis is becoming more common in North America but is usually associated with immunocompromised patients or immigrant populations. Musculoskeletal disease is the result of hematogenous spread, typically from the lungs. Perhaps half of all cases of musculoskeletal tuberculosis affect the spine. The body of L1 is the site most commonly affected, but involvement of multiple contiguous levels is frequent, and involvement of the cervical and thoracic region, posterior elements, and SI joints is known to occur. The infection usually begins in the anterior aspect of the vertebral body at an end plate. Infection may spread by extending into the disc space, along the subligamentous space, or into the paraspinal soft tissues (Fig. 16.14). Paravertebral psoas abscesses may burrow into the groin or thigh.

> Musculoskeletal tuberculosis affects the spine in 50% of cases.

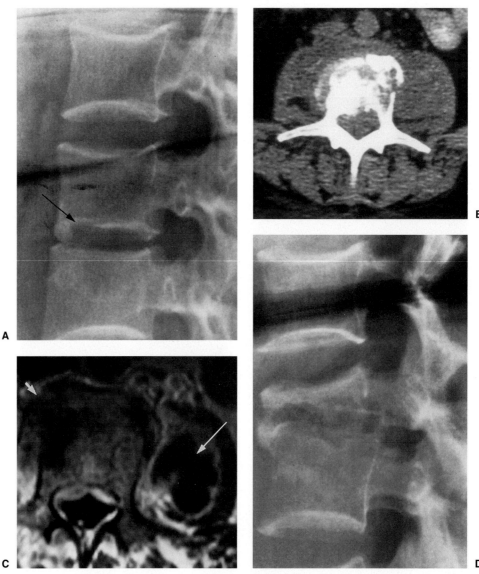

A   **B**   **C**   **D**

Figure 16.14 Tuberculosis spondylitis. *A*. Radiograph at presentation shows loss of height at the L3-L4 disc level and early inferior end-plate destruction at L3 (*arrow*). *B*. CT shows bone destruction and paraspinal inflammation. *C*. Axial T2-weighted MRI shows paraspinal inflammatory mass (*short arrow*) with left psoas muscle abscess (*long arrow*). *D*. Radiograph after 1 month shows further destruction of L3.

Tuberculosis may spread to the joints, resulting in a granulomatous synovial infection that requires synovial biopsy or joint aspiration for diagnosis. In the usual situation, the process is monarticular, and there is osteomyelitis adjacent to the involved joint. The classic radiographic appearance is juxta-articular osteoporosis, peripherally located erosions, and gradual joint space narrowing. However, multifocal disease, periostitis, sclerosis, and large soft tissue abscesses may occur.

Tuberculous osteomyelitis may result from contiguous spread from an adjacent joint or from hematogenous spread. The ends of long bones are typically involved, and there may be multiple sites of involvement within the same bone or dispersed throughout the skeleton. On radiographs, osteolysis, erosions, and osteoporosis are the dominant features (Fig. 16.15). Soft tissue extension with burrowing abscesses may be present, but reactive bone formation is sparse or absent. On MRI, the region of involvement has low signal on T1-weighted images and high signal on T2-weighted images, with enhancement after gad-

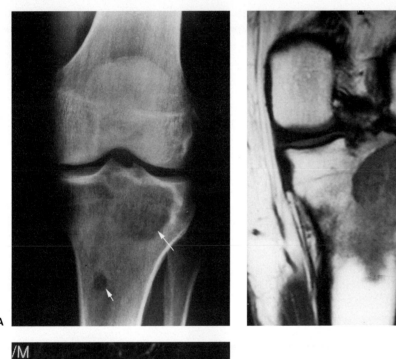

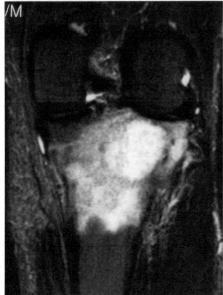

Figure 16.15 Tuberculosis osteomyelitis. *A.* AP radiograph of the proximal tibia shows a dominant rounded, lucent lesion (*long arrow*) in the epiphysis with a smaller daughter lesion (*short arrow*) distally. Reactive bone formation is sparse. *B.* Coronal T1-weighted MRI shows low signal in the lesion with an incomplete margin (*arrow*). *C.* Coronal T2-weighted MRI shows high signal within the lesion and surrounding marrow edema.

olinium injection. Periosteal reactive bone and subperiosteal involvement tend to be absent, unlike acute pyogenic osteomyelitis.

FUNGAL INFECTIONS

Fungal infections are caused by dimorphic pathogenetic organisms. The mycelial form of the organism produces infectious spores that may be inhaled and converted to yeast-like pathogens in the host. The entire range of fungal infections that occurs in the lungs may also involve the musculoskeletal system, especially coccidioidomycosis, histoplasmosis, and blastomycosis. The infections are often low grade and chronic but may become virulent when host defenses are compromised. Opportunistic infections such as candidiasis may also occur in immunocompromised individuals. Radiologic features of fungal osteomyelitis include osteolysis with discrete or permeated margins, surrounding sclerosis that is less florid than in bacterial infections, and variable amounts of periosteal reaction (Fig. 16.16). Extensive bone sclerosis and formation of sequestra are unusual. Fungal septic arthritis has a nonspecific appearance with soft tissue swelling, diffuse joint space loss, and central and marginal erosions of bone. The progression of disease is slower and the host bone reaction milder than pyogenic infections.

> Extensive bone sclerosis and formation of sequestra are unusual in fungal osteomyelitis.

CELLULITIS

Cellulitis is diffuse purulent inflammation of the loose subcutaneous soft tissues. The process may disseminate along anatomic planes. The early clinical presentation of cellulitis—particularly in children—is virtually identical to that of early osteomyelitis, but direct extension of cellulitis through the cortex of adjacent bone into the marrow space to cause osteomyelitis occurs only occasionally. On radiographs, cellulitis is evident as soft tissue swelling and obliteration of normal tissue planes, the same early radiographic features of osteomyelitis. If a gas-forming organism is involved, soft tissue gas may be present (Fig. 16.17). The three-phase bone scan can distinguish between cellulitis and osteomyelitis. On immediate postinjection flow images (radionuclide angiogram) and on blood pool images (obtained 5 minutes after injection, reflecting distribution of radionuclide in the vascular space), both cellulitis and osteomyelitis show diffusely increased soft tissue uptake. However, on delayed images (obtained 2 hours after injection), cellulitis shows no focal abnor-

> If a gas-forming organism is involved, soft tissue gas may be present.

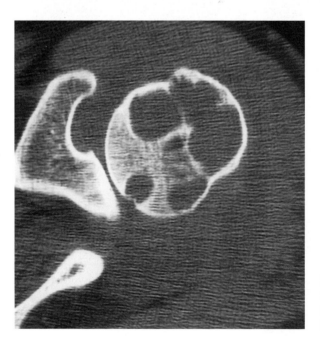

Figure 16.16 Candidal osteomyelitis of the humerus. CT shows focal bone destruction and minimal reactive change.

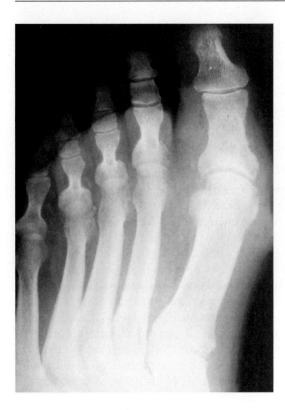

Figure 16.17 Cellulitis involving the great toe in a diabetic foot. Note soft tissue swelling, gas, and interdigital vascular calcifications.

mality, but osteomyelitis shows focal tracer uptake in bone at the site of infection. MRI and CT are also highly accurate in delineating soft tissue infections. On MRI, cellulitis is evident as reticular subcutaneous edema and enhancement after gadolinium injection (Fig. 16.18). Edema and enhancement of the underlying fascia, muscle, or bone are indicative

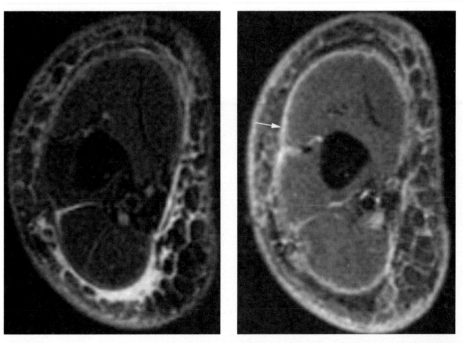

A

B

Figure 16.18 Cellulitis and fasciitis of the arm. *A.* Axial T2-weighted fat-suppressed MRI shows edema infiltrating the subcutaneous fat and superficial fascia. *B.* Axial T1-weighted fat-suppressed MRI after gadolinium injection shows enhancement (*arrow*) of the subcutaneous tissues and of the superficial fascia.

of fasciitis, myositis, and osteomyelitis, respectively. If present, soft tissue abscesses show rim enhancement after gadolinium injection. Soft tissue gas is more difficult to identify on MRI than CT.

Noninfectious subcutaneous edema—as might occur after a bite from a spider or snake or after an allergic reaction to a bee sting—results in soft tissue edema. The radiologic appearance is similar to infectious cellulitis except gas formation and abscess formation do not occur. Osteomyelitis of the underlying bone does not occur.

NECROTIZING FASCIITIS

Necrotizing fasciitis is an uncommon, deep soft tissue infection caused by group A streptococci. Known in the lay literature as the disease caused by "flesh-eating bacteria," necrotizing fasciitis has a mortality rate of approximately 25%. Although it occurs more frequently in diabetics, intravenous drug abusers, immunosuppressed patients, and patients at risk for other infections, it may also occur in young and previously healthy patients, including athletes. The abdominal wall, extremities, and perineum are the most common sites of involvement, and necrotizing fasciitis may occur with streptococcal toxic shock syndrome. Both direct implantation of bacteria through a break in the skin and hematogenous spread may occur. Patients present with severe local pain, skin changes, and systemic toxicity. Radiographs of necrotizing fasciitis in the extremities may show extensive subcutaneous edema and gas (Fig. 16.19). The gas may track along fascial planes. On CT, gas in the soft tissues is more easily identified than on radiographs. Diffuse thickening of the skin, edema of the subcutaneous tissues, thickening of the fascia, and fluid collections are other features of CT. On MRI, involved fascial planes have low signal on T1-weighted images and high signal on T2-weighted images. Enhancement of the fascia after gadolinium injection is indicative of inflammation, whereas lack of enhancement is indicative of tissue necrosis.

> Necrotizing fasciitis has a mortality rate of approximately 25%.

> Enhancement of the fascia after gadolinium injection is indicative of inflammation, whereas lack of enhancement is indicative of tissue necrosis.

PYOMYOSITIS

Pyomyositis is caused by *S. aureus* in approximately 90% of cases; most of the remaining cases are caused by *Streptococcus*. Because healthy muscle is resistant to hematogenous infections, pyomyositis usually is found in the presence of predisposing conditions such as local trauma, nutritional deficiency, immunocompromise, or con-

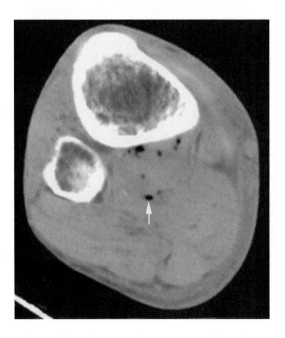

Figure 16.19 Necrotizing fasciitis in the deep posterior compartment of the leg. Axial CT slice shows muscle edema and bubbles of gas (*arrow*).

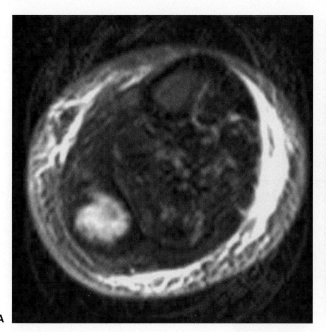 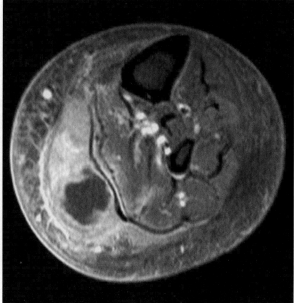

A   B

Figure 16.20 Pyomyositis with abscess in the soleus muscle of the leg of an immunosuppressed patient. *A.* Axial T2-weighted MRI shows heterogeneous high signal in a lesion in the soleus with extensive subcutaneous edema and obliteration of the normal fat between the muscle fascicles. *B.* Axial T1-weighted fat-suppressed postgadolinium MRI shows enhancement of the superficial posterior compartment and the rim of the abscess.

current infections elsewhere. Pyomyositis is relatively unusual outside the tropics. Imaging by sonography, CT, or MRI shows extensive inflammation and abscess formation (Fig. 16.20). Direct extension to bone may occur. The definitive diagnosis is made by aspiration and culture.

GAS GANGRENE

Clostridial contamination of traumatic wounds may produce extensive tissue damage and gas formation in devitalized tissues (gas gangrene). The causative agent, *Clostridium perfringens,* is widely distributed in nature. Unlike deep group A streptococcal infections, clostridial infections spare the fascia but cause rapid necrosis of muscle. Clostridial myositis is an acute, rapidly progressive, invasive infection of muscle that often results in myonecrosis and systemic toxicity. Exotoxins elaborated by the bacteria promote the rapid spread of infection by destroying healthy tissue and interfering with normal host responses. Clostridial myonecrosis has a classic radiographic appearance of extensive feather-like linear collections of gas that are widely dispersed throughout the affected muscles (Fig. 16.21). Therapy for clostridial myonecrosis includes surgery, antibiotics, and hyperbaric oxygen, with reported mortality rates of 5% to nearly 30%.

Extensive feather-like linear collections of gas within muscle are characteristic of clostridial myonecrosis.

PARASITIC INFESTATION

Cysticercosis—infestation by the larval form of the pork tapeworm—may cause dense, widespread calcifications in the muscular tissues. Calcification is a late finding that is seen years after infestation. Larval death evokes a foreign body reaction that causes localized tissue necrosis with caseation. The calcifications may be up to 3 cm in size and tend to be oriented with the muscle fibers. Parasitic infestation with other worms is unusual in the United States except among immigrants from endemic tropical regions of the world.

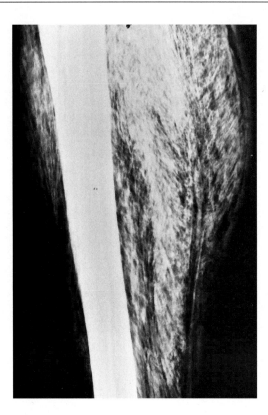

Figure 16.21 Clostridial myonecrosis with widespread dissection of gas along muscle fibers, resulting in a feathery appearance.

LEPROSY

Leprosy is a chronic granulomatous infection of the skin, peripheral nerves, mucous membranes, and other organs. It becomes evident after a lengthy incubation. Caused by *Mycobacterium leprae,* the disease is virtually unknown in the United States except among immigrants from Africa, South America, and parts of Asia. The most common radiographic abnormalities in leprosy are related to involvement of the peripheral nerves. Atrophic neuropathic osteoarthropathy may result from denervation and repetitive minor injury. On radiographs, findings may include atrophy, resorption, and tapering of the ends of the bones, particularly of the digits of the hands and feet. Involvement is generally asymmetric. Leprous periostitis, osteitis, and osteomyelitis occur, but they do so infrequently. There is a propensity for the development of squamous cell carcinoma at sites of cutaneous ulcerations. There is an increased risk of developing lymphoma and leukemia.

HUMAN IMMUNODEFICIENCY VIRUS INFECTION AND ACQUIRED IMMUNODEFICIENCY SYNDROME

Osteomyelitis in AIDS may be caused by common as well as opportunistic organisms.

Infection with HIV devastates cellular-mediated immunity, leading inexorably to AIDS and death. Musculoskeletal manifestations are less common than manifestations in the central nervous system, the gastrointestinal tract, and the lungs. These include infections, neoplasms, and rheumatologic conditions. Osteomyelitis may be caused by common and opportunistic organisms, including *S. aureus, Salmonella,* tuberculosis, fungus, and *Rochalimaea henselae* (the rickettsial species that causes bacillary angiomatosis). Bacterial myositis and septic arthritis may also be caused by common and opportunistic organisms. Non-Hodgkin lymphoma has an incidence 60 times greater in AIDS patients than in the general population. Primary and secondary involvement of the marrow is common. Kaposi sarcoma also may metastasize to bone. Anemia is common in HIV-positive patients and leads to reconversion of fatty (yellow) marrow to hematopoietic (red) marrow. Polymyositis and inflammatory arthritis have been reported in AIDS patients.

MARROW AND STORAGE DISEASES

The bone marrow is one of the largest organs of the body. Confined to the intramedullary space of bone, it consists of a meshwork of trabecular bone with fat cells, myeloid cells, reticulum cells, and supporting structures. At birth, the marrow cavities of tubular bones, flat bones, and vertebrae have a predominance of hematopoietic cells. With advancing age, the hematopoietic marrow regresses and is replaced by fatty marrow, beginning distally in the extremities and progressing to encompass incompletely the pelvis, spine, and cranium. The process may reverse (marrow reconversion) when there is an increased demand for hematopoiesis, as may occur in anemia or replacement of normal hematopoietic marrow by a pathologic process.

Radiographic findings of marrow disorders are indirect and nonspecific. When chronic marrow space expansion occurs in the growing skeleton, adaptive bone changes may occur during the development of the bone. Actual enlargement of the marrow space alters the normal bony contours; such changes do not occur acutely nor do they occur in the adult. The best method for direct imaging of the bone marrow is MRI. Because marrow is a conglomeration of different tissues, the appearance on MRI may vary, with the composition of the marrow as well as with the particular technical parameters. In general, fatty marrow has the predominant signal characteristics of fat, and hematopoietic marrow has signal characteristics more similar to muscle. Nuclear scans with technetium-99m (^{99m}Tc) sulfur colloid or ^{99m}Tc-methylene diphosphonate can provide physiologic assessments of the reticuloendothelial marrow elements and the surrounding bone, respectively.

> The best method for direct imaging of the bone marrow is MRI.

MUCOPOLYSACCHARIDOSES

The mucopolysaccharidoses are a spectrum of hereditary diseases resulting from various enzyme deficiencies in the metabolism of mucopolysaccharides. The individual diseases are differentiated by clinical features, inheritance, and specific biochemical defect, but all of them result in deposits of abnormal metabolites in the central nervous system, marrow space, and other sites. Dwarfism is common to all, and they have similar radiographic features that are collectively referred to as *dysostosis multiplex*. These features include macrocephaly with premature closure of the sagittal suture, hypoplastic paranasal and mastoid sinuses, a J-shaped sella, canoe paddle–shaped ribs, focal thoracolumbar kyphosis, and a distinctive hypoplastic "spinnaker sail" vertebra in the upper lumbar region with an inferior beak (Fig. 16.22). The diaphyseal and metaphyseal regions of the long bones are expanded, there is delayed epiphyseal ossification and cortical thinning, the iliac wings are flared with narrow supra-acetabular portions, and the metacarpals are short and wide with tapered ends.

> The various mucopolysaccharidoses have similar radiographic features that are collectively referred to as *dysostosis multiplex*.

GAUCHER DISEASE

The prototype for the lipid storage diseases is Gaucher disease (glucocerebroside lipidosis). In this autosomal-recessive condition, deficiency of glucocerebrosidase results in the progressive accumulation of histiocytes laden with glucocerebroside lipids in the bone marrow and other organs and tissues. Secondary changes in bone are observed. The classic radiographic finding is the Erlenmeyer flask deformity, which is undermodeling of the metaphysis due to marrow space packing (Fig. 16.23). Cortical thinning by endosteal erosion and osteopenia are additional radiographic abnormalities that may be evident. Osteonecrosis of the femoral head is a common association; this event is usually bilateral. After prolonged enzyme replacement therapy with macrophage-targeted glucocerebrosidase (glucosylceramidase), marrow composition, bone mass, and bone morphology revert toward normal.

> Osteonecrosis of the femoral head is common in Gaucher disease.

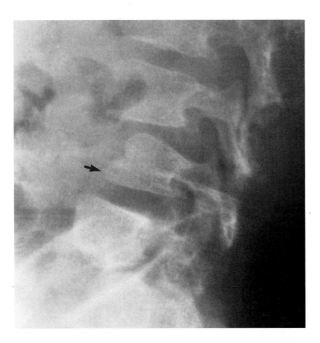

Figure 16.22 Hunter syndrome (mucopolysaccharidosis II). Lateral lumbar spine radiograph at 11 years of age shows hypoplastic "spinnaker sail" vertebra with inferior beak (*arrow*).

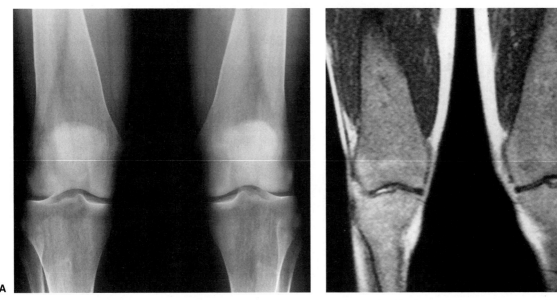

Figure 16.23 Gaucher disease. *A.* AP radiograph of both knees shows Erlenmeyer flask deformities of the femurs and tibias. *B.* Coronal T1-weighted MRI shows uniform replacement of the fatty marrow.

OSTEONECROSIS (AVASCULAR NECROSIS, ASEPTIC NECROSIS)

Most bones have a dual blood supply. The periosteum has a rich network of vessels that supplies the periosteal portion of the cortex. The endosteal blood supply enters through one or more nutrient arteries and supplies the marrow, the trabecular bone, and the endosteal portion of the cortex. Portions of bone that are covered with articular cartilage or enclosed within joint capsules have no periosteum and therefore have only an endosteal blood supply, leaving them more vulnerable to ischemic infarction.

FEMORAL HEAD

The femoral head is the most important clinical site of osteonecrosis. Men are affected more often than women (by 4:1), and the usual age range of patients is 30 to 70 years. The typical presentation is abrupt onset of hip pain without trauma. In 50% of cases, bilateral involvement is present; bilateral disease is usually asymmetric.

Osteonecrosis begins with interruption of the blood supply to the femoral head. The precise event that initiates the loss of circulation may be unknown, although a large number of clinical conditions appear to be associated with it (Table 16.1). One possible event is an increase in intraosseous pressure within the femoral head; when this pressure exceeds the perfusion pressure, blood flow stops. Ischemic necrosis of the marrow and bone follows with the onset of pain, but radiographs are normal. Intramedullary pressure measurements of the proximal femur are elevated. The typical distribution of infarction is a wedge-shaped region under the weight-bearing surface of the femoral head. The articular cartilage itself remains viable because its nutrition is derived from the synovial fluid. After infarction, the avascular area becomes revascularized from the periphery, and creeping substitution of devitalized bone occurs. When repair begins, plain films may show an increase in bony density around the periphery of the infarction. This increased peripheral density may slowly progress centrally as repair proceeds. Sometimes, the dead bone is incompletely resorbed, and a sclerotic zone remains indefinitely (Fig. 16.24). Because this repair process involves both resorption and replacement of bone, the mechanical strength may decrease transiently, and subchondral insufficiency fractures may result. Insufficiency fractures of the subchondral bone may be recognized by a crescentic lucent zone that separates the

Table 16.1: Clinical Conditions Associated with Osteonecrosis of the Femoral Head in Adults

Unilateral		Bilateral
	Commonly associated conditions	
Idiopathic		Alcoholism
Trauma		Corticosteroids
Surgery		Idiopathic
	Uncommonly associated conditions	
Gout		Arteriosclerosis
Hemophilia		Caisson disease
Infection		Cushing disease
		Gaucher disease
		Hemoglobinopathy
		Systemic lupus erythematosus
		Pancreatitis
		Pheochromocytoma
		Rheumatoid arthritis

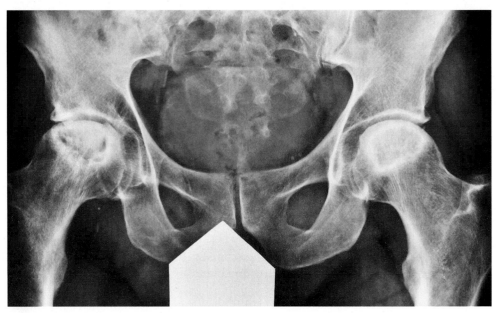

Figure 16.24 Osteonecrosis of the right femoral head with collapse of the articular surface. The left femoral head is also osteonecrotic.

fragment. This late segmental collapse of the femoral head may lead rapidly to deformity and secondary osteoarthritis of the hip.

Early osteonecrosis is best demonstrated by MRI. The region of osteonecrosis is evident as a loss of the normal bright marrow signal on T1-weighted MRI (Figs. 16.25 and 16.26).

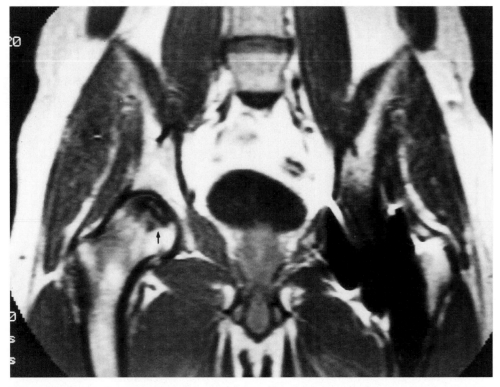

Figure 16.25 MRI of osteonecrosis of the right femoral head. Abnormally low signal is present in the superior weight-bearing quadrant of the right femoral head (*arrow*), corresponding to the segment of devascularization. The overall morphology of the head is normal. The left hip has a metallic prosthesis, hence the abnormal signal on that side.

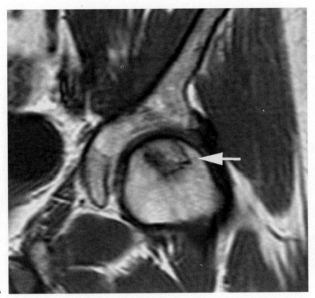
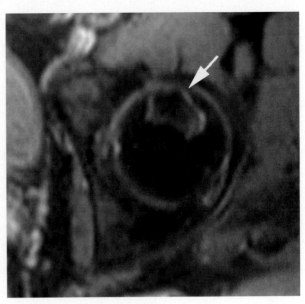

A   B

Figure 16.26 Osteonecrosis of the femoral head. *A.* Coronal T1-weighted MRI shows serpentine low signal (*arrow*) surrounding the region of osteonecrosis. *B.* Axial T2-weighted fat-suppressed MRI shows subchondral collapse (*arrow*).

Characteristically, the region of involvement is the superior weight-bearing quadrant of the femoral head. If marrow edema is present in the femoral head and sometimes femoral neck, then the osteonecrosis is acute or subacute. Hip effusion is commonly present. As the osteonecrosis begins to remodel, edema and revascularization results in the "double line" sign. On T2-weighted MRI, the region of osteonecrosis is circumscribed by a peripheral zone of high signal and an adjacent outer zone of low signal. MRI can also depict late osteonecrosis and subchondral collapse of the femoral head. The radionuclide bone scan may initially show loss of radionuclide accumulation in the avascular stage with subsequent variable increases in accumulation in the reparative stage (Fig. 16.27). The nuclear scan is less sensitive than MRI

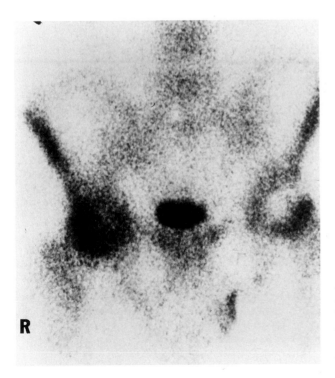

Figure 16.27 Bone scan of bilateral osteonecrosis of the femoral heads. The left head is photopenic, indicating devascularization. The right head is hot, indicating repair.

and gives poor anatomic detail. The common asymmetric bilaterality of osteonecrosis of the femoral head may complicate interpretation of the bone scan. The most sensitive test for early osteonecrosis of the femoral head is intramedullary pressure measurement.

Initial treatment of osteonecrosis is controversial. Many physicians perform a procedure to decompress the femoral head, usually by drilling a hole in the lateral cortex through the neck and into the head. Others wait for signs of deformity and osteoarthrosis and then propose a prosthesis.

SPONTANEOUS OSTEONECROSIS OF THE KNEE

Spontaneous osteonecrosis of the knee (SONK) is typically found in adult women older than 50 years of age who present with persistent knee pain and tenderness. The medial femoral condyle is most commonly involved, but the lateral femoral condyle or even the tibial plateau may be affected. The condition appears to be self-limited, with resolution within a few months, but subchondral collapse may lead to secondary osteoarthritis. Radiographs may be normal, but if subchondral collapse occurs, then sclerosis, subchondral lucency, flattening of the condyle, and eventual secondary degenerative joint disease may be seen. On MRI, the affected region initially shows a geographic area of signal abnormality, with decreased signal on T1-weighted images and increased signal on T2-weighted images (Fig. 16.28). As the area becomes revascularized and remodels, the region of osteonecrosis becomes better defined by low signal around the periphery. If the lesion progresses to subchondral collapse, the condyle may become flattened, and overlying articular cartilage may be lost.

OTHER SITES

Osteonecrosis has been described at various sites in the skeleton. The pathophysiology is the same regardless of site and follows the stages described above: ischemia, revascularization, repair, deformity, and osteoarthrosis. Examples include osteonecrosis of the humeral head (Fig. 16.29), osteonecrosis of the lunate (Kienböck disease) (Figs. 16.30 and 16.31), and osteonecrosis of the second metatarsal head (Freiberg infraction) (Fig. 16.32). On MRI, medullary infarcts are usually multiple and have a diagnos-

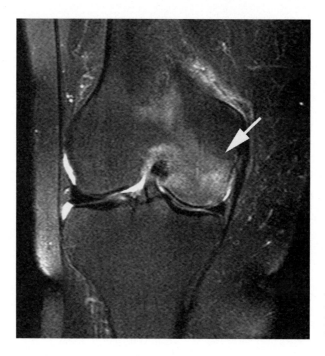

Figure 16.28 Spontaneous osteonecrosis of the knee. Coronal STIR MRI shows high signal (*arrow*) in the medial femoral condyle.

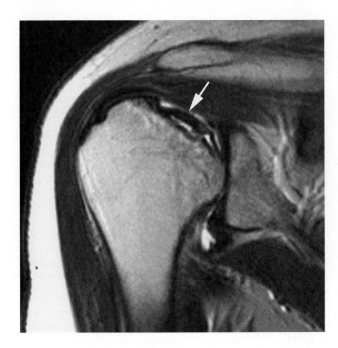

Figure 16.29 Osteonecrosis of the humeral head. Coronal T1-weighted MRI shows subchondral collapse (*arrow*) of the humeral head.

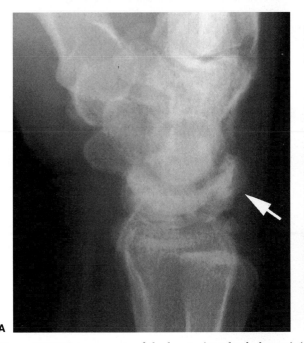

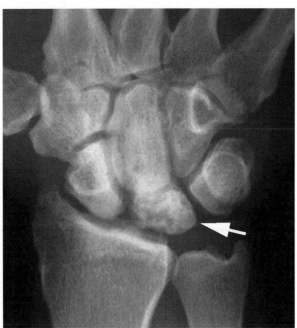

A

B

Figure 16.30 Osteonecrosis of the lunate (Kienböck disease) (*arrows*). *A.* Lateral radiograph. *B.* PA radiograph.

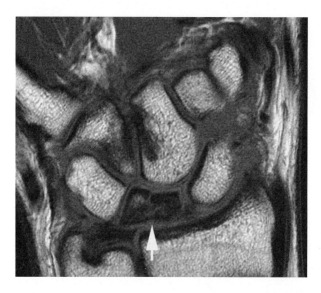

Figure 16.31 Osteonecrosis of the lunate (Kienböck disease). Coronal T1-weighted MRI shows sclerosis and deformity of the lunate (*arrow*).

tic appearance. They have an irregular, serpiginous, sharply defined low signal border on T1-weighted and PD images (Fig. 16.33). If there is a surrounding zone of high signal on T2-weighted MRI, then the infarcts are acute or subacute. This zone of high signal on T2-weighted images corresponds to the margin of revascularization and remodeling. Contemporaneous radiographs are often normal, but the infarcted marrow may eventually calcify (Fig. 16.34). This dystrophic calcification in infarcts may resemble the mineralized matrix of an endosteal cartilage tumor.

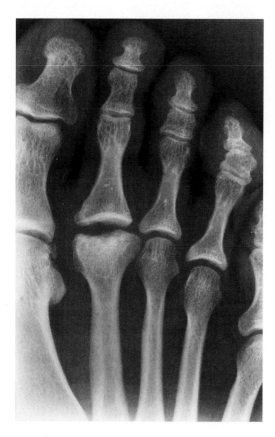

Figure 16.32 Osteonecrosis of the head of the second metatarsal (Freiberg infraction).

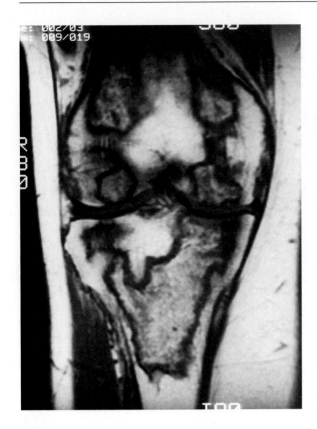

Figure 16.33 Medullary bone infarcts. Coronal T1-weighted MRI shows infarcts in the femur and tibia.

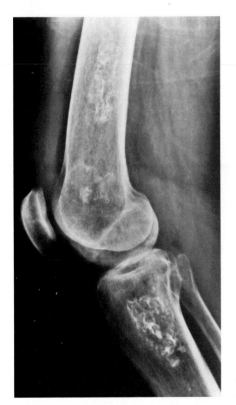

Figure 16.34 Calcified marrow infarcts in the femur and tibia.

OSTEOCHONDROSES

The osteochondroses are a group of heterogeneous conditions in which there is osteonecrosis of a growing epiphysis or apophysis. These are described in Chapter 14.

HEMATOLOGIC DISEASES

SICKLE CELL ANEMIA

Sickle cell disease is caused by an inherited structural defect in hemoglobin that leads to red cell dysfunction. The radiologic features of sickle cell disease in bone are the result of bone marrow hyperplasia, vascular occlusion, and osteomyelitis. Hyperplasia of the bone marrow expands the marrow space. Vascular occlusion results in osteonecrosis. Any portion of any bone may be involved; frequent sites include the medullary space of long bones, growing epiphyses, and the hands. Multiple small infarcts sustained over a period of years may result in sclerotic bones (Fig. 16.35). New periosteal bone apposed to necrotic cortex may result in a double layer of cortex that has been likened to tram tracks (Fig. 16.36). Involvement of growing epiphyses leads to growth disturbances (Fig. 16.37); if the femoral head is involved, the pathophysiologic events and sequelae are indistinguishable from those of Legg-Calvé-Perthes disease. A growth disturbance in the vertebral body leads to development of H-shaped vertebrae (Fig. 16.38). Localized infarctions of bone with repair or dystrophic calcification result in focal areas of bony sclerosis scattered about the skeleton. Hemochromatosis may follow repeated transfusions of blood (Fig. 16.39).

Patients with sickle cell disease have a high incidence of osteomyelitis. Unlike hematogenous osteomyelitis in other situations, the infection in sickle cell disease is most frequent at the diaphysis of the long bones, where the oxygen tension is lowest. In approximately 50% of cases, *Salmonella* species or mixed flora are the causative organisms (their presence is exceedingly unusual under any other circumstance); the remaining cases are usually caused by *Staphylococcus* species. Chronicity and recurrence are common. Osteomyelitis may be difficult to differentiate from infarction on both clinical and radiologic

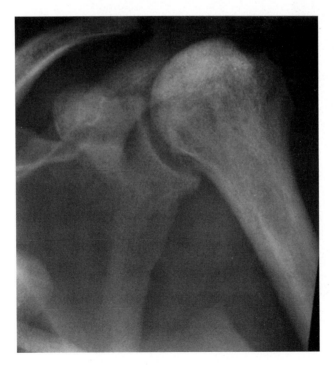

Figure 16.35 Sickle cell disease with diffuse sclerosis of the humerus from multiple small infarcts.

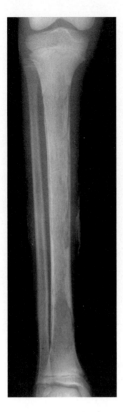

Figure 16.36 Sickle cell disease with osteonecrosis of the tibial shaft.

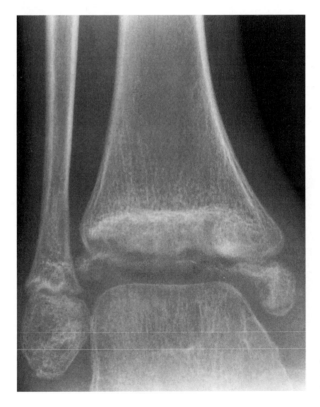

Figure 16.37 Sickle cell disease with osteonecrosis of the distal-tibial epiphysis.

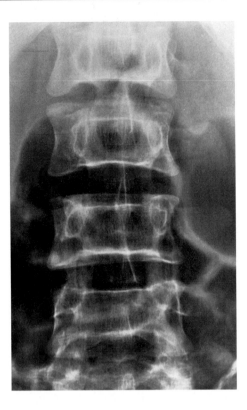

Figure 16.38 Sickle cell disease with H-shaped vertebral bodies from infarctions during development.

grounds; either one can be a complication of the other. The radiographic signs of osteomyelitis are superimposed on whatever preexisting bone changes are present from the sickle cell disease.

THALASSEMIA

Thalassemia comprises a group of disorders caused by inherited abnormalities of globin production that lead to ineffective hematopoiesis and anemia. The defect is in the synthesis

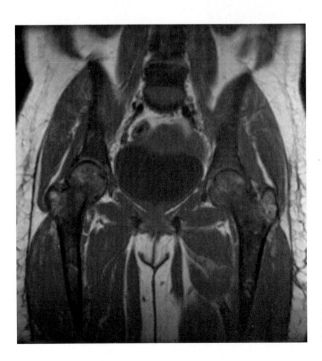

Figure 16.39 Sickle cell hemochromatosis. Coronal T1-weighted MRI of the pelvis shows marrow replacement.

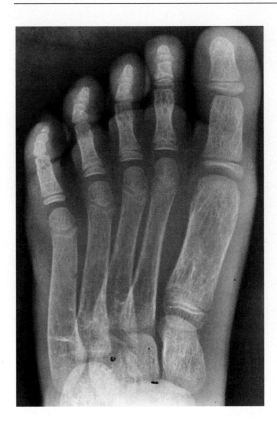

Figure 16.40 Thalassemia with manifestation in the foot. The marrow spaces are packed with hematopoietic elements, causing the bones to have thin, scalloped cortices without much medullary structure.

of one of the globin chains. There are many types of thalassemia that are distinguished on the basis of the specific globin chain affected and the particular molecular defect present. The radiologic findings of thalassemia in bone result from marrow hyperplasia and marrow space expansion. These lead to growth disturbances, modeling deformities from marrow space packing (Fig. 16.40), and premature closure of the growth plate. Localized bone infarcts and insufficiency fractures occur occasionally. Secondary hemochromatosis may follow repeated transfusions of blood. Bone marrow transplant may be curative and should lead to regression of the skeletal abnormalities.

HEMOPHILIA

Classic hemophilia is a bleeding diathesis caused by a sex-linked hereditary deficiency of coagulation factor VIII. Hemophilia B (Christmas disease) is a hereditary deficiency of factor IX, and hemophilia C is a hereditary deficiency of factor XI. The clinical features are similar, and the radiologic manifestations are indistinguishable. Approximately 90% of hemophiliac patients have spontaneous or traumatic hemarthrosis involving the large joints, often in repeated episodes. The hemarthroses are monarticular in 70% of cases. The knee is most commonly affected, followed in frequency by the elbow or ankle (Fig. 16.41). Different joints may become involved in succession, leading to polyarticular involvement. During an acute bleed, joint effusion and osteoporosis may be seen. Chronic or repeated hemorrhage leads to synovial hypertrophy and chronic inflammation. As the abnormal synovium extends across the articular surface, the cartilage is dissolved, leading to degenerative changes. Subchondral cyst formation is common, and overgrowth of the epiphyses results from chronic hyperemia; the younger the age at which these events begin, the more severe the changes. Secondary degenerative joint disease follows the destruction of the articular cartilage (Fig. 16.42). Intraosseous bleeding and the subsequent inflammatory reaction that clears the hemorrhage may create radiolucent defects in bone called *pseudotumors*. Repeated bleeding into a pseudotumor may cause it to recur and enlarge, simulating malignancy (Fig. 16.43). When such a pseudotumor is large enough to contain several

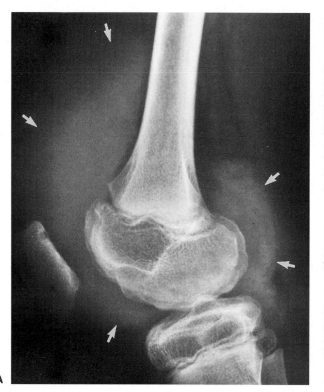
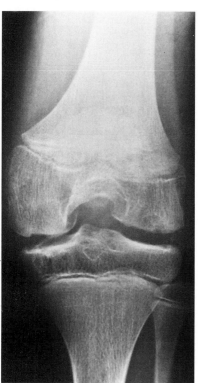

Figure 16.41 Hemophiliac knee. *A.* Lateral radiograph shows marked synovial hypertrophy and effusion (*arrows*) with epiphyseal overgrowth. *B.* AP radiograph shows squaring of the condyles and degenerative changes.

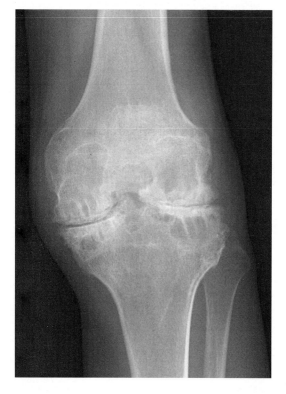

Figure 16.42 Hemophiliac knee. AP radiograph shows overgrowth of the epiphyses, widening of the intercondylar notch, and secondary degenerative changes.

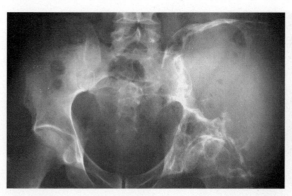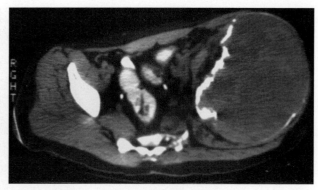

A
B

Figure 16.43 Hemophilia with pseudotumor in the pelvis. *A.* AP radiograph of the pelvis shows a large, expansile, lucent lesion involving the left iliac wing. *B.* CT scan shows heterogeneous attenuation within the mass without calcification.

units of blood, life-threatening hemorrhage is possible. Many hemophiliacs have been infected with HIV during transfusions with contaminated blood products.

MISCELLANEOUS CONDITIONS

SARCOIDOSIS

Sarcoidosis is a multisystem disease of unknown etiology characterized by the presence of noncaseating granulomas. Although the predominant site of involvement is the pulmonary system, sarcoidosis may involve the joints in approximately 10% of cases. Sarcoidosis most often causes transient migratory polyarticular arthralgias without radiographic findings. A chronic granulomatous arthritis leading to chronic noncaseating granulomatous inflammation of the synovium develops in only a few patients. Granulomas within or adjacent to the bone may result in punched-out cortical erosions or central lytic lesions with nonaggressive features within the medullary cavity. The fingers and toes are the typical sites of involvement (Figs. 16.44 and 16.45). The characteristic appearance caused by the presence of multiple granulomatous lesions has been described as lace-like.

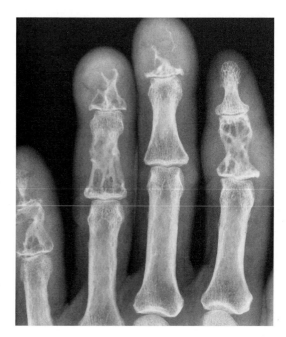

Figure 16.44 Sarcoidosis in the hand with lace-like appearance.

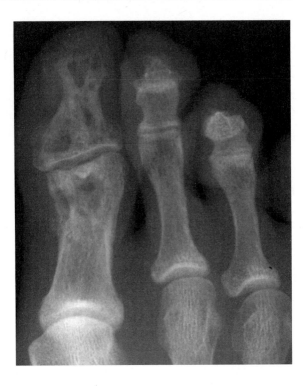

Figure 16.45 Sarcoidosis in the foot.

INFANTILE CORTICAL HYPEROSTOSIS

Infantile cortical hyperostosis (Caffey disease) is a condition of young children in which widespread, florid periostitis is seen at multiple sites, especially the mandible, ribs, clavicles, ulnas, and tibias (Fig. 16.46). Apposition of thick, mature periosteal new bone may be evident as tender, palpable lumpiness on clinical examination. The onset is usually around 2 months of age, but it is always before 5 months of age. Irritability and local inflammatory signs may be present. The condition, is in most cases, self-limited and benign, and the bones remodel over a period of months to years. The cause of infantile cortical hyperostosis is thought to be infectious or postinfectious, although this has not been shown conclusively. There is a familial tendency in some cases. The differential diagnosis includes accidental and intentional trauma and multifocal osteomyelitis. The absence of fractures helps exclude trauma, and the absence of joint effusions and bone destruction helps exclude osteomyelitis.

HYPERTROPHIC OSTEOARTHROPATHY

Hypertrophic osteoarthropathy is a combination of generalized periostitis and digital clubbing. In approximately 5% of cases, the condition is inherited and called *primary hypertrophic osteoarthropathy* or *pachydermoperiostosis*. In 95% of cases, hypertrophic osteoarthropathy is secondary to other—often pulmonary—disease. Bronchogenic carcinoma is the most common cause of secondary hypertrophic osteoarthropathy, and approximately 5% of cases of bronchogenic carcinoma have secondary hypertrophic osteoarthropathy. Periostitis, the hallmark of this condition, is found in multiple sites, usually beginning in the diaphysis of the long bones and extending toward the metaphysis (Fig. 16.47). Increased vascular perfusion of the affected bones and overgrowth of vascular connective tissues surrounding the bones, joints, and tendons appear to precede the periostitis. The clinical presentation is pain and swelling in the affected extremities. The pathogenesis of secondary hypertrophic osteoarthropathy is unknown; possibilities described in the literature include a humoral factor, a neurogenic mechanism, and hypervascularity.

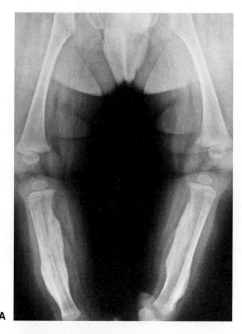

A

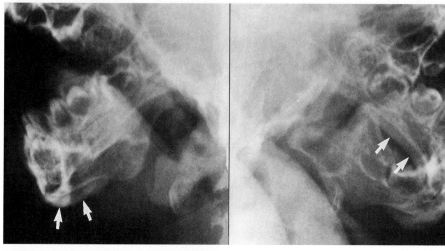

B

Figure 16.46 Infantile cortical hyperostosis in a 5-month-old boy. *A.* Thick, periosteal new bone is present along both tibias. *B.* Thick, periosteal new bone is present along the mandible (*arrows*).

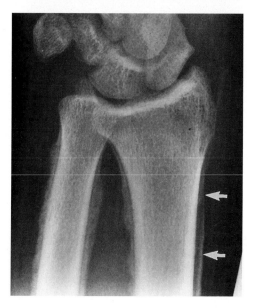

Figure 16.47 Secondary hypertrophic osteoarthropathy (*arrows*) in a patient with lung cancer.

SOURCES AND READINGS

Berquist TH, ed. *MRI of the musculoskeletal system*, 4th ed. Philadelphia: Lippincott Williams & Wilkins, 2001.

Brothers TE, Tagge DU, Stutley JE, et al. Magnetic resonance imaging differentiates between necrotizing and nonnecrotizing fasciitis of the lower extremity. *J Am Coll Surg* 1998;187(4):416–421.

Green RJ, Dafoe DC, Raffin TA. Necrotizing fasciitis. *Chest* 1996;110:219–229.

Henkin RE, Boles MA, Dillehay GL, et al., eds. *Nuclear medicine*. St. Louis: Mosby–Year Book, 1996.

Hermann G, Pastores GM, Abdelwahab IF, et al. Gaucher disease: assessment of skeletal involvement and therapeutic responses to enzyme replacement. *Skeletal Radiol* 1997;26:687–696.

Hirsch R, Miller SM, Kazi S, et al. Human immunodeficiency virus-associated atypical mycobacterial skeletal infections. *Semin Arthritis Rheum* 1996;25:347–356.

Lew DP, Waldvogel FA. Osteomyelitis. *N Engl J Med* 1997;336:999–1007.

Modic MT, Masaryk TJ, Ross JS. *Magnetic resonance imaging of the spine*, 2nd ed. St. Louis: Mosby, 1994.

Rosenthal DI, Doppelt SH, Mankin HJ, et al. Enzyme replacement therapy for Gaucher disease: skeletal responses to macrophage-targeted glucocerebrosidase. *Pediatrics* 1995;96:629–637.

Schmid MR, Kossmann T, Duewell S. Differentiation of necrotizing fasciitis and cellulitis using MR imaging. *AJR Am J Roentgenol* 1998;170(3):615–620.

Seal DV. Necrotizing fasciitis. *Curr Opin Infect Dis* 2001;14:127–132.

Steinbach LS, Tehranzadeh J, Fleckenstein JL, et al. Human immunodeficiency virus infection: musculoskeletal manifestations. *Radiology* 1993;186:833–838.

Tehranzadeh J, Wong E, Wang F, et al. Imaging of osteomyelitis in the mature skeleton. *Radiol Clin North Am* 2001;39:223–250.

Trueta J. *Studies in the development and decay of the human frame*. Philadelphia: WB Saunders, 1968.

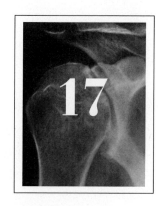

POSTSURGICAL IMAGING

IMAGING TECHNIQUES

Viewing images of postsurgical orthopedic patients can be mind-numbing if one does not understand the surgery that was performed. This chapter describes the imaging of the musculoskeletal system after a variety of orthopedic operations. Imaging after fracture treatment is described in Chapter 6.

The standard diagnostic imaging techniques for the musculoskeletal system can be applied to postsurgical patients. Many operations are guided by the use of intraoperative fluoroscopy or radiographs. Standard radiographs are generally obtained immediately after surgery to document the postoperative results. At follow-up visits, radiographs are obtained to monitor healing and to screen for complications. When extensive hardware has been implanted, nonstandard, obliquely positioned radiographs—or even radiographs positioned under fluoroscopy—may be necessary to project the hardware away from the bone, allowing it to be visualized. More specialized techniques are generally reserved for problem solving. CT can be used to evaluate the progress of healing when radiographs are equivocal, especially in the presence of complex anatomy and hardware. Streak artifacts on CT result from the high x-ray attenuation by metal (Fig. 17.1). Improvements in CT scanners and reconstruction algorithms and in orthopedic hardware materials have reduced the impact of these artifacts. On MRI, extensive artifacts are caused by metallic implants (Fig. 17.2). Large implants may distort the surrounding magnetic field and cause the computer to distort the anatomy around the implants. Even when no hardware has been left behind, artifacts may be present from microscopic metallic particles introduced by instruments. These artifacts tend to be minimized on T1-weighted images but become more extensive ("bloom") on T2-weighted or inversion recovery images (Fig. 17.3). However, previous surgery and orthopedic implants are not contraindications to MRI, and MRI may provide useful information in many situations. Arthrography should be considered when there is a question of joint infection or other postsurgical joint abnormality. Stress views

CT can be used to evaluate the progress of healing when radiographs are equivocal, especially in the presence of complex anatomy and hardware.

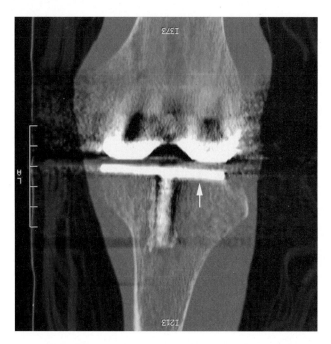

Figure 17.1 Coronal reconstruction of CT scan through total knee replacement shows severe artifact from the presence of metal, yet the metal–bone interface (*arrow*) of the tibial component is clearly visible.

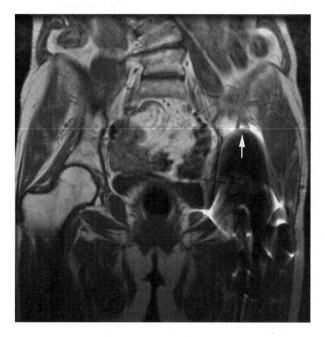

Figure 17.2 Coronal T2-weighted MRI of the pelvis with major metal artifact on the left side due to the presence of a total hip replacement. The computer has located the artifact (*arrow*) well above the actual location of the replacement.

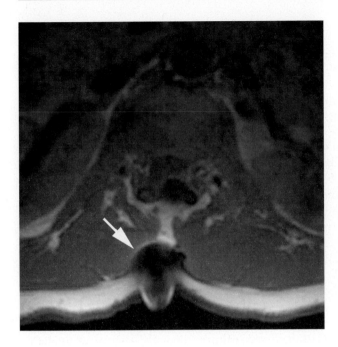

Figure 17.3 MRI with metal artifact from metal surgical instruments. T1-weighted axial spine MRI shows very dark areas (*arrow*) overlying the skin and the left posterolateral spinal canal in this patient with laminectomy. There were no actual metal clips or other implants present.

or examination under fluoroscopy may document motion at sites where none was intended. The radionuclide bone scan is useless in the immediate postoperative period because of tracer uptake at the surgical site. The intensity of tracer accumulation returns toward normal after approximately 6 months, at which time bone scan may be obtained when indicated (Fig. 17.4). Imaging with labeled leukocytes or gallium-67 may be helpful when there is a question of infection.

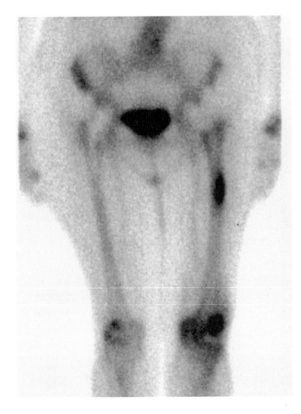

Figure 17.4 Anterior view of radionuclide bone scan of a patient with bilateral total hip replacements. A stress fracture was present in the lateral femoral cortex on the left.

OSTEOTOMY

An osteotomy is any operation that involves a surgical cut through bone. Osteotomies are commonly performed to change the alignment, length, or shape of a bone. For example, a fracture malunion with angular deformity may be revised by an osteotomy that realigns the fragments. Osteotomies may be described by their site and the direction of change in the distal fragment. A valgus osteotomy of a long bone realigns the distal fragment into valgus relative to its original alignment. A lateral displacement osteotomy repositions the distal fragment laterally. Changes in rotational alignment may also be made; these are called *rotational osteotomies*. Shortening is accomplished by the removal of bone. Lengthening may be accomplished by displacement of overlapping fragments by the insertion of bone graft or by bone distraction using an external fixator. The fixation and healing of osteotomies are similar to that of fractures, and the hardware devices used to treat fractures are applicable (see Chapter 6). Complications of healing are rare.

Osteotomies are also used to alter the alignment and biomechanics of joints. A high tibial valgus osteotomy is a common treatment for severe medial compartment osteoarthritis with varus deformity (Fig. 17.5). By realigning the tibial shaft, the varus deformity is corrected, and the mechanical axis of the knee is restored. This has the effect of reducing the weight-bearing stress on the diseased medial compartment and redistributing some of it to the lateral compartment. Distal femoral varus osteotomies can correct valgus deformities at the knee from lateral compartment osteoarthritis. Similarly, angular or rotational osteotomies of the proximal femur alter the major weight-bearing portion of the femoral head in the treatment of hip dysplasia, early osteoarthritis, or similar conditions. An innominate osteotomy may be used to deepen the acetabulum.

A bunion is a symptomatic protrusion at the medial aspect of the head of the first metatarsal that is the result of a valgus deformity of the great toe and a varus deformity of the first metatarsal (also called *hallux valgus primus varus*). Tension along the flexors and extensors of the great toe acts like bowstrings to increase the angular deformities. The condition may be painful and is often compounded by the difficulty of fitting shoes. Surgical

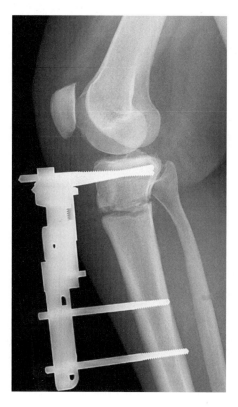

Figure 17.5 High tibial valgus osteotomy with external fixator.

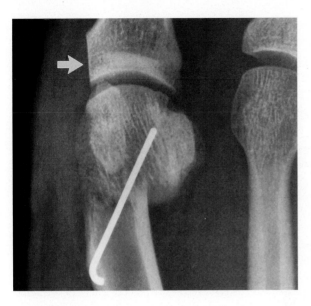

Figure 17.6 Bunion repair with shortening and displacement osteotomy of the first metatarsal, fixed by K-wire. Also note osteotomy of the proximal phalanx of the great toe (*arrow*).

correction involves not only removing the bony prominence but also—more important—realigning the great toe with its flexors and extensors. Commonly, the first metatarsal is shortened, and the head is displaced laterally (Fig. 17.6).

ARTHRODESIS

An arthrodesis is a surgical fusion of a joint. An intra-articular arthrodesis is accomplished by resecting the joint and fixing the ends of the articulating bones together. Internal or external fixation may be used as well as bone graft. A healed and remodeled arthrodesis has a continuous cortex and trabecular structure across the site. Adaptive changes may occur in adjacent joints in response to the loss of motion. Joint pain in arthritis can be eliminated by synovectomy and arthrodesis. Common sites for arthrodesis include the fingers, for treatment of arthritis; the wrist, for treatment of arthritis or posttraumatic instability; and the subtalar joint, for treatment of posttraumatic arthritis. One of the more common arthrodeses involving the foot is the triple arthrodesis, in which the subtalar joints, calcaneocuboid joint, and talonavicular joints are arthrodesed (Fig. 17.7). In the setting of arthritis, it may sometimes be difficult to distinguish an arthrodesis from a bony

In the setting of arthritis, it may sometimes be difficult to distinguish an arthrodesis from a bony ankylosis (joint fusion caused by disease).

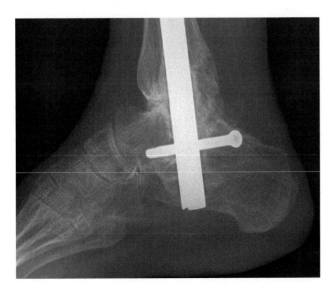

Figure 17.7 Ankle arthrodesis with locked intramedullary rod fixation.

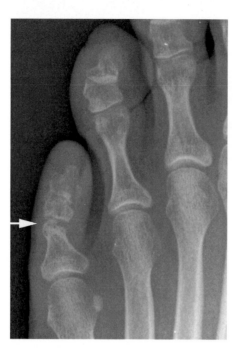

Figure 17.8 Resection arthroplasty of the interphalangeal joint (*arrow*) of the fifth toe.

ankylosis (joint fusion caused by disease). An extra-articular arthrodesis is accomplished by establishing a bony bridge across a joint that prevents motion without actually resecting the joint itself. Some spine fusions involve an extra-articular arthrodesis. An epiphysiodesis, a surgical fusion of an open growth plate, may be performed for correction of growth discrepancy.

ARTHROPLASTY

An arthroplasty is a surgical repair of a joint. Resection arthroplasty involves excision of one or both of the articular surfaces, leaving the ends of the bone to articulate with each other. Because the joint is not fixed, a pseudoarthrosis develops, preserving motion. Common sites for resection arthroplasty include the toes and hip. Many toe deformities result from soft tissue contractures. Reducing the length of the bone through resection arthroplasty eliminates the effect of contractures (Fig. 17.8). Resection arthroplasty may also be performed with resection of a small bone at a painful joint such as the trapezium from the first carpometacarpal (CMC) joint (Fig. 17.9). At the

Common sites for resection arthroplasty include the toes and the hip.

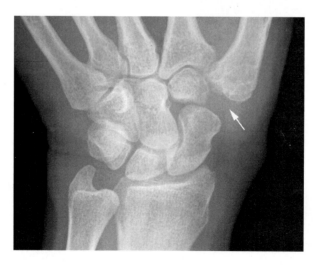

Figure 17.9 Resection arthroplasty of the first carpometacarpal joint (*arrow*).

hip, a resection arthroplasty is called a *Girdlestone procedure*. Replacement arthroplasty involves replacing one or more articular surfaces with a prosthesis (discussed in the section Joint Replacement).

JOINT REPLACEMENT

Prosthetic joint replacements are the most common elective orthopedic operations performed in the United States. A total joint replacement arthroplasty replaces both sides of the joint with prosthetic components. A hemi-arthroplasty replaces one side of the joint with a prosthesis.

MATERIALS AND TECHNIQUES

Metal, polyethylene, and cement are commonly used in manufacturing joint replacements. Metal components—usually titanium or a cobalt-chromium alloy—are used for strength and stiffness. The fatigue strength of these metals under cyclic loading is such that *in vivo* failure is rare. Ultra-high-molecular-weight polyethylene is used for concave articular surfaces such as the acetabulum, tibial plateau, and glenoid fossa. This material is denser and stiffer than the polyethylene used in common kitchenware and is manufactured to have high resistance to abrasive wear. A metal back is often used to provide mechanical support. Polyethylene is radiolucent—like other plastics—but the presence of a metal back, especially at the acetabulum, may obscure the polyethylene on radiographs. Many polyethylene components have embedded metal markers that indicate their position on radiographs. Bone cement (polymethylmethacrylate or methylmethacrylate) is a rapidly polymerizing acrylic plastic that is used as an adhesive to fix metallic or polyethylene components to bone. Cement is rendered radiopaque during manufacture by the addition of barium sulfate. Ceramics recently have been introduced for use as articular surfaces, usually as femoral heads in total hip replacements (THRs). For the small joints of the hands and feet, silicone rubber prostheses may be used. Recently, polycarbonate plastic components have been introduced for use in the hand.

> Polyethylene is radiolucent.

Implanted metal components are often fixed into bone with cement. Bubbles in the cement that might act as stress risers are removed before use by centrifugation or vacuum chamber, and the cement is injected into the medullary space under high pressure. A polyethylene plug at the bottom of the prepared cavity creates a closed space and prevents flow of cement down the medullary canal. Metal prostheses that are implanted without cement may have a mechanical press fit that provides immediate stability and a specially textured surface (porous coat) that allows ingrowth of bone or fibrous tissue, providing eventual long-term fixation. A high degree of precision is ensured at surgery through the use of jigs, cutting guides, and mock-ups that allow the surgeon to achieve a perfect geometric fit between bone and prosthetic component. Screws temporarily secure some cementless components until bone ingrowth occurs. Hydroxyapatite crystals applied to the surfaces of cementless metal components during manufacturing may improve biologic fixation in bone. The crystalline coating of the prosthesis is directly incorporated into the molecular structure of the host bone.

Because different materials deform to different degrees under mechanical loading (their stiffness is different), shear stresses develop at the interfaces, particularly between bone and metal or bone and cement. A layer of fibrous tissue that grows into these interfaces helps dissipate the forces by redistributing them over a greater surface area. This layer is similar to the periodontal ligament that cushions the teeth in the softer cancellous bone of the jaws. The fibrous layer may be visible on radiographs as a fine lucency (no more than 2 mm thick) between bone and cement or bone and metal. An additional area of increased stress is the interface between cement and metal; microscopic motion may occur at this interface, but no gap should be seen.

HIP REPLACEMENT

Hemi-arthroplasties are used for disease of the proximal femur in which the acetabulum is relatively normal.

There are several general types of hip replacements. A cup arthroplasty resurfaces the articular surface of the femoral head with a metal cup (Fig. 17.10). Hemi-arthroplasties of the hip replace the femoral head. Simple femoral prostheses compose a single metal component with a stem that is fitted into the medullary canal and a head that articulates with the native acetabulum (Fig. 17.11). Bipolar femoral prostheses have a metal femoral component comprising a stem and a head and an acetabular component comprising a metal socket with a polyethylene liner. The metal socket articulates with the native acetabulum, and the head of the femoral component articulates with the polyethylene liner. Although the acetabular component is not fixed, most of the motion takes place between the head and liner, preserving the native acetabular cartilage (Fig. 17.12). Hemi-arthroplasties are used for disease of the proximal femur in which the acetabulum is relatively normal. For example, a femoral neck fracture complicated by osteonecrosis might be managed with a bipolar femoral prosthesis. A bipolar prosthesis may be converted to a THR with interchangeable components. A THR has both femoral and acetabular components that replace the native articular surfaces (Fig. 17.13). Most currently implanted prostheses have a metal acetabular component with a polyethylene liner that forms the articular surface. The components may be fixed to the bone with or without cement. Some surgical approaches require an osteotomy of the greater trochanter for exposure; it is usually reattached with wires or cables. If a nonunion develops, a lurching gait disturbance results. If a gluteal soft tissue release is used for surgical exposure, the gluteal musculature may be reattached to the greater trochanter with sutures, screws with washers, or soft tissue anchors. Bone graft and specialized hardware may be inserted to buttress a deficient proximal femur or acetabulum.

The most common early complication of THR is dislocation (Fig. 17.14), sometimes occurring as the patient is being transferred from the operating room table to a gurney for transport to the recovery room (Table 17.1).

Heterotopic bone formation after THR is common; it may occasionally interfere with motion (Fig. 17.15).

Osteolysis in total joint replacements is usually caused by foreign body granulomatous reaction. The mechanical friction of metal on polyethylene abrades microscopic particles

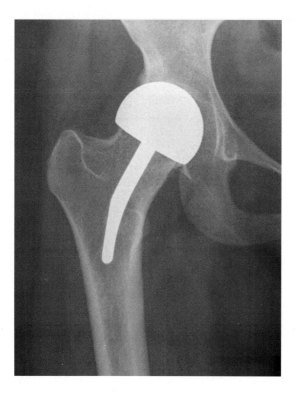

Figure 17.10 Cup arthroplasty of the hip.

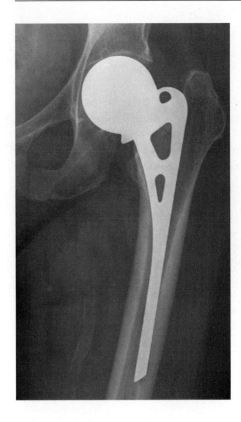

Figure 17.11 Austin-Moore femoral endoprosthesis.

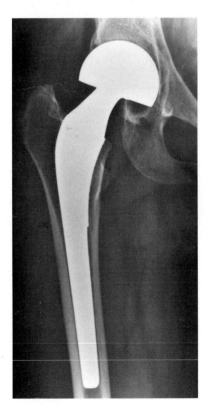

Figure 17.12 Cementless bipolar femoral endoprosthesis.

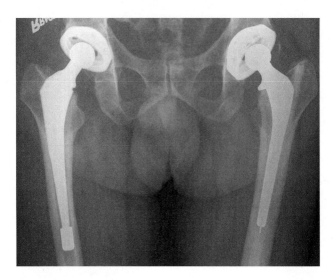

Figure 17.13 Bilateral total hip replacements. The prosthesis on the right side is noncemented. The prosthesis on the left side has a cemented femoral component and a noncemented acetabular component.

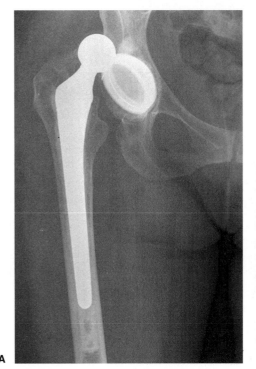

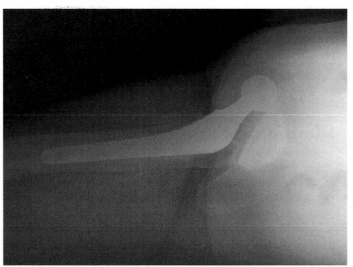

A   B

Figure 17.14 Dislocated total hip replacement. *A.* AP radiograph shows lateral and superior dislocation. *B.* True lateral radiograph shows anterior dislocation with external rotation.

Table 17.1: Complications of Joint Replacement

Fracture
Dislocation
Polyethylene wear or failure
Osteolysis
Metallosis
Infection
Loosening
Stress fracture
Neurovascular injuries
Thromboembolism

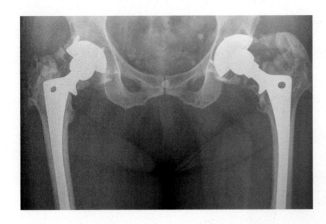

Figure 17.15 Heterotopic ossification in bilateral total hip replacements.

of polyethylene, which incite an osteolytic granulomatous foreign body reaction. Migration of polyethylene debris and its accompanying reaction along cement–bone or metal–bone interfaces—often in the form of a thin membrane—may eventually cause gross loosening. Massive localized osteolysis may also occur; these lesions are filled with the same polyethylene foreign body reaction that causes component loosening. Polyethylene osteolysis usually progresses slowly over many years. Debris may pass through lymphatics to regional lymph nodes. Because the radiolucent polyethylene liners of total joint replacements are responsible for the joint space on radiographs, thinning or gross failure of the polyethylene is evident on radiographs as narrowing of the joint space (Fig. 17.16). Some newer prostheses have eliminated the polyethylene acetabular liner from their designs, replacing it with metal or ceramic liners. Their prostheses therefore have ceramic-on-ceramic or metal-on-metal bearing surfaces.

> Microscopic particles of polyethylene may incite an osteolytic granulomatous foreign body reaction that leads to loosening of components.

Radiographic findings that suggest loosening of prosthetic components include widening of the lucent zone at the cement–bone or metal–bone interfaces to greater than 2 mm, migration of components from their original positions, development of a lucent gap between metal and cement, cement fracture, periosteal reactive bone, and osteolysis (Figs. 17.17 and 17.18). Any gap between metal and cement is abnormal. A gap of more than 2 mm between bone and metal or bone and cement is abnormal. However, a component may not be clinically loose or symptomatic until the gap surrounds the component completely. With radiography, only the interface that is in tangent to the x-ray beam can be confidently assessed. Fragmentation of cement appears to be the result of mechanical failure rather than a biologic process.

> Any gap between metal and cement is abnormal.

KNEE REPLACEMENT

A total knee replacement (TKR) has a bicondylar femoral component, a tibial component, and usually a patellar component (Fig. 17.19). The tibial and patellar components have polyethy-

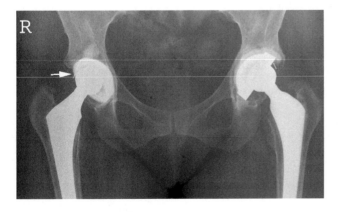

Figure 17.16 Polyethylene failure in total hip replacement. AP radiograph shows the right femoral head is asymmetrically located within the acetabular component (*arrow*).

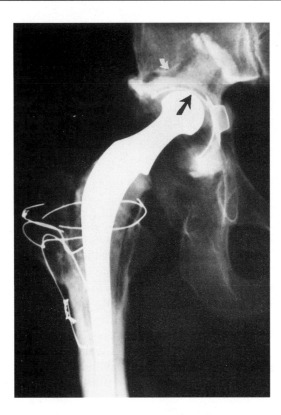

Figure 17.17 Failed total hip replacement with gross failure of the acetabular liner (*black arrow*), loosening, and osteolysis (*white arrow*).

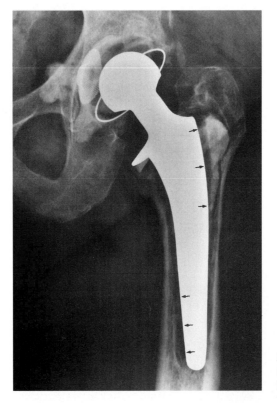

Figure 17.18 Loose cemented total hip replacement with failure of the cement–metal bond of the femoral component (*arrows*).

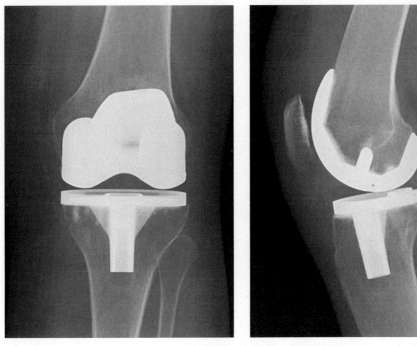

A   B

Figure 17.19 Bicondylar total knee replacement. *A.* Lateral radiograph. *B.* AP radiograph.

lene articular surfaces. Unconstrained TKRs depend on the muscles and ligaments of the knee for stability. If the soft tissue supports of the knee are poor, a constrained (hinged) prosthesis may be used. Because the normal knee rotates as it flexes, hinged TKRs have a second articulation comprising a metal post that inserts into a polyethylene socket that allows rotation.

The bone stock of the tibia is sometimes deficient because of previous high tibial osteotomy; bone graft may be used to supplement it (Fig. 17.20). The surgical approach for

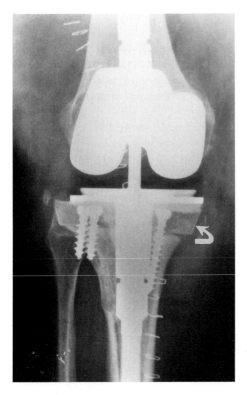

Figure 17.20 Posterior cruciate ligament–substituting total knee replacement with bone graft (*arrow*).

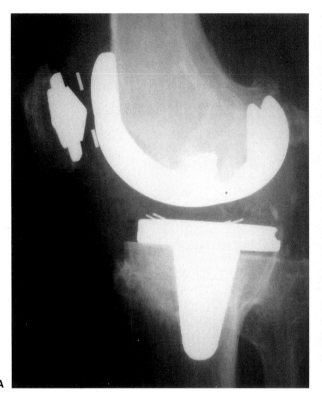 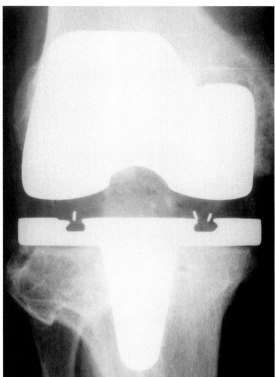

Figure 17.21 Total knee replacement with meniscal bearings. *A.* Lateral radiograph. *B.* AP radiograph.

placement of a TKR is anterior and usually requires sacrifice of the anterior cruciate ligament (ACL). Some designs also require sacrifice of the posterior cruciate ligament (PCL), and these prostheses incorporate a mechanism that replaces its function. In these PCL-substituting TKRs, a post extends vertically from the tibial component and fits into a slot in the condylar component. In flexion, the post restrains the condylar component from sliding anteriorly over the tibia, substituting for the PCL. Cement is typically used as a surface adhesive to fix the components to bone. The ideal alignment of the tibial articular surface is parallel to the floor; this is best demonstrated on standing radiographs. Some designs incorporate meniscal bearings that move with flexion and extension, attempting to duplicate more closely the normal kinematics of the knee (Fig. 17.21).

In knee replacement, cement is typically used as a surface adhesive to fix the components to bone.

A unicondylar TKR is used when there is significant, symptomatic disease of either the medial or lateral compartment but relative preservation of the other compartments. Both sides of the joint of the involved compartment are replaced (Fig. 17.22). The components are typically cemented in place. The bearing surface is polyethylene. The stability of these prostheses depends on the inherent stability of the host knee; the surgery can be accomplished with preservation of both the ACL and PCL. The cost is lower than a bicondylar TKR, and the rehabilitation is typically easier. The long-term results are less predictable, because intervening disease of the remaining compartments often leads to revision to a bicondylar TKR.

Most complications of knee replacements involve the patellar component (Fig. 17.23). Major trauma to limbs with prosthetic joints may result in fractures and dislocations. When fractures occur, they usually begin at a bone–metal interface that acts as a stress riser (Fig. 17.24).

Polyethylene wear and gross fragmentation of the polyethylene bearing surface of the tibia may occur (Fig. 17.25). Polyethylene wear can be recognized on radiographs as loss of joint space on weight-bearing views. Some polyethylene inserts have metal wires embedded within them, and displacement of these wires signifies displacement of the polyethy-

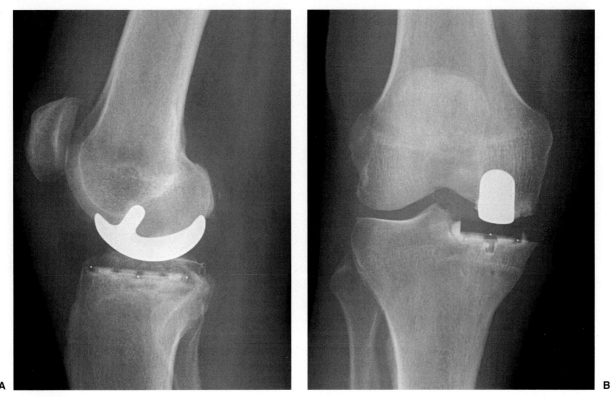

A

B

Figure 17.22 Unicondylar total knee replacement with cemented polyethylene tibial component. *A.* Lateral radiograph. *B.* AP radiograph.

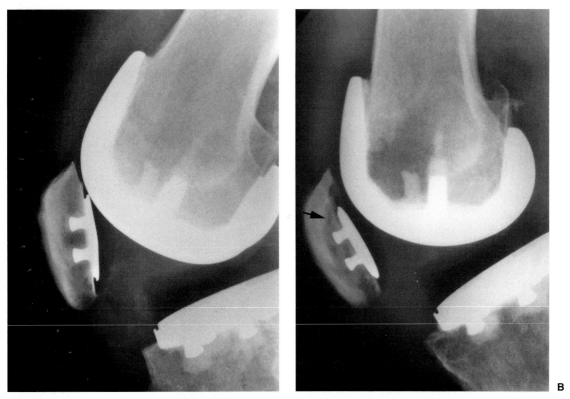

A

B

Figure 17.23 Total knee replacement with loosening of patellar component. *A.* Postoperative radiograph. *B.* Follow-up radiograph several months later shows resorption of bone at the cement–bone interface of the patellar component (*arrow*).

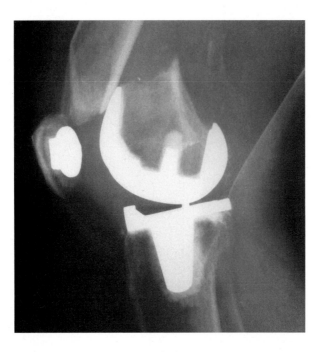

Figure 17.24 Fracture of femur through stress riser at the superior edge of the femoral component.

lene. Polyethylene loss from the patellar component is difficult to recognize without axial (sunrise) patellar radiographs.

Metal particles are also found around joint implants and may be carried to regional lymph nodes. Synovial discoloration is common around prostheses (seen at revision arthroplasty, not on imaging), and the deposition of metal particles has been associated with synovitis (Fig. 17.26). Other biologic effects of metallosis are suspected but not proved.

Osteolysis may occur around TKRs, similar to the situation at the hip (Fig. 17.27).

Infection is an uncommon complication that often requires arthrocentesis for diagnosis.

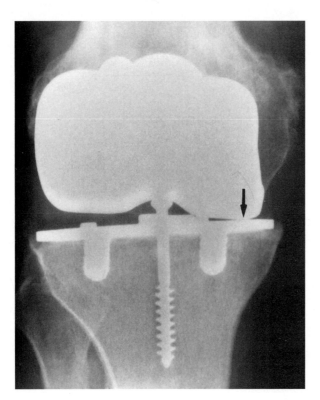

Figure 17.25 Total knee replacement with polyethylene thinning in the medial compartment (*arrow*).

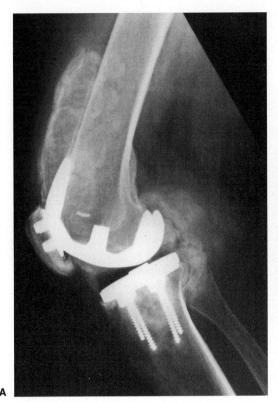
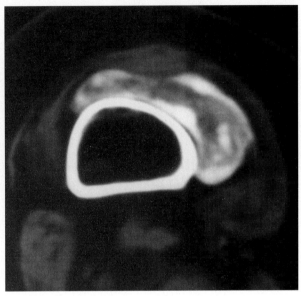

A   B

Figure 17.26 Total knee replacement with metallosis. *A.* Lateral radiograph shows increased radiodensity within the knee capsule, most visible in the suprapatellar recess and the posterior aspect of the joint. *B.* Axial CT scan shows metal deposition within the synovium of the suprapatellar recess.

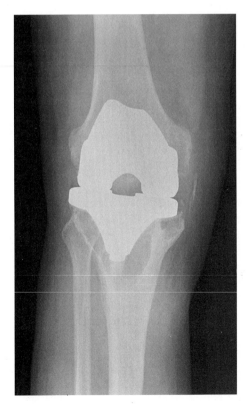

Figure 17.27 Osteolysis around the tibial component of a total knee replacement.

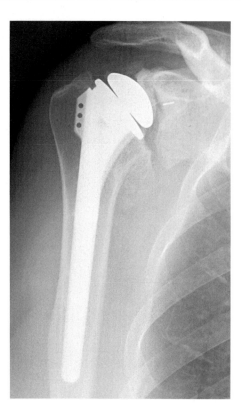

Figure 17.28 Total shoulder replacement in rheumatoid arthritis.

Soft tissue swelling with a new effusion is a typical but nonspecific radiographic sign of infection. If organisms are not cultured from the joint fluid at arthrocentesis, an open synovial biopsy may be necessary. Infection of a prosthesis typically leads to its removal.

SHOULDER REPLACEMENT

Shoulder replacement may be used to treat incapacitating arthritic pain. Shoulder prostheses are unconstrained, serving only to resurface the glenohumeral joint (Fig. 17.28). They depend on the stability provided by the native soft tissues. A typical shoulder replacement has a metal humeral component with a head and an intramedullary stem, as well as a polyethylene glenoid component. Simple humeral head replacements may be used after resection of the native humeral head for problems such as tumors, osteonecrosis, or severe fracture-dislocations (Fig. 17.29).

ELBOW REPLACEMENT

Elbow replacement is sometimes performed in patients with advanced rheumatoid arthritis (Fig. 17.30). In the past, constrained hinged prostheses were used, but these tended to loosen because there was no provision for rotational motion of the forearm. More recent implants are less constrained and permit rotational motion; these may dislocate, however. When there is isolated proximal radioulnar disease, a resection arthroplasty rather than a joint replacement may be performed.

WRIST REPLACEMENT

Arthroplasties of the wrist are usually reserved for patients with deformities from inflammatory arthritis. Total wrist prostheses with metal components and polyethylene articular surfaces are available; placement of these devices requires resection of the proximal carpal row, and results are not consistently good (Fig. 17.31). An alternative type of arthroplasty

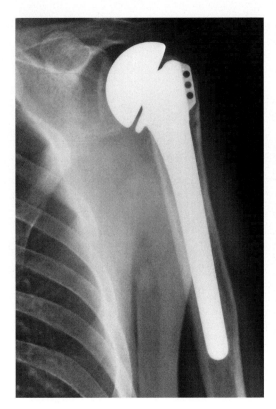

Figure 17.29 Hemi-arthroplasty of shoulder.

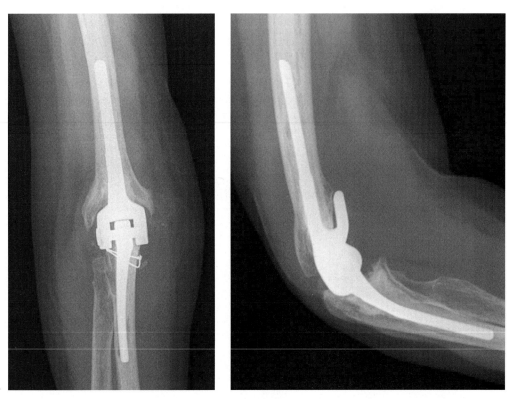

A

B

Figure 17.30 Total elbow replacement. *A.* Lateral radiograph. *B.* AP radiograph.

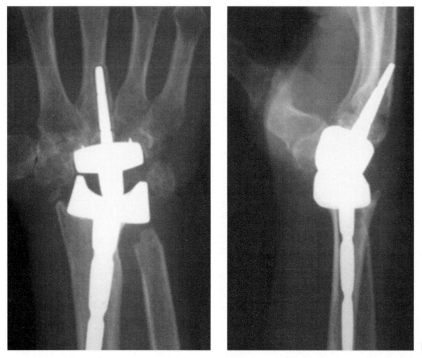

Figure 17.31 Total wrist replacement. *A.* PA radiograph. *B.* Lateral radiograph.

is resection of the joint and implantation of a two-ended silicone plug into the resulting gap (Fig. 17.32). In the wrist, silicone rubber implants may also be used to replace the scaphoid or lunate. Resection arthroplasty may also be used at the wrist, in which the scaphoid, lunate, and triquetrum are resected, leaving the distal carpal row to articulate

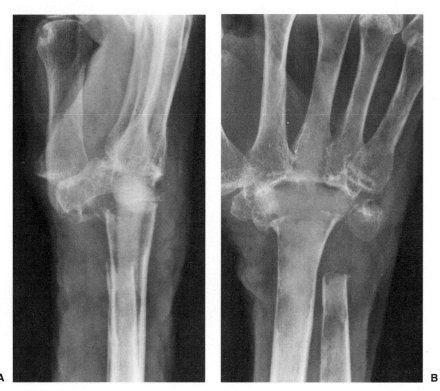

Figure 17.32 Silastic wrist replacement. *A.* Lateral radiograph. *B.* AP radiograph.

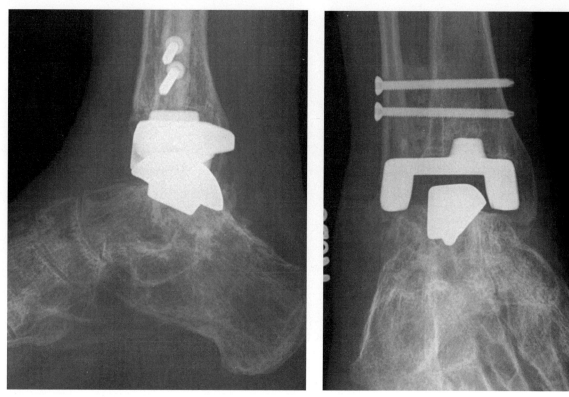

A   B

Figure 17.33 Total ankle replacement. *A.* Lateral radiograph. *B.* AP radiograph.

with the distal radius. In general, arthrodesis of the wrist has been favored over replacement arthroplasty because arthrodesis has fewer complications.

ANKLE REPLACEMENT

Arthroplasties of the ankle are usually reserved for patients with severe pain from degenerative arthritis, often posttraumatic. Total ankle prostheses with metal components and polyethylene articular surfaces are available, but long-term follow-up has been sparse (Fig. 17.33). In general, arthrodesis of the ankle has been favored over replacement arthroplasty because arthrodesis has fewer complications.

SMALL JOINT REPLACEMENT

At small non–weight-bearing joints, a small implant may be inserted (but not fixed) into the ends of the bone after the articular cortex has been removed (Fig. 17.34). These implants are usually made of radiopaque silicone rubber (Silastic, polymeric silicone substances). These implants maintain the proper length of the digit while still allowing limited motion because they are flexible and may have a piston-like motion in and out of the bone. Common sites for silicone implants include the proximal and distal radioulnar joint, the carpus, the metacarpophalangeal (MCP) and interphalangeal (IP) joints of the hand, and the metatarsophalangeal (MTP) joint of the great toe. Possible complications (Table 17.2) include mechanical fragmentation of the implant, migration of the prosthesis or its fragments, and silicone-associated synovitis. Polycarbonate prostheses for small joints have recently become available (Fig. 17.35).

MTP joint replacement may be performed for osteoarthritis at the great toe. Silastic implants are typically used.

Prostheses for temporomandibular joint replacement may replace the articular surface of the mandibular condyle or the entire joint (Fig. 17.36). These are typically used for severe symptoms from osteoarthritis.

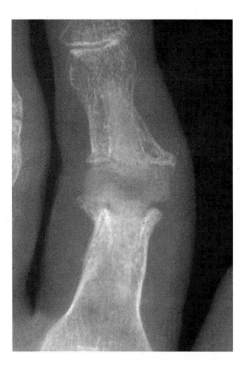

Figure 17.34 Silastic arthroplasty at the proximal interphalangeal joint (rheumatoid arthritis).

Table 17.2: Complications of Silicone Prostheses

Implant fracture
Infection
Implant dislocation
Synovitis
Recurrent deformity
Mechanical fragmentation of implant
Migration of prosthesis or its fragments

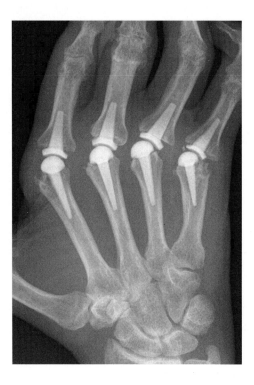

Figure 17.35 Polycarbonate metacarpophalangeal joint prostheses.

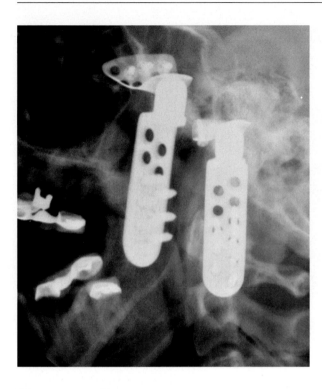

Figure 17.36 Bilateral total temporomandibular joint replacements.

TUMOR RESECTION

Bone lesions may be resected piecemeal or en bloc. Incisional procedures involve cutting through the lesion itself and, typically, removing it in pieces. Curettage is a procedure of scooping out the contents of a lesion using an instrument called a *curet*. Sometimes, physical or chemical treatments, such as cryotherapy, are applied to the surgical bed in an effort to eradicate residual lesional tissue. Reconstruction after curettage is typically packing with bone chips (Fig. 17.37) or methylmethacrylate cement (Fig. 17.38).

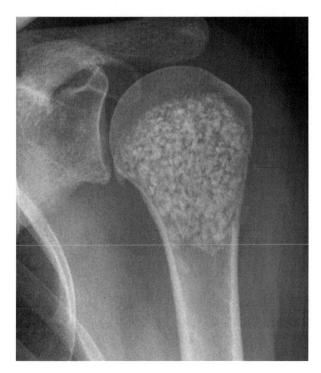

Figure 17.37 Bone chips packing site of curettage for enchondroma.

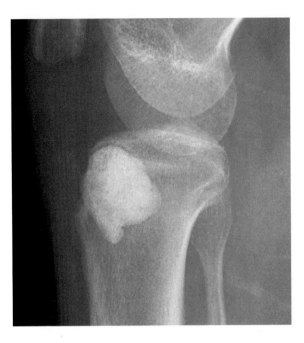

Figure 17.38 Methylmethacrylate cement in curettage site.

Resorbable calcium sulfate bone graft substitute is an alternative to bone chips or methylmethacrylate cement for filling curettage defects.

A recent alternative to packing bone defects with bone chips or methylmethacrylate cement is the use of calcium sulfate bone graft substitute, a resorbable material that acts as a scaffold for formation of new bone. As new bone forms, the calcium sulfate is resorbed by the body. Over a period of 2 or 3 months, the radiopaque material disappears and is replaced by a faint rim of new bone formation that continues to grow and remodel after the bone graft substitute is gone (Fig. 17.39). The calcium sulfate pellets may also be impregnated with antibiotics for use in an infected bone defect.

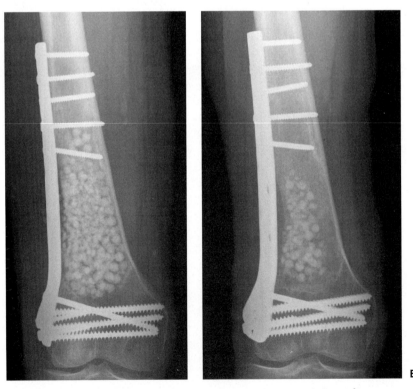

Figure 17.39 Bone graft substitute with progressive incorporation. *A.* Immediate postoperative radiograph. *B.* Radiograph 2 months after surgery.

Excisional resections typically remove the lesion en bloc. A marginal excision cuts around the gross margin of the lesion and may leave microscopic residua. A wide excision removes a cuff of normal tissue in continuity with the lesion and is intended to provide tumor-free margins. Segmental resections remove part of a limb but leave the distal portion. Amputations sacrifice the distal portion of an entire extremity and are named for the level at which the limb is transected. For example, a below-knee amputation is an amputation of the leg at the level of the proximal tibia. It is possible for an amputation to be incisional or excisional depending on the level of the amputation relative to the tumor site. Saucerization is a procedure in which the medullary cavity is exposed widely, typically for drainage of a bone abscess.

A wide excision removes a cuff of normal tissue around the lesion to provide tumor-free margins.

TRANSPLANTATION

Tissue that is transplanted within the same individual is called *autograft*; tissue transplanted from one human to another is *allograft* (homograft); and tissue transplanted from one species to another is *xenograft* (heterograft). Bone for autografts is commonly obtained from the iliac crest, distal radial metaphysis, ribs, or fibula, depending on the site of surgery and the type of bone graft required. Allograft bone is usually obtained from a bone bank. Banked bone may be obtained from living donors or from cadavers. Living donors typically donate femoral heads that have been resected incidental to hip replacement surgery. Cadaver bone is harvested from donors under aseptic conditions by traveling surgical teams maintained by regional bone banks. The tissue must be harvested within 24 hours of death before bacterial skin contamination becomes unacceptably high. Careful donor selection and microbial cultures of the harvested tissue reduce the risk of transmission of infectious diseases. Depending on the planned use of the tissue, the harvested bone may include ligament and tendon insertions and articular cartilage. The tissue is sterilized by irradiation or gas treatment. Repeated washings during processing to remove the marrow and storage in the frozen or freeze-dried state render the bone tissue hypoallergenic. Immunosuppression of recipients is not necessary. When banked allograft bone is needed, an appropriate graft can be chosen from a radiographic catalog of available tissue.

Allograft bone is usually obtained from a bone bank.

Bone graft can stimulate osteogenesis, fill defects, provide mechanical stability, and form a scaffold for creeping substitution. Common uses include spine fusion, cyst packing, long-bone replacement, osteoarticular replacement, and treatment for fracture and fracture nonunion. Bone-forming cells may be transplanted with the graft itself (if an autograft) or inducted from local mesenchymal cells. Bone tissue can be implanted as a powder, slurry (morselized bone), chips or fragments, intercalary segments or blocks, or entire intact structures, including an articular surface (Fig. 17.40). When large allografts are used, the biologic effect is similar to an organ transplant rather than a tissue transplant. Direct remodeling of large allografts that begins at the graft-host junction may ultimately encompass the entire implant after months or years. Graft failure is recognized when there is progressive resorption of the graft or failure to unite to the host bone. The alternative to a massive allograft is often a modular total joint replacement (Fig. 17.41).

Bone tissue can be implanted as a powder, slurry (morselized bone), chips or fragments, intercalary segments or blocks, or entire intact structures, including an articular surface.

Soft tissues such as tendons may also be harvested, banked, and used as implants, particularly for ligament reconstruction. Autograft or allograft tendons are avascular when implanted but undergo a complex biologic process called *ligamentization* in which there is graft necrosis, revascularization, cellular repopulation, collagen deposition, and, finally, graft remodeling and maturation. This process takes 1 to 3 years and is analogous to creeping substitution in bone remodeling. The intra-articular injection of living chondrocytes from cell culture into patients with joint disease is a promising new transplantation technique.

Cruciate ligament tears are typically reconstructed with graft material. One common autograft for ACL is the central third of the infrapatellar tendon, with the bony attachments on either end. This graft is threaded through a tunnel that is drilled through the femur and tibia and secured with interference screws. The interference screws compress the bony portions of the graft against the tunnel walls (Fig. 17.42). Other grafts used for ACL repair

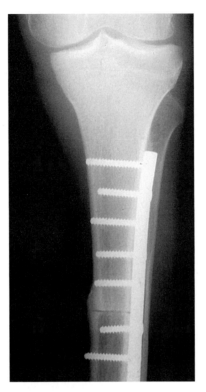

Figure 17.40 Massive proximal osteoarticular tibial allograft for tumor reconstruction.

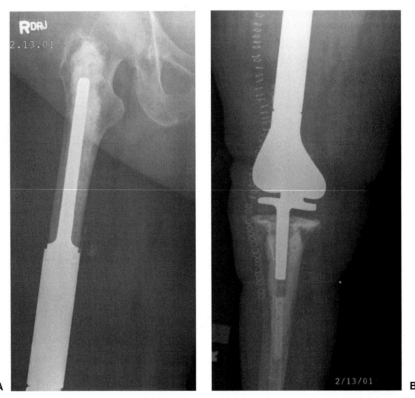

Figure 17.41 Modular total joint replacement for tumor reconstruction. *A.* Hip. *B.* Knee.

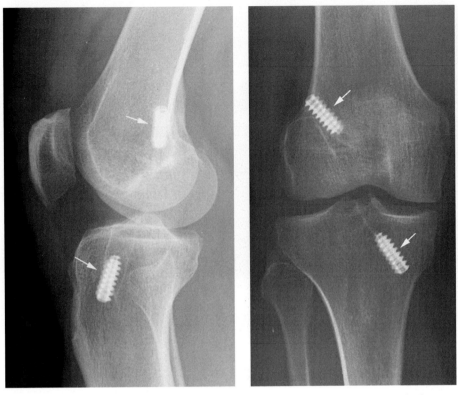

A   B

Figure 17.42 Anterior cruciate ligament repair with interference screws securing the bony ends (*arrows*) of the graft. *A.* Lateral radiograph. *B.* AP radiograph.

include autograft or allograft hamstring tendons (semitendinosus and gracilis) and synthetic materials such as polytetrafluoroethylene (Gore-Tex). Hamstring tendon grafts are usually fixed to bone by screws with washers. Radiographs can assess the position of hardware or bony portions of a graft. MRI can be used to visualize the graft itself (Fig. 17.43) and is useful when graft failure is suspected (Fig. 17.44).

Reimplantation of a traumatically amputated limb or appendage is made possible by rapid transport of victims to a medical center and microsurgical techniques. In cases in which critical structures such as the thumb or multiple fingers of the dominant hand have been lost, a func-

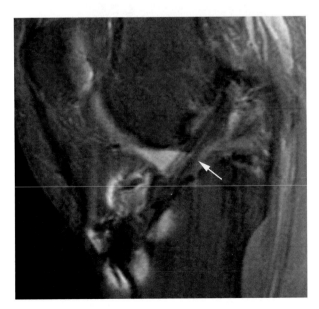

Figure 17.43 Sagittal PD-weighted fat-suppressed MRI of intact anterior cruciate ligament graft (*arrow*).

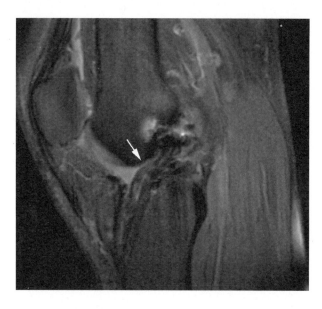

Figure 17.44 Sagittal T2-weighted fat-suppressed MRI of anterior cruciate ligament graft (*arrow*) with impingement.

tional hand may be reconstructed by reimplanting other digits such as toes. Lengthening the bone with external fixators may be combined with implantation in a multistage procedure.

SOFT TISSUE OPERATIONS

A soft tissue release is performed by surgically dividing a soft tissue structure. The flexor retinaculum, for example, is incised in a carpal tunnel release. Tendon transfer may be performed by mobilizing the bony insertion of a tendon (by osteotomy) and reattaching it in a different location or by releasing the tendon and reattaching it to another soft tissue structure. Transfer of the insertion of the infrapatellar tendon may be performed to treat problems related to abnormal patellar tracking. Tendon transfers around the hip may improve function in spastic neuromuscular conditions such as cerebral palsy. Soft tissue structures without integral bone segments may be attached to bone with sutures (sometimes metallic), bone staples, screws with washers, or soft

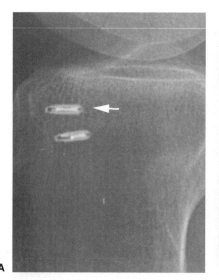
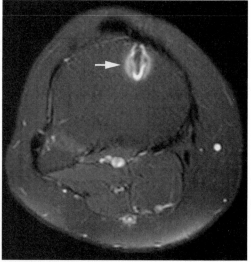

Figure 17.45 Soft tissue anchors used for fixation of patellar tendon transfer (*arrows*). *A.* Lateral radiograph. *B.* Axial T2-weighted fat-suppressed MRI.

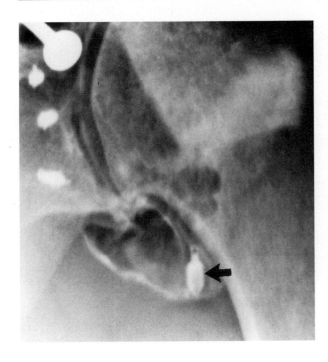

Figure 17.46 Anterior shoulder repair with loose soft tissue anchor (*arrow*) demonstrated by arthrography to be intracapsular.

tissue anchors (Fig. 17.45). Operations that involve only the soft tissues may not be evident on postsurgical radiographs. For example, shoulder reconstructions—usually soft tissue operations performed to correct instability or to repair the rotator cuff—generally repair the shoulder capsule (capsuloplasty) or a torn rotator cuff. In cases in which metallic fixation is used, radiographs may be helpful in documenting the position of hardware (Fig. 17.46). Arthrography, CT, and MRI often retain their usefulness in imaging the reconstructed shoulder (Fig. 17.47).

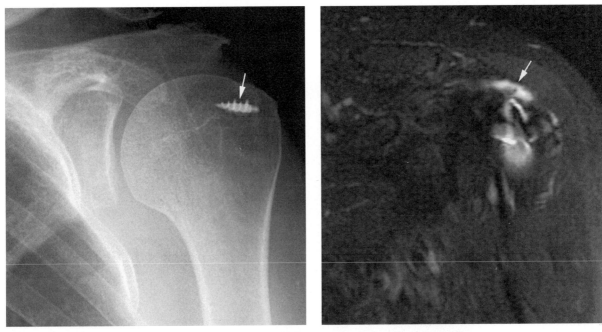

A

B

Figure 17.47 Recurrent rotator cuff injury after surgery. *A.* AP radiograph shows metallic soft tissue anchor (*arrow*) in humerus. *B.* Oblique coronal T2-weighted fat-suppressed MRI has artifact from anchor, but retracted supraspinatus tear (*arrow*) is evident.

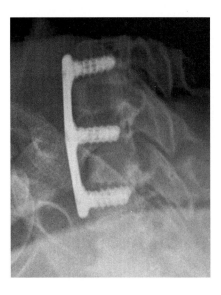

Figure 17.48 Postoperative radiographs of an anterior fusion of C5 to C7 with internal fixation and bone graft.

Spine Fusion

Surgical fusion of the spine is performed in various circumstances. Long-term stability of spinal fusion depends on bony fusion, not instrumentation. Instrumentation and external braces (orthoses) provide immediate postoperative stability. Anterior fusion involves removal of the intervertebral disc joints, and sometimes other structures, with insertion of bone graft (Fig. 17.48). Anterior fusions are performed in the cervical region after removal of herniated discs from an anterior approach. Posterior fusions may include wiring or instrumentation and placement of onlay bone grafts after preparation of the host surfaces by decortication, resection of facet joints, and so forth. Posterolateral or intertransverse fusion is used in the lumbar region, where the transverse processes and other posterior elements are incorporated into the posterior fusion. Most thoracic and lumbar spine fusions use a combined anterior and posterior approach. Pedicle screws inserted posteriorly are attached to rods. Removal of the disc material from the involved levels is followed by insertion of bone graft material. Blocks of allograft bone may be used; alternatively, fusion cages filled with morselized bone graft may be inserted (Fig. 17.49). Follow-up films of spinal fusions should document healing and incorporation of graft

Most cervical spine fusions use either an anterior or a posterior approach.

Most thoracic and lumbar spine fusions use a combined anterior and posterior approach.

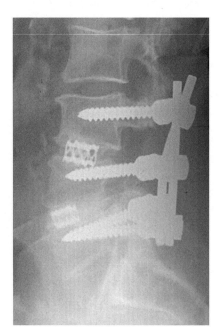

Figure 17.49 Lumbar spine fusion with pedicle screws, rods, and anterior fusion cages.

Table 17.3: Complications of Spinal Fixation

Incorrect diagnosis
Inaccurate identification of nerve root or disc level
Intraoperative
    Injury to spinal cord, nerve roots, dura, vessels, or soft tissue
    Malpositioned or migrated hardware
Postoperative
    Hematoma
    Cord edema
    Disc herniation
    Hardware failure or migration
    Pseudoarthrosis

material, maintenance of postsurgical alignment, and integrity of wires and instrumentation. Pseudoarthrosis, the most common complication (Table 17.3), is more likely to occur if excessive motion at the fusion site is present. It may be suspected when there is localized pain, motion, or loss of correction or fixation. If standard radiographs are unrevealing, CT with coronal, sagittal, or three-dimensional reconstructed images may be helpful in demonstrating the presence or lack of bony bridging at sites of arthrodesis. Lateral views in flexion and extension may reveal abnormal motion.

SCOLIOSIS SURGERY

Spinal fusion for arrest and partial correction of severe or progressive scoliosis may be performed with various implants by posterior and anterior approaches. The instrumentation used for correction of scoliosis applies loads to the spine either axially or transversely. Axial loading may be applied by distraction or compression. These devices are typically combined with arthrodesis of the involved vertebrae and bone grafting. Incorporation of the bone graft provides long-term stability to the spine, so that late failures of the hardware are not necessarily important.

Late failures of hardware in spine fusions for scoliosis may be unimportant if the bony fusion remains intact.

The original Harrington instrumentation for arrest of scoliosis consisted of a thick distraction rod with opposite-facing hooks on each end that was placed on the concave side to distract the curve and a thin, threaded compression rod on the convex side to pull it together. The hooks of the compression rod opened toward each other.

Axial compressive forces on the convex side can be applied to the anterior column by a tension device coupled to the vertebral bodies. A Dwyer device consists of screws fixed into several contiguous vertebral bodies on the convex side of the curve that are connected by a cable threaded through a window in the screw heads (Fig. 17.50). The cable is tightened to provide a corrective bending moment. A Zielke device is similar to the Dwyer device but uses a threaded rod instead of a cable.

Transverse corrective force can be applied by wires threaded about the laminae (sublaminar wiring) or through the spinous processes and anchored to a rod. Luque rods (L-rods) may be used as an anchor; the segmental wiring is typically at every level. Segmental wiring for transverse corrective forces can also be anchored to Harrington distraction rods. Luque and Harrington distraction rods may be mixed in particular patients for a combined approach with both axial and transverse corrective forces (Fig. 17.51).

Three-dimensional correction that uses both axial and transverse forces is possible with Cotrel-Dubousset and similar double-rod multiple hook instrumentation. This apparatus consists of thick compression and distraction rods with multiple pairs of hooks at several levels and transverse connecting rods. The compression and distraction rods are knurled, and the hooks are fixed by set screws (Fig. 17.52).

Three-dimensional corrections may also be obtained using variations and combinations of techniques, including combined anterior and posterior instrumentation, L-rods

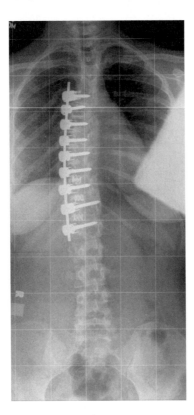

Figure 17.50 Anterior spinal fusion for congenital scoliosis with a Dwyer device extending over nine vertebral levels.

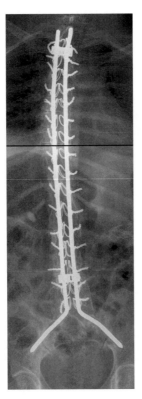

Figure 17.51 Anterior and posterior spinal fusion for idiopathic scoliosis with Luque rods and segmental wiring around the lamina.

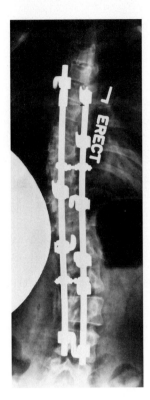

Figure 17.52 Spinal fusion for idiopathic scoliosis with Cotrel-Dubousset instrumentation (knurled rods with hooks fixed by set screws).

combined with hooked rods, segmental wiring combined with multiple hooks, pedicle screws combined with hooks, and so forth. Telescoping rods for treatment of children with significant remaining growth potential are also available (Fig. 17.53).

Neurologic damage is an uncommon but known risk in scoliosis surgery. The early postsurgical complication is hook dislodgment. A late complication is failure of the spinal

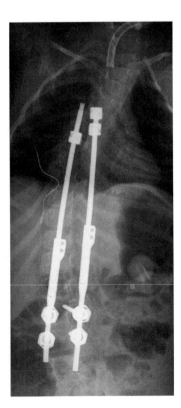

Figure 17.53 Spinal fusion in a child for scoliosis with telescoping rods.

fusion, leading to fatigue failure of the instrumentation. If the fusion is solid, breakage of the instrumentation often has little clinical significance.

SOURCES AND READINGS

Adams JC, Stossel CA. *Standard orthopedic operations: a guide for the junior surgeon*, 4th ed. Philadelphia: Churchill Livingstone, 1992.

Berquist TH. *Imaging atlas of orthopedic appliances and prostheses*. Philadephia: JB Lippincott Co, 1994.

Henkin RE, Boles MA, Dillehay GL, et al., eds. *Nuclear medicine*. St. Louis: Mosby–Year Book, 1996.

Hoppenfeld S, Zeide MS. *Orthopaedic dictionary*. Philadelphia: JB Lippincott Co, 1994.

Hunter TB, Bragg DG, eds. *Radiologic guide to medical devices and foreign bodies*. St. Louis: Mosby, 1994.

Mohaideen A, Nagarkatti D, Banta JV, et al. Not all rods are Harrington—an overview of spinal instrumentation in scoliosis treatment. *Pediatr Radiol* 2000;30:110–118.

Petty W. *Total joint replacement*. Philadelphia: WB Saunders, 1997.

Phillips WC, Kattapuram SV. Prosthetic hip replacements: plain films and arthrography for component loosening. *AJR Am J Roentgenol* 1982;138:677–682.

Shellock FG, Morisoli S, Kanal E. MR procedures and biomedical implants, materials, and devices: 1993 update. *Radiology* 1993;189:587–599.

Smith SE, Estok DM 2nd, Harris WH. 20-year experience with cemented primary and conversion total hip arthroplasty using so-called second-generation cementing techniques in patients aged 50 years or younger. *J Arthroplasty* 2000;15:263–273.

Tomford WW. *Musculoskeletal tissue banking*. New York: Raven Press, 1993.

Weissman BNW, Sledge CB. *Orthopedic radiology*, 2nd ed. Philadelphia: WB Saunders, 2002.

DIAGNOSTIC AND INTERVENTIONAL PROCEDURES

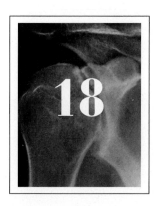

18

INFORMED CONSENT

Informed consent should be obtained before performing any invasive procedure on a patient. The process of informed consent should include a description of the procedure in layperson's terms, followed by an explanation of the benefits, risks, and alternatives (Table 18.1). The patient should indicate that he or she understands what he or she has been told and that he or she consents to the procedure. An explicit opportunity for the patient to ask questions should be provided. The patient, the radiologist, and a witness should sign a consent form. The consent form documents that the patient has given informed consent; it does not represent the informed consent itself, which is typically given verbally. A statement that informed consent was obtained should be included in the radiologic report of the procedure, and at some institutions it may be considered sufficient for documentation for minor procedures (e.g., joint aspiration) without the use of the consent form.

A patient may withdraw informed consent during a procedure.

ANESTHESIA AND SEDATION

Local anesthesia at the skin can be accomplished with 1% lidocaine, except in patients with an allergy to lidocaine. A skin wheal should be raised. Mixing sodium bicarbonate with lidocaine buffers the lidocaine and greatly reduces the sudden burning sensation in the skin that occurs as lidocaine is infiltrated into the skin. Deep injection of local anesthetic is generally not necessary for arthrography or other injections.

> **Table 18.1: Informed Consent for Single-Contrast Arthrography and MR Arthrography of a Joint**
>
> Description
>> A needle is passed through your skin into the [specify] joint. A mixture of contrast medium and gadolinium is injected into the joint. The needle is removed. We take a few x-rays, and then we move you to the MRI suite for an MRI scan. The fluid we inject will eventually be removed from your body by your kidneys; the fluid is clear so you won't notice it. The U.S. Food and Drug Administration has not specifically approved gadolinium for injection into the joints; however, we have found it to be safe and effective.
>
> Benefits
>> We are doing this to get images of your [specify] joint that will help us let your doctor know what might be wrong with your [specify] joint. The internal structure of the [specify] joint is complex, and some structures are difficult to see—even with MRI—unless we fill the joint with something that will make them easier to see.
>
> Risks
>> Because we are passing a needle from the outside to the inside, there is a risk of introducing an infection. The risk is very low because we use a sterile technique.
>>
>> Because we are placing a sharp object into your body, there may be some pain or discomfort, and there is a risk of bleeding. (Ask for history of bleeding disorders or blood thinners, including aspirin and anticoagulants.) We will use local anesthetic at the site of injection to minimize any pain. The needle is small enough that the risk of significant bleeding is very low. We will also be avoiding any large blood vessels.
>>
>> As with any medication or substance that is injected into your body, there is always a risk of an adverse reaction. Although adverse reactions to either contrast medium or gadolinium are very rare when injected into a joint, a reaction is always possible. (Ask for history of drug allergies and reactions to contrast medium or gadolinium.) Adverse reactions to contrast medium and gadolinium that have been reported range from a mild rash to difficulty breathing, heart trouble, and even death. Most of these reactions occurred after injection into the bloodstream; we will be injecting your joint, not your veins.
>
> Alternatives
>> We could do the MRI without injecting contrast and gadolinium, but it would be less accurate for certain types of disorders, one of which your doctor thinks you might have.
>>
>> We could do the MRI after we inject gadolinium into your veins, but it might be less accurate than the MRI arthrogram for certain types of disorders, one of which your doctor thinks you might have.
>>
>> We could do no procedure at all, but your doctor might not be able to determine what is wrong with your [specify] joint and, therefore, might not be able to treat it properly.
>>
>> If you do not want us to perform this procedure now, we can always reschedule it.
>
> Understanding
>> Do you understand the procedure we are planning to perform on you?
>>
>> Do you have any questions about it?
>
> Documentation
>> To document that we have explained this procedure and that you understand the benefits, risks, and alternatives, please sign this consent form.

Conscious sedation or general anesthesia is rarely, if ever, necessary for the performance of arthrography. However, musculoskeletal biopsy can be painful, particularly if normal bone must be traversed to gain access to the lesion. For most patients, small amounts of fentanyl and midazolam given intravenously alone or in combination typically provide sufficient sedation for the procedure to be completed in relative comfort. A radiology nurse can administer the medications and monitor the patient under the supervision of the radiologist. Physicians should follow their institutions' guidelines for the administration of conscious sedation.

During conscious sedation, a radiology nurse should be available to administer the medications and monitor the patient.

General anesthesia is occasionally used. In select circumstances, such as small children undergoing technically demanding procedures or radiofrequency ablation, general anesthesia is essential. An anesthesiologist or nurse anesthetist working under the direct supervision of an anesthesiologist should be present.

IMAGING GUIDANCE

The procedures described in this chapter are performed under fluoroscopic or CT guidance. Joint injections and aspirations in the limbs can be performed easily using single-plane fluoroscopic equipment. Injections around the spine are best performed using C-arm or biplane fluoroscopic equipment, although it is possible to perform epidural injections using single-plane fluoroscopic equipment. Biopsies are easiest to perform under CT guidance. CT fluoroscopy is another option for imaging guidance at some institutions. Ultrasound may be used for localization of soft tissue lesions or fluid collections. MRI guidance has not yet found a role in musculoskeletal procedures.

ARTHROGRAPHY

Arthrography is a procedure in which contrast medium is injected directly into a joint, followed by imaging. Conventional arthrography and CT arthrography typically involve the injection of iodinated contrast medium with or without air, followed by radiographic imaging or CT scanning, respectively. MR arthrography typically involves the injection of gadolinium, followed by MRI. Potential complications of arthrography are listed in Table 18.2.

Occasionally, the referring physician may request intra-articular injection with bupivacaine, a long-acting anesthetic, for both diagnostic and therapeutic purposes. If the patient's symptoms are relieved by the injection, the result supports intra-articular pathology as a cause of the patient's symptoms. The patient may then be considered for procedures such as total joint replacement.

CONTRAST MIXTURE FOR MAGNETIC RESONANCE ARTHROGRAPHY

For MR arthrography, a solution of gadolinium is injected into the joint. The radiologist and patient should both be aware that the U.S. Food and Drug Administration has approved commercially available preparations of gadolinium MR contrast agents for intravenous injection but not for intra-articular injection. Therefore, disclosure of this off-label use is necessary. There have been no reported complications or adverse reactions to intra-articular injection of gadolinium. The gadolinium is cleared from the joints by lymphatics and veins and excreted by the kidneys.

A 0.5% solution of gadolinium is optimal for intra-articular use. As a paramagnetic contrast agent, gadolinium is most conspicuous on MRI using T1-weighted pulse sequences with fat suppression. Although adding iodinated contrast medium to the gadolinium mixture decreases the signal intensity of the gadolinium on T1-weighted sequences, this effect is small and has not been shown to affect the interpretation of images in clinical practice. The addition of iodinated contrast medium allows one to document with certainty the space into which the contrast mixture has been injected. One can also perform a conventional single-contrast arthrogram at the same time. The addition of epinephrine to the mixture will delay the resorption of the contrast mixture, providing a period of approximately 2 hours during which the MRI examination can be completed.

> Disclosure to the patient of the off-label use of gadolinium for MR arthrography is necessary.

Table 18.2: Complications of Arthrography
Infection
Bleeding
Adverse reaction to contrast medium
Vasovagal syncope
Synovitis

To prepare the contrast mixture for MR arthrography, begin with a 100-mL bag of normal saline, to which 1 mL of gadolinium contrast agent is added. The saline and gadolinium are thoroughly mixed by shaking the bag. Using a 20-mL syringe, 10 mL of the saline-gadolinium mixture is withdrawn. Using the same syringe with the saline-gadolinium mixture already in it, add 10 mL of nonionic contrast and 0.3 mL of 1:1,000 epinephrine. The contents of the syringe should be thoroughly mixed. It is now ready for use.

An alternate method of preparing the contrast mixture for MR arthrography begins with 10 mL of normal saline drawn into a 20-mL syringe. To this syringe, 0.1 mL of gadolinium contrast agent is added using a 1-mL tuberculin syringe. Using the same syringe with the saline-gadolinium already in it, add 10 mL of nonionic contrast and 0.3 mL of 1:1,000 epinephrine. The contents of the syringe should be thoroughly mixed. It is now ready for use.

SHOULDER

I use an anterior approach to the glenohumeral joint using fluoroscopic guidance. After informed consent, the patient is positioned supine with the shoulder externally rotated. A small sandbag placed on the palm of the hand reminds the patient to keep the shoulder rotated and still. The site of injection is localized using fluoroscopy (Fig. 18.1), and the skin is marked. A sterile field is prepared at the site of injection. The skin is cleansed with povidone-iodine solution and the shoulder is draped. It is helpful to ask the patient to look away, as the drape commonly extends to the lower face. For an arthrogram, I use a 22-gauge 3.5-in. spinal needle. I try to place the needle tip at the medial edge of the humeral articular surface, halfway between the superior and inferior margins of the joint. The needle is kept absolutely vertical and inserted straight down through the skin into the joint. Because the needle bevel tends to steer the needle tip in the direction away from the side of the bevel, I rotate the needle 180 degrees every 5 mm of advancement to keep it straight. The needle will begin to encounter resistance as it meets the subscapularis tendon. If you stop here, you will inject the subcoracoid bursa. Keep pushing, and the needle will pop through the tendon and will be inside the joint. The contrast-gadolinium solution should flow into the joint with no resistance until it begins to distend. Contrast should flow immediately away from the needle tip and begin to outline the inside of the joint (Fig. 18.2). The capacity of a normal adult shoulder is approximately 12 mL in a woman and 15 mL in a man.

> When the needle is correctly positioned within the joint, there should be no resistance when contrast is injected.

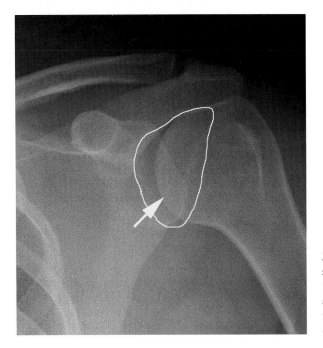

Figure 18.1 Scout radiograph of the shoulder showing the needle insertion site (*arrow*) using an anterior approach. The location of the anterior portion of the capsule is indicated by the line.

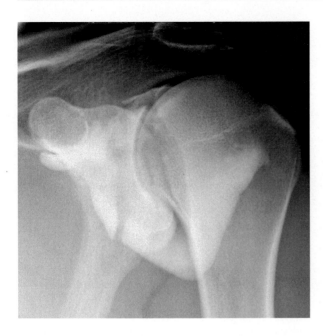

Figure 18.2 Radiograph of the shoulder shows successful injection of iodinated contrast medium and gadolinium mixture.

The shoulder should be exercised lightly before imaging. Full-thickness rotator cuff tears are recognized by contrast flowing into the subdeltoid-subacromial bursa, outlining the rotator cuff (Fig. 18.3). Identifying and characterizing the site of tear is difficult on conventional arthrography.

For identification of labral tears, MR or CT arthrography should be performed.

ELBOW

Arthrography of the elbow should be performed in conjunction with MRI or CT. The patient is placed in the prone position on the fluoroscopic table with the arm above the head. The elbow is flexed 90 degrees and the thumb is pointed up. The injection is made at the articulation of the radial head with the capitellum (Fig. 18.4). I use a 22-gauge 1.5-in. hypodermic needle for injection into the elbow joint. When the needle tip is located within the joint capsule, contrast should flow immediately away from the needle tip and begin to outline the joint (Fig. 18.5). The capacity of the normal adult elbow is approximately 8 mL in a woman and 10 mL in a man.

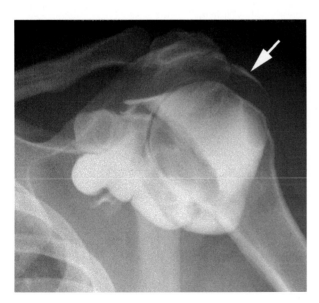

Figure 18.3   Single-contrast arthrogram of the shoulder shows that contrast has passed into the subdeltoid-subacromial bursa (*arrow*), indicating a full-thickness rotator cuff tear.

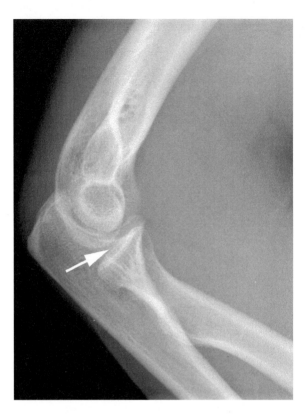

Figure 18.4 Scout radiograph of the elbow shows the needle insertion site (*arrow*) using a lateral approach.

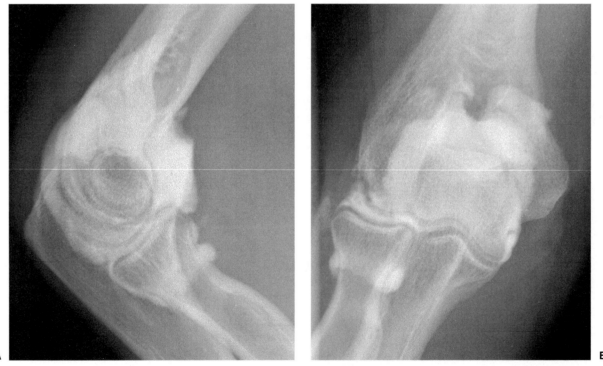

Figure 18.5 Elbow arthrogram. Lateral (*A*) and AP (*B*) radiographs show successful injection of mixture of iodinated contrast medium and gadolinium.

WRIST

The patient should be positioned supine, with the wrist at the side, next to the hip. It is helpful to place a sponge underneath the wrist so that it is slightly flexed and maintained in a pronated position.

Approach to the radiocarpal compartment is dorsal, between the scaphoid and distal radius. The dorsal edge of the distal radius can be palpated at the crook between the tendons of the extensor pollicis longus and the index slip of the extensor digitorum. This crook is just medial (toward the ulna) to the anatomic snuff box, on the medial side of the extensor pollicis longus tendon. On the scout radiograph, the needle location for vertical dorsal approach is between the scaphoid and the radius (Fig. 18.6).

For injection into the wrist joints, I use a 22- or 23-gauge 1.5-in. hypodermic needle. The needle should be inserted vertically until it passes into the joint. If bone is encountered, it is the dorsal lip of the radius, and the needle should be directed slightly distally to pass over the radius. Once passed, it should be brought to the vertical again and inserted into the joint. When the needle tip is located within the joint capsule, contrast should flow immediately away from the needle tip and begin to outline the joint (Fig. 18.7). A small radiocarpal joint may hold 5 mL; a large one may hold 8 mL.

The distal radioulnar joint may be approached from the dorsal aspect using a vertically oriented needle. The wrist should be rotated slightly until the superior and inferior margins of the sigmoid notch of the radius (the fossa on the medial aspect of the distal radius that articulates with the distal ulna to form the distal radioulnar joint) are overlapping. I use a 25-gauge 1-in. butterfly or hypodermic needle. The needle should be directed at the lateral edge of the distal ulna. A distal radioulnar joint may hold 1 to 2 mL.

Approach to the midcarpal compartment is vertical. The wrist should be positioned so that the four corners of the capitate, hamate, lunate, and triquetrum meet to form a cross. The needle should be inserted vertically at the four corners. The needle will enter the midcarpal compartment immediately, and intra-articular position can be confirmed by injec-

The wrist has three separate compartments.

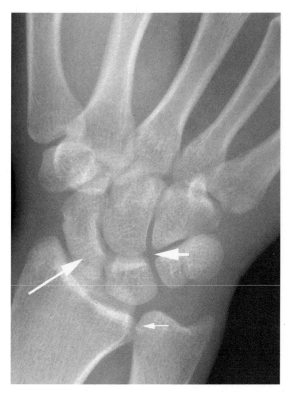

Figure 18.6 Scout radiograph of the wrist shows the needle insertion sites using a dorsal approach. Recommended approaches for the radiocarpal compartment (*long arrow*), the distal radioulnar joint (*small arrow*), and the midcarpal compartment (*short arrow*) are indicated.

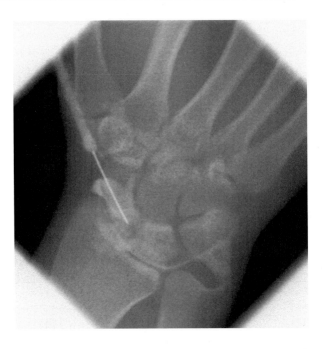

Figure 18.7 Radiograph of the wrist shows successful injection of iodinated contrast medium and gadolinium mixture into the radiocarpal compartment.

tion of contrast. If the needle is inserted too far, opacification of the flexor tendon sheaths may be demonstrated.

If contrast flows from one compartment to another, an abnormal tear or perforation is generally present (Fig. 18.8).

HIP

Identify the femoral vessels before attempting to inject the hip.

For injection into the hip joint, a 22-gauge 3.5-in. spinal needle is used. I use an anterior approach to the hip capsule. After identifying the femoral vessels, I make a direct vertical approach to the medial cortex of the proximal femur at the head–neck junction. If the femoral vessels are in the way, or if there is abdominal pannus, rotation of the patient away from the side being injected moves the femoral vessels medially and projects the femoral neck into better profile. The hip capsule is large and extends from the acetabulum distally

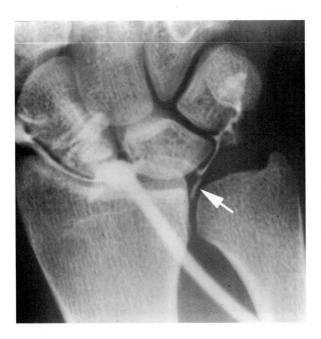

Figure 18.8 Single-contrast arthrogram of the wrist with injection of the radiocarpal compartment shows that contrast has passed into the distal radioulnar joint (*arrow*), indicating a tear or perforation of the triangular fibrocartilage complex, and the midcarpal compartment, indicating a tear or perforation of the scapholunate or lunatotriquetral ligaments.

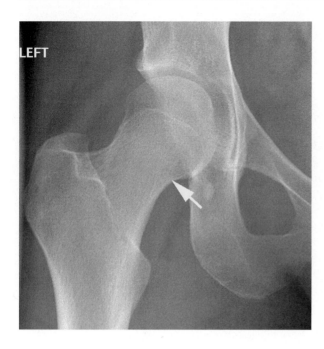

Figure 18.9 Scout radiograph of the hip shows the needle insertion site (*arrow*) using an anterior approach. The femoral vessels should be located before insertion of the needle.

to the midportion of the femoral neck; therefore, vertical placement of the needle anywhere over the proximal femur will allow intra-articular injection (Fig. 18.9). The two pitfalls in anterior vertical approaches to the hip are placing the needle too superficially and too deeply. Superficial needle placement may result in an injection into the iliopsoas bursa or tendon sheath, in which case the contrast will extend linearly along the axis of the femoral neck (inferior-lateral to superior-medial). Deep needle placement may result in intraosseous injection, in which case the contrast will collect at the tip of the needle. When the needle tip is located within the joint capsule, contrast should flow immediately away from the needle tip and begin to outline the posterior portion of the capsule around the femoral neck (Fig. 18.10). An oblique anterior approach along the axis of the femoral neck and a lateral

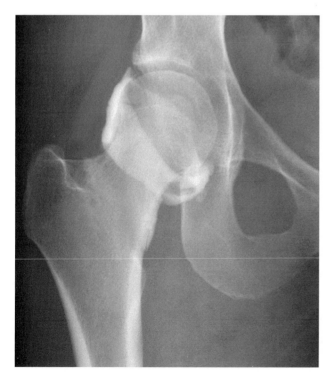

Figure 18.10 Radiograph of the hip shows successful injection of iodinated contrast medium and gadolinium mixture.

approach to the femoral neck are alternative methods. The adult hip joint holds approximately 15 mL.

KNEE

For injection into the knee joint, a 22-gauge 1.5-in. hypodermic needle is used. I use a lateral approach to injecting the knee joint, using superficial landmarks. The needle is placed between the patella and the patellofemoral groove of the femur at the midpoint of the patella. This site is easier to access if the knee is fully extended and the patella is manually subluxated laterally, so that the needle can be inserted deep to the patellar articular cartilage (Fig. 18.11). Placement of the needle is generally done without fluoroscopic guidance, but the injection of contrast can be followed with fluoroscopy. The injection should occur with no resistance, and contrast should flow away from the needle tip—generally, inferiorly along the patellofemoral groove—initially pooling in the knee joint posteriorly (Fig. 18.12). If contrast stays around the needle tip, the injection is typically into the prefemoral fat, and the needle should be withdrawn and directed toward the patellar cartilage and the feet. The capacity of the adult knee joint is approximately 20 mL.

Knee arthrography can be combined with CT as an alternative to MRI.

Knee arthrography can be especially useful in a postoperative meniscus when followed by cross-sectional imaging, particularly with CT. The inherent signal abnormality present within a postoperative meniscus may make detection of a recurrent meniscal tear difficult on unenhanced MRI. The use of a multidetector CT scanner to acquire a three-dimensional dataset with submillimeter slices allows for excellent spatial resolution. The addition of iodinated contrast material into the joint before scanning affords excellent contrast between meniscus and joint cavity. Wrapping of the suprapatellar recess to promote contrast collection near the joint line follows the injection of 20 to 30 mL of iodinated contrast material into the joint. Normal and postoperative menisci appear hypodense, whereas a recurrent or new meniscal tear allows the abnormal passage of contrast material into the substance of the meniscus. An additional benefit of high-resolution CT arthrography is the ability to detect the presence of cartilage defects (Fig. 18.13).

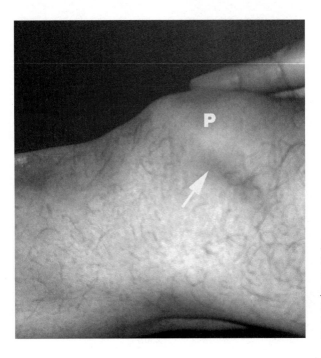

Figure 18.11 Photograph shows surface landmarks for insertion of the needle into the knee joint (*arrow*), just below the laterally subluxated patella (P). If the patient is obese, fluoroscopy may be necessary to confirm the location of the needle tip.

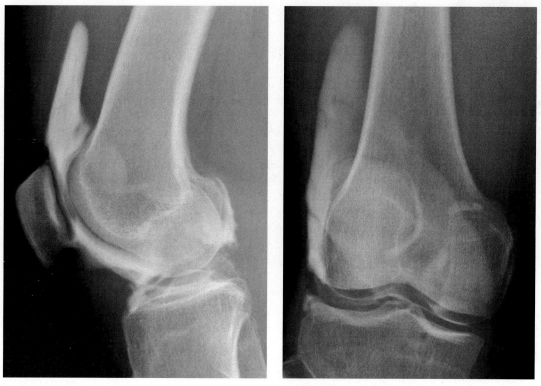

Figure 18.12 Successful injection of contrast medium into the knee joint. *A,B.* Lateral and PA spot radiographs show the normal distribution of contrast medium within the knee joint.

ANKLE

For injection into the ankle joint, a 22-gauge 3.5-in. spinal needle is used. Injection of the ankle joint (tibiotalar joint) is made through an anterior approach. The dorsalis pedis artery is identified, and the site of injection is chosen lateral to this. The foot is plantar flexed to open up the anterior aspect of the ankle joint. Fluoroscopic guidance in the lateral projection can be used to follow the needle to the joint. The injection should occur without resistance, with contrast flowing away from the needle tip and pooling initially in the dependent portion of the joint. The ankle joint holds approximately 10 mL.

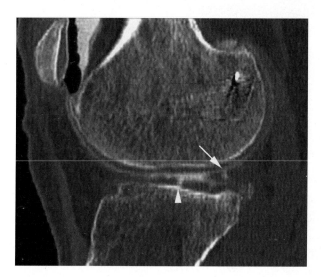

Figure 18.13 CT arthrogram of the knee. Sagittal CT reconstruction through the knee shows a recurrent medial meniscal tear (*arrow*) and tibial cartilage defect (*arrowhead*).

JOINT ASPIRATION

Joint aspirations under fluoroscopic guidance are generally performed in the setting of suspected joint infection. A larger needle (18- to 20-gauge) is used than would be typical for joint injection, because pus and normal synovial fluid are more viscous than contrast medium. Cells and other particulate matter are commonly present in infected joint fluid. The approach to the various joints is similar to that used for arthrography or injection. However, care must be taken to avoid passing the needle through areas of cellulitis because of the risk of introducing bacteria into an uninfected joint. An acutely infected joint will typically produce bloody or grossly purulent fluid that is under pressure. If no fluid can be aspirated, the intra-articular position of the needle tip can be confirmed with the injection of a small amount of contrast medium. The joint should be irrigated with nonbacteriostatic (preservative-free) saline and the saline aspirated. For a large joint, inject 10 mL of saline and expect to reaspirate 1 mL. Any material aspirated from a joint in the setting of suspected infection should be delivered to the bacteriology lab for gram stain, aerobic and anaerobic bacterial cultures, wet prep and fungus culture, and acid-fast stain and mycobacterium culture.

When performing arthrocentesis, avoid passing the needle through an area of cellulitis.

The post-replacement hip joint is the most commonly requested site of arthrocentesis. I prefer an anterior approach with the needle directed toward the medial edge of the femoral neck component at the head-neck junction. When the needle tip scrapes the metal of the prosthesis, it is in the joint (Fig. 18.14). The hip joint pseudocapsule after hip replacement will extend from the bony portion of the acetabulum to the bony portion of the femur, encompassing the entire exposed metal portion of the prosthesis. If a joint effusion is present, joint fluid can be aspirated with the needle positioned anywhere along the femoral component. However, in the absence of effusion, the capsule may be tightly applied to the femoral component, and it may be necessary to place the needle alongside the metal. An additional aid once the needle is in place is to flex the hip, tightening the posterior capsule and increasing the redundancy of the anterior capsule. Fluid may also be shifted more anteriorly within the joint, in better range of the needle.

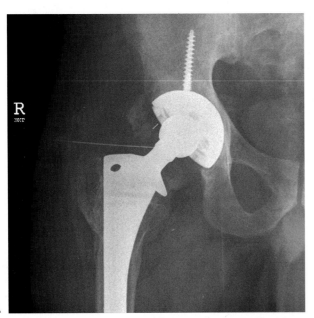
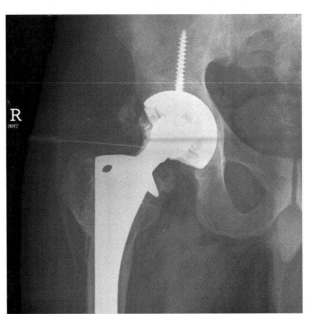

A

B

Figure 18.14 Arthrocentesis of total hip replacement. *A.* Spot radiograph of the hip after insertion of the needle. *B.* Spot radiograph after injection of contrast medium for confirmation of position.

PERCUTANEOUS COMPUTED TOMOGRAPHY–GUIDED BIOPSY

Percutaneous CT-guided biopsy is used as an alternative to an open surgical procedure for the purpose of obtaining tissue for histologic, cytologic, or microbiologic diagnosis. Potential complications of percutaneous needle biopsy are listed in Table 18.3.

LYTIC BONE LESIONS

Lytic bone lesions can typically be sampled without drilling through bone (Fig. 18.15). For a purely lytic lesion, fine-needle aspiration using a 22-gauge Chiba needle (Cook Inc., Bloomington, Indiana) placed coaxially through a 19-gauge Chiba needle is appropriate. If the cortex of bone is partially intact, or the lesion has mixed lytic and sclerotic features, an 18-gauge Franseen needle can be used. The Franseen needle is a front-cutting core biopsy needle with a stylet that has a triangular cutting tip and a cannula that has three cutting teeth. It can be maneuvered through small amounts of bone and can be used to obtain a core. A 22-gauge Chiba needle will fit coaxially through an 18-gauge Franseen needle.

> A 22-gauge Chiba needle placed coaxially through a 19-gauge Chiba needle can be used to sample most lytic bone lesions.

SCLEROTIC BONE LESIONS

Sclerotic bone lesions or lesions protected by intact cortical bone require a bone-cutting needle for access (Fig. 18.16). The needles I prefer are the Ackerman trephine needle and the Bonopty eccentric drill. A number of other bone biopsy needles are available and can be used effectively. Both instruments will produce small bone fragments that are compacted into a plug of bone that resembles a core.

The needle path should be planned in conjunction with the orthopedic surgeon who may be performing a tumor resection and may need to resect the biopsy tract along with the tumor because of the risk of tumor recurrence along the tract. For long bones, the approach is generally orthogonal to the cortex of the bone, avoiding neurovascular structures and joints, and taking the most direct route. For the posterior elements of the spine, a direct posterior approach may be used. For cervical vertebral bodies, the approach is anterolateral, just medial to the carotid sheath (Fig. 18.17). For thoracic vertebral bodies, the approach is posterior through the pedicles or intercostovertebral (posterolateral adjacent to the costovertebral joints) (Fig. 18.18). For lumbar vertebral bodies or the intervertebral disc space, the approach is transpedicular or posterolateral (Figs. 18.19 through 18.21). The nerve root should be explicitly identified and avoided through a posterolateral approach. At the level of the transverse process, the nerve root can be avoided; at other levels, the nerve root may be encountered if it is not identified and avoided. Some areas are difficult or unsafe to approach, including the face, base of the skull, upper cervical spine, and ischium.

> In malignant disease, the biopsy tract must be resected with the tumor.

Table 18.3: Complications of Percutaneous Needle Biopsy

Infection
Bleeding
Nerve root injury
Pseudoaneurysm
Vasovagal syncope
Complex regional pain syndrome (reflex sympathetic dystrophy)
Tumor seeding along needle tract

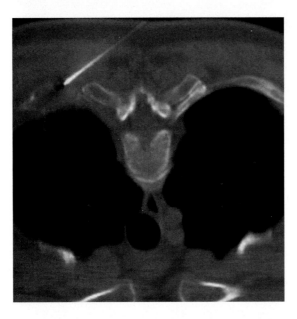

Figure 18.15 CT-guided biopsy of a rib mass. A tangential approach to the chest wall has been used to avoid the possibility of pneumothorax.

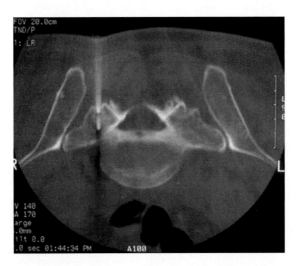

Figure 18.16 CT-guided biopsy of a small, sclerotic lesion in the sacral ala. A trephine needle has been used to obtain a biopsy from a sclerotic lesion in the right sacral ala.

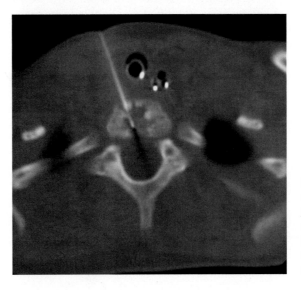

Figure 18.17 CT-guided biopsy of the cervical spine using an anterior approach. An approach between the trachea and carotid sheath is made with a 19-gauge Chiba needle, and the fine-needle aspiration is performed through a coaxially placed 22-gauge Chiba needle.

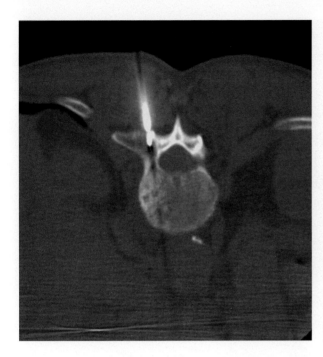

Figure 18.18 CT-guided biopsy of a thoracic vertebral body using a transpedicular approach. A trephine needle has been used to gain access to the lesion, but the diagnostic specimen was obtained with a coaxially placed 19-gauge Chiba needle.

The Ackerman biopsy needle set (Cook Inc., Bloomington, Indiana) consists of a 12-gauge skin perforator, a 12-gauge needle guide with a 14-gauge trocar-pointed stylet, and long and short 14-gauge trephine needles with blunt obturators. It is available in long and short lengths. In the United States, the manufacturer has marked the sterile packages for one-time use, but because of their high cost and their durability, many hospitals treat Ackerman needle sets as surgical instruments and resterilize them for repeated use.

A short (5-mm) skin wound is made using a no. 11 scalpel blade. The skin perforator should be inserted to the hub. The needle guide, with trocar-point stylet in place, should be inserted under CT guidance and directed to the lesion. The needle is then advanced with a twisting motion over the stylet until it is firmly seated against the periosteum. After removal of the stylet, local anesthetic can be injected through the needle guide into the

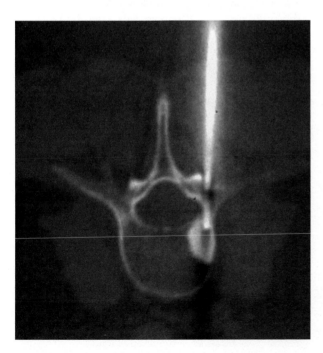

Figure 18.19 CT-guided biopsy of a sclerotic lumbar vertebral body lesion using a transpedicular approach.

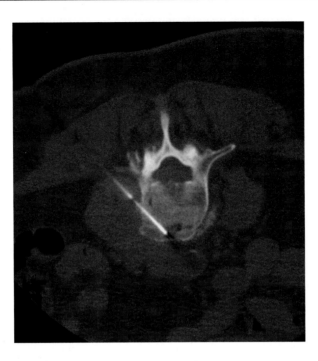

Figure 18.20 CT-guided biopsy of a lumbar vertebral body using a posterolateral approach.

periosteum. The short trephine needle, with the obturator removed, is inserted coaxially through the needle guide, taking care to maintain the position of the needle guide against the periosteum. The trephine needle is operated by clockwise rotation with firm, steady pressure against the bone. The trephine needle has a tendency to "walk," or change in position, as the initial rotations are made, and so great care should be taken to maintain the position of the needle guide as the trephine needle is rotated. Once the trephine begins to cut into the bone, it becomes stable, and greater pressure can be used. The position of the needle should be periodically checked by CT. The needle should be periodically withdrawn and the plug of bone pushed out using the blunt obturator. If the bone plug is impacted in the needle, it has a tendency to pop out of the needle suddenly and ricochet out of the sterile field. The short trephine needle protrudes 1 cm beyond the needle guide, and the long trephine needle protrudes 2 cm beyond. After the biopsy is complete, the stylet should be reinserted into the needle guide and the entire instrument removed.

The Elson bone biopsy needle set (Cook Inc., Bloomington, Indiana) includes trephine needles that are similar to the Ackerman biopsy set. The introducer needle is a 22-gauge trocar-pointed needle with a removable hub. Once the introducer has been passed

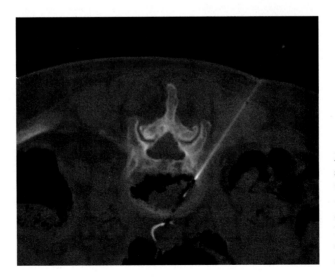

Figure 18.21 CT-guided biopsy of a lumbar disc space using a posterolateral approach. A 22-gauge Chiba needle has been passed coaxially through an 18-gauge Franseen needle. Gas has been drawn into the space after the aspiration of fluid.

through the skin to the lesion, the hub is removed, and the needle guide—consisting of an outer 12-gauge cannula with a tapered, inner 14-gauge cannula—is passed over the introducer needle coaxially until it is firmly seated against the periosteum. The introducer and inner cannula are removed, and the biopsy is performed with the short and long trephine needles.

The Bonopty Penetration Set (Radi Medical Systems, Uppsala, Sweden) is an eccentric drill and cannula. The 15-gauge drill has an eccentric tip, allowing it to cut a larger hole that permits the passage of the 14-gauge cannula. This arrangement allows one to perform a biopsy through any thickness of bone, limited only by the length of the drill. A Bonopty biopsy set is a front-sampling needle that may be placed through the penetration set. It is also possible to pass the Bonopty instrument through the 12-gauge needle guide of an Ackerman needle set.

SOFT TISSUE LESIONS

Soft tissue biopsy can be accomplished with fine-needle aspiration, front-cutting core biopsy, and side-cutting core biopsy, depending on the circumstance. For fine-needle aspiration, I prefer a 22-gauge Chiba needle, typically used coaxially through a 19-gauge Chiba needle or an 18-gauge Franseen needle. The 22-gauge needle should be 5 cm longer than the larger-gauge outer needle to allow adequate throw. The Franseen needle itself can be used to obtain a soft tissue core biopsy. The side-cutting core biopsy needle that I prefer is the spring-loaded, semi-automatic Temno gun (Alliance Healthcare, McGaw Park, Illinois) or similar devices.

EPIDURAL STEROID INJECTION

Epidural injections of steroids and local anesthetics are performed for relief of back pain, including refractory back pain of unknown origin. Patients will generally be evaluated by a spine surgeon and imaged with MRI before referral. Indications and contraindications are listed in Table 18.4. The epidural space is a potential space between the dural sac and the ligamentum flavum that contains the nerve roots and their dural investment, extending from the foramen magnum to the sacral hiatus. Access to the whole epidural space can be gained via a caudal or a translaminar approach. We inject a mixture of methylprednisolone diluted in preservative-free saline and bupivacaine (Table 18.5).

For the caudal approach to the epidural space, a 22-gauge spinal needle is placed in the midline through the sacral hiatus into the epidural space (Fig. 18.22). The sacral hiatus can often be palpated just above the natal cleft. It can be identified on fluoroscopy just below the S4 spinous process. Biplane fluoroscopy is necessary to localize the needle position. On the lateral projection, the needle should project over the spinal canal (Fig. 18.23); on the frontal projection, the needle should project in the midline. Nonionic contrast medium should be injected to confirm position (sacral epidurography); the contrast

Access to the whole epidural space may be gained via a caudal or translaminar approach.

Table 18.4: Indications and Contraindications for Epidural Steroid Injection

Indications
    Back pain caused by spinal stenosis
    Back pain caused by disc herniation with or without sciatica
    Refractory back pain of uncertain etiology
Contraindications
    Uncorrectable coagulopathy or bleeding diathesis
    Superficial infection along the needle path
    Contrast allergy (can premedicate with corticosteroids)

Table 18.5: Therapeutic Agents for Epidural, Nerve Root, and Joint Injections

Epidural injection (caudal or translaminar approach)
    Methylprednisolone, 80 mg, suspended in normal saline to a total volume of 5 mL
    Bupivacaine, 5 mL of 0.25% solution
Nerve root injection (transforaminal epidural injection), per root
    Methylprednisolone, 20 mg
    Bupivacaine, 1 mL of 0.25% solution
Large joint (elbow, shoulder, hip, knee, ankle)
    Methylprednisolone, 80 mg, suspended in normal saline to a total volume of 5 mL
    Bupivacaine, 5 mL of 0.25% solution
Small joint (sacroiliac joint, facet joint, wrist, hand, or foot)
    Methylprednisolone, 20 mg
    Bupivacaine, 1 mL of 0.25% solution

medium should flow away from the needle tip and outline the sacral plexus (Fig. 18.24). Some patients have a prominent venous plexus within the spinal canal, and care should be taken to avoid intravenous injection. The needle should be repositioned, usually anteriorly, until the tip is in the epidural rather than the intravenous space. If the epidural space cannot be accessed by this method, then a translaminar or a transforaminal approach should be used.

For the translaminar approach to the epidural space, we generally choose a lower lumbar level that is not involved by spinal stenosis or disc herniation. In elderly patients or patients with extensive degenerative disease, the caudal approach may be preferred. The needle is inserted in the interlaminar space deep to the lamina but superficial to the thecal sac. The needle is inserted to the inferior bony margin of the lamina and then "walked off." This is achieved by gently retracting the needle a few millimeters while also shifting the needle a few millimeters toward the edge of the bone and then readvancing the needle back to its original depth. This method can accomplish the task of minor needle repositioning to the very edge of a narrow portion of cortical bone such as a laminar margin. Once the needle is at the edge of the cortical bone, it is very gently advanced toward the spinal canal. By checking continuously for resistance to injection, the epidural space can be localized

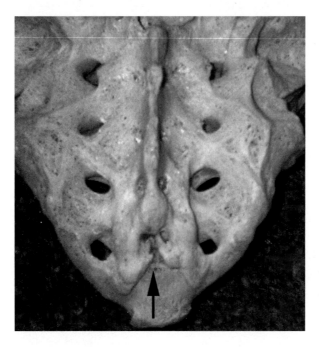

Figure 18.22 Photograph of skeleton showing sacral hiatus and proper needle placement site (*arrow*) for epidural injection using caudal approach.

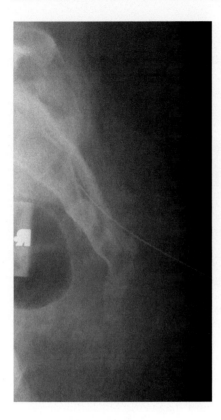

Figure 18.23 Lateral radiograph documenting needle placement through the sacral hiatus.

when resistance to injection suddenly disappears. Care must be taken to avoid puncture of the thecal sac.

After the injection, we monitor the patient for a few minutes and assess the response to the local anesthetic. Immediate and marked response is common; however, some

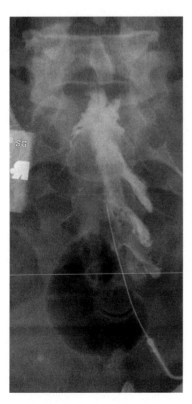

Figure 18.24 Contrast in the epidural space after caudal needle placement.

patients do not respond. If three epidural steroid injections spaced over several weeks do not provide relief, additional injections are unlikely to provide relief, and the patient is returned to the referring physician. Patients are instructed not to engage in vigorous physical activity or operate dangerous machinery (e.g., automobiles) until the day after the injection, to avoid accidental injury in the rare event that minor leg anesthesia could occur and interfere with these activities.

NERVE ROOT BLOCK (TRANSFORAMINAL EPIDURAL STEROID INJECTION)

Injections into the vicinity of exiting nerve roots are performed for diagnosis and control of radicular pain. The thoracic and lumbar nerve roots exit the spinal canal through the neural foramina just inferior to the pedicle. Under fluoroscopic or CT guidance, a 22-gauge spinal needle can be advanced through a slightly oblique posterior approach or a posterolateral approach to the inferior margin of the pedicle, so that the tip is positioned at the anterior-superior aspect of the neural foramen (Figs. 18.25 and 18.26). Frequently, radicular paresthesias will be elicited as the needle reaches the appropriate position. An alternative method is to put a gentle bend at the needle tip, away from the side of the bevel. This allows the needle to be steered, and a curved needle course with the skin insertion point lateral to the transverse processes can be used. Lateral fluoroscopy is necessary to document the correct positioning of the needle tip. When nonionic contrast is injected, the nerve root should be outlined, and contrast should flow proximally into the epidural space. For a diagnostic block, lidocaine or Sensorcaine can be injected to determine whether sensation from that nerve root is responsible for the patient's pain. For a therapeutic block, bupivacaine and methylprednisolone are injected. We generally do not perform more than two nerve root blocks in a single session. The S1 nerve root is difficult to access using fluoroscopy but easy to access using CT (Fig. 18.27).

> Radicular paresthesias may be elicited as the needle reaches the appropriate position for a nerve root injection.

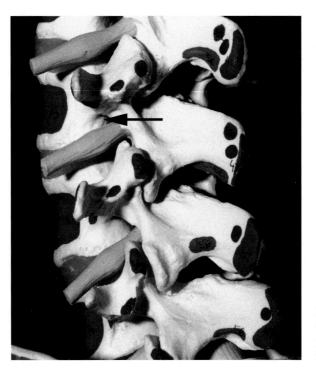

Figure 18.25 Photograph of skeleton showing proper needle tip placement (*arrow*) for nerve root injection.

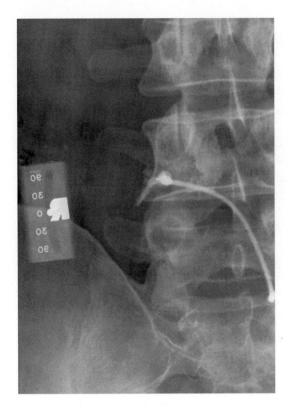

Figure 18.26 Fluoroscopy-guided lumbar nerve root injection.

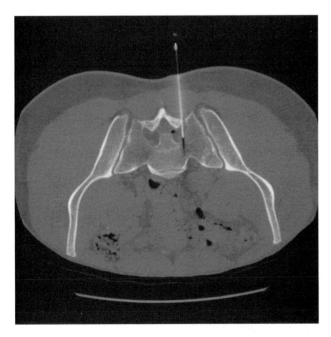

Figure 18.27 CT-guided injection of S1 nerve root.

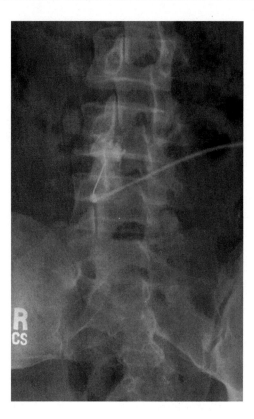

Figure 18.28 Fluoroscopy-guided lumbar facet joint injection using a posterior approach.

FACET JOINT INJECTION

Facet joint injections are performed for pain control and for diagnosis. In the cervical and thoracic regions of the spine, the joint spaces of the articular facet joints are relatively flat and oriented in an oblique coronal plane. In the lumbar region, where the majority of these procedures are performed, the joint spaces become more complex, often with a curved shape that is in the sagittal plane posteriorly and in the coronal plane anteriorly. The orientation of the facet joints may change from the top to the bottom of the lumbar spine. Although the joint spaces can be seen with the patient in the oblique position, access to the joint is often easier with the patient in the prone position. The presence of osteophytes may impede access to the joint. However, the goal is not to place the needle into the joint space, but rather to place the needle into the joint capsule or at least in the immediate vicinity (Fig. 18.28). Review of cross-sectional images of the facets to be injected will help guide the best percutaneous approach to the joint.

The presence of osteophytes may impede access to the facet joints.

We use a 22-gauge 3.5-in. spinal needle for most patients; for obese patients, a 22-gauge 5-in. or 7-in. spinal needle may be necessary.

NONUNION AND PARS DEFECT INJECTION

Injections of fracture nonunions and pars defects are generally performed for diagnosis. The typical question in these situations is whether a patient's symptoms will be alleviated by surgical stabilization. The approach is made under fluoroscopic or CT guidance, depending on the location, using a 22-gauge spinal or Chiba needle (Fig. 18.29). Local anesthetic is injected into the site. If the patient's symptoms are alleviated, surgical stabilization is much more likely to be successful than if symptoms are unchanged. There is not a consistent correlation between the response to injection and the results of surgery, and the value of the procedure is controversial.

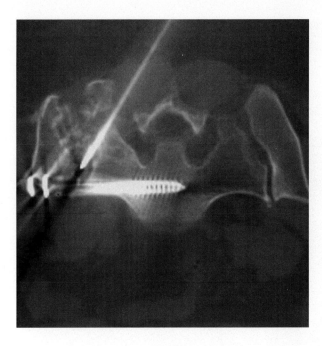

Figure 18.29 CT-guided injection of pelvic nonunion. A 22-gauge spinal needle has been placed into a painful fracture nonunion of the right iliac wing. Injection of bupivacaine ameliorated the patient's symptoms.

SACROILIAC JOINT INJECTION

Sacroiliac joint injections are performed for pain control and for diagnosis. I prefer to use CT guidance, although fluoroscopy may be used instead. A 22-gauge 3.5-in. spinal needle is directed into the posterior aspect of the synovial portion of the joint (Fig. 18.30). Depending on the specific anatomy of the sacroiliac joint, a vertical or oblique path to the joint may be required.

DISCOGRAPHY

Discography is a diagnostic procedure in which contrast is injected into the nucleus pulposus of an intervertebral disc in an attempt to reproduce the patient's pain. If the injection does

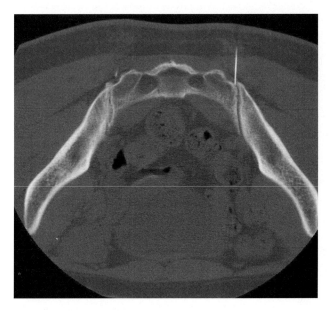

Figure 18.30 CT-guided sacroiliac joint injection.

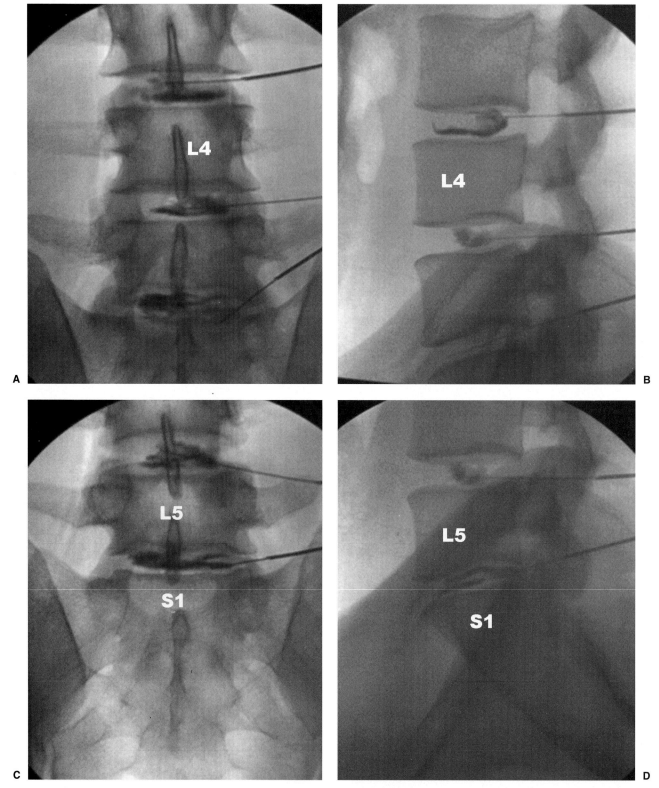

Figure 18.31 Fluoroscopy-guided lumbar discogram. *A,B.* AP and lateral radiographs of the upper lumbar spine show injections into normal intervertebral discs at L3-L4 and L4-L5. *C,D.* AP and lateral radiographs of the lumbosacral junction show injection into abnormal intervertebral disc at L5-S1.

reproduce the pain, then surgical excision of that disc with fusion is more likely to be successful than if the pain is not reproduced. The procedure is most commonly performed in the lumbar region. The correlation of discography results with surgical results in the literature ranges from good to poor, but techniques and outcome measures of both discography and surgery are difficult to compare across studies.

The nucleus pulposus is generally accessed under guidance by a C-arm fluoroscope using a posterolateral approach, with the needle insertion on the side opposite the symptoms (Fig. 18.31). As with other procedures described in this chapter, there are several methods. In general, the needle should always be placed in the same plane as the disc. For the straight coaxial approach, an 18- or 19-gauge needle is inserted midway between the vertebral end plates and just ventrolateral to the superior articulating process (ear of the "Scottie dog"). The needle tip is left just at the edge of the disc. A 22-gauge needle is placed coaxially through the 18- or 19-gauge needle and advanced into the center of the nucleus; this may be painful. A change in resistance can usually be felt as the needle passes through the gritty-feeling annulus fibrosis into the nucleus. The 22-gauge needle can also be inserted directly into the nucleus without using a coaxial guide; it can also be curved and steered so that the path from skin to disc is curved rather than straight. Multiple levels are typically done at the same time, and all needles can be placed before any injections are performed. The injections should be made without the patient knowing exactly which disc is being injected. An asymptomatic (control) level should be included. Nonionic myelographic contrast is used. The injection should be made slowly under fluoroscopic visualization until firm resistance (end point) is met; if there is firm resistance initially, the needle tip may still be in the annulus. A normal lumbar disc can accommodate 1.5 to 3.0 mL of contrast. If there is no firm end point, the annulus is generally not intact, but the injection may be continued in an attempt to reproduce symptoms. If severe pain is encountered at any time during the injection, the injection should be stopped.

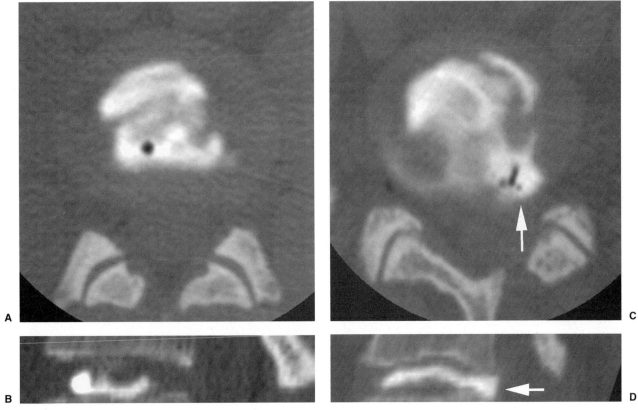

Figure 18.32 CT of the lumbar spine after discography. *A.* Axial scan at L3-L4 shows normal discogram. *B.* Sagittal CT reformation shows normal discogram. *C.* Axial scan at L4-L5 shows leakage of contrast through a radial tear (*arrow*). *D.* Sagittal CT reformation shows the contrast filling the tear (*arrow*).

After injection of each level, the location and intensity of any pain should be ascertained from the patient. In particular, the patient should be asked whether the pain resulting from the injection is his or her usual pain in distribution, quality, and intensity. Involuntary signs of pain such as body posturing, facial grimacing, or vocalization should be noted. Some authors inject local anesthetic into symptomatic discs in an attempt to extinguish the pain; if the pain does disappear, it is considered additional evidence that the disc injected is symptomatic.

Because discitis is a known complication of discography, 1 g of cefazolin is given intravenously immediately after the procedure as prophylaxis.

Imaging after injection should include AP and lateral radiographs and axial CT in the plane of each injected disc with coronal and sagittal reformations (Fig. 18.32).

> Discitis is a known complication of discography.

PERCUTANEOUS VERTEBROPLASTY

Vertebroplasty is a technique of injecting methylmethacrylate cement into a vertebral body fracture for the purposes of fracture stabilization and pain control. Indications include osteoporotic compression fractures, pathologic compression fractures, and aggressive vertebral body hemangioma (Table 18.6). Patient selection is important for a positive response to the procedure. Indicators of a positive response include a recent history of compression fracture (within a few weeks), point tenderness at the involved vertebra, hot bone scan, and marrow edema on MRI. Patients who are improving on medical therapy and patients with acute trauma are not candidates for vertebroplasty. Additionally, the presence of spinal stenosis is a relative contraindication. In such cases, there is not only an increased danger of worsening the stenosis by the vertebroplasty procedure, but one should also consider that the stenosis itself may be the cause of the patient's symptoms. Joint efforts in consultation with the patient and the spine surgeon may be helpful to assess for the most likely cause of pain and the most prudent treatment options. Vertebroplasty will not restore loss of height resulting from compression fractures, nor will it correct a kyphotic deformity. Patients and referring physicians may mistake vertebroplasty for kyphoplasty, an investigational procedure performed by some spine surgeons that requires general anesthesia and surgical exposure of the spine. Kyphoplasty is similar to vertebroplasty (see below) but involves the addition of an inflatable balloon before the addition of methylmethacrylate in an attempt to restore height to the vertebral body. Complications of vertebroplasty are listed in Table 18.7.

> Patients who are improving on medical therapy and patients with acute trauma are not candidates for vertebroplasty.

The patient is placed in the prone position and local anesthetics and conscious sedation are used as appropriate. A bone-cutting trocar-cannula needle system is used for placement into the vertebral body through a transpedicular or posterolateral approach, using fluoroscopic guidance. The methylmethacrylate is supplied with a sealed mixing system and injector specifically for vertebroplasty. A small amount of barium powder is added to

---

Table 18.6: Indications and Contraindications for Percutaneous Vertebroplasty

Indications
    Painful, recent osteoporotic compression fracture not improving on medical therapy
    Painful neoplastic vertebral destruction (with or without fracture)
    Painful vertebral fracture associated with osteonecrosis
Contraindications
    Infection
    Acute, traumatic fracture
    Uncorrectable coagulopathy or bleeding diathesis
    Radiculopathy
    Cord compression
    Complete vertebral collapse

Table 18.7: Complications of Vertebroplasty

Pulmonary embolism, death
Spinal cord compression
Infection
Pain
Systemic methylmethacrylate toxicity
Disc extrusion of cement

the methylmethacrylate powder monomer before adding the hardener. The methyl-methacrylate is injected under fluoroscopic guidance, filling the vertebral body. One or two injections can be made into each vertebral body. A postprocedure CT may be obtained to document the distribution of methylmethacrylate (Fig. 18.33). Oral analgesics may be

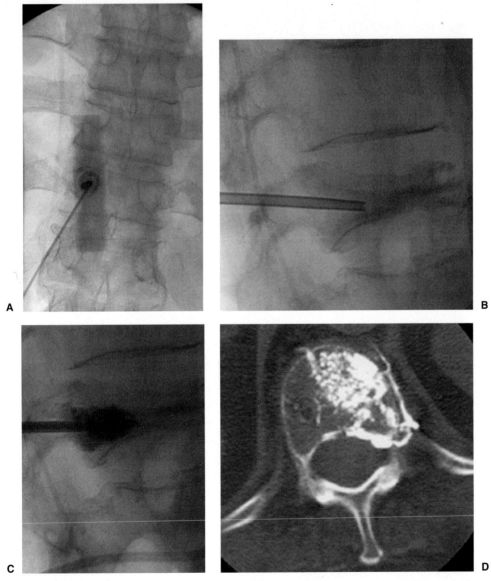

Figure 18.33 Fluoroscopy-guided vertebroplasty. *A,B.* PA and lateral spot radiographs show place-ment of the cutting needle into the compressed vertebral body through a transpedicular approach. *C.* Lateral spot radiograph shows injection of methylmethacrylate into the vertebral body. *D.* CT scan after vertebroplasty shows distribution of methylmethacrylate within the vertebral body.

given while the patient lies flat in bed with the back straight for at least 2 hours, allowing the methylmethacrylate to harden. The patient should be carefully monitored during this time, with particular attention to the neurologic evaluation of the lower extremities.

RADIOFREQUENCY ABLATION

Radiofrequency ablation and pulsed radiofrequency ablation of focal bone and soft tissue lesions uses radiofrequency (microwave) energy delivered through an electrode that is inserted percutaneously under imaging guidance. Deposition of microwave energy results in heating of the tissues (similar to microwave cooking), causing coagulative necrosis. This technique can be used to perform permanent nerve and ganglion blocks for treatment of chronic pain disorders after a successful diagnostic block. Radiofrequency ablation has also become a standard therapy for osteoid osteoma (Fig. 18.34) and is used successfully for other small, focal bone lesions. Radiofrequency ablation is also used as an adjunct to chemotherapy and radiotherapy for treatment of bone and soft tissue metastases (Fig. 18.35).

Radiofrequency ablation is performed under general anesthesia. The lesion is localized under CT, and a percutaneous CT-guided biopsy is obtained. Once the diagnosis has been established, the radiofrequency electrode is passed coaxially through the needle guide of the biopsy needle into the lesion. The volume of tissue that is ablated is spheric; the diameter of the sphere depends on the exact electrode used. For bone lesions, the diameter of ablation is approximately 1 cm, so that accurate placement of the active tip of the electrode is essential. It is generally necessary to pass the electrode completely through the lesion. Once the position has been confirmed and the needle guide retracted away from the active tip of the electrode, the lesion is heated to 90°C for (however many) minutes. The electrode may then be withdrawn and the patient recovered from anesthesia. Symptomatic response to the treatment is generally evident within 1 or 2 days.

Percutaneous radiofrequency ablation has become one of the standard treatments for osteoid osteoma.

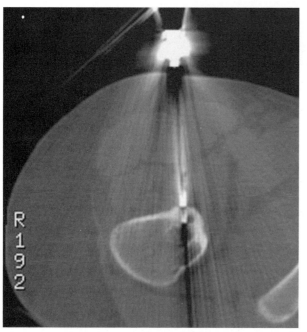
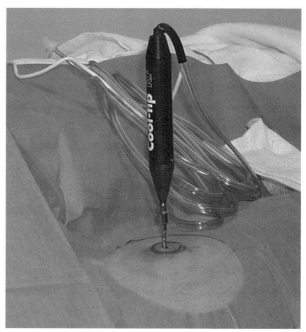

A   B

Figure 18.34 CT-guided radiofrequency ablation of an osteoid osteoma. *A.* Axial CT scan shows a trephine needle drilled into an osteoid osteoma in the cortex of the proximal femur. *B.* Photograph shows the radiofrequency electrode inserted through the needle guide into the lesion.

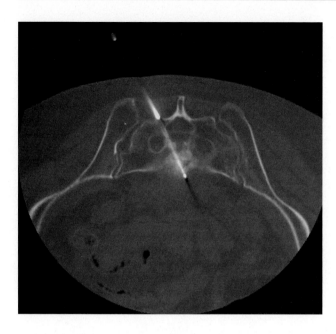

Figure 18.35 CT-guided radiofrequency ablation of a bone metastasis in the sacrum.

SOURCES AND READINGS

Barr JD, Barr MS, Lemley TJ, et al. Percutaneous vertebroplasty for pain relief and spine stabilization. *Spine* 2000;25:923–928.

Freiberger RH, Kaye JJ. *Arthrography*. New York: Appleton Communication, 1979.

Gangi A, Dietemann JL, Mortazavi R, et al. CT-guided interventional procedures for pain management in the lumbosacral spine. *Radiographics* 1998;18:621–633.

Hau MA, Kim JI, Kattapuram S, et al. Accuracy of CT-guided biopsies in 359 patients with musculoskeletal lesions. *Skeletal Radiol* 2002;31:349–353.

Hodge JC. *Musculoskeletal imaging: diagnostic and therapeutic procedures*. Basel: Karger Landes, 1997.

Link S, el-Khoury GY, Guilford WB. Percutaneous epidural and nerve root block and percutaneous lumbar sympatholysis. *Radiol Clin North Am* 1998;36:509–521.

Maldjian C, Mesgarzadeh M, Tehranzadeh J. Diagnostic and therapeutic features of facet and sacroiliac joint injection. Anatomy, pathophysiology, and technique. *Radiol Clin North Am* 1998;31:497–508.

Murtagh R. The art and science of nerve root and facet block. *Neuroimaging Clin North Am* 2000;10:465–477.

Schellhas KP. Diskography. *Neuroimaging Clin North Am* 2000;10:579–596.

Williams, AL. Murtagh FR. *Handbook of diagnostic and therapeutic spine procedures*. St. Louis: Mosby, 2002.

INDEX

Note: Page numbers followed by *t* indicate tables; those followed by *f* indicate figures.